OLLI P. HEINONEN, M.D., M.Sc.

DENNIS SLONE, M.D.

SAMUEL SHAPIRO, F.R.C.P.

Drug Epidemiology Unit
Boston University Medical Center

BIRTH DEFECTS AND DRUGS IN PREGNANCY

with

Leonard F. Gaetano, B.Ch.E.
Stuart C. Hartz, Sc.D.
Allen A. Mitchell, M.D.
Richard R. Monson, M.D.
Lynn Rosenberg, M.S.
Victor Siskind, Ph.D.

David W. Kaufman, B.A., Editor

Publishing Sciences Group, Inc.
Littleton, Massachusetts

1977

Library of Congress Cataloging in Publication Data

Heinonen, Olli P
  Birth defects and drugs in pregnancy.

  Bibliography: p.
  Includes index.
  1. Fetus, Effect of drugs on the. 2. Deformities—
Causes and theories of causation. 3. Teratogenic
agents. 4. Collaborative Perinatal Study. I. Slone,
Dennis, joint author. II. Shapiro, Samuel, 1931-
joint author. III. Title.
RG627.S56   618.3'2   75-16094
ISBN 0-88416-034-3

1977. Publishing Sciences Group, Inc.

The data presented in this book are from the Collaborative Perinatal Project (CPP) of the National Institute of Neurological and Communicative Disorders and Stroke. The following institutions participated in the CPP: Boston Lying-In Hospital; Brown University; Charity Hospital, New Orleans; Children's Hospital of Buffalo; Children's Hospital of Philadelphia; Children's Hospital Medical Center, Boston; Columbia-Presbyterian Medical Center; Johns Hopkins Hospital; Medical College of Virginia; New York Medical College; Pennsylvania Hospital; University of Minnesota Hospitals; University of Oregon Medical School; and University of Tennessee.
This study was supported by a contract (N01-NS-2-2322) with the National Institute of Neurological and Communicative Disorders and Stroke, the U.S. Public Health Service, and a contract (223-75-3036) with the Food and Drug Administration.

Printed in the United States of America.

International Standard Book Number: 0-88416-034-3

Library of Congress Catalog Card Number: 75-16094

Contents

Drugs in Pregnancy

Evaluation of Drugs in Relation to Malformations

Drugs as Potential Teratogens
The Need for Surveillance

Appendices

Preface

Between 1958 and 1965, under the auspices of the National Institute of Neurological and Communicative Disorders and Stroke, a prospective study of over 50,000 pregnancies was undertaken with the main objective of determining whether there are factors during pregnancy or delivery that are related to the risk of cerebral palsy or other neurological outcomes. This study ultimately became known as the Collaborative Perinatal Project. Among many items of data obtained, drug use was recorded during pregnancy, and birth defects identified in the children were recorded subsequently. With the growing realization that drugs are sometimes teratogenic, it became mandatory to evaluate the data from that perspective. In 1970, our group was assigned this task.

The purpose of this book is to present data on drugs used by 50,282 gravidae in relation to the birth defects identified in the children. The achievement of this objective was difficult and complicated. Prior to commencing analysis, it was necessary to verify and reclassify much of the data concerning factors other than drugs; to verify and reclassify many of the recorded birth defects; and most importantly of all, to make a detailed assessment of the drug exposure data, much of which had to be re-recorded and assigned new code numbers after original records were scrutinized.

The analytical tasks were also complicated. We were required to analyze several hundred drugs against many categories of malformations, as well as individual malformations. This involved, quite literally, thousands of comparisons. It was possible, and even likely, that each comparison would have its own unique set of covariate predictive factors related both to drugs and outcomes, that could introduce confounding bias into the analyses. We decided, in these circumstances, to adopt a conservative analytical strategy by taking into account all identifiable predictor variables for the larger malformation categories. If spurious positive associations, and their implications, were to be avoided, the analyses could thus be rigorously controlled in a standard way without having to determine, for each individual comparison, whether any of the variables were also related to drug exposure. This, in turn, required reliance in much of the work on multivariate statistical methods since many of the malformation outcomes appeared to have multiple risk factors which themselves were interrelated. Many of the decisions concerning how to select factors for inclusion in the multivariate analyses, and in other analyses, depended to a greater or lesser extent on judgment. When in doubt about whether any particular factor should be selected, we generally opted for selection.

In this cohort, it is clear that there was no common drug teratogen analogous to thalidomide. A no less important question, however, is whether there may not have been commonly used drugs that were less dramatically teratogenic to humans, either in terms of their potency, or in terms of the uniqueness of the defects that they caused. The public health implications of such "concealed" drug teratogens could well be even more grave than that of a drug like thalidomide,

since their effects can easily go undetected. Even here, the results in this study were generally reassuring. Certainly, some suspicions have been raised, and these are alluded to in the appropriate places. But, as we will stress time and again throughout this book, they are no more than suspicions and they require confirmation.

There was no major epidemic of malformations during the years of recruitment to the study. This, however, was more a matter of good fortune than anything else: drug use over the recruitment period increased. We doubt whether the quality of the pregnancies was thereby improved—and certainly, to the extent that drugs may be *potentially* teratogenic, the women were taking greater and greater risks.

This volume does not only contain information concerning drugs in relation to malformations. Material is presented that should be of interest to scientists concerned with all aspects of teratology, and particularly to epidemiologists engaged in exploring birth defects whether from the perspective of hypothesis generation, or that of hypothesis testing. There is a full classification and description of the malformations that were identified in the cohort. A large number of risk factors are analyzed in relation to birth defects both in univariate settings, as well as in more rigorously controlled multivariate settings.

Obviously, since the primary purpose of this study was to evaluate *drugs* as risk factors, the exploration of the role of other risk factors was sometimes, of necessity, incomplete. Nevertheless, we believe this book adds substantially to what is known about the general epidemiology of birth defects. It also provides quantitative information, much of it not previously available, concerning relationships between birth defects. With regard to hypotheses, it confirms, and elaborates in quantitative terms, what is known about relationships between factors such as single umbilical artery and birth defects. It raises, again in quantitative terms, many hypotheses concerning risk factors; some previously suspected, but without quantitative information, and some not previously suspected. Certain findings may warrant further research in this cohort and elsewhere. Perhaps the most important conclusion to emerge with regard to the general epidemiology of malformations is that the etiology of birth defects appears to be multifactorial, and that it is the exception, rather than the rule, for any birth defect to have a single cause.

Specialized readers may be interested in much of the material presented here while for others this book may be of use primarily as a reference volume to be consulted as the need arises. A physician noting that a malformed child was exposed to a certain drug may wish to compare his observation with the experience in this cohort. Workers carrying out formal epidemiological investigations may wish to estimate required sample sizes, or compare their results with ours, and so on. When this book is used for reference purposes, we believe readers will be assisted in evaluating the data if they consult Chapters 1 to 5, 18 and 19, and 34 and 35. At minimum, a quick reading of Chapter 19 will assist in evaluating the chapters that follow.

In recent decades, the literature on malformations, and on chemical and drug teratogens, particularly in an experimental setting, has become vast. Here we have made no more than a cursory attempt to keep pace. Instead, we wish to refer readers to a number of excellent publications. Foremost, of course, is the outstanding work on congenital malformations by Warkany.[1] We have found his book to be indispensable. Wilson, in *Environment and Birth Defects*,[2] provides a larger background in which drugs can be viewed in context. His comments on experimental drug teratogens, as well as drug teratogenicity in humans, are thoughtful and authoritative. Tuchmann-Duplessis[3] has reviewed his large experience spanning many years, as well as that of other workers, concerning drug teratogens, and he has also reviewed some of the evidence in human populations. Shepard[4] has undertaken the task of reviewing and cataloging much of the literature. He and his associates have summarized virtually all of the reports connecting drugs and malformations that are more than merely anecdotal. Most recently, Mirkin[5] and his collaborators have reviewed the topic with special emphasis on placental, fetal, and perinatal pharmacology.

Among the most critical issues in this work was the choice of appropriate statistical methods. The initial idea of modifying established multivariate techniques for the purposes of this study was first proposed by Dr. Stuart Hartz, and then explored by him and Ms. Lynn Rosenberg. Later, they were joined by Dr. Victor Siskind, who also explored certain theoretical matters. Mr. Jerome Cornfield gave advice regarding this aspect of the work.

It is our pleasure to acknowledge the help of many people. We would particularly like to thank various members of our staff who were at one or another time engaged in this project. It is impossible to name them all, but we must mention

[1]Warkany, J.: *Congenital Malformations: Notes and Comments*. Chicago: Year Book Medical Publishers, Inc., 1971.

[2]Wilson, J.G.: *Environment and Birth Defects*. New York: Academic Press, 1973.
[3]Tuchmann-Duplessis, H: *Drug Effects on the Fetus*. Sydney: Adis Press. Acton, Mass.: Publishing Sciences Group, Inc., 1975.
[4]Shepard, T.H.: *Catalog of Teratogenic Agents*. Baltimore: Johns Hopkins University Press, 1973.
[5]Mirkin, B.L. (ed.) *Perinatal Pharmacology and Therapeutics*. New York: Academic Press, 1976.

Ms. Cynthia DaRu, Ms. Virginia Vida, Ms. Marguerite Angeloni, R.N., Ms. Kathleen McMahon, Ms. Barbara Pascoe, Dr. Dean MacLaughlin, Ms. Deborah Kuyamjian, Dr. Micha Levy, Mr. Kurt Johnston, Ms. Nancy Ferrell, Ms. Diane Chase, and Ms. Carol Enseki.

We owe a special debt of gratitude to Ms. Virginia Bucciaglia, R.N., without whose endurance and dedication this study could never have been completed.

We also wish to acknowledge the advice and help of Dr. Ernest B. Hook of the Birth Defects Institute, New York Department of Health, and Dr. Olli Miettinen of the Harvard School of Public Health.

Various members of the Collaborative Perinatal Project gave us unstinting help. Again, all of them cannot be named, but we wish to mention the director of the Collaborative Perinatal Project, Dr. Joseph Drage. Mrs. Annie Litz, R.N., of the Perinatal Branch staff in Bethesda provided invaluable assistance in reviewing thousands of records and Mrs. Barbara Katz and Dr. Kinne McCabe were helpful and patient with our numerous inquiries. In the first years, our collaboration with the Collaborative Perinatal Project was initiated by Dr. Heinz Berendes and Mr. William Weiss. One group of persons perhaps deserves the greatest credit. We refer to the nurses, technicians, physicians, pathologists, and others who were responsible for the work in the field. We believe the data attest to the excellence of that work.

In this sort of enterprise publishers are long-suffering; Dr. Frank Paparello, our publisher, was obliged to be more long-suffering than most. There are no words that can adequately convey our gratitude for his patience and assistance.

Olli P. Heinonen, M.D., M.Sc.

Dennis Slone, M.D.

Samuel Shapiro, F.R.C.P.

CHAPTER 1

The Teratogenic Role of Drugs in Humans

Since Gregg's classical demonstration in 1941 that maternal rubella infection could cause malformations in humans,[1] it has become increasingly evident that the mammalian embryo is subject to a variety of environmental influences which can have deleterious effects upon its development. Birth defects represent a complex interplay of genetics and environment. Probably, such interplay is always present, but it is sometimes possible to identify a predominant causal factor. Wilson has estimated that approximately 25% of developmental defects are primarily genetic or chromosomal in nature, about 10% are caused by known environmental factors, and fully 65% arise from unknown causes.[2]

Since the thalidomide disaster,[3-5] attention has been focused on drugs as potential teratogens. In animal experiments, it has been demonstrated that numerous drugs and chemical substances cause malformations, but in only a few instances has it been possible to provide proof of their adverse effects on human embryogenesis. Clearly, extrapolation from animal experiments to humans is difficult.

This book presents the results of an epidemiological investigation of the possible teratogenic role of drugs, as used in a cohort of over 50,000 mother-child pairs recruited in 12 centers in the United States during the years 1959 to 1965. The data are part of a large-scale study known as the Collaborative Perinatal Project (CPP).[6] The purpose of this book is to evaluate whether there are associations between drugs taken during pregnancy and malformations in the offspring. This chapter presents a brief review of some known environmental causes of birth defects in humans. It also discusses certain principles of experimental teratology as they bear on non-experimental studies in human populations. Finally, some epidemiological principles of relevance to the present study are considered.

Known Environmental Causes of Birth Defects in Humans

Physical

The first environmental agent shown to be teratogenic in humans was ionizing radiation.[7] During the 1920s, it was discovered that pregnant women treated with therapeutic doses of radiation for pelvic malignancy gave birth to children with serious defects, including central nervous and skeletal defects, microcephaly, and mental retardation.[8,9] Similar defects were observed in fetuses exposed to radiation at Hiroshima and Nagasaki.[10,11] There is also evidence that low doses of diagnostic radiation are associated with childhood cancer.[12] It is now generally agreed that exposure of pregnant women to X-rays should, if possible, be avoided.

Biological

Of the identified biological causes of malformations, the classical teratogen is the rubella virus.[1] A large proportion of fetuses born to mothers who had clinical rubella during the early months of pregnancy were malformed.[2,7] Similarly, cytomegalovirus and herpesvirus hominis[2,7] have been shown to cause fetal abnormalities.

Chemical (Other Than Drugs)

Perhaps the most well-documented chemical teratogen in humans is methyl mercury.[13] This chemical, contaminating coastal waters, has been shown to be responsible for a congenital form of Minamata disease. The affected babies were born to mothers who ate large amounts of contaminated fish, even though many of the mothers were not themselves affected. Suspicion has also been focused on lead, selenium, cigarette smoke, and a variety of pesticides and industrial solvents.[2]

Drugs

Prior to the thalidomide disaster during the early 1960s, it was commonly believed that the placental barrier effectively protected the fetus from drugs given to the mother.[2,14] However, since that time, a large number of associations between drugs and birth defects have been reported. Only a few of these associations are universally accepted as causal:

Thalidomide The evidence implicating thalidomide as a teratogen is overwhelming,[2,14] and the experience with the drug demonstrates the need for caution in extrapolating from animal models to humans. No evidence of a teratogenic effect was seen when thalidomide was tested in certain animals prior to its release for clinical use. In pregnant women, exposure to even a single dose, from the 20th to the 35th day after conception, produced a rather unique syndrome characterized principally by deformities of the arms, legs, and face, often together with more widespread deformities. Subsequently, teratological effects similar to those produced in humans were demonstrated in certain primates.[2,14] Other laboratory animals were relatively insensitive to the teratologic potential of thalidomide — and these animals included those most commonly used in laboratory tests, such as mice, rats, and rabbits. It seems reasonable to assume that laboratory experience with primates might, on the whole, more closely approximate anticipated human experience. But even this assumption is questionable.[2,14] Clearly, several different species, including primates, should be tested in the laboratory; but, ultimately, it is unlikely there is any substitute for careful documentation of the occurrence of malformations in relation to drug exposure in human populations.

Since one powerful teratogen has been identified in humans, and since it was only identified at the expense of several thousand malformed children, there can be no question about the need for epidemiological surveillance of human populations.

Steroid Hormones Early exposure to high doses of androgenic hormones leads to masculinization of female fetuses.[2] *In utero* exposure to stilbestrol likely leads to an increased risk of vaginal cancer in women some 10 or more years later.[15,16]

Folic Acid Antagonists and Other Cytotoxic Drugs Antineoplastic drugs usually lead to abortion; of those fetuses that do survive to term, about 20% to 30% are malformed.[2,17]

Tetracyclines These drugs have been shown to have a strong affinity for developing osseous and dental tissue. There is unequivocal evidence that tetracyclines cause dental staining.[18]

Thalidomide, steroid hormones, antineoplastic drugs, and tetracyclines represent instances in which the evidence to implicate drugs as teratogens in human populations is reasonably convincing. However, there is a large list of suspected drugs, based on laboratory observations, epidemiological studies, and case reports.[2,14,19] At appropriate points in this book, some of these drugs will be referred to in relation to the findings in this study.

Some Principles of Experimental Teratology As They Bear on Non-Experimental Studies in Humans

As previously stated, there are great difficulties in generalizing from animal experiments to humans. However, certain general principles are relevant:

Different animal species react differently to environmental exposures. Factors known to be teratogenic in animals may have no association with birth defects in humans, or vice versa. However, when a factor causes birth defects in animals — especially, if many species are involved — and shows an association in humans, this must be taken as at least presumptive reflection of a causal connection.

The developmental state of the fetus at exposure is an important determinant of outcome. Most defects arise early in fetal life, during organogenesis. Thus, when epidemiological methods are used to evaluate a possible association of a factor with birth defects, the time of exposure in pregnancy should be determined — and the principal concentration of any research effort must be on exposure occurring early in pregnancy. In fact, when a late exposure is found to be associated with a defect that can, presumably, only arise during early embryogenesis, a causal explanation is suspect. Some defects, however, may arise at any time during pregnancy (e.g., congenital cataract, pyloric stenosis). A proper evaluation of such outcomes requires that exposures at any time during pregnancy be examined.

Specific agents act in specific ways to cause abnormal development. If biological pathways are analogous in humans and animals (e.g., folic acid antagonists), a causal inference is strengthened.

The nature of an agent determines its access to developing tissues. If an agent readily crosses the placental barrier in animals and in humans, and if it is shown to be teratogenic in animals, an association in humans may well be causal.

The dose of an agent is an important determinant of its effect. In animals, most teratogens show a dose-response relationship which may be time-dependent. However, some do not. In human populations, the precision of recorded drug dosage and time of exposure in epidemiological studies such as the Collaborative Perinatal Project is usually not great; thus, while the presence of a dose-response relationship is generally a strong point favoring an inference of causality, the absence of such a relationship is not necessarily of particular value. If an association is present, but a dose-response relationship is not, a causal inference may nevertheless be justifiable.

The teratogenic effect of an agent should be reproducible. If an association between an exposure and a defect is to be regarded as causal in humans, it must be seen in at least two, and preferably more than two, independent studies. This is desirable if only to eliminate chance as an explanation for any observed association (or absence of association). Even then, several epidemiological studies do not guarantee that all non-causal associations will be properly identified. Similar methodological faults, biases, and confounding factors can be present in more than one study. Nevertheless, when different investigators, having different biases and using different approaches to study different populations, identify similar associations, a causal inference is strengthened.

Some Epidemiological Considerations

The remarks that follow are intended as an introduction to the epidemiological principles underlying the study described in this book. An attempt has been made to avoid unnecessarily complicated technical descriptions.

In general, the study of the causes of birth defects in animals is experimental. An agent is assigned at random to a group of animals, and the frequency of subsequent defects in the offspring is compared to the frequency in a control group. The dose and time of administration of the agent can be specified with precision. The causal nature of the association seen can be readily accepted. In non-experimental epidemiological studies, the situation is quite different. The example of thalidomide will be considered first since the effects of this drug illustrate some of the more important issues.

For ease of identification as a drug teratogen, thalidomide can be considered an "ideal" drug. Identification would have been hindered if all of the following conditions were not met.

- Given a pregnant woman's exposure to thalidomide during the susceptible period of embryogenesis, the risk of having a defective child was many times greater than when no exposure took place.
- Thalidomide was used as a sedative or hypnotic. It is unlikely that anxiety or insomnia are themselves risk factors for bearing a malformed child.
- The most prominent component of the thalidomide syndrome, phocomelia, is easily and precisely diagnosed.
- There was an epidemic of the syndrome whose onset and termination corresponded with the introduction and removal of the drug. Before the epidemic, phocomelia was extremely rare.

Identification of other drugs as teratogens can be far more complex. As a further example, assume insulin causes cleft anomalies. (It must be stressed that this is only an assumption.)

- If diabetes mellitus also causes clefts, evaluation of the separate effects of the disease and the drug used to treat it becomes a very difficult matter. If insulin were used for a wide variety of indications, separate evaluation of the drug according to each indication might afford insight into whether or not suspicion should remain focused on the drug rather than on some underlying condition that provokes its use. However, insulin is hardly used for conditions other than diabetes. Therefore, the problem can only be studied if there are comparable diabetic women not using insulin. Such comparable women do not exist because their disease is less severe.

- Since insulin-dependent diabetics are, for practical purposes, only able to bear children if they take the drug, and since the prevalence of diabetes in women of child-bearing age is relatively stable, there can be no identifiable epidemic.
- Compared with phocomelia, cleft anomalies are much more common. Therefore, an association of the same proportion as the thalidomide disaster might go undetected because clinicians would not be so readily alerted to the possibility that something unusual is happening.
- It is a relatively simple matter to identify an agent which almost inevitably causes malformations. The methodological difficulties are considerably greater if an agent, although it damages the fetus, does so less frequently than does thalidomide.

The complexity of these considerations presents the epidemiologist with formidable difficulties in making a general evaluation of various drugs taken by pregnant women. The identification of teratogens that may be less potent than thalidomide and that may cause malformations that are less obvious than those caused by thalidomide is likely to be particularly difficult. In addition, it is equally important to avoid raising suspicions of causality when they are not justified.

Having stated the broad problems, we will now review the epidemiological issues in greater detail.

The Collaborative Perinatal Project is a cohort study. The exposure of interest was determined prior to the birth of the child. The rates of birth defects were measured in children born to exposed women and in children born to non-exposed women. A condition of a causal association is that the rate of malformed children born to exposed women is higher than the corresponding rate among non-exposed women.

In epidemiological studies, one of the principal concerns is possible bias. In the present setting, two general types of bias deserve special consideration. Each can produce false associations between an exposure and a defect, and each can obscure a true association.

Observation Bias In a cohort study, the most serious type of observation bias arises when the occurrence of birth defects is measured differently in children of exposed and non-exposed women.

A basic technique used to prevent or minimize observation bias is "blindness." If the person who diagnoses birth defects does not know which mothers were exposed and which mothers were not, observation bias is less likely. This was the rule in the Collaborative Perinatal Project. Objectivity is also ensured when the outcome is beyond dispute (e.g., anencephaly).

Similarly, observation bias is present if drug exposure is ascertained differently when the risk of malformations is different. In cohort studies, this is not usually a major problem, although its possible existence requires careful consideration.

Confounding Bias Confounding bias arises when some third factor (or set of factors) either is responsible for an indirect association between an exposure and a defect or conceals a direct one. There is a great potential for confounding bias in all epidemiological studies. To minimize false inferences, it is imperative to make every effort to control confounding. While observation bias can be controlled relatively simply in a cohort study, confounding can arise from many sources, and its nature can be complex and subtle. Even more importantly, confounding may not even be suspected.

In studies of the relationship between drugs and birth defects, an important source of confounding bias is the reason for the administration of the drug. The underlying maternal condition is of necessity associated with the drug because the drug is prescribed for the condition. If the condition is also a cause of some defect (or if it merely reflects some more basic cause), an indirect association will be present.

There are two basic strategies used to minimize confounding bias. The first is to control potential confounding from certain sources in the design of the study. For example, rubella is a strong risk factor for malformations, and it may provoke exposure to certain drugs. In the present study, comparability with respect to rubella has been achieved by excluding mother-child pairs in which either the mother or the neonate had clinical rubella. Thus, confounding bias from diagnosed rubella has been avoided by design.

The second strategy is to allow for potential confounding in the analysis. This can be accomplished by a variety of methods, including stratification, standardization, and multivariate techniques. These methods have in common the objective of achieving comparability between exposed and non-exposed groups; selection of one of the analytical options depends on the data at hand.

Chance   Associations between an exposure and an outcome may occur by chance. If it can be assumed that chance and cause are the only possibilities in a given experimental study, tests of statistical significance may be used to evaluate the role of chance. Tests of statistical significance play a major role in the evaluation of data from experimental studies. In non-experimental studies the possible existence of confounding bias must be considered in the evaluation of any association. Since it is never possible to rule out confounding bias with complete confidence, it is never possible to measure with precision the effects of chance. For this reason, the interpretation of tests of statistical significance in non-experimental studies must be carried out with extreme caution.

Limitations to interpreting statistical significance will be stressed repeatedly in this book. In the Collaborative Perinatal Project, information on a large variety of drugs taken in pregnancy and on a large variety of outcomes was obtained. In the analyses, many thousands of comparisons were carried out. Clearly, a number of "statistically significant" associations were bound to arise by chance; without recourse to other data, there is no way to identify which associations might be explicable on this basis, and which may be causal.

Measures of Association   The most useful measure, and the one used throughout this book, is the point estimate of *relative risk*, which is often presented together with its 95% confidence intervals. The relative risk is the ratio of the rate of a defect in exposed children to the rate in non-exposed children. The confidence intervals are estimates of the extent to which the relative risk could, by chance, have been greater or less than the value actually estimated. If the lower 95% confidence limit of a relative risk is greater than 1.0, this implies that the association is unlikely to be due to chance. These measures, taken together, can give an impression of the stability of the relative risk, as well as its relative size. The advantage of using the relative risk as an estimator of association is that it affords insight into the magnitude of the association and thus enables a judgment of the extent to which the risk can be reduced if the causal factor is removed.

Concluding Remarks

Experimental work with animals can be suggestive, but never conclusive, that a drug may be teratogenic to humans. In human populations, we are limited to what can be learned by means of epidemiological methods. Certain drugs, if they are potent enough as teratogens, and striking enough in their effects, can be relatively easily identified — an obvious example being thalidomide. Other drugs which are less potent, but nevertheless teratogenic, and which cause defects that are important but not unusual, are more difficult to identify. If there are any undetected teratogenic drugs currently in use, they may well be of the latter type. If they are to be detected, complex and careful epidemiologic analysis is mandatory. Even then, the conclusions that can be drawn on the basis of only one study must be considered as purely tentative.

The data from the Collaborative Perinatal Project presented here must be viewed in this context. A battery of epidemiological and statistical methods have been used to screen a large number of drugs against a variety of malformation outcomes. At the outset it is worth stressing the complexity of the issues and the tentativeness of any identified associations — even if these persist after rigorous analysis. None of the associations presented in this book should be regarded as anything more than hypotheses requiring independent confirmation.

CHAPTER 2

The Collaborative Perinatal Project

Design, Recruitment, and Data Collection

The idea of carrying out a prospective study of factors in pregnancy related to cerebral palsy and other forms of damage to the central nervous system, eventually known as the Collaborative Perinatal Project, was first mooted in the early 1950s. As the project developed, its scope was increased until, ultimately, it was designed to collect data on a large number of antenatal and perinatal events in the mothers and postnatal events in the children. The scope of the study was extended far beyond that of determining causes of cerebral palsy. The detailed evolution of this large and ambitious project — perhaps the largest of its kind ever undertaken — has already been described.[1,2] In the present context, it is relevant that information on drugs used by the gravidas was recorded prior to delivery, and that detailed data on malformations in the offspring were collected. There was thus an opportunity to carry out an epidemiological evaluation of drugs as potential teratogens.

Fourteen university-affiliated hospitals were involved in the study. In 10 centers the obstetric and pediatric departments were in the same hospital and in Boston and Philadelphia they were in separate hospitals; thus, 12 medical centers participated in collecting data. Recruitment of the study participants lasted seven years, extending from January 2, 1959 to December 31, 1965.

Selection of the Participants

Participants were selected from among pregnant women admitted to collaborating hospital clinics. The selection procedures were not uniform in all hospitals; they were modified because of considerations such as the capacity of each center to commit its resources to the study for 15 years or more, the degree of interference with the different routines of the maternity clinics, and the individual interests of researchers in each institution.

The sampling frame was designed to ensure roughly equal recruitment of White and Black women, but no *a priori* ethnic exclusions were stipulated. In order for women to be placed in the sampling frame, a variety of constraints were imposed in all antenatal clinics. Common disqualifications were a woman's intention to leave the locality soon, certain areas of residence, and delivery on the same day as first registration into the study — "walk-in" cases. With these pre-set limitations, there were 132,560 gravidas in the sampling frame available for study before the local selection schemes for entry were applied.

In two of the hospitals all presenting gravidas in the sampling frame were enrolled; in nine hospitals systematic selection was based upon the terminal digit of the record number, the woman's day of birth, or some similar selection device; in one hospital, random selection was used. If a woman had more than one pregnancy at a collaborating hospital within the stipulated time limits, she could be admitted as a participant more than once.

Depending on the special interests of collaborating physicians in individual centers, it was permissible, to an agreed extent, to enroll and collect data as a routine part of the study for certain specified groups — for example, one special group consisted of all gravidas under 16 years of age seen at the Johns Hopkins Hospital, Baltimore. Apart from this special group, for gravidas registered according to the principal scheme of the study, the sampling ratio was approximately two out of five eligible pregnancies at that hospital.

A total of 58,282 pregnancies were registered. Of these, 2,622 were members of special groups, 298 were "walk-ins", and 55,908 conformed strictly with the general selection rules. The correctly selected proportion of women registered into the study in each hospital ranged from 14% to 100% of those initially available in the sampling frame. In each of the participating institutions, the sample correctly enrolled in the study did not differ with regard to age, ethnic group, marital status, or weeks of gestation at admission as compared with the total group of women who initially formed the sampling frame.[1]

Over 2,000 correctly selected registrants refused to participate. In addition, a small number of gravidas moved and could not be traced. Sometimes, for one reason or another, information concerning labor, delivery, or the child could not be obtained. In all, refusals and losses to follow-up amounted to 2,977 mother-child pairs (5.3%), which reduced the sample from 55,908 to 52,931. While there were no statistically significant differences between the non-responders and responders with regard to age, ethnic group, marital status, and weeks of gestation at registration, the non-responders were, overall, slightly more often well-educated, married, and over the age of 35 years. These differences were, however, not consistent by hospital.

There were 954 pregnancies (1.7%) that terminated in spontaneous abortion, therpeutic abortion, ectopic pregnancy, or hydatidiform mole before the 20th week after the last menstrual period. This reduced the study cohort to 51,977 mother-child pairs.

Finally, for the purposes of the analyses reported in this book, certain exclusions, representing a total of 1,695 pregnancies (3.3%), were stipulated for the following overlapping reasons: twin and triplet pregnancies (1.2%); mother's ethnic group other than White, Black, or Puerto Rican (1.0%); important pertinent data (e.g., maternal age, diseases and/or complications of pregnancy, sex of child) not available (1.0%); and clinically evident maternal rubella during pregnancy and/or congenital rubella syndrome in the offspring (0.2%).

After all exclusions, 50,282 mother-child pairs in which the pregnancy lasted five lunar months or longer, including children who survived or died during the follow-up period, were available for analysis.

Data Collection

Information routinely collected included data on the mother's social and medical background, co-existing diseases, and complications of pregnancy. Similarly, data concerning the child's birth, development, any diseases that occurred, and any congenital defects that were noted were also collected, according to systematic design, up to the eighth birthday. Information on the child's siblings, father, and other relatives was also obtained.

On entry to the study, usually while visiting the participating clinic the first time during the pregnancy, each woman was interviewed by a specially trained examiner to obtain medical, genetic, and social data. Specifically with regard to medications, the women were questioned about current drug use as well as drug use extending back beyond the date of the last menstrual period. Detailed, structured forms were used, and the data collection procedure was guided by use of extensive manuals (available on request from the Perinatal Research Branch, National Institute of Neurological and Communicative Disorders and Stroke, National Institutes of Health, Bethesda, Maryland 20014). Initially at monthly visits to the clinic, and then at shorter intervals during the last trimester, interviewers and obstetricians continued to collect data. The completed study forms were then reviewed and compared with hospital records for completeness by another person. If the woman had received medical attention before entry into the study, further information on events taking place prior to registration was acquired from "non-study" physicians and from hospitals to complement and verify certain items of interview data. Completed forms were once more edited in the study hospital, this time by attending medical personnel. The assembled material was then sent to a central facility where it was processed into computer files. Various precautionary measures were taken to prevent coding and punching errors in the massive flow of data. In addition, certain computer procedures were routinely used to identify and correct obvious mistakes in the original computer files.

Information on the offspring was collected from birth and processed in a similar manner. The first period of systematic data collection covered the baby's stay in hospital. Among other things, the baby was examined by a pediatrician every day during the first week after delivery, or weekly if the child remained in the hospital longer. In addition to the detailed forms, a summary for the nursery period was produced locally.

The mother was interviewed for what was termed an "interval history" when the child was 4, 8, 12, 18 and 24 months old and, thereafter, annually. If, in the interim, the child had been taken to a physician or a hospital, further data about the child's illness were acquired from these sources. An extensive, standardized pediatric examination was performed on the children at the age of one year. The response rate for the one-year examination was 91% in the surviving children. For most of the remaining children, an interval history was available. Finally, of 2,227 children who were stillborn, or who died before the fourth birthday (4.4% of the cohort), 81% came to autopsy; the autopsy rate did not vary appreciably according to the age at death.

Preparation of the Collaborative Perinatal Data for Analysis

The main purpose of the Collaborative Perinatal Project was, and is, to evaluate factors in pregnancy as they may relate to cerebral palsy and other forms of damage to the central nervous system. The collection of data pertinent to the drug/ malformation axis was, in context, tangential to the main purpose of the study. It was therefore to be expected that the material would have to be extensively reorganized before analysis of drugs as potential teratogens could commence. The principal steps were to evaluate and re-classify the drug exposure information; to evaluate and, to some extent, re-classify the malformation data; and to reorganize data on a large number of pregnancy-related variables.

Drug Exposure Data

Several hundred different pharmacological entities, alone or in various combinations, were taken by the pregnant women. In the original CPP drug dictionaries, drugs were classified according to either their generic or brand names. The tally for any given generic compound did not include instances in which the compound was an ingredient in a multiple-component product. Often, only the brand name was coded; for some of the brand name drugs, the individual components had not been determined. For example, there were literally hundreds of preparations, each having a separate code number and containing various mixtures of aspirin, phenacetin, or caffeine, with or without antihistamines, barbiturates, tranquilizers, and sympathomimetic amines, as well as other

substances. An even more difficult problem arose because there were instances when a variety of brand name drugs, usually used for roughly the same indications but having different ingredients, were assigned the same code number.

The CPP did not collect information on vitamins or iron preparations (unless they were received parenterally) or antacids because it was judged that these agents would be used by practically all of the participants.

It became clear that for the purposes of this study, it would be necessary to reorganize the drug data. Each ingredient was identified and coded according to its generic name. Also exact ascertainment of the drug exposures required inspection of a large proportion of the original records to determine the actual brand name drugs used, so that their components could be coded. Ultimately, over 8,000 records had to be inspected.

Before final code numbers could be assigned, it was necessary to adopt a standard nomenclature. American names were used wherever they existed, and names were generally shortened to include only the active ingredient. The nomenclature was taken from the following sources, in preferential order:

1. *The United States Pharmacopeia*, 18th Revision (1970)[3]
2. *U.S.A.N. 10, 1961-1971 Cumulative List*, and *1974 Supplement*[4]
3. *The National Formulary*, 13th Edition (1970)[5]
4. *The International Pharmacopeia*, 2nd Edition (1967) and *Supplement* (1971)[6]
5. *I.N.N.* (1971)[7]
6. *American Drug Index*, 1975[8]
7. Any other official source, such as *The British Pharmacopeia*
8. *The Merck Index*, 8th Edition (1968)[9]

After the actual drugs used were identified, as accurately as possible, and names were standardized, the next task was to classify them. The classification ultimately used in this study was based on conventional pharmacological considerations, the indications for drug use, and how commonly the various drugs were used. The full classification is given in Appendix 3.

Malformations

A large array of malformations were recorded. Some of these were of minor importance and their recording was likely to vary substantially because of the subjective judgment of individual observers, in which case such malformations were ignored. For example, accessory nipples were deemed trivial; also, rates of accessory nipple, by hospital, were extremely variable, suggesting that there was indeed a substantial subjective component to its diagnosis. Other examples of this type included cleft uvula and dislocation of the fifth toe.

The remaining malformations, affecting 3,248 children, represent the outcomes considered in this study. With some exceptions regarding cardiovascular defects (to be noted shortly), the malformations were those identified in the following categories: stillborn children born to pregnancies lasting at least five lunar months; liveborn children during the first year of life, whether or not they died during that year; and children who died between the first and fourth birthday.

Malformations were considered to be accurate when an individual diagnosis was recorded in at least two of the following independent computer files: nursery period summary; summary of the period after discharge from the nursery up to and including the examination carried out at one year of age; and the autopsy file. Alternatively, when the diagnoses were not identical in the various files, or when they were recorded in only one of them, the original case records were reviewed by hand and the malformation was only considered acceptable if the record was

unequivocal. Several hundred records were reviewed for this purpose.

As mentioned previously, malformations of the cardiovascular system were ascertained using methods that were somewhat different and which have been described elsewhere in detail.[10] These methods included detailed review of all files for diagnoses of definite or possible congenital heart disease; detailed searches of medical clinic files in each hospital to ensure that no cardiovascular abnormalities escaped recording in the routine data forms of the CPP; re-examination, by a qualified cardiologist, of all children who were even suspected of having a cardiovascular defect; re-examination of the preserved hearts in 35% of autopsied children together with a detailed review of the original autopsy report (in consultation with the pathologist who originally did the autopsy); and inclusion of a small number of children in whom cardiovascular defects were first diagnosed only after the age of four years. The cardiovascular malformations were probably determined more accurately and completely than any others in the cohort.

A full listing of the malformations analyzed in the study is given in Appendix 2. Initially, hospital distributions of all malformations with adequate numbers were compared to determine whether any of them showed grossly variable rates. Comparisons were made separately for each ethnic group. Six malformations were found in which there was considerable variability in the hospital rates, but which were nonetheless deemed important. These anomalies, designated as "non-uniform" malformations, were inguinal hernia, clubfoot, cleft gum, pectus excavatum, urethral obstruction, and abnormalities of the hands and fingers. The six malformations have in common the characteristic that they can, at one extreme, be so mild that there may be a substantial subjective component to their diagnosis while, at the other extreme, they can be serious. For example, pectus excavatum can be simply a "cosmetic" defect, or it can lead to crippling and even fatal cardiopulmonary disease. Thus, the variability of the hospital rates probably reflects the range of severity of these malformations, the most severe of which are unmistakable, and the least severe of which tend to be diagnosed largely on a subjective basis.

Combining the non-uniform malformations with other more evenly distributed malformations would greatly complicate the analysis; variability among the twelve hospitals would have to be controlled. On the other hand, it is not justifiable to ignore the non-uniform malformations. Accordingly, the strategy adopted in this study has been to deal with the uniform and non-uniform malformations separately in all but the initial analyses.

There were 2,277 children with one or more uniform malformations. The malformations in these 2,277 children were divided along two axes. The first axis comprised three categories: major and minor malformations and tumors, which were not designated as either major or minor. Major malformations were defined as being either life-threatening, requiring major surgery, or having serious cosmetic effects. Each uniform malformation was considered by the medically qualified investigators in this study and deemed to be either major or minor (Appendix 2). The second axis along which the 2,277 children with uniform malformations were divided was based on a series of anatomical classes, together with syndromes and tumors. It should be noted that tumors were retained as a separate category in both classifications.

Other Study Variables

A large number of data items other than drugs or malformations were re-corded for each mother-child pair. Some of these were judged to be of no interest for present purposes and were ignored (e.g., size of community of birthplace of the gravida). The factors retained for analysis were classified as follows:

- Administrative data, such as hospital, number of antenatal visits
- Personal characteristics of the mother, such as age, ethnic group
- Characteristics and survival of the offspring
- Reproductive history of the mother
- Characteristics and complications of the pregnancy
- Environmental factors such as cigarettes or X-rays
- Genetic factors such as family history of malformations

All maternal diseases present during pregnancy were automatically selected for inclusion in the analysis. Other factors were chosen on the basis of existing suspicion in the medical literature of an adverse effect on normal embryogenesis (e.g., smoking status). Some were chosen because of biological similarities with reported risk factors — for example, since hypoxia is believed to interfere with the normal development of the fetus, complications of pregnancy that may intermittently simulate this condition, such as vena cava syndrome, were considered. Certain factors were chosen for their intrinsic interest (e.g., social class), and some were chosen for technical reasons (e.g., hospital).

For each item, distributions of the recorded values (e.g., maternal age, birthweight) were scrutinized. In addition, data were checked for internal consistency. Questionable or conflicting values were checked in the original source documents. The initial scrutiny indicated that it was necessary to check and correct only a small proportion of the material, and the corrections were mostly of minor importance. Nevertheless, the total number of records that had to be processed obviously increased as the number of factors under scrutiny increased. In the case of the recorded date of the last menstrual period, approximately 4% of the cohort required correction. Erroneous dates showed clear concentration around the New Year.

A considerable effort was made to ensure the greatest possible completeness of the data. Often, data on the same or on a similar item were available from more than one source. For example, the genetic history obtained for each child contained information on stillborn siblings and half-siblings: this information could be used to substitute for missing information in the mother's reproductive history. An additional method used to minimize the amount of missing information was to examine successive data in women who registered into the study during more than one pregnancy. For example, if during the current pregnancy the gravida did not have a recorded smoking history, but it was known from a later pregnancy that she had never smoked, this was considered to apply to all pregnancies; likewise, if the mother's height was only recorded once, this variable was applied to all the registered pregnancies.

Generally, missing information was randomly distributed, but there were some exceptions. Placental weight and the number of umbilical arteries were unknown during the earlier years because routine registration of these variables was only introduced after the study had been in progress for some time. Thus, unknown values of these variables were clearly not random with respect to time of entry. To give another example, there were some women enrolled in the study because their gestation period exceeded twenty weeks, who, in clinical terms, had spontaneous abortions often only a day or two after registration. Understandably, it was quite common for a large proportion of the data items concerning these pregnancies to be missing. However, as mentioned earlier, it was

unusual for crucial information to be missing, and only 484 mother-child pairs to whom this applied had to be excluded.

The principal analytical method adopted in this study required that the values of all variables be classified in categories. Maternal age, for example, was classified by half-decade from below the age of 15 years to 45 years and over. In general, extreme values were considered to be of particular interest and were kept in separate categories; otherwise, relatively broad categories were created.

All categories were created without knowledge of how any of the malformations were distributed in each of them. This also held true with regard to the distribution of drug use in the various categories.

Even after rejecting certain variables as being of no interest in the present study, a large number still needed to be considered as potentially confounding factors. Since none of the maternal diseases were rejected in this way, to determine which of them should be retained in the final analyses, the following procedure was adopted: Each disease was evaluated in relation to the set of 2,277 children with uniformly distributed malformations. For each disease, the overall malformation rate in children whose mothers had the disease was compared with the rate in children born to mothers who did not. If the ratio of the two rates was close to unity (relative risk approximately 1.0), this was taken to indicate lack of association between the disease in question and uniform malformations. The same procedure was adopted for major malformations, minor malformations, malformations classified by anatomical site, syndromes, and tumors. These comparisons were, in all instances, carried out separately within each ethnic group. If any one or more of the outcomes showed a substantial positive or negative deviation from a relative risk of 1.0, the disease under consideration was retained for further analysis. Diseases not as-

14

sociated with any of the outcomes were omitted from further analysis since it was judged that they were unlikely to have a confounding influence on drug/malformation associations.

In summary, before it was possible to commence analysis of drugs taken in pregnancy in relation to malformations, a great deal of work had to be done in reorganizing the data. The reorganization included recoding of drug data; organization of the drug data into a suitable classification; verification of the malformation data as well as classification of the material to suit the present purposes; and evaluation and classification of a large series of variables to be taken into account as potentially confounding factors.

CHAPTER 3

Data Analysis

Summary

For the benefit of readers who are not interested in the intimate details of the methodology, the main features of the analysis will be summarized.

Our objective was to explore the relationships between exposure during pregnancy to various drugs and the subsequent appearance in the offspring of various classes of malformations (outcomes). It was necessary to ensure, as far as possible, that confounding (the influence of third factors, or covariates, on rates of both drug use and malformations) neither exaggerated nor obscured such relationships. For those malformation classes containing adequate numbers of affected children, an attempt was made to control confounding in advance by the use of the following strategy.

We selected a set of covariates (i.e., maternal health conditions, factors in pregnancy or characteristics of the infant other than malformation status) which together best identified pregnancies at high risk for the outcome in question. We began by examining for each covariate in turn, and without reference to any other covariate, its association with the outcome. To this end, we compared the observed outcome rates in the various categories of the covariate. The covariates which showed at least some evidence of association were then together subjected to linear discriminant function analysis.

The latter procedure determined which covariates retained their predictive power in the presence of the others; those failing to do so were discarded. Using the set of covariates which survived this screening process, we fitted a mathematical model for outcome risk in the absence of drug effects to the data; the average of the fitted risks over those pregnancies in which a given drug exposure occurred is in effect an estimated outcome rate for this group, adjusted for the influence of the covariates but not for drug use. The ratio of the observed rate for each such exposed group to the corresponding adjusted rate — a standardized relative risk (or more precisely an adjusted relative risk) — served in this study as the principal measure of the strength of association between each sufficiently common outcome and each drug. Approximate confidence limits for it were computed in every case. As a check, unadjusted ratios of rates, or ratios adjusted for only one or two factors, were also examined for every drug-outcome combination, including now the less common malformation categories and individual defects.

Introduction

The analytic problem with which we are confronted is, in principle, straightforward: to assess the effect of each of one class of factors, the exposure variables, on each of a class of outcome events, in the presence of a third, "nuisance" class of factors, or covariates, which may themselves be risk factors for one or more of the outcomes.

The first class of factors comprises exposure to or avoidance of certain drugs, vaccines, and others by the gravida. A typical outcome event from the second class of factors would be the occurrence in the offspring of a specific malformation or of at least one of a specific group of malformations. Examples of covariates from the third class of factors are maternal age,

ethnic group, and health conditions during pregnancy.

In practice, this three-way classification is not entirely clear-cut; there are drugs — e.g., insulin, anticonvulsants, antihypertensives — which are both exposure variables of interest and indicators of health conditions in the mother, while certain factors — such as infant survival — have some of the properties of both outcome variables and covariates. Such issues will be given due consideration in their proper places.

Some of these covariates may be linked antecedently to both the outcome event and exposure to a drug and so give rise to a "spurious" association between them. This phenomenon is called confounding, a concept central to much of epidemiologic methodology and covered in most standard textbooks. For present purposes, a few simple but realistic examples may best serve to illustrate how confounding could lead to erroneous conclusions. The first case concerns an artefactual association between exposure to killed polio virus in the first four lunar months of pregnancy and subsequent fetal loss.[1] Here the confounding variable is gestational age at the first recorded antenatal visit. The study cohort in this instance is one in which pregnancies lasting less than 20 weeks had not yet been excluded. Among 6,941 women exposed to killed polio virus early in pregnancy, the rate of fetal loss was 3.7%, whereas in the non-exposed group the rate was 2.4%. When these rates are recalculated separately for those women who entered the study in the first trimester of their pregnancies and those who entered at a later stage, a different picture emerges: the early-entry group shows a 4.2% loss-rate among exposed women compared to 4.9% among the non-exposed, while for the late entrants these values are 1.6% and 1.8%, respectively. Women who are under medical care early in pregnancy are more likely to receive vaccines at that stage, while women whose first antenatal clinic visit was late in pregnancy have fetuses who have, with few exceptions, survived at least to that point.

A more subtle issue arises when one attempts to evaluate the teratogenicity of drugs used to treat chronic disease — for instance, anticonvulsants. Suppose that certain types of malformations occur more frequently in the children of treated or untreated epileptic women than in those of healthy mothers (i.e., that epilepsy is itself a risk factor for these malformations). Then the fact that phenytoin, for example, is used mainly to treat epilepsy implies that exposure to this drug will be found to be associated with higher malformation rates, whether or not it is itself deleterious to the developing fetus. In other words, the effects of exposure and of disease are mutually confounded at least to some degree.[2,3]

Apart from the analytic aspects, we are faced with the necessity of presenting in concise, comprehensible form the results of the analysis, which involves several dozen outcomes (malformations) and several hundred pharmaceutical compounds. The statistical index of the effects of a given exposure on a given outcome which seems best to meet our various needs is relative risk. In its crudest form relative risk is merely the ratio of the frequency or risk of the outcome event among those exposed to a drug to the risk among the non-exposed; it takes no account of possible confounding variables. The crude relative risk could equivalently be defined as the ratio of the observed number of outcome events among the exposed to the number which one would expect if the outcome rate among the non-exposed applied throughout the cohort. Note that if the exposed group happened to comprise a small fraction of the total cohort, one could, without great error, compute the expected number on the basis of the overall cohort rate.

In view of what has been said in previous paragraphs, it is clearly advisable to obtain a "standardized" index of effect (i.e., one which is as free of the effects of confounding as possible). As described below, we do this by incorporating in advance the effects of all the important risk factors into the calculation of the expected number of outcome events.

A related phenomenon, not always easily distinguished from confounding, is effect-modification.[4,5] Here the association of drug and malformation would not be a reflection of the common influence of other variables, or at any rate would persist after confounding had been controlled. However, the strength of the association varies with the levels of a third, modifying factor, or group of factors. It might happen, for instance, that a drug was almost without effect on malformation rates in younger women but was a powerful teratogen in elderly gravidae. If the effects of some drug were modified so strongly as to be protective against malformation in one group of women and teratogenic in another, the methodology we have employed might well fail to detect the association between drug and malformation. We do not believe that such occurrences are at all common in practice. On the other hand, once a connection between drug exposure and outcome has been established beyond reasonable doubt, closer examination of the data would soon uncover any significant effect-modification which might be present.

When only a limited number of covariates are involved and not too many analyses have to be performed, adequate techniques have long been available for mitigating the effects of any confounding that may be — and in a non-experimental study often is — present. Among these techniques are various standardization procedures in which the data are first cross-classified into strata by all combinations of the confounding variables, analysis of variance of transformed rates, analysis of variance of logits, and analysis of covariance for continuously scaled covariates and outcome variables.[6-8] With the development of computer technology, large-scale prospective epidemiological studies such as the CPP have become feasible. One could now, in principle at least, collect, store, organize, retrieve, and analyze huge volumes of information; in practice, this would be possible only at the expense of introducing a greater degree of heterogeneity into the study material. In addition, many factors are recognized as potentially relevant to the outcome of interest, both as possible etiological agents themselves and as sources of confounding.

This is not the place to review the wealth of methods developed in response to various aspects of the problem of data analysis for cohort studies or to argue their respective merits. We will content ourselves in this chapter with describing the various complementary statistical techniques that were actually employed in this study. Some techniques are familiar to most investigators and are employed in familiar ways. Other procedures were either specially developed to meet our data-analytic and descriptive needs or involve potentially controversial applications of existing methods. Where some justification has seemed necessary, arguments are advanced.

It is convenient to start by describing a mathematical model for risk of malformation used extensively in this investigation — viz., the multiple logistic risk function (MuLoRF). Various workers have given details of its properties, general appropriateness, and relation to discriminant function analysis.[6,9,10] First suppose that k covariates $X_1, \ldots, X_k$ are risk factors for ("predict") some outcome, and that in a "subject" (a mother-child pair) the values $x_1, \ldots, x_k$ are observed. We will call this vector of observed values the "profile" of the subject. The MuLoRF model postulates that the probability or risk that the outcome occurs, given the profile $x_1, \ldots, x_k$, is of the form

$$p(x_1, \ldots, x_k) = [1 + \exp[-\beta_0 - \sum_{i=1}^{k} \beta_i x_i]]^{-1} \quad (1)$$

The k + 1 coefficients, $\beta_0, \beta_1, \ldots, \beta_k$, are, of course, unknown and are estimated from the data on maximum likelihood principles, using an iterative algorithm.

In principle, the procedure we have followed may now be briefly sketched, with amplification, qualification, and discussion to follow. An outcome and a drug to be studied are chosen; the set of covariates relevant to the outcome are identified; their coefficients, $\beta_0, \ldots, \beta_k$ in (1), are estimated from either (a) those subjects not exposed to the drug, or (b) the entire cohort of subjects but ignoring all information on exposure to the drug; finally, the estimated MuLoRF's are computed for all exposed subjects and summed. We now have an estimate of the number of outcomes that would be expected among exposed subjects if the hypothesis that the drug had no effect were true. The ratio of the observed number of outcomes among the exposed to this expected value is a standardized relative risk (SRR). Values of the SRR appreciably different from unity indicate a strong association between drug and outcome, over and above any associations which might be due to other risk factors in the MuLoRF.

This methodology is especially effective when the number of children affected by one or more malformations in a given class is fairly large. It is less effective, relative to its cost, for outcomes, particularly the many single malformations, which occur with lower frequency. Moreover, it could be postulated that some of the many factors taken into account were links in a (causal) chain connecting exposure to outcome. Such a situation would give rise to the phenomenon known as overcontrolling, which we discuss in a later section.

For these reasons, we used in addition a simpler screening procedure, in which less strenuous attempts to eliminate confounding were made: for each drug-malformation combination a crude relative risk was computed, as well as two relative risks standardized by different (sets of) covariates. The first standardization was by the single factor, institution of birth; the second was by a set of covariates which varied in its detailed composition among outcomes, but was principally a combination of ethnic group, survival status of the child, and the presence of at least one of a subset of antenatal maternal factors.

At least the first-level associations were thus detected, unless negative confounding from other sources was still acting to obscure such relationships — surely a rather remote contingency. Where data on associations between individual drugs and most single malformations are presented, the hospital-standardized relative risk is the one used.

Selection of Risk-Function Variables

In order to control confounding, it is enough to consider only those variables related to exposure as well as to outcome. In the present study there are a great many drugs and covariates and a fair number of outcomes. To determine for every outcome and every drug just which covariates are appropriate, in that they introduce at least some confounding, would be a vast exercise in futility. To circumvent this problem we employed the above adaptation of the MuLoRF analysis, rather than an existing approach; if all the factors which predict the event to any substantial degree were included in the risk function, confounding could not occur whichever drug was being investigated. Subject to certain restrictions discussed later, the same estimated MuLoRF, with the same subset of covariates, could therefore be used repeatedly to obviate confounding with re-

spect to the great majority of exposure factors.

On the other hand, it would hardly be feasible from a computational point of view to take more than a limited number of covariates into consideration when computing probabilities of outcome from (1). An additional if rather minor point is that, as can be shown, the inclusion in the MuLoRF of factors unrelated to outcome will, in general, increase the variance of the estimates of risk. One of the first practical steps once the data had been prepared was thus to select those covariates most closely related to a particular outcome and hence best able to predict it.

In choosing these factors, we employed clinical judgment and carefully evaluated the data. First, frequencies of the outcome in question at each level of every factor were compared. Once the obviously unrelated or weakly related factors had been eliminated, the coefficients of a linear discriminant function (LDF) of the remaining variables were calculated and examined.

To forestall the criticism that the LDF is not theoretically applicable to the dichotomous or categorical variables with which we are mainly concerned, we would merely point out that the making of probability statements — as in significance testing, posterior distributions, and the like — are not of interest here.[11] On the other hand, the sizes of the LDF coefficients, both absolute and after division by their standard errors, are a measure of the relative predictive importance of each of the factors in the presence of the others. This approach has incidentally yielded valuable insights, reported under other headings, into the epidemiology of various malformations.

It should be noted in passing that the objectives of controlling confounding in order to study drug effects and those of exploring other aspects of teratology do not always coincide. It could well happen that somewhat different sets of factors

20

would be appropriate to each of them. And there are other considerations. As already mentioned, inclusion of variables of the ambiguous type mentioned earlier — partly covariates, partly outcomes — may lead to overcontrolling, perhaps through being links in a "causal" chain. Two of the most important such factors are birthweight and infant survival. Exposure variables which reflect maternal health present other sorts of difficulties. We will return to these important topics in later sections.

In the majority of cases variables have been brought into the LDF and subsequently the MuLoRF in a dichotomous (zero-one) form, even though originally they may have been measured on a quantitative scale, as with age or length of gestation, or coded ordinally with increasing severity, like certain antenatal health conditions. Other factors, although dichotomously coded from the outset, had had of necessity a third category, "unknown," assigned to them. Our method of recoding variables clearly needs explanation.

First, note that a useful, if crude, classification can be made by distinguishing the factors in which all categories have, medically speaking, equal status among themselves from those factors in which one or more categories are in some way more "healthy" or "normal" than others. Examples of the former, which we define as "unordered," are ethnic group or religion; examples of the latter are length of gestation, occurrence of vaginal bleeding, exposure to X-rays, and even age (in that both very young girls and women over 35 years are thought to be at greater risk for unfavorable pregnancy outcomes). Among most factors of this second type, the majority of subjects falls into the normal category or categories, one notable exception being the occurrence of vomiting in pregnancy: it might be considered healthier not to vomit, but, at least in this cohort, about two-thirds of the pregnant women did.

We have usually not scrupled to combine the "unknown" category with whichever category of known values it most resembled with respect to frequency of outcome. There is here an underlying assumption — which we have no trouble accepting — that the absence from the record of this portion of the data does not in itself tell us something about the gravida or her child which is both of importance and not conveyed by other, known factors. In other words, we believe that, within a factor, the category of missing values has little epidemiological significance per se, and is composed of subjects with roughly the same distribution of variable values as in the cohort as a whole; the data themselves by and large lend support to this contention. This situation arises in part from the way in which the data were prepared for analysis (see Chapter 2).

Under these circumstances, combining the unknown with the normal group, where it exists, will produce at most a small amount of misclassification with respect to the factor in question, mainly of the false-negative type, with negligible effects on bias or statistical power. Among the unordered factors and factors without a large normal category, there were generally either very few unknowns or none at all.

When unordered categorical variables at more than two levels (for instance, ethnic group) had to be considered, the usual practice of assigning a dummy zero-one variable to each level but one was initially adopted. Later LDF analysis sometimes indicated that categories could be combined. With respect to the quantitatively scaled variables, the data rarely revealed anything approaching a monotonic trend in outcome rates across the domain of the variable. If any effect at all was present, it commonly showed up as stable, random fluctuations in frequency of outcome within a fairly wide "normal" range, and higher but unstable rates in the comparatively small group of subjects falling outside this range. In some of such cases, the dichotomy "normal" versus "abnormal" seemed to describe the variation most satisfactorily; in other cases, a pair of dichotomies, "low" versus "normal" and "high" versus "normal," appeared necessary. Where it seemed justified by the data, one or two additional ordinal values (i.e., the values 2, 3) were assigned to extreme factor categories. In one instance, birthweights below 1,500 gm were assigned the value 3; weights in the ranges 1,500 to 1,999 gm and 2,000 to 2,499 gm, the values 2 and 1, respectively; and weights of 2,500 gm or above, the value zero. In all cases care was taken that the recoding should not upset any existing monotonic relationships among the covariates themselves.

Apart from considerations of effectiveness from a data-analytic point of view, restricting each selected covariate to a limited number of variable values resulted in a substantial saving in computation costs. Moreover, as pointed out in the next section, the coefficients of these covariates now have a particularly simple practical interpretation.

The Multiple Logistic Risk Function Procedure

Suppose that one particular outcome is being studied and that the set of variables which predict it has been selected. The next step is to estimate the coefficients, $\{\beta_i\}$ in (1). The considerations determining whether one uses the entire cohort for this purpose or, alternatively, omits the exposed group, and the statistical consequences of this choice, merit separate discussion. It should be emphasized again that in the former case no provision is made in the formulation of the MuLoRF for a variable or coefficient representing exposure to any drug, and that in the estimation process information on this aspect is ignored.

In several of our manipulations, and in particular in the estimation procedure,

there is an implicit assumption, which we attempt to justify later on, that the pregnancies can be treated as statistically independent for most practical purposes, despite the fact that some 16% of pregnant women appear more than once in the cohort.

For efficient solution of the maximum likelihood equations for the $\{\beta_i\}$, good initial values are required. A convenient set of these is provided by the LDF coefficients.[12] But some care is necessary. In general, when the outcome probabilities $p(x_1, \ldots, x_k)$ are all rather small, the dominant term in the linear combination of variables in the MuLoRF is β_0, the term which is always present. Suppose that the LDF coefficient of some zero-one variable was of the same order of magnitude as the initial β_0, but of opposite sign. Those individuals positive for this variable would then be assigned initial probabilities near $\frac{1}{2}$, a value which could well be much too large. If more than a small proportion of individuals were so affected, the first few cycles of the Newton-Raphson procedure might result in considerable oscillation, and convergence would be slow. It is our experience that judicious trimming of such initial estimates, and a little common sense, usually takes care of the problem.

Once calculated, the coefficients were combined with each individual profile in turn to derive a distribution of estimated risks over the cohort (or over that portion used in the estimation process). Formal methods of testing the goodness-of-fit of the MuLoRF are available, but since the theoretical adequacy of the logistic model was of little practical interest to us, we used instead a less formal approach. We ranked the subjects by MuLoRF value and compared the observed number of events in each decile or two-percentile stratum with its expectation as computed from the MuLoRF. An example is given in Chapter 5. The model was accepted as satisfactory if the agreement between observed and expected numbers was reasonably close, especially at the higher risks, and if, moreover, the ratios of observed malformation rates and of calculated risks at the two extremes of the distribution were both large, showing that the factors chosen discriminated well between subjects at high and at low risks.

The MuLoRF coefficients have a meaningful interpretation in their own right: since the outcome probabilities, $p(x_1, \ldots, x_k)$ in (1) are for the most part rather small, the exponential term dominates the denominator of the risk function, whence

$$p(x_1, \ldots, x_k) = \exp(\beta_0) \exp(\beta_1 x_1) \ldots \exp(\beta_k x_k)$$

If now a variable, say the first, is dichotomous, the outcome probability when the variable takes the value 1 (i.e., when the factor is present) is about $\exp(\beta_1)$ times the probability when the factor is absent. In other words, the coefficient β_1 is to a first approximation the natural logarithm of the relative risk for the first factor, after allowing for the effects of the other factors in the risk function. For variables taking more than two values, the relevant part of this statement would be modified to read " . . . relative risk per unit deviation from zero." More accurately, $\exp(\beta_1)$ is the relative odds for the first factor, which is known to be close to the relative risk when the outcome is rare.

The central step in the analysis consists of comparing the number of events occurring among the subset of individuals exposed to a given drug to the sum, over the subset, of the estimated risks. This sum is the MuLoRF estimate of the expected number of antenatally exposed children with the malformation in question on the hypothesis that exposure is without effect. Using the entire cohort for the purposes of estimating the coefficients, we were able in this way to screen a great many pharmacological entities, mostly with usage rates below 10%. For the handful of preparations

used more frequently, there is a danger that the SRR may be biased towards unity. This problem is discussed in the next section.

When only a limited number of drugs are of interest, perhaps after preliminary screening, an alternative method of analysis can be used. In this procedure, one treats the drug exposures as additional risk-function variables on the same footing as the original covariates. In this way the interrelationships among the drugs themselves, and between the drugs and the covariates, can be explored. As explained above, relative risks for drug exposures can now be computed from the estimated MuLoRF coefficients.

We have performed three such analyses for the outcomes, central nervous cardiovascular,[13] and musculoskeletal malformations, introducing in each case those drugs which appeared to be associated with the outcome in question. In no case were the coefficients of the covariates appreciably altered (see Chapter 34). We have not deemed it necessary to reanalyze in this way any associations between drug and malformation class presented in this volume.

When a great many comparisons are to be made, one must clearly be wary of the results of conventional significance testing. We have therefore been content to provide a pair of limits on either side of the SRR with nominal confidence coefficient of roughly 95%. Since the complications of multiple testing are present also in the construction of confidence intervals, these limits are to be regarded as being mainly for guidance in any particular case.

These pseudo-confidence intervals were constructed, for given outcome and risk factor, according to the following simple principles. In the "large-sample" case, the natural logarithm of the SRR was taken to be a normally distributed random variable whose asymptotic standard error could be derived from the data and to which the usual confidence-interval theory applied. In the "small-sample" case, the observed number of events among the exposed subjects was treated as the only random variable of interest, the variance of the estimate of the expected number being regarded for this purpose as negligible. Specifically, if the observed number did not exceed 20, it was assumed to have a binomial distribution with unknown mean and "sample size" equal to the number exposed to the drug; 95% confidence limits for a binomial mean can be simply derived from the analogous limits for a Poisson mean, which are readily accessible in tabular form.[14] By dividing the expected number into these two limits, one obtains the desired approximate confidence interval for the SRR. Some heuristic justification, with further discussion, is given in an appendix to this chapter.

The Use of the Entire Cohort in Estimation*

When testing the effects of exposure to a drug, one should theoretically exclude from the estimation cohort all subjects exposed to that drug. Failure to do so would bias the SRR towards unity, since the model, (1), is fitted (i.e., obliged to conform) to the exposed group as part of the whole. (For remarks on a related issue, see, for example, Truett et al.[15] and Brunk et al.[16]) Let the exposed subjects comprise a fraction, ζ, of the entire cohort, and let ρ be the "true" relative risk; rough asymptotic arguments (which assume that the distributions of profiles in the exposed group and in the entire cohort are not too dissimilar) show that the expectation of the SRR under this procedure will be something like $\rho/\{1 + \zeta(\rho-1)\}$ provided neither ζ nor $|\rho-1|\zeta$ is too large.

On the other hand, it would be patently impracticable to estimate the coef-

---

* The derivation of certain results quoted in this section and the next is outlined in the appendices at the end of this chapter.

ficients anew for every drug of interest, using only those individuals whose records do not indicate that it was used. It might seem a feasible alternative to omit from the estimating cohort all subjects known to have ingested any drug during pregnancy, but only about 6% of that cohort would be left over (see Chapter 18).

In the current study the vast majority of drugs was used by less than 10% of the population; it is clear that for these the bias in the SRR is very unlikely to be large enough to obscure a genuine effect of medical significance. With respect to the more common drugs, one can, as a guideline, equate the confidence limits calculated with the exposed included in the estimating cohort to the above expression for the approximate expectation of the SRR. Thus if c were the value of a confidence limit calculated without regard to bias, a corrected value, less affected by bias, would be $(1-\zeta)c / (1-\zeta c)$. One could decide on the basis of this new pair of limits whether a fresh analysis, in which the exposed group was omitted from the estimated cohort, would be worth the effort.

Note that the damping effect of the bias increases with ζ, but that, as a counterbalance, the relative risk is estimated with greater precision, and the confidence interval is shorter, as the number in the exposed group becomes larger.

A more serious case arises when a drug is used only in the treatment of a disease occurring in pregnant women. A classic example is insulin and insulin-dependent diabetes. Suppose that the drug being studied, rather than the disease for which it was used, were the teratogen. The disease would then appear to be a risk factor for the malformation in question and would be one of the risk-function variables selected. Since exposure occurs only among women with the disease, the rest of the cohort is effectively irrelevant from the point of view of bias. The previous approximate formula for the expectation of the SRR would now apply with ζ being the (possibly appreciable) fraction of exposed subjects among the diseased. Should the group of exposed subjects coincide with the group of diseased subjects ($\zeta = 1$), the expectation of the SRR would be from the formula, unity. No drug effect, however strong, could be detected, as is otherwise obvious. Frequently, of course, there will be competing drugs, or the drug may be used more widely, and this will tend to reduce the bias. Special methods will usually be called for when this sort of drug is involved.

The SRR is the ratio of two random quantities which can be shown to have positive covariance when the estimating cohort contains the exposed subjects. In fact, when the exposure is unrelated to outcome (i.e., $\rho = 1$), the covariance of the numerator and the denominator is, to the first order of approximation, equal to the variance of the denominator. From the well-known formula for the variance of a ratio,[17] it is clear that the variance of the SRR is smaller when the exposed group is included than it would be if the latter were omitted. However, since the ratio of the variance of the expected value (the denominator) to that of the observed number (the numerator) is of the same order of magnitude as ζ, the proportion of drug users, the gain is not a very important one.

Statistical Independence of Pregnancies

One could hardly claim that what happens to a woman during one pregnancy is biologically independent of the occurrences during another, although in fact even successive pregnancies of a woman will be far from identical. Moreover, her drug usage may vary greatly from pregnancy to pregnancy. For the purposes of statistical analysis, in particular for the application of the MuLoRF procedure, a weaker form of independence is quite adequate. Thus, consider a woman appearing t times in the cohort and define the Bernoulli (zero-one) variables, Y_j, j = 1, 2, . . . , t, which take the value 1 if the jth pregnancy results in a specific outcome event and is zero otherwise; write $\underline{x}_j$ for the woman's profile on the jth pregnancy. It suffices for most analytic purposes that

$$\Pr \{Y_1 = y_1, \ldots, Y_t = y_t | \underline{x}_1, \ldots, \underline{x}_t\}$$

$$\doteq \prod_{j=1}^{t} \Pr \{Y_j = y_j | \underline{x}_j\} \quad (2)$$

i.e., that, conditional on the profiles, the joint probability of the Y's is at least approximately equal to the product of their conditional marginal probabilities.

For those malformations, notably polydactyly, in which the genetic component is strong, this relationship probably will not hold at all; although if the profiles included variables describing family malformation histories, the discrepancy would be appreciably reduced.

If (2) did not hold, one would expect a positive correlation between pregnancies of the same mother, implying a greater number of malformed children than expected among women appearing more than once in the cohort. The expectation would be computed by summing the risks estimated from the MuLoRF over the re-entrants according to the appropriate probabilistic rules (see Appendix 3.3). In the following analysis, we ignored the risk functions and have calculated an expected number of malformed children from the observed rates, either overall or within ethnic group and, where appropriate, hospital grouping. This has then been compared with the number of malformed children actually born to women entering the cohort more than once.

In the particular cohort under study (in which, it should be recalled, multiple births have been excluded), 5,467 women appeared just twice, 1,154 three times, 188 four times, 33 five times, and 3 six times; 61 bore 2 malformed children each, while another 2 bore 3 malformed children each. Among the offspring of these 63 women, there were 24 cases in which 2 siblings were afflicted by the same malformation, either alone or together with other malformations: the malformation in question was, in 13 cases, polydactyly; in 7 cases, inguinal hernia; in 2 cases, hypospadias; and in 1 case each, pectus excavatum and syndactyly.

A total of 3,248 malformed children were born to the women in the cohort in 50,282 pregnancies; if the pregnancies were independent, one would estimate the overall probability of bearing a malformed child as 0.0646. Substituting this into the formula in Appendix 3.3, one obtains for the expected number of women bearing two malformed children, the value 41.71, with standard error equal to 6.43. Taking ethnic group into account, one gets 42.64 and 6.50, respectively. Similarly, the expected number of women bearing three malformed children is 0.55, with standard error 0.74, or, on a race-specific basis, 0.62 with standard error 0.79. The race-specific expected number of sibling pairs with polydactyly is 0.95, the expected values for syndactyly and hypospadias being 0.09 and 0.15, respectively. Taking into account both ethnic and hospital group (see Chapter 17), one gets 2.28 as the expected number of sibling pairs with inguinal hernia.

The discrepancy between observed and expected is thus about 20 for all malformations taken together. This is largely accounted for by malformations with known genetic component, principally polydactyly, and with some contribution from syndactyly and hypospadias, and by inguinal hernia. Inguinal hernia, like pectus excavatum, is a malformation exhibiting appreciable interhospital variability in its recorded frequency, suggesting a substantial subjective component in the diagnosis (see Chapter 17). Such malformations have been considered separately.

As remarked earlier, the above excess of observed over expected would have been greatly reduced had family malformation history been allowed for, as was done in the main analyses. These considerations suggest that the assumption of statistical independence of pregnancies is unlikely to lead us into serious error, at least as far as physical malformations are concerned.

The problem could have been avoided altogether by including only a single pregnancy per woman, perhaps the first, or a random one, in our cohort. In view of the foregoing, the consequent loss of some 17% of the information seemed too high a price to pay. On the other hand, more detailed evaluation of findings involving malformations with a large familial component might well require some such selection procedure.

The Problem of Overcontrolling

Certain covariates which are associated with higher malformation rates, and are therefore candidates for inclusion in the MuLoRF, have themselves some of the characteristics of outcomes, notably in that they are observed in the products of conception at the termination of the pregnancy.[18] Examples are infant survival, birthweight, placental weight, and presence of a single umbilical artery. The argument in favor of controlling the effect of such factors is that their presence may reflect, or be correlated with, maternal health conditions on which we have inadequate information and which may influence drug use.

On the other hand, if drug exposure, covariate, and outcome are linked in a complex "causal" chain,[5,19] controlling with respect to the covariate may wholly or partially obscure a genuine effect of exposure. This phenomenon is known as overcontrolling. (Words such as "cause" or "causal" are to be interpreted here in a rather loose sense: for instance, fetal death could be said to "cause" malformations in that, in the present study, it led in most cases to autopsy and hence to more thorough detection of birth defects.)

A now classic example of the problems of interpretation which can arise in the presence of overcontrolling is the relation of smoking in pregnancy to perinatal mortality in the offspring.[18] In several studies the children of smokers were observed to experience a greater frequency of stillbirth and neonatal death than the children of non-smokers; when birthweight was taken into consideration, however, this was no longer the case. Nevertheless, the association between smoking and mortality cannot legitimately be judged spurious on that account.

Analysis shows that of all the likely ways in which exposure, covariate, and outcome could be causally interconnected in this body of data, the only pattern which could lead to serious underestimation of the influence of drug exposure is the one in which the drug effect is expressed solely or principally through the intervention of the controlled covariate. Thus, suppose a drug were instrumental in the agenesis of one of the umbilical arteries, which in turn led to the development of fetal abnormalities. Controlling the effects of the factor, single umbilical artery, would give a SRR of unity (apart from sampling errors) unless the drug had in addition a teratogenic effect expressed through other pathways. In practice, the single-path action with intervening variable described above is probably not very common; where there are several avenues of possible drug influence, the bias due to overcontrolling will usually be slight, particularly when the frequencies of such intervening control variables are low.

One other likely pattern that may bias the SRR towards unity is the one in which the outcome itself has a strong influence on the covariate. The presence in the developing fetus of certain types of abnormality may, for example, retard sub-

sequent growth, so that such children would be appreciably lighter on average than unaffected infants. However, unless the outcomes in question were frequent and their effect on the covariate powerful, this source of bias would not be unduly troublesome.

As already mentioned, the highest malformation rates are observed in autopsied infants; on the other hand, many types of malformations threaten viability. The covariate, infant survival, may thus be an element in both the patterns described above. It was decided not to consider this factor as a potential risk-function variable for any outcome. Extensive investigations on the outcome, considered in Chapter 5 ("Malformations with Similar Frequencies in the Hospitals"), had shown that no conclusion concerning the strength of an association between this outcome and a drug would be substantially different whether survival were included among the MuLoRF variables or not.

Other covariates of this ambiguous nature, notably single umbilical artery and low birthweight, do appear in the risk functions of many of the malformation classes. When a crude relative risk significantly greater than unity is substantially reduced by MuLoRF standardization, the reason might be adequate control of confounding or it might be overcontrolling (or both). An investigator should carefully examine the list of risk factors taken into consideration and use medical judgment to decide whether overcontrolling has played any important part.

We do not believe there are any instances of associations appreciably attenuated by overcontrolling (see Chapter 34). However, the ingredients on which a possible distorting judgment could be made are all present in this book: SRRs are given, and crude relative risks, if not displayed, are easily computed, while the factors that went into constructing risk-function models are listed and discussed in the chapters dealing with the malformation classes.

Appendix 3.1: Confidence Limits for the SRR

NB. A given exposure factor and a given outcome are implied throughout this section; unless otherwise stated, reference is to, and summations are over, the subjects (mother-child pairs) in the exposed group; the confidence coefficient, say 95%, is also to be taken as fixed.

Define: G: number of outcome events in the exposed group

π_j: the risk (probability of outcome event) for the jth subject in the absence of a drug effect; this risk depends on the subject's profile

S_m: $\sum_j \pi_j^m$

Then $E(G) = S_1$, $Var(G) = S_1 - S_2 < E(G)$; when the π_j are all small, $S_2 << S_1$, and G is to a first approximation Poisson with mean S_1. To a better approximation, G is binomial with the same mean, and "sample size" N^*, say, the integer for which the variances most closely agree, so that $N^* \doteq S_1^2/S_2 \le M$, where M is the size of the exposed group.

Suppose now that in the presence of a drug effect the risk for the jth subject is $\rho\pi_j$, i.e. that the relative risk is ρ. $E(G) = \rho S_1$; clearly (approximate) confidence limits for the mean of the distribution of G can be converted into (approximate) confidence limits for ρ by dividing by S_1 or by $\hat{S}_1$, say, an estimate of S_1 whose variance is small compared to that of G.

In the MuLoRF analysis, this will be so if M is small compared to the size of the cohort, unless the exposed subjects are, as a group, very different from the others. Note that even if $Var(\hat{S}_1)$ is small, N^* (which is independent of ρ) may nevertheless be estimated with low precision. In practice, N^* will rarely be very different from M.

One can show that, when the observed value of a binomial variable with sample size N, say, is g, a good approximation to the upper confidence limit of the mean is

$$\lambda_{U,g} - 1/2\lambda_{U,g}(\lambda_{U,g} - g)/N$$

and to the lower limit,

$$\lambda_{L,g} - 1/2\lambda_{L,g}(g - 1 - \lambda_{L,g})/N,$$

where $\lambda_{U,g},(\lambda_{L,g})$ is the analogous upper (lower) confidence limit for a Poisson mean.[20] The latter quantities are easily accessible; if N^* and S_1 were known, confidence limits for ρ could be calculated with little error from the above result. Note that the length of the interval for a binomial mean is an increasing function of N, and furthermore that if the exposed group is part of the estimating cohort, it can be shown that (asymptotically) $Var(G/\hat{S}_1) \le Var(G)/S_1^2$. Thus, if we take G to be bionomial with sample size M, and $\hat{S}_1$ to be of negligible variance, we may construct by the above method confidence intervals for ρ which are adequate, but, if anything, a trifle too long. When the exposed group comprises a rather larger fraction of the whole, $Var(\hat{S}_1)$ becomes less negligible, and other approximate methods may be more appropriate.

Appendix 3.2: Results on Variance and Bias of the Estimate of Expected Number of Outcome Events

Let G, S_1, M, and ρ be as in Appendix 3.1; let the size of the (estimating) cohort be N, and $\zeta = M/N$. Assume that there are only $R \le M$ distinct profiles, x_r; that among the subjects in the exposed group there are m_r profiles of the rth type, so that

$$\sum_{r=1}^{R} m_r = M;$$ and that the cohort has

n_r of the rth type, $\sum_{r=1}^{R} n_r = N$. Put $z_r = m_r/n_r$. The risk, π_j in the previous

28

section, is now assumed to be of the MuLoRF type, i.e., $\pi_j = p(\underline{x}_r) \equiv p_r$, if the jth subject has the profile, $\underline{x}_r$; thus, $S_1 = \sum_r m_r p_r$: let $\hat{S}_1$, $\hat{p}_r$, etc., be estimates derived from the cohort.

It can be shown that, if $\rho = 1$,

$$\text{Var}(\hat{S}_1) \simeq \underline{u}'I^{-1}\underline{u}, \text{ where } \underline{u}$$
$$= \sum_{r=1}^{R} m_r p_r (1 - p_r)\underline{x}_r \text{ and } I \text{ is}$$

the symmetric information matrix for the estimates of

$\beta_0, \ldots, \beta_k$, i.e. $\left\{-E\left(\dfrac{\partial^2 L}{\partial \beta_i \partial \beta_j}\right)\right\}$; also
$$\text{Var}(G) = \sum_r m_r p_r (1 - p_r), \text{ the}$$

element in $\underline{u}$ corresponding to β_0. Now the first column of I is $\sum_r n_r p_r (1 - p_r)\underline{x}_r = \underline{v}$, say. Thus $\underline{v}'I^{-1}\underline{v} = \sum_r n_r p_r (1 - p_r) = v_0$, say. If $z_r = \zeta$, all r, then $\underline{u} = \zeta\underline{v}$, $\text{Var}(\hat{S}_1) \simeq \zeta^2 v_0$, while $\text{Var}(G) = \zeta v_0$, i.e., $\text{Var}(S_1)/\text{Var}(G) \simeq \zeta$ under these circumstances. If $z_r \neq \zeta$ for some r, it can be shown that the ratio $\text{Var}(\hat{S}_1)/\text{Var}(G)$ is increased.

In the above derivation, it was immaterial whether the exposed group formed part of the estimating cohort or not. Suppose now that it does form part, and that the restriction, $\rho = 1$, has been removed. The outcome probability for a subject in the exposed group will be assumed to be ρp_r, if the profile in question is $\underline{x}_r$. From the estimating equations for $\beta_0, \ldots, \beta_k$ it follows that

$$\sum_r n_r x_{ri} E(\hat{p}_r) = \sum_r (n_r - m_r)x_{ri} p_r$$
$$+ \rho\sum_r m_r x_{ri} p_r = \sum_r n_r\{1 + (\rho - 1)z_r\}x_{ri} p_r,$$

for $i = 0, 1, \ldots, k$, where x_{ri} is the ith element of $\underline{x}_r$.

Now even if $z_r = \zeta$, all r, it is not exactly the case that $E(\hat{p}_r) = \{1 + (\rho - 1)\zeta\}p_r$, since the p_r and $\hat{p}_r$ are subject to additional constraints among themselves imposed by the logistic form. However, if ζ and $|\rho - 1|\zeta$ are both small, the result holds approximately.

Appendix 3.3: Statistical Independence of Pregnancies: Some Elementary Theory

Definitions:

m_t: the number of women appearing just t times in the cohort

$B_j^{(t)}$: the event that the jth such woman bore a malformed child

$\chi_j^{(t)} = 1$ if $B_j^{(t)}$ occurs, $= 0$ if not

T: the number of women who bore a malformed child on two separate entries

$\underline{x}_{jr}$: profile (vector of predictor variables) of the jth woman on her r^{th} entry

$p(\underline{x}_{jr})$: probability, given $\underline{x}_{jr}$, that a malformation occurs

If the pregnancies are independent, conditionally on the profiles, then

$$E\{\underline{x}_j^{(2)}\} = p(\underline{x}_{j1})\,p(\underline{x}_{j2}) = P\{B_j^{(2)}\}$$

$$E\{x_j^{(3)}\} = p(\underline{x}_{j1})\,p(\underline{x}_{j2})\{1 - p(\underline{x}_{j3})\}$$
$$+ p(\underline{x}_{j1})\{1 - p(\underline{x}_{j2})\}p(\underline{x}_{j3})$$
$$+ \{1 - p(\underline{x}_{j1})\}p(\underline{x}_{j2})\,p(\underline{x}_{j3}) = P\{B_j^{(3)}\},$$

and similarly for $t = 4, 5, \ldots$ From the definitions,

$$T = \sum_{t \geq 2} \sum_{j=1}^{m_t} \chi_j^{(t)}, \quad E(T) = \sum_t \sum_j P\{B_j^{(t)}\},$$
$$\text{Var}(T) = \sum_t \sum_j P\{B_j^{(t)}\}[1 - P\{B_j^{(t)}\}],$$

since clearly the pregnancies of different women are independent.

If the dependence of the probabilities on the profiles is ignored, so that $p(\underline{x}_{jr}) \equiv p$, say,

$$P\{B_j^{(t)}\} \equiv P\{B^{(t)}\} = \binom{t}{2}p^2(1 - p)^{t-2}$$

$$E(T) = \sum_t m_t P\{B^{(t)}\}, \quad \text{Var}(T)$$
$$= \sum_t m_t P\{B^{(t)}\}[1 - P\{B^{(t)}\}].$$

Note that if p is very small, $\text{Var}(T) = E(T)$

The extension to the case of a malformed child born on three separate entries is straightforward, with, mutatis mutandis,

$$E(T) = \sum_t m_t \binom{t}{3}p^3(1 - p)^{t-3}.$$

CHAPTER 4

The Women, Their Offspring, and The Malformations

This chapter is intended as a general introduction to Chapters 5 to 17. It briefly describes characteristics of the 50,282 mother-child pairs forming the cohort, with particular emphasis on the malformed children.

Characteristics of the Mothers and Their Offspring

The 50,282 gravidas (more precisely, the pregnancies from which the children in the study cohort were born) included 22,811 Whites, 24,030 Blacks, and 3,441 Puerto Ricans. Their mean age was 24.1 years overall; 24.7 years in Whites, 23.7 years in Blacks, and 23.6 years in Puerto Ricans. The mean socioeconomic index was 4.7 (5.7, 3.8, and 3.8).[1,2] The proportion of nulliparous women was 30% (32%, 28%, and 30%). The mean time of registration into the study was 21.6 weeks from the first day of the last menstrual period (approximately 19 to 20 weeks after conception), and the mean duration of the entire pregnancy from the last menstrual period was 276 days (279, 272, and 275). While the mother-child pairs represented 50,282 children, some mothers had more than one pregnancy in the study, and the total number of mothers was 41,796: 84% of the women had one pregnancy registered in the study, 5,467 women were registered twice, 1,154 three times, 188 four times, 33 five times, and 3 six times.

The average weight at birth was 3,131 gm (3,521; 3,019; 3,114), and 50.8% of the children were males. At the end of the postnatal observation period, 95.5% of the children were alive; there were 798 stillbirths (1.6%), 806 neonatal deaths (1.6%), 384 infant deaths (0.8%), and 239 childhood deaths (0.5%).

The Malformations

There is no general agreement about what constitutes a malformation. In this study, children were considered to be malformed when they had structural defects at or soon after birth, including tumors and syndromes that tend to be prominently associated with structural defects. Certain insignificant defects, such as accessory nipple, were excluded as explained in Chapter 2.

In total, there were 3,248 malformed children (64.6 per 1,000) having, among them, 4,446 malformations. Of these, 2,277 children comprised the set with malformations showing uniform rates by hospital, and 1,128 children comprised the set with non-uniform malformations. Among the 3,248 with malformations, 157 had both uniform and non-uniform malformations.

The overall malformation rate of 6.5% is rather high[3] and can probably be explained by the following circumstances. In this study, all children born after five or more lunar months of gestation were considered, whether live or dead. In addition, the children were followed for one to four years, resulting in recording of malformations that were diagnosed only after the neonatal period.

The remainder of this chapter describes briefly the way in which the malformations were classified. In subsequent sections of this book, the results of the study are organized with a number of objectives. One objective is to show how malformations in the different organ systems relate to each other, both within and between the various systems. Another objective is to present risk factors for malformations other than drugs. Quite aside from possible drug effects, these factors are intrinsically of interest. The most important objective, of course, is to show how drugs, as risk factors, relate to malformations when the allowance is made for confounding.

Malformations With Uniform Hospital Distributions Table 4.1 indicates the way in which the 2,277 children with uniform malformations were classified. Two

Table *4.1*

Classification of Children With Malformations Showing Uniform Rates by Hospital

Malformation Class	No. of Children	Rate/1,000
Any malformation	2,277	45.3
Major malformations	1,393	27.7
Minor malformations	898	17.9
Central nervous	266	5.3
Cardiovascular	404	8.0
Musculoskeletal	717	14.3
Respiratory	218	4.3
Gastrointestinal	301	6.0
Genitourinary	463	9.2
Eye and ear	121	2.4
Syndromes	176	3.5
Tumors	164	3.3

Table *4.2*

Classification of Children With Malformations Showing Non-Uniform Rates by Hospital

	No. of Children	Rate/1,000
Any non-uniform malformation	1,128	22.4
Inguinal hernia	683	13.5
Clubfoot	192	3.8
Pectus excavatum	92	1.8
Urethral obstruction	68	1.4
Cleft gum	110	2.2
Abnormal hands and fingers	10	0.2

principal and overlapping classifications were used. The first was based on severity; the children were categorized according to whether they had major or minor malformations. Tumors were not classified as either major or minor. The second classification was based on the anatomical site of the deformity, giving seven classes, with syndromes and tumors forming two further classes. Those children with any of the malformation entities listed in Table 4.1 represent the 12 principal outcome groups in this study. The details of the specific malformations that constituted the classes are given in Appendix 2.

In Chapters 5 to 16 the relationships between the study variables and classes of uniform malformations are presented. In Chapter 5 *all* of the factors retained for study are described in relation to the malformed children whether or not the factors happened to be associated with that specific outcome. In subsequent chapters dealing with other classes of malformations, the general rule is to present only those factors that were associated with the outcome under consideration. Sometimes an exception is made if absence of association for some factor seems to be of general interest. It should be noted that while the factors were always analyzed in their original categories, for the purposes of presentation categories have been combined where convenient. After the results of the initial analyses are presented, the results based on multivariate analysis are described.

Malformations With Non-Uniform Hospital Distributions Table 4.2 lists the six non-uniform malformations, affecting a total of 1,128 children. Inguinal hernia (rate, 13.5 per 1,000) was the most commonly diagnosed specific malformation in the entire cohort. At the other extreme, abnormal hands and fingers were diagnosed in only 10 children (0.2 per 1,000). Clubfoot, pectus excavatum, urethral obstruction, and cleft gum had intermediate rates. Detailed data on how the non-uniform malformations were distributed in the 12 institutions are given in Chapter 17. Factors related to non-uniform malformations are presented in the same chapter.

Malformations Possibly Arising During Late Embryogenesis On embryological grounds, it is likely that most malformations can only arise during early embryogenesis. It is at least possible, however, that some malformations may also arise at later stages in the development of the fetus.[3] Appendix 1 describes a subset of malformations that were judged to be of this type, together with related factors. Appendix 1 follows the same format as the chapters dealing with malformation classes.

CHAPTER 5

Malformations With Similar Frequencies in the Hospitals

In this chapter detailed consideration will be given to the 2,277 children (45.3 per 1,000) with malformations showing reasonably uniform hospital distributions. To simplify the analytical procedures, the children with exclusively non-uniform malformations will be considered separately. In this study, all of the selected factors have been evaluated in relation to all of the principal malformation entities. In this chapter only, all of these factors will be described whether or not associations were found. In subsequent chapters, factors will only be alluded to where associations exist, or where the matter appears to be of some general interest.

Interrelationships Among Malformations

Among the 2,277 children, there was a total of 3,282 malformations. In Table 5.1, these children are classified according to whether they had major or minor malformations, or tumors, which were not classified as either major or minor. There were 1,393 of the 2,277 children (61%) with major malformations, while 898 (39%) had minor malformations. In Table 5.2, the children are classified according to the type of malformations. It should be noted that tumors appear in both this and the previous classification. Musculoskeletal malformations occurred in 717 children (31%), and cardiovascular malformations occurred in 404 (18%). The

Table **5.1**

Distribution of Malformed Children by Severity of Malformation and by Ethnic Group (Rates per Thousand)

	White (n=22,811)		Black (n=24,030)		Puerto Rican (n=3,441)		Total (n=50,282)	
	No.	**Rate**	**No.**	**Rate**	**No.**	**Rate**	**No.**	**Rate**
Major malformations	748	32.79	551	22.93	94	27.32	1,393	27.70
Minor malformations	302	13.24	560	23.30	36	10.46	898	17.86
Tumors	88	3.86	66	2.75	10	2.91	164	3.26
Any malformations or tumors[1]	1,050	46.03	1,097	45.65	130	37.78	2,277	45.28

[1]Categories not mutually exclusive

Table **5.2**

Distribution of Malformed Children by Malformation Class and by Ethnic Group (Rates per Thousand)

	White (n=22,811)		Black (n=24,030)		Puerto Rican (n=3,441)		Total (n=50,282)	
Malformation Class	**No.**	**Rate**	**No.**	**Rate**	**No.**	**Rate**	**No.**	**Rate**
Central nervous	131	5.74	109	4.54	26	7.56	266	5.29
Cardiovascular	197	8.64	180	7.49	27	7.85	404	8.04
Musculoskeletal	268	11.75	418	17.39	31	9.01	717	14.26
Respiratory	117	5.13	87	3.62	14	4.07	218	4.34
Gastrointestinal	168	7.36	120	4.99	13	3.78	301	5.99
Genitourinary	189	8.29	161	6.70	16	4.65	366	7.28
Eye and ear	54	2.37	55	2.29	12	3.49	121	2.41
Syndromes	92	4.03	74	3.08	10	2.91	176	3.50
Tumors	88	3.86	66	2.75	10	2.91	164	3.26
Any malformations or tumors[1]	1,050	46.03	1,097	45.65	130	37.78	2,277	45.28

[1]Categories not mutually exclusive

least common categories of malformations were defects of the eye and ear (121 children, 5%) and tumors (164, 7%, of which 24 were malignancies). Overall, malformation rates were similar in Whites (46.0 per 1,000) and Blacks (45.7 per 1,000), and lower in Puerto Ricans (37.8 per 1,000). However, it should be noted that rates for various categories differed among the ethnic groups. For example, musculoskeletal deformities were more common in Black children (17.4 per 1,000, compared with 11.8 per 1,000 in Whites, and 9.0 per 1,000 in Puerto Ricans). Specific ethnic differences will be dealt with in detail in the relevant chapters.

In Table 5.3 the malformed children have been classified into mutually exclusive categories according to whether they

Table **5.3**

Distribution of Malformed Children by Major Malformations, Minor Malformations, and Tumors

Types of Malformation	No. of Children	Rate/1,000
Major only	1,222	24.3
Major and minor (not tumor)	147	2.9
Major and tumor (not minor)	19	0.4
Major, minor, tumor	5	0.1
Minor and tumor	2	0.0
Minor only	744	14.8
Tumor only	138	2.8
Total	2,277	45.3

had major malformations, minor malformations, tumors, or combinations. Of the 2,277 children, 1,222 (54%) had major malformations only, a rate of 24.3 per 1,000; 744 (33%) had minor malformations only, a rate of 14.8 per 1,000; and 138 (6%) had tumors only, a rate of 2.8 per 1,000. The rate of major and minor malformations, occurring in the same child, was 2.9 per 1,000 (147 children), and all remaining combinations had extremely low rates.

In Table 5.4, children with major and minor malformations (classification not mutually exclusive) are considered in terms of whether they had single or multiple anomalies. There were 1,393 children with major malformations (28 per 1,000), and 898 with minor malformations (18 per 1,000). Of the 1,393 with major

Table **5.4**

Distribution of Malformed Children by Number of Major and Minor Malformations[1]

No. of Malformations	Malformed Children				
	Major			Minor	
	No.	%		No.	%
1	995	71.4		856	95.3
2	224	16.1		31	3.5
3	71	5.1		6	0.7
4	48	3.4		4	0.4
5	25	1.8		1	0.1
6	9	0.6		0	
7	7	0.5		0	
8	2	0.1		0	
9	5	0.3		0	
10	2	0.1		0	
11	2	0.1		0	
12	2	0.1		0	
13	1	0.1		0	
Total	1,393	100.0		898	100.0

[1]There were no children with multiple tumors.

malformations, 71.4% had only one such malformation. The remainder had two (16.1%) or more associated major malformations. Among the 898 children with minor malformations, 95.3% had only one such malformation. The remainder had two (3.5%) or more associated minor malformations. Thus, major malformations were considerably more often multiple than were minor malformations.

In Table 5.5, the children are tabulated by malformation class according to whether they had only one malformation or more than one malformation within the same class. The malformation classes are not mutually exclusive. Cardiovascular malformations occurred most commonly as multiple entities, as compared with other malformation classes: 25.7% of children with cardiovascular malformations had more than one cardiovascular anomaly. Central nervous and genitourinary anomalies were also quite often multiple (24.4% and 19.1%, respectively). There were no instances of more than one tumor occurring in the same child, and only 2.8% of children with various syndromes were identified as having more than one syndrome.

The proportions of children with major malformations, minor malformations,

and combinations, within each of the anatomical classes, are given in Table 5.6. In this table tumors are not considered because they were not classified as either major or minor. The proportion of children in each class who had only major malformations ranged from 38.3% for genitourinary anomalies to 100% for syndromes. Over 90% of children with cardiovascular or central nervous anomalies had major defects.

In Table 5.7 the occurrence of multiple malformations both within and across malformation classes is examined. Children with tumors most commonly had single malformations (84.1%), closely followed by children with musculoskeletal anomalies (82.0%). Single malformations were least common among children with syndromes (40.3%). With respect to multiple malformations occurring in more than one class, there was considerable variability in the proportions, the highest being 59.7% for children with syndromes. This latter proportion included all five children (shown in Table 5.5) who had more than one syndrome. The proportion of malformations in other classes was also high for children with respiratory malformations (41.7%) and central nervous malformations (36.5%). It was

Table **5.5**

Overlapping Between Malformation Classes

Malformation Class*	Children with Only One Malformation in the Class		Children with More than One Malformation in the Class		Total Number of Malformed Children in the Class	
	No.	%	No.	%	No.	%
Central nervous	201	75.6	65	24.4	266	100.0
Cardiovascular	300	74.3	104	25.7	404	100.0
Musculoskeletal	646	90.1	71	9.9	717	100.0
Respiratory	200	91.7	18	8.3	218	100.0
Gastrointestinal	258	85.7	43	14.3	301	100.0
Genitourinary	296	80.9	70	19.1	366	100.0
Eye and ear	108	89.3	13	10.7	121	100.0
Syndromes	171	97.2	5	2.8	176	100.0
Tumors	164	100.0	0	0.0	164	100.0

*Categories not mutually exclusive

Table **5.6**

"Major-Minor" Distribution of Malformed Children by Malformation Class[1]

Malformation Class[2]	Children with Major Malformations		Children with Major and Minor Malformations		Children with Minor Malformations		Total Number of Children	
	No.	%	No.	%	No.	%	No.	%
Central nervous	249	93.6	7	2.6	10	3.8	266	100.0
Cardiovascular	365	90.3	23	5.7	16	4.0	404	100.0
Musculoskeletal	296	41.3	26	3.6	395	55.1	717	100.0
Respiratory	159	72.9	5	2.3	54	24.8	218	100.0
Gastrointestinal	176	58.5	21	7.0	104	34.5	301	100.0
Genitourinary	140	38.3	7	1.9	219	59.8	366	100.0
Eye and ear	70	57.8	7	5.8	44	36.4	121	100.0
Syndromes	176	100.0	0	0.0	0	0.0	176	100.0

[1]Tumors not included (164 children)
[2]Categories not mutually exclusive

Table **5.7**

Single and Joint Occurrence of Malformations by Class

Malformation Class	Single Malformation Only		Two or More Malformations Occurring Exclusively within the Same Malformation Class		Malformations Also Occurring in Other Malformation Classes	
	No.	%	No.	%	No.	%
Central nervous	144	54.1	25	9.4	97	36.5
Cardiovascular	229	56.7	59	14.6	116	28.7
Musculoskeletal	588	82.0	41	5.7	88	12.3
Respiratory	125	57.3	2	0.9	91	41.7
Gastrointestinal	196	65.1	18	6.0	87	28.9
Genitourinary	245	66.9	24	6.6	97	26.5
Eye and ear	83	68.6	7	5.8	31	25.6
Syndromes	71	40.3	0	0.0	105	59.7
Tumors	138	84.1	0	0.0	26	15.9

lowest for those with musculoskeletal malformations (12.3%) and intermediate for the remainder. Finally, with regard to two or more malformations occurring exclusively within the same malformation class, the proportions were similar for children in all but one of the classes (varying from 5.7% to 9.4%). The exception was cardiovascular anomalies: 14.6% of children whose cardiovascular system, *exclusively*, was affected had more than one cardiovascular defect. This proportion of 14.6% can be considered in relation to the *total* proportion of cardiovascular anomalies that were multiple (25.7%): by subtraction, 11.1% of cardiovascular anomalies, in addition to being multiple, were also associated with anomalies in other malformation classes.

Table 5.8 examines the question of

Table **5.8**

Children Having Malformations in Other Classes According to Single and Multiple
Malformations Within Each Referent Class

Malformation Class		No. of Children	Children with Malformations in Other Classes	
			No.	%
Central nervous	Single	201	57	28.4
	Multiple	65	40	61.5
Cardiovascular	Single	300	71	23.7
	Multiple	104	45	43.3
Musculoskeletal	Single	646	58	9.0
	Multiple	71	30	42.3
Respiratory	Single	200	75	37.5
	Multiple	18	16	88.9
Gastrointestinal	Single	258	62	24.0
	Multiple	43	25	58.1
Genitourinary	Single	296	51	17.2
	Multiple	70	46	65.7
Eye and ear	Single	108	25	23.1
	Multiple	13	6	46.2
Syndromes	Single	171	100	58.5
	Multiple	5	5	100.0
Tumors	Single	164	26	15.8
	Multiple	0	0	0.0

whether severe maldevelopment in one organ system occurs simultaneously with maldevelopment in other systems. The malformed children are divided according to whether the malformations within each referent class were single or multiple, and according to whether they had malformations in other classes. For example, of the 717 children with musculoskeletal malformations, 646 had only one and 71 had more than one musculoskeletal malformation. Of the 646 children with only one musculoskeletal deformity, 58 had malformations occurring in other classes (9.0%), and the corresponding number among the 71 children with multiple musculoskeletal deformities was 30 (42.3%). Of the children with tumors (there were no multiple tumors), 15.8% had other malformations as well. Apart from tumors, proportions of children who had malformations in more than one class were considerably higher when the malformations in the referent class were multiple. Over 40% of children with more than one class-specific deformity also had malformations elsewhere. For single malformations in the referent class, the percentages of malformations in other classes ranged from 15.8 to 28.4.

Table 5.9 specifies the extent to which other organ systems are affected when maldevelopment is present in a particular system. Syndromes tended particularly to be associated with cardiovascular malformations; 27.3% of children with syndromes were thus affected. In the entire table, there were no other proportions as high as this. In contrast to syndromes, respiratory malformations generally

38

Table **5.9**

Single and Joint Occurrence of Malformations by Class

| | Children with Class-Specific Malformations Only | | Children with Other Malformations | | | | | | | | | | | | | | | | | TOTAL |
| | | | Central Nervous | | Cardio-vascular | | Musculo-skeletal | | Respi-ratory | | Gastro-intestinal | | Genito-urinary | | Eye and Ear | | Syn-dromes | | Tumors | | |
	No.	%	No.	%	No.	%	No.	%	No.	%	No.	%	No.	%	No.	%	No.	%	No.	%	No.
Central nervous	169	(63.5)	—	—	22	(8.3)	28	(10.5)	30	(11.3)	25	(9.4)	28	(10.5)	10	(3.7)	37	(13.9)	7	(2.6)	266
Cardiovascular	288	(71.3)	22	(5.4)	—	—	26	(6.4)	32	(7.9)	42	(10.4)	34	(8.4)	10	(2.5)	48	(11.9)	4	(1.0)	404
Musculoskeletal	629	(87.7)	28	(3.9)	26	(3.6)	—	—	37	(5.2)	26	(3.6)	30	(4.2)	10	(1.4)	25	(3.5)	6	(0.8)	717
Respiratory	127	(58.3)	30	(13.7)	32	(14.7)	37	(17.0)	—	—	33	(15.4)	36	(16.5)	5	(2.3)	29	(13.3)	3	(1.4)	218
Gastrointestinal	214	(71.1)	25	(8.3)	42	(13.9)	26	(8.6)	33	(11.0)	—	—	39	(13.0)	4	(1.3)	19	(6.3)	2	(0.7)	301
Genitourinary	269	(73.5)	28	(7.7)	34	(9.3)	30	(8.2)	36	(9.8)	39	(10.7)	—	—	6	(1.6)	21	(5.7)	6	(1.6)	366
Eye and ear	90	(74.4)	10	(8.3)	10	(8.3)	10	(8.3)	5	(4.1)	4	(3.3)	6	(5.0)	—	—	6	(5.0)	3	(2.5)	121
Syndromes	71	(40.3)	37	(21.0)	48	(27.3)	25	(14.2)	29	(16.5)	19	(10.8)	21	(11.9)	6	(3.4)	—	—	5	(2.8)	176
Tumors	138	(84.1)	7	(4.3)	4	(2.4)	6	(3.7)	3	(1.8)	2	(1.2)	6	(3.7)	3	(1.8)	5	(3.0)	—	—	164

tended to be associated with relatively high proportions of malformations in all of the remaining classes. Malformations of the central nervous system were more prominently related to deformities of the eye and ear (3.7%) than were the other classes. In addition, central nervous malformations were quite prominently related to syndromes (13.9%), respiratory anomalies (11.3%), and musculoskeletal deformities (10.5%). Other features of note were rather prominent associations between gastrointestinal and cardiovascular deformities (13.9%), and between genitourinary and gastrointestinal deformities (10.7%).

One further point needs to be made: association in one direction did not necessarily imply an equivalent degree of association in the reverse direction. For example, as already mentioned, the most prominent relationship in the table was that of associated cardiovascular defects which occurred in 27.3% of children with syndromes. The reverse relationship was not as striking: 11.9% of children with cardiovascular malformations had syndromes, and the proportions of children with syndromes were higher in those who had central nervous malformations (13.9%) and respiratory malformations (13.3%).

The preceding observations will now be summarized: major malformations accounted for about 60% of the affected children, and these malformations also tended to be multiple more commonly than minor malformations. Musculoskeletal and cardiovascular anomalies represented the most common malformation classes. The proportions of major malformations varied by class, being highest for children with syndromes and lowest for those with musculoskeletal anomalies. Cardiovascular malformations were most commonly multiple: almost 30% of the affected children had multiple cardiovascular anomalies. Multiple anomalies occurring in more than one class were present in almost 60% of

children with syndromes and in over 40% of children with respiratory malformations. Less than 20% of children with musculoskeletal malformations or tumors had malformations in other classes as well; in the remaining classes the rates were intermediate, all of them being above 20%. Cardiovascular and central nervous anomalies were common in children with syndromes. Multiple malformations within one class strongly predisposed to malformations within other classes.

Risk Factors for
Uniform Malformations

Administrative Data

Institution (Table 5.10) The largest number of pregnancies was seen in Boston (11,356), and this institution has been used as the reference category with the relative risk set at 1.0. There was little variability in the rates among the 12 institutions; the relative risks varied from 0.7 to 1.2. This has occurred by design since, as pointed out before, malformations showing considerable hospital variability have been considered separately.

Ordinal Number of Entry into the Study (Table 5.11) In 41,796 instances, the studied pregnancy was the only one registered, and the remaining 8,486 pregnancies represented second to sixth registrations. Since for each malformation rate the denominator was the number of pregnancies, rather than the number of mothers, it is important to determine the degree to which the ordinal number of entry of the pregnancy was related to the risk of having a malformed child. The table shows that the risk was uniform for the first to the third ordinal entry. For the fourth to the sixth ordinal entries (263 pregnancies), the relative risk for having a malformed child was 1.4.

Duration of Pregnancy at Registration (Table 5.12) The bulk of the mothers was first registered into the study when the pregnancy had reached five to eight

Table **5.10**

Distribution of Malformed Children by Institution

Location of Institution	No. of Children	Malformed Children		Relative Risk
		No.	Rate/1,000	
Boston, MA	11,356	541	48	1.0*
Buffalo, NY	2,291	129	56	1.2
New Orleans, LA	2,507	122	49	1.0
New York, NY (N.Y. Medical)	4,248	136	32	0.7
New York, NY (Columbia)	2,046	113	55	1.2
Baltimore, MD	3,397	159	47	1.0
Richmond, VA	3,058	136	44	0.9
Minneapolis, MN	2,934	131	45	0.9
Portland, OR	2,966	118	40	0.8
Philadelphia, PA	9,382	438	47	1.0
Providence, RI	2,681	113	42	0.9
Memphis, TN	3,416	141	41	0.9

*Reference category

Table **5.11**

Distribution of Malformed Children by Ordinal Number of Entry to the Study

Ordinal Number of Entry	No. of Children	Malformed Children		Relative Risk
		No.	Rate/1,000	
1	41,796	1,886	45	1.0*
2–3	8,223	375	46	1.0
4–6	263	16	61	1.4

*Reference category

lunar months of gestation. For White and Black mothers, the rates were similar regardless of the time of entry, so that the relative risks were all close to unity. For Puerto Ricans, the relative risks were high for both early (1.3) and late (1.4) entries.

Number of Antenatal Visits (Table 5.13) The relative risk among 8,624 women who attended for antenatal examinations fewer than five times was 1.3.

Year of Last Menstrual Period (Table 5.14) Among White and Black children conceived during the years 1958 to 1965

there was no evidence to suggest secular changes in the malformation rates. Because of small numbers, rates were rather unstable in Puerto Rican children, but no consistent trend was evident.

Calendar Month of Last Mentrual Period (Table 5.15) There were no obvious seasonal trends consistently present in the three ethnic groups.

Personal Characteristics
of the Mother

Ethnic Group (Table 5.16) Race-specific rates have been given in several tables wherever deemed appropriate.

Table **5.12**

Race-Specific Distribution of Malformed Children by Duration of Pregnancy at Registration

	Duration of Pregnancy at Registration (lunar months)	No. of Children	Malformed Children		Relative Risk
			No.	Rate/1,000	
White	1–4	8,400	404	48	1.0
	5–8	11,015	524	48	1.0*
	≥9	3,396	122	36	0.8
Black	1–4	4,269	192	45	1.0
	5–8	16,263	744	46	1.0*
	≥9	3,498	161	46	1.0
Puerto Rican	1–4	766	34	44	1.3
	5–8	2,334	80	34	1.0*
	≥9	341	16	47	1.4

*Reference category

Table **5.13**

Distribution of Malformed Children by Number of Antenatal Visits

No. of Antenatal Visits	No. of Children	Malformed Children		Relative Risk
		No.	Rate/1,000	
1–4	8,624	478	55	1.3
5–9	20,964	893	43	1.0*
≥10	20,694	906	44	1.0

*Reference category

Table **5.14**

Race-Specific Distribution of Malformed Children by Year of Mother's Last Menstrual Period (LMP) (Rates per Thousand)

Year of LMP	No. of Children	White (n = 22,811)		Black (n = 24,030)		Puerto Rican (n = 3,441)		Total (n = 50,282)	
		No.	Rate	No.	Rate	No.	Rate	No.	Rate
1958	1,877	31	36.0	38	42.6	7	55.6	76	40.5
1959	5,735	119	45.2	114	41.8	14	37.2	247	43.1
1960	7,285	131	40.4	167	47.2	23	45.5	321	44.1
1961	7,441	151	45.2	174	49.3	29	50.5	354	47.6
1962	8,216	172	48.3	175	43.9	21	31.1	368	44.8
1963	7,986	166	47.9	199	49.3	13	27.0	378	47.3
1964	7,817	178	48.9	159	43.0	13	27.1	350	44.8
1965	3,925	102	49.3	71	43.5	10	45.0	183	46.6
Total	50,282	1,050	46.0	1,097	45.7	130	37.8	2,277	45.3

Table **5.15**

Race-Specific Distribution of Malformed Children by Month of Mother's
Last Menstrual Period (LMP) (Rates per Thousand)

Month of LMP	No. of Children	White (n = 22,811)		Black (n = 24,030)		Puerto Rican (n = 3,441)		Total (n = 50,282)	
		No.	Rate	No.	Rate	No.	Rate	No.	Rate
January	4,185	89	48.0	102	49.8	7	24.9	198	47.3
February	4,075	77	41.7	87	44.2	8	31.0	172	42.2
March	4,136	90	49.4	101	49.0	12	47.2	203	49.1
April	4,154	81	42.7	98	49.2	15	56.4	194	46.7
May	4,194	79	41.9	89	44.3	11	36.9	179	42.7
June	4,118	87	45.2	68	35.7	9	31.1	164	39.8
July	3,817	88	48.6	84	48.1	9	34.7	181	47.4
August	4,001	86	44.7	84	47.1	10	33.9	180	45.0
September	4,049	80	43.1	74	39.1	11	37.2	165	40.8
October	4,539	95	47.3	96	43.5	9	27.8	200	44.1
November	4,412	108	53.8	108	51.2	9	30.3	225	51.0
December	4,602	90	45.6	106	46.0	20	61.7	216	46.9
Total	50,282	1,050	46.0	1,097	45.7	130	37.8	2,277	45.3

Table **5.16**

Distribution of Malformed Children by Ethnic Group

	No. of Children	Malformed Children		Relative Risk
		No.	Rate/1,000	
White	22,811	1,050	46	1.0
Black	24,030	1,097	46	1.0*
Puerto Rican	3,441	130	38	0.8

*Reference category

While it is well known that there are certain malformations that show considerable racial variability, this was not evident overall among White or Black children: the malformation rates for 22,811 pregnancies in White women and 24,030 pregnancies in Black women were both 46 per 1,000, while the rate was somewhat lower (38 per 1,000) in 3,441 Puerto Rican women, giving a relative risk of 0.8.

Mother's Age at Registration (Table 5.17) In all ethnic groups, although numbers were rather small, the rates were elevated for pregnancies occurring in mothers aged less than 15 years, when compared with the most common age group of 20 to 24 years. The relative risks ranged from 1.2 to 2.8. At the other extreme, the malformation rate was again higher in children born to women over the age of 39 years: the relative risks ranged from 1.3 to 5.1.

Socioeconomic Status (Table 5.18) The malformation rates according to six categories of socioeconomic status are

Table **5.17**

Race-Specific Distribution of Malformed Children by Mother's Age at Registration

	Mother's Age	No. of Children	Malformed Children		Relative Risk
			No.	Rate/1,000	
White	≤14	25	3	120	2.6
	15–19	4,049	137	34	0.7
	20–24	9,012	411	46	1.0*
	25–29	5,208	249	48	1.0
	30–34	2,726	151	55	1.2
	35–39	1,405	76	54	1.2
	40–44	369	22	60	1.3
	≥45	17	1	59	1.3
Black	≤14	394	21	53	1.2
	15–19	6,584	285	43	1.0
	20–24	8,109	366	45	1.0*
	25–29	4,638	209	45	1.0
	30–34	2,610	122	47	1.0
	35–39	1,343	60	45	1.0
	40–44	339	31	91	2.0
	≥45	13	3	231	5.1
Puerto Rican	≤14	10	1	100	2.8
	15–19	842	26	31	0.9
	20–24	1,354	48	35	1.0*
	25–29	746	29	39	1.1
	30–34	319	15	47	1.3
	35–39	136	8	59	1.7
	40–44	34	3	88	2.5
	≥45	0	0	0	—

*Reference category

given.[1] Among 465 pregnancies in White mothers with unknown socioeconomic status, the relative risk was 1.3. All remaining relative risks were close to unity.

Marital Status (Table 5.19) The race-specific malformation rates according to whether the mothers were single, married, or "other" (widowed, divorced, common-law marriage) gave no evidence that marital status was related to the risk of having a malformed child.

Religion (Table 5.20) Compared with Protestants, among White children whose mothers' religion was unknown, the relative risk was 1.5. However, the corresponding value for Black children was 0.6. All the remaining relative risks were close to unity. (A large proportion of

the 1,441 White women whose religion was categorized as "other" were Jewish.)

Prepregnant Weight, Height, and Ponderal Index (Tables 5.21, 5.22) Among the various categories of weight and height, malformation rates showed only slight variation. Relative risks were elevated in the middle category of ponderal index in White and Black women. However this proved to be a function of age.

Characteristics and Survival of the Offspring

Birthweight (Table 5.23) Low birthweight was among those factors most strongly associated with a high malformation rate. The table gives the race-specific malformation rates for four

*Table **5.18***

Race-Specific Distribution of Malformed Children by Mother's Socioeconomic Status (SES)

	SES (Scale of 0–10)	No. of Children	Malformed Children		Relative Risk
			No.	Rate/1,000	
White	≤ 1.9	661	26	39	0.9
	2–3.9	4,381	204	47	1.0
	4–5.9	6,639	304	46	1.0*
	6–7.9	6,533	311	48	1.0
	≥ 8.0	4,132	177	43	0.9
	Unknown	465	28	60	1.3
Black	≤ 1.9	2,968	139	47	1.1
	2–3.9	9,750	455	47	1.1
	4–5.9	7,740	323	42	1.0*
	6–7.9	2,772	141	51	1.2
	≥ 8.0	445	23	52	1.2
	Unknown	355	16	45	1.1
Puerto Rican	≤ 1.9	262	10	38	1.0
	2–3.9	1,598	60	38	1.0
	4–5.9	1,168	44	38	1.0*
	6–7.9	345	14	41	1.1
	≥ 8.0	33	1	30	0.8
	Unknown	35	1	29	0.8

*Reference category

*Table **5.19***

Race-Specific Distribution of Malformed Children by Mother's Marital Status

	Marital Status	No. of Children	Malformed Children		Relative Risk
			No.	Rate/1,000	
White	Single	1,125	43	38	0.8
	Married	20,079	935	47	1.0*
	Other	1,607	72	45	1.0
Black	Single	6,172	266	43	0.9
	Married	15,063	690	46	1.0*
	Other	2,795	141	50	1.1
Puerto Rican	Single	250	7	28	0.7
	Married	2,556	101	40	1.0*
	Other	635	22	35	0.9

*Reference category

Table **5.20**

Race-Specific Distribution of Malformed Children by Mother's Religion

		No. of Children	Malformed Children		Relative Risk
			No.	Rate/1,000	
White	Protestant	9,031	408	45	1.0*
	Roman Catholic	11,943	562	47	1.0
	Other	1,441	53	37	0.8
	Unknown	396	27	68	1.5
Black	Protestant	20,620	932	45	1.0*
	Roman Catholic	2,833	142	50	1.1
	Other	366	17	46	1.0
	Unknown	211	6	28	0.6
Puerto Rican	Protestant	279	13	47	1.0*
	Roman Catholic	3,136	116	37	0.8
	Other	6	0	—	—
	Unknown	20	1	50	1.1

* Reference category

Table **5.21**

Distribution of Malformed Children by Mother's Prepregnant Weight and Height

		No. of Children	Malformed Children		Relative Risk
			No.	Rate/1,000	
Weight	≤ 39	372	20	54	1.2
(kg)	40–79	46,164	2,061	45	1.0*
	≥ 80	2,718	144	53	1.2
	Unknown	1,028	52	51	1.1
Height	≤ 149	2,947	138	47	1.0
(cm)	150–169	39,483	1,772	45	1.0*
	170–189	5,525	250	45	1.0
	Unknown	2,327	117	50	1.1

*Reference category

categories of birthweight ranging from less than 1.5 to 2.5 kg or more. There was a steady increase in the rates as birthweight decreased. This was most striking in children born to White mothers, among whom the malformation rate was 40 per 1,000 in the highest birthweight category, as against 188 per 1,000 (relative risk 4.7) in children weighing less than 1.5 kg. The corresponding contrast for children born to Black mothers was 41 per 1,000 as against 105 per 1,000 (relative risk 2.6). Among Puerto Ricans numbers were small in the low-weight categories. Nevertheless, there was more than a trebling of the malformation rate in children weighing less than 2 kg.

Sex of the Child (Table 5.24) The

Table **5.22**

Distribution of Malformed Children According to the Prepregnant Ponderal Index of the Mother

Race	Ponderal Index (weight × 1,000)/(height)^2	No. of Children	Malformed Children		Relative Risk
			No.	Rate/1,000	
White	≤ 1.9	6.185	279	45	1.0
	2.0–2.4	11,134	486	44	1.0*
	2.5–2.9	2,668	134	50	1.2
	3.0–3.4	724	44	61	1.4
	3.5–3.9	225	9	40	0.9
	≥ 4.0	88	4	45	1.0
	Unknown	1,787	94	53	1.2
Black	≤ 1.9	6,118	286	47	1.0
	2.0–2.4	11,249	505	45	1.0*
	2.5–2.9	4,043	177	44	1.0
	3.0–3.4	1,344	72	54	1.2
	3.5–3.9	396	23	58	1.3
	≥ 4.0	178	6	34	0.8
	Unknown	702	28	40	0.9
Puerto Rican	≤ 1.9	870	32	37	0.9
	2.0–2.4	1,590	62	39	1.0*
	2.5–2.9	524	18	34	0.9
	3.0–3.4	121	2	17	0.4
	3.5–3.9	23	1	43	1.1
	≥ 4.0	7	1	143	3.7
	Unknown	306	14	46	1.2

*Reference category

Table **5.23**

Race-Specific Distribution of Malformed Children by Child's Birthweight

	Birthweight (grams)	No. of Children	Malformed Children		Relative Risk
			No.	Rate/1,000	
White	≤ 1,499	357	67	188	4.7
	1,500–1,999	288	39	135	3.4
	2,000–2,499	1,201	102	85	2.1
	≥2,500	20,965	842	40	1.0*
Black	≤ 1,499	602	63	105	2.6
	1,500–1,999	606	54	89	2.2
	2,000–2,499	2,259	147	65	1.6
	≥2,500	20,563	833	41	1.0*
Puerto Rican	≤ 1,499	57	5	88	2.8
	1,500–1,999	66	11	167	5.3
	2,000–2,499	244	18	74	2.4
	≥2,500	3,074	96	31	1.0*

* Reference category

Table **5.24**

Distribution of Malformed Children by Sex of Child

	No. of Children	Malformed Children		Relative Risk
		No.	Rate/1,000	
Male	25,542	1,293	51	1.3
Female	24,740	984	40	1.0*

*Reference category

respective malformation rates in male and female children were 51 and 40 per 1,000.

Birth Order (Table 5.25) The malformation rates showed only slight and inconsistent variation according to the birth order ranking of the child.

Survival of the Child (Table 5.26) Failure to survive was strongly associated with high malformation rates: the relative risks for malformations in stillbirths,

neonatal deaths, and childhood deaths among White children ranged from 6.1 to 8.1. The corresponding range of relative risks among Black children was 3.4 to 6.5. While the relative risks were all increased for Puerto Rican children (4.4 to 15.0), they fluctuated rather widely because of small numbers.

Autopsy (Table 5.27) Compared to children who died but did not come to

Table **5.25**

Race-Specific Distribution of Malformed Children by Birth Order of Child

	Birth Order[1]	No. of Children	Malformed Children		Relative Risk
			No.	Rate/1,000	
White	1	7,388	341	46	1.0*
	2–3	9,430	388	41	0.9
	4–5	4,016	222	55	1.2
	6–7	1,410	68	48	1.0
	8–9	427	26	61	1.3
	≥ 10	140	5	36	0.8
Black	1	6,740	297	44	1.0*
	2–3	8,805	414	47	1.1
	4–5	4,798	211	44	1.0
	6–7	2,254	113	50	1.1
	8–9	931	37	40	0.9
	≥ 10	502	25	50	1.1
Puerto Rican	1	1,038	38	37	1.0*
	2–3	1,494	53	35	1.0
	4–5	601	28	47	1.3
	6–7	215	5	23	0.6
	8–9	66	4	61	1.7
	≥ 10	27	2	74	2.0

*Reference category
[1]Determined by number of prior liveborn and stillborn siblings

Table **5.26**

Race-Specific Distribution of Malformed Children by Survival of the Child

	Survival of Child	No. of Children	Malformed Children		Relative Risk
			No.	Rate/1,000	
White	Stillbirth	327	74	226	6.1
	Neonatal death	302	91	301	8.1
	Infant death	130	38	292	7.8
	Childhood death	91	26	286	7.6
	Survived	21,961	821	37	1.0*
Black	Stillbirth	407	52	128	3.4
	Neonatal death	450	91	202	5.3
	Infant death	229	57	249	6.5
	Childhood death	134	27	201	5.3
	Survived	22,810	870	38	1.0*
Puerto Rican	Stillbirth	64	8	125	4.4
	Neonatal death	54	14	259	9.1
	Infant death	25	8	320	11.2
	Childhood death	14	6	429	15.0
	Survived	3,284	94	29	1.0*

*Reference category

autopsy, the relative risks for White and Black children who were autopsied were 1.7 and 1.6, respectively.

Reproductive History of the Mother

Prior Pregnancies (Table 5.28) The malformation rates were similar for widely varying numbers of prior pregnancies.

Prior Premature Births (Table 5.29) Only among women who had previously given birth to three or more premature children was there an increase in the malformation rate (relative risk, 1.3).

Prior Fetal or Neonatal Loss (Table

Table **5.27**

Race-Specific Distribution of Dead Malformed Children by Presence of Autopsy Report

	Autopsy Report	No. of Children	Malformed Children		Relative Risk
			No.	Rate/1,000	
White	Present	674	199	295	1.7
	Absent	176	30	170	1.0*
Black	Present	1,008	202	200	1.6
	Absent	213	26	122	1.0*
Puerto Rican	Present	128	29	227	0.9
	Absent	29	7	241	1.0*

*Reference category

Table **5.28**

Distribution of Malformed Children by History of Prior Pregnancies

No. of Prior Pregnancies[1]	No. of Children	Malformed Children		Relative Risk
		No.	Rate/1,000	
None	14,168	617	44	1.0
1–2	18,629	823	44	1.0*
3–4	9,802	457	47	1.1
5–6	4,614	226	49	1.1
≥ 7	3,069	154	50	1.1

*Reference category
[1]Includes abortions

5.30) The relative risks according to history of prior abortion, stillbirth, and neonatal death were 1.1, 1.2, and 1.4, respectively.

Characteristics and Complications of the Pregnancy

Duration of Pregnancy (Table 5.31) The race-specific malformation rates according to four categories of duration of pregnancy are given. With a duration of 9 to 10 lunar months as the reference, the relative risks increased as duration decreased. For the shortest pregnancies, the relative risks ranged from 2.1 to 3.9. The effect was more prominent among White mothers. Postmature pregnancies were also associated with an increased malformation rate; the relative risks for pregnancies lasting more than 10 lunar months ranged from 1.3 to 2.0.

Placental Weight (Table 5.32) The table gives the malformation rates according to four categories of placental weight. The relative risk increased with decreasing placental weight, being 3.1 for the lowest category (less than 200 gm).

Single Umbilical Artery (Table 5.33) It is well known that single umbilical artery is strongly associated with a high malformation rate. The race-specific rates confirm the association in this study. The number of umbilical arteries was not recorded during the earliest part of the study; there were 5,090 infants for whom this was unknown. Relative risks, given

Table **5.29**

Distribution of Malformed Children by History of Prior Premature Births

No. of Prior Premature Births	No. of Children	Malformed Children		Relative Risk
		No.	Rate/1,000	
Prior births not premature	26,707[1]	1,192	45	1.0*
1	5,443	259	48	1.1
2	1,677	75	45	1.0
≥ 3	901	53	59	1.3
No prior liveborn	15,554	698	45	1.0

*Reference category
[1]Includes 952 unknowns

Table **5.30**

Distribution of Malformed Children by History of Prior Fetal or Neonatal Loss

	No. of Children	Malformed Children		Relative Risk
		No.	Rate/1,000	
Prior abortion	9,135	458	50	1.1
No prior abortion[1]	26,979	1,202	45	1.0*
No prior pregnancy	14,168	617	44	1.0
Prior stillbirth	2,837	156	55	1.2
No prior stillbirth[2]	32,280	1,445	45	1.0*
No prior pregnancies 20 weeks or over	15,165	676	45	1.0
Prior neonatal death	2,174	134	62	1.4
No prior neonatal death[3]	32,554	1,445	44	1.0*
No prior liveborn	15,554	698	45	1.0

*Reference category
[1]Includes 108 unknowns
[2]Includes 179 unknowns
[3]Includes 947 unknowns

single umbilical artery, were 3.4, 5.5, and 5.2 in White, Black, and Puerto Rican children, respectively.

Signs of Toxemia (Table 5.34) A hierarchical classification was created: (1) eclampsia, (2) uncontrolled chronic hypertension (BP $\geq$ 160/110 mm Hg after LM 6), (3) controlled chronic hypertension (without BP $\geq$ 160/110 mm Hg after LM 6), (4) acute hypertension (BP $\geq$ 160/110 mm Hg arising for the first time after LM 6), (5) proteinuria, (6) generalized

Table **5.31**

Race-Specific Distribution of Malformed Children by Duration of Pregnancy

	Length of Gestation (lunar months)	No. of Children	Malformed Children		Relative Risk
			No.	Rate/1,000	
White	5–6	178	29	163	3.9
	7–8	896	91	102	2.4
	9–10	21,293	901	42	1.0*
	$\geq$ 11	444	29	65	1.5
Black	5–6	354	31	88	2.1
	7–8	2,147	142	66	1.6
	9–10	21,068	898	43	1.0*
	$\geq$ 11	461	26	56	.1.3
Puerto Rican	5–6	27	3	111	3.3
	7–8	249	17	68	2.0
	9–10	3,075	104	34	1.0*
	$\geq$ 11	90	6	67	2.0

*Reference category

Table **5.32**

Distribution of Malformed Children by Placental Weight

Placental Weight (grams)	No. of Children	Malformed Children		Relative Risk
		No.	Rate/1,000	
≤ 199	388	51	131	3.1
200–299	2,095	161	77	1.8
≥ 300	41,385	1,769	43	1.0*
Unknown	6,414	296	46	1.1

*Reference category

Table **5.33**

Race-Specific Distribution of Malformed Children by Number of Umbilical Arteries

	No. of Umbilical Arteries	No. of Children	Malformed Children		Relative Risk
			No.	Rate/1,000	
White	One	219	34	155	3.4
	Two	20,351	918	45	1.0*
	Unknown	2,241	98	44	1.0
Black	One	107	26	243	5.5
	Two	21,399	938	44	1.0*
	Unknown	2,524	133	53	1.2
Puerto Rican	One	15	3	200	5.2
	Two	3,101	120	39	1.0*
	Unknown	325	7	22	0.6

*Reference category

Table **5.34**

Distribution of Malformed Children by Signs of Toxemia[1]

	No. of Children	Malformed Children		Relative Risk
		No.	Rate/1,000	
Eclampsia	22	3	136.4	3.0
Uncontrolled chronic hypertension (BP ≥ 160/110 after LM 6)	283	20	70.7	1.6
Controlled chronic hypertension (without BP ≥ 160/110 after LM 6)	386	25	64.8	1.4
Acute hypertension (BP ≥ 160/110 after LM 6)	930	61	65.6	1.5
Proteinuria	1,213	64	52.8	1.2
Generalized edema	11,425	479	41.9	0.9
None	36,023	1,625	45.1	1.0*

*Reference category
[1]This classification is hierarchical—for example, a pregnancy complicated by uncontrolled chronic hypertension is classified as such, even though proteinuria and edema may also be present.

edema, (7) none. Thus, for example, a pregnancy complicated by uncontrolled chronic hypertension was classified as such even though proteinuria and edema might also have been present. The following classification of hypertension, conforming as closely as possible with the recommended classification of the American Committee of Maternal Welfare[2] with definitional additions of the American College of Obstetricians and Gynecologists,[3] has been adopted: hypertension was defined as a systolic blood pressure of 160 mm Hg or greater and/or a diastolic pressure of 110 mm Hg or greater. Chronic hypertension was considered to be present if there was a history of earlier hypertension when not pregnant, together with at least one of the following: hypertension detected before the seventh lunar month, or persistence of hypertension after delivery. It was also considered to be present in the absence of a prior history, if hypertension was detected before the seventh lunar month and if it persisted after delivery.

Table 5.34 gives the malformation rates according to the seven categories of toxemia. For a small sample of 22 mothers with eclampsia, the relative risk was 3.0. For the three categories which include hypertension, the relative risks were between 1.4 and 1.6. Among pregnancies complicated by proteinuria only, the relative risk was 1.2. For 11,425 pregnancies with generalized edema only, the relative risk was 0.9.

The data suggest that eclampsia, the various other hypertensive complications of pregnancy, and possibly proteinuria are each related to the risk of giving birth to a child with any of malformations designated as uniform. There is a suggestion of a monotonic gradation of risk for these factors. On the other hand, there is no evidence, based upon a large sample of women with generalized edema, that this factor is related to the risk of having a malformed child.

Vomiting During Pregnancy and Hyperemesis (Table 5.35) There was no evidence that vomiting or a diagnosis of hyperemesis gravidarum was associated with malformations. Vomiting, in particular, occurred in a majority of the pregnancies, and based on these very substantial numbers, the relative risk was 1.0.

Incompetent Cervix (Table 5.35) Based on small numbers, the relative risk was 1.4.

Vaginal Bleeding (Table 5.35) The mal-

Table **5.35**

Distribution of Malformed Children by Various Complications of Pregnancy

	No. of Children	Malformed Children		Relative Risk*
		No.	Rate/1,000	
Vomiting during pregnancy	33,341	1,500	45	1.0
Hyperemesis gravidarum	540	24	44	1.0
Incompetent cervix	184	12	65	1.4
Vaginal bleeding				
1st trimester	3,668	182	50	1.1
2nd trimester	2,546	145	57	1.3
3rd trimester	6,980	326	47	1.0
Hydramnios	694	84	121	2.7
Tight true cord knot	108	6	56	1.2
Hemorrhagic shock	99	15	152	3.4
Vena cava syndrome	144	10	69	1.5

*For each condition, the reference category consists of those without that condition.

formation rates were only slightly elevated for 13,194 pregnancies that were complicated by vaginal bleeding. The relative risk was highest (1.3) for bleeding that occurred during the second trimester; it was barely increased when bleeding occurred during the first trimester.

Hydramnios (Table 5.35) The malformation rate among children born to mothers with hydramnios was elevated, giving a relative risk of 2.7.

Tight Cord Knot (Table 5.35) Based on small numbers, the relative risk was 1.2.

Hemorrhagic Shock (Table 5.35) The relative risk for this complication was 3.4. Some two-thirds of the events were due to placenta previa and/or placental separation.

Vena Cava Syndrome (Table 5.35) Positional shock was recorded in 144 pregnancies. The malformation rate was 69 per 1,000, giving a relative risk of 1.5.

Placental Factors (Table 5.36) The table gives the malformation rates for pregnancies complicated by marginal sinus rupture, abruptio placentae, placenta previa, and placental infarcts more than 3 cm in diameter (smaller placental infarcts were not associated with malformations). The numerators and denominators for each of the factors were sufficiently large to ensure stable rates. All four factors were positively related to malformations, with the relative risks ranging from 1.4 to 2.0. The latter relative risk occurred in pregnancies complicated by abruptio placentae.

Weight Change During Pregnancy (Table 5.37) Most mothers gained in excess of 7.4 kg, although the median weight gain was lower among Black mothers. With respect to malformations, trends in the data were inconsistent: among White mothers there was evidence to suggest that the malformation rate was inversely related to weight gain. For those who lost weight or failed to gain, the relative risk was 1.6. No such trend was evident among Black or Puerto Rican mothers. Subdivision into a larger number of categories of weight gain failed to reveal evidence of a trend, even among Black or Puerto Rican mothers who lost weight. One curious feature is that for those pregnancies in which the degree of weight change was unknown, the malformation rates were consistently elevated in each of the ethnic groups, with relative risks ranging from 1.2 to 1.4.

Diabetes (Table 5.38) This table gives the malformation rates for pregnancies associated with established or suspected diabetes. The classification in the table is hierarchical and is based upon duration and severity. There were 98 pregnancies in which the disease was known to have been present for at least five years. In 96 pregnancies, the disease had been present for less than 5 years, but required treatment. The least severe category comprised 142 pregnancies, all untreated, in which a clinical diagnosis was recorded. The relative risk for the most severe diabetic category was 4.1, and for treated

Table **5.36**

Distribution of Malformed Children by Placental Factors

	No. of Children	Malformed Children		Relative Risk*
		No.	Rate/1,000	
Marginal sinus rupture	639	45	70	1.6
Abruptio placentae	1,030	92	89	2.0
Placenta previa	317	20	63	1.4
Placental infarct ≥ 3 cm diameter	1,501	92	61	1.4

*For each condition, the reference category consists of those without that condition.

Table **5.37**

Race-Specific Distribution of Malformed Children by Weight Change During Pregnancy

	Weight Change (kg)	No. of Children	Malformed Children		Relative Risk
			No.	Rate/1,000	
White	Lost/no change	305	21	69	1.6
	Gained ≤ 7.4	4,707	251	53	1.2
	Gained ≥ 7.5	17,124	744	43	1.0*
	Unknown	675	34	50	1.2
Black	Lost/no change	509	20	39	0.9
	Gained ≤ 7.4	6,334	327	52	1.2
	Gained ≥ 7.5	16,298	697	43	1.0*
	Unknown	889	53	60	1.4
Puerto Rican	Lost/no change	106	3	28	0.8
	Gained ≤ 7.4	933	35	38	1.0
	Gained ≥ 7.5	2,099	78	37	1.0*
	Unknown	303	14	46	1.2

*Reference category

Table **5.38**

Distribution of Malformed Children by Maternal Diabetes Mellitus

	No. of Children	Malformed Children		Relative Risk*
		No.	Rate/1,000	
Treated diabetes ≥ 5 years	98	18	184	4.1
Treated diabetes < 5 years	96	9	94	2.1
Untreated diabetes or keto-acidosis	142	7	49	1.1
No diabetes	49,946	2,243	45	1.0*

*Reference category

diabetes lasting less than 5 years, it was 2.1. For the untreated group, the relative risk was 1.1. Thus there appeared to be a monotonic trend in the malformation rate according to the severity of the diabetes.

Thrombosis or Thrombophlebitis (Table 5.39) There was no evidence that this complication of pregnancy was related to the risk of having a malformed child (relative risk, 0.8).

Functional Cardiovascular Disorders (Table 5.39) This category comprised, almost in its entirety, women in whom var-ious arrhythmias or electrocardiographic abnormalities were recorded. An elevated malformation rate was present (relative risk, 1.7).

Anemia (Table 5.39) Anemia was recorded as a clinical diagnosis in 11,761 pregnancies (23.4%). We chose not to examine subcategories of anemia, but only to evaluate whether the clinical diagnosis of anemia, overall, was associated with malformations. There was no evidence of such association (relative risk, 0.9).

Hyperthyroidism (Table 5.39) Based

Table **5.39**

Distribution of Malformed Children by Selected Diseases of the Mother During Pregnancy

	No. of Children	Malformed Children		Relative Risk*
		No.	Rate/1,000	
Thrombosis/phlebitis	144	5	35	0.8
Functional cardiovascular disorders	314	24	76	1.7
Anemia	11,761	504	43	0.9
Hyperthyroidism	87	7	80	1.8
Endocrine disease other than diabetes, hypothyroidism or hyperthyroidism	1,537	90	59	1.3
Syphilis	918	54	59	1.3
Urinary tract infection (fever ≥ 100.4°F)	709	36	51	1.1
Hematuria (≥ 15 RBC/HPF)	1,059	65	61	1.4
Convulsive disorder	294	24	82	1.8
Convulsions during pregnancy	131	11	84	1.9
Bacterial infection (after 4th lunar month)	899	51	57	1.3
Septic shock	9	2	222	4.9

*For each disease, the reference category consists of those without that disease.

on 87 pregnancies complicated by this condition, the relative risk was 1.8.

Other Endocrine Disorders (Table 5.39) Apart from diabetes or hormonal disturbances of the thyroid gland, there were 1,537 pregnancies in which a disturbance of endocrine function was recorded. Nearly all of these represented women in whom there was thought to be some hormonal inbalance. As a rule, detailed biochemical documentation was not available. For this category, the relative risk was 1.3.

Syphilis (Table 5.39) For 918 pregnancies in which syphilis (mostly inactive) was diagnosed, the relative risk was 1.3.

Urinary Tract Infection (Table 5.39) This diagnosis was only accepted if, in addition to there being evidence of bacteriuria, pyuria, or hematuria, the temperature was at least 100.4°F. The relative risk was 1.1.

Hematuria (Table 5.39) This diagnosis was only accepted if there was a red cell count of at least 15 cells per high power field. The relative risk was 1.4.

Convulsive Disorder (Table 5.39) Convulsive disorder in this study represents either those mothers who had epilepsy before they became pregnant, or alternatively, those mothers who had a convulsive disorder diagnosed during the current pregnancy that was not attributed to eclampsia. There were 294 affected gravidas with a relative risk of 1.8; in 131 of these there were one or more convulsive episodes during pregnancy (relative risk, 1.9).

Bacterial Infection and Septic Shock (Table 5.39) For 899 pregnancies in which a diagnosis of bacterial infection was made after the fourth lunar month, and for 9 pregnancies complicated by septic shock, the relative risks were 1.3 and 4.9, respectively. Bacterial infection in early pregnancy was not associated with malformations.

Coagulation Defects (Table 5.40) Among 55 pregnancies complicated by various coagulation defects, the relative risk was 3.6. Based on small numbers, relative risks were elevated for

Table **5.40**

Distribution of Malformed Children by Coagulation Defects in the Mother

	No. of Children	Malformed Children		Relative Risk
		No.	Rate/1,000	
Low plasma fibrinogen only	37	7	189	4.2
Low plasma fibrinogen together with other coagulation defects	3	1	333	7.4
Other coagulation defects	15	1	67	1.5
Any coagulation defect	55	9	164	3.6
No coagulation defect	50,227	2,268	45	1.0*

*Reference category

low plasma fibrinogen with or without other coagulation defects, as well as for coagulation defects not affecting fibrinogen levels.

Environmental Factors

Cigarette Smoking (Table 5.41) There was little variability in the race-specific malformation rates, regardless of smoking status. All relative risks were at or close to unity. In this study, when women had stopped smoking, they were asked to state the age at which they stopped. If the age during the current pregnancy was the same, smoking status could not be determined and was classified as uncertain.

Pelvic or Abdominal X-Ray Exposure (Table 5.42) Among 11,400 mothers exposed to pelvic or abdominal X-rays during pregnancy, the relative risk was 1.2.

Exposure to Rubella (Table 5.43) Mother-child pairs in which the mothers and/or the newborn had clinically evident rubella were excluded. There remained 1,987 pregnancies in which the

Table **5.41**

Race-Specific Distribution of Malformed Children by Maternal Cigarette Smoking

	Cigarette Smoking (no./day)	No. of Children	Malformed Children		Relative Risk
			No.	Rate/1,000	
White	Never/Ex/Uncertain	11,334	533	47	1.0*
	≤ 14	5,100	219	43	0.9
	15–29	4,951	235	47	1.0
	≥ 30	1,426	63	44	0.9
Black	Never/Ex/Uncertain	14,776	684	46	1.0*
	≤ 14	7,026	312	44	1.0
	15–29	1,913	86	45	1.0
	≥ 30	315	15	48	1.0
Puerto Rican	Never/Ex/Uncertain	2,487	98	39	1.0*
	≤ 14	698	24	34	0.9
	15–29	212	6	28	0.7
	≥ 30	44	2	45	1.2

*Reference category

Table **5.42**

Distribution of Malformed Children by Pelvic and/or Abdominal X-Ray Exposure During Pregnancy

| Pelvic and/or Abdominal X-Ray Exposure | No. of Children | Malformed Children | | Relative Risk |
		No.	Rate/1,000	
Present	11,400	590	52	1.2
Absent	38,882	1,687	43	1.0*

*Reference category

Table **5.43**

Distribution of Malformed Children by Maternal Exposure to Rubella Infection During Pregnancy

| Rubella Exposure | No. of Children | Malformed Children | | Relative Risk |
		No.	Rate/1,000	
1st trimester	535	29	54	1.2
2nd trimester	869	47	54	1.2
3rd trimester	583	22	38	0.8
None	48,295	2,179	45	1.0*

*Reference category

mothers were recorded as having been exposed to rubella. For pregnancies exposed before the seventh lunar month, the relative risk was 1.2; for those exposed thereafter, the relative risk was 0.8.

Genetic Factors

Consanguinity of Maternal Grandparents (Table 5.44) There were eight malformed children born to 136 gravidas in which the mother's parents were known to be related (second cousins or closer), giving a relative risk of 1.3.

Consanguinity of the Child's Parents Table 5.44) In 112 pregnancies, the parents were either second cousins or more closely related. The relative risk was 1.4.

Malformed Parents (Table 5.45) A history of malformations in either the mothers or the fathers was associated with elevated malformation rates in the children, giving relative risks of 1.5 and 1.8, respectively. Data on malformations in the fathers were generally obtained by interviewing the mothers, except when the father agreed to be interviewed, which was uncommon.

Malformed Siblings (Tables 5.46, 5.47) There was a monotonic increase in the malformation rate according to the number of prior affected siblings, with relative risks of 1.4, 2.1, and 3.3 for one, two, and three or more malformed siblings, respectively (Table 5.46). Malformations in prior siblings were classified as displayed in Table 5.47. The relative risks ranged from 1.4 to 2.4.

Rh and ABO Incompatibility and Erythroblastosis (Table 5.48) There were

58

Table **5.44**

Distribution of Malformed Children by Consanguinity

	No. of Children	Malformed Children		Relative Risk*
		No.	Rate/1,000	
Mother's parents second cousins or closer	136	8	59	1.3
Child's parents second cousins or closer	112	7	63	1.4

*For each of the above, the reference category consists of those with a negative family history of consanguinity.

Table **5.45**

Distribution of Malformed Children by History of Maternal or Paternal Malformation

	No. of Children	Malformed Children		Relative Risk*
		No.	Rate/1,000	
Congenital malformation in child's mother	1,168	79	68	1.5
Congenital malformation in child's father	664	47	71	1.8

*For each of the above, the reference category consists of those with a negative parental history. Histories were unknown in 1,087 mothers and 4,880 fathers.

Table **5.46**

Distribution of Malformed Children by History of Malformation in Prior Siblings

	No. of Children	Malformed Children		Relative Risk
		No.	Rate/1,000	
Congenital malformation in one prior sibling	3,319	203	61	1.4
Congenital malformation in two prior siblings	347	32	92	2.1
Congenital malformation in three or more prior siblings	57	8	140	3.3
Prior siblings not malformed	30,613[1]	1,321	43	1.0*
Firstborn child	15,166	676	45	1.0

*Reference category
[1] Includes 780 unknowns

Table **5.47**

Distribution of Malformed Children by History of Selected Malformations in Prior Siblings

Malformation in Prior Sibling(s)	No. of Children	Malformed Children		Relative Risk*
		No.	Rate/1,000	
Cleft palate	106	11	103.8	2.4
Clubfoot	291	17	58.4	1.4
Cardiac malformation	329	22	66.9	1.5
Head/spine	466	32	68.7	1.6
Miscellaneous other malformations[2]	1,301	77	59.2	1.4
Prior siblings not malformed	30,613[1]	1,321	43.2	1.0*
Firstborn child	15,166	676	44.6	1.0

*Reference category
[1]Includes 808 unknowns
[2]Not including malformations of fingers and toes

Table **5.48**

Distribution of Malformed Children Classified by Rh and ABO Incompatibility and Erythroblastosis

		No. of Children	Malformed Children		Relative Risk
			No.	Rate/1,000	
Erythroblastosis	Present (Rh)	266	17	64	1.4
	Present (ABO)	162[1]	10	62	1.4
	Absent	49,479	2,233	45	1.0*
	Unknown	375	17	45	1.0
Rh incompatibility	Present	3,286	144	44	1.0
	Absent	44,210	2,008	45	1.0*
	Unknown	2,786	125	45	1.0
ABO incompatibility	Present	9,729	413	42	1.0
	Absent	36,325	1,562	43	1.0*
	Unknown	4,228	302	71	1.7

*Reference category
[1]Includes seven cases of varieties of erythroblastosis other than Rh or ABO

266 infants in whom a diagnosis of erythroblastosis due to Rh incompatibility was made, and there were 162 in whom the incompatibility was of the ABO type. The relative risks were both 1.4.

There were substantial numbers of infants whose blood was incompatible with the mothers' blood according to various categories of Rh and ABO, but who were not recorded as having erythroblastosis. Relative risks for all of these categories were at or close to unity. One curious feature was an increase in the malforma-

60

tion rate among mother-child pairs in which the ABO status was unknown (relative risk, 1.7).

Multivariate Analysis

In the preceding pages, those variables identified as risk factors for having a malformed child have been described. However, no data concerning the relationships among these factors have been given. When complex interrelationships among risk factors may be present, one efficient way of controlling their influence on each other is by multivariate analysis.

At this point it would be helpful to recapitulate the steps taken in identifying those risk factors selected for inclusion in the multivariate analyses. Considerations underlying the choice of these variables included relative risk, sample size, and medical judgement as to their possible importance.

The next step was to determine whether each selected variable, identified on univariate analysis, remained a risk factor when all covariate risk factors were simultaneously controlled. This step was accomplished by using linear discriminant function analysis. Such analysis resulted in the elimination of some variables whose effects were accounted for by their covariates. The remaining variables represented those risk factors which independently continued to contribute to the risk of having a malformed child when due allowance for the influence of the covariates was made. Finally, the risk factors not eliminated by the preceding steps were included in a multiple logistic regression model used to determine the contribution made by each factor when all other factors were simultaneously controlled. A detailed description of the analytical procedures is presented in Chapter 3.

After selecting the risk factors, we combined the categories to reduce their number as much as possible, whenever the rates were reasonably similar. Ordinal scaling was applied only if the malformation rate was monotonically related to ordered categories of a given variable (e.g., values of 0, 1, 3 were assigned to decreasing ranges of birthweight). In all other circumstances, binary scaling (0,1) was used.

Based on the results of linear discriminant function analysis, six variables were eliminated by one or more of their covariates and have not been included in the multiple logistic regression model: (1) high ordinal number of entry to the study; (2) history of prior abortion, stillbirth, or neonatal death; (3) low placental weight; (4) vaginal bleeding; (5) urinary tract infection or hematuria; and (6) bacterial infection after the fourth lunar month. Low placental weight is a good example of how an apparently strong risk factor, identified in univariate analysis, was eliminated in multivariate analysis. The most strongly associated covariate of low placental weight was low birthweight, and the latter factor accounted for most of the association between malformations and low placental weight.

Table 5.49 lists the factors retained in the multiple logistic risk function model. The estimated standardized relative risk for each factor is a function of the estimated risk function coefficient (for details, see Chapter 3). The relative risks derived in this way are adjusted for the concomitant effects of the other factors. Thus, a coefficient of 0.4 implies something like a 50% increase in risk of bearing a malformed child; a coefficient of 0.7 or 1.1 implies a doubling or tripling, respectively, of the risk. The precision with which a coefficient is estimated is measured by its standard error; a ratio of coefficient to standard error of less than 2 is conventionally taken to suggest that even an apparently strong factor effect may be a chance phenomenon, whereas large ratios indicate that the estimate is probably reliable.

Table **5.49**

Factors Related to the Risk of a Malformed Child Based Upon Multiple Logistic Risk Function Analysis

	Estimated Risk Function Coefficient	Standard Error of Coefficient	Estimated Standardized Relative Risk
Single umbilical artery	1.42	0.15	4.1
Birthweight less than 1,500 gm	1.23	0.07	3.1
Malformed sibling ≥ three	1.08	0.15	2.9
Hydramnios	0.87	0.13	2.4
Treated maternal diabetes, duration ≥ 5	0.86	0.27	2.4
Convulsive disorder	0.55	0.22	1.7
Coagulation defect in the mother	0.53	0.39	1.7
Hemorrhagic shock during pregnancy	0.50	0.31	1.6
Duration of pregnancy ≥ 11 lunar months	0.44	0.13	1.6
Maternal age ≥ 40 years	0.42	0.14	1.5
Vena cava syndrome	0.40	0.34	1.5
Maternal age ≤ 14 years	0.33	0.21	1.4
Syphilis	0.29	0.14	1.3
Male infant	0.28	0.04	1.3
Functional cardiovascular disorders	0.28	0.22	1.3
Abruptio placentae	0.25	0.12	1.3
Endocrine disorder other than hypothyroidism, hyperthyroidism, or diabetes mellitus	0.22	0.11	1.2
Placental infarcts ≥ 3 cm in diameter	0.22	0.11	1.2
Proteinuria, hypertension, and/or eclampsia	0.19	0.08	1.2
Pelvic and/or abdominal x-ray exposure during pregnancy	0.12	0.05	1.1

Table 5.49 shows that those factors most strongly linked to the uniform malformations, with relative risks greater than three, were single umbilical artery (4.1) and low birthweight (3.1). Both findings were statistically significant, as evidenced by the ratios of the coefficients to their standard errors. Factors with relative risks between two and three were as follows: at least three prior malformed siblings (2.9), hydramnios (2.4), and treated maternal diabetes of at least five years' duration (2.4), all of which were statistically significant. Of the remaining factors, the following were statistically significant: convulsive disorder (1.7); duration of pregnancy at least 11 lunar months (1.6); maternal age at least 40 years (1.5); syphilis (1.3); male infant (1.3); abruptio placentae (1.3); endocrine disorder other than hypothyroidism, hyperthyroidism, or diabetes (1.2); large

placental infarct (1.2); signs of toxemia (1.2); and maternal pelvic or abdominal X-ray exposure during pregnancy (1.1).

A cautionary note is appropriate. It should be stressed that it remains desirable to confirm the results in other bodies of data. It should also be stressed that the risk factors listed in Table 5.49 are ranked according to the strength of their association with uniform malformations in terms of their relative risk estimates. However, it is essential to examine not only the relative risk, but also the frequency with which each risk factor occurs, if the contribution made by each factor toward the risk of the outcome is to be properly assessed. Thus, a common factor having a low relative risk may contribute more to the outcome than an uncommon factor with a high relative risk.

In Table 5.50, the mother-child pairs

Table **5.50**

Distribution of Observed and Expected Numbers of Malformed Children by Multiple Logistic Risk Function Scores

Risk Score Percentile[1]	Observed Number of Malformed Children	Expected Number of Malformed Children
99–100	173	179.0
97–98	119	112.5
95–96	92	93.5
93–94	80	80.9
91–92	66	69.8
Subtotal (91-100)	530	535.7
81–90	290	290.3
71–80	218	235.8
61–70	228	208.1
51–60	184	190.1
41–50	173	190.1
31–40	201	183.7
21–30	163	153.7
11–20	142	144.3
1–10	148	145.2
Total	2,277	2,277.0

[1]Each decile contains 5,025 pregnancies, except the lowest which contains 5,057 pregnancies.

have been ranked in descending order of risk score as derived from the multiple logistic analysis. The highest decile has been divided into two percentile strata, each containing 1,005 pairs. In the remainder of the table, the observed and expected numbers are given by decile, each containing 5,025 pairs, except for the lowest decile which contains 5,057. In each of the strata, the correspondence between the observed and expected numbers is reasonably close. In addition, the procedure appears to discriminate quite well between high and low risk. This is indicated by the size of the ratio of numbers in the top decile of risk to numbers in the lowest (greater than 3).

At this point the later application of the model in evaluating drugs can be illustrated with some hypothetical examples. For all 50,282 mother-child pairs, the overall expected malformation rate is 44 per 1,000. Assume that a hypothetical drug is given exclusively to 2,010 mothers in the top four percentiles of risk and that the observed number of malformed children is 293. This gives a malformation rate of 146 per 1,000, or an unadjusted relative risk of 3.3 (146/44). Nevertheless, there is no justification for an inference of causality since the observed number of malformations in the children exposed *in utero* to the drug is, in fact, identical to the expected number when the appropriate risk factors are taken into account: the standardized relative risk is 1.0. In actually carrying out multivariate analysis in this way, a non-causal association would be eliminated.

Conversely, if all of the 5,057 mothers in the lowest decile of risk were exposed to another hypothetical drug and there were 146 malformed children born to those mothers, the malformation rate would be 29 per 1,000. The unadjusted relative risk in this case would be 0.7 (29/44). Once again, a "protective" effect of the drug cannot be inferred, since the adjusted relative risk is 1.0. Even more important, if a malformation rate of 44 per 1,000 were observed for this group of pregnancies, the adjusted relative risk would not be 1.0, but 1.5 — indicating a 50% greater risk of developing a malformation, given drug exposure. Without taking the negative confounding that exists into account, this association would go undetected.

CHAPTER 6

Major Malformations

All malformations with uniform hospital distributions were arbitrarily categorized as major or minor. Major malformations were defined as those which were potentially life-threatening or which were major cosmetic defects. Such malformations would be expected to be diagnosed in a reasonably consistent manner.

Among the 50,282 children, there were 1,393 (27.7 per 1,000) with 2,216 major malformations. As seen in Table 6.1, major malformations were most common in White children (32.8 per 1,000), intermediate in Puerto Ricans (27.3 per 1,000), and least common in Black children (22.9 per 1,000).

Risk Factors for Major Malformations

Administrative Data

Number of Antenatal Visits (Table 6.2) Children whose mothers had fewer than five antenatal visits had a higher rate of major malformations than did those who had five or more visits (relative risk, 1.3).

Year of Last Menstrual Period (Table 6.3) Among children conceived during the years 1958 to 1965, there was no evidence to suggest secular changes in the rate of major malformations.

Month of Last Menstrual Period (Table 6.4) There were no obvious seasonal trends in the rate of major malformations.

Table **6.1**

Distribution of Children with Major Malformations by Ethnic Group

	No. of Children	Rate/1,000
White	748	32.79
Black	551	22.93
Puerto Rican	94	27.32
Total	1,393	27.70

Table **6.2**

Distribution of Children with Major Malformations by Number of Antenatal Visits

No. of Antenatal Visits	No. of Children	Children with Major Malformations		Relative Risk
		No.	Rate/1,000	
1–4	8,624	292	34	1.3
5–9	20,964	536	26	1.0*
≥10	20,694	565	27	1.0

*Reference category

Table **6.3**

Distribution of Children with Major Malformations by Year of Mother's Last Menstrual Period (LMP)

Year of LMP	No. of Children	Children with Major Malformations	
		No.	Rate/1,000
1958	1,877	50	26.6
1959	5,735	157	27.4
1960	7,285	184	25.3
1961	7,441	225	30.2
1962	8,216	223	27.1
1963	7,986	226	28.3
1964	7,817	218	27.9
1965	3,925	110	28.0
Total	50,282	1,393	27.7

Table **6.4**

Distribution of Children with Major Malformations by Month of
Mother's Last Menstrual Period (LMP)

Month of LMP	No. of Children	Children with Major Malformations	
		No.	Rate/1,000
January	4,185	126	30.1
February	4,075	91	22.3
March	4,136	123	29.7
April	4,154	125	30.1
May	4,194	100	23.8
June	4,118	103	25.0
July	3,817	119	31.2
August	4,001	113	28.2
September	4,049	102	25.2
October	4,539	119	26.2
November	4,412	136	30.8
December	4,602	136	29.5
Total	50,282	1,393	27.7

Characteristics of the Mother

Mother's Age at Registration (Table 6.5) Major malformations were increasingly common in children born to women aged 30 and above. In Whites, relative risks ranged from 1.2 for women aged 30 to 34 years to 1.8 for women aged at least 40 years. In Blacks, the range was 1.2 to 3.4, with a relative risk of 7.3 for women of at least 45 years, based on two malformed children. In Puerto Ricans, the relative risks ranged from 1.3 for women aged 25 to 29 years to 3.6 for women aged 40 to 44 years.

Mother's Prepregnant Weight and Height (Table 6.6) There was no association of major malformations with height; children born to relatively low-weight and relatively high-weight women had an increased risk of a major malformation, with relative risks of 1.3 and 1.2, respectively. Among children of women with unknown weight or height, the relative risk was 1.4.

Characteristics of the Offspring

Birthweight (Table 6.7) In White and Black children, the risk of major malfor-

mations increased monotonically with decreasing birthweight. Relative risks ranged from 2.3 (Whites) and 2.4 (Blacks) for children weighing between 2,000 and 2,499 gm, to 4.4 (Whites) and 3.9 (Blacks) for children weighing less than 1,500 gm. The rates among Puerto Rican children were unstable because of small numbers, but were elevated in all categories of low birthweight.

Sex of Child (Table 6.8) Major malformations were slightly more common in White males and in Black males. Thus, the relative risk for White and Black males was 1.2.

Survival of the Child (Table 6.9) Major malformations were frequently associated with the death of the child. Given stillbirth, neonatal death, infant death, and childhood death, the relative risks among Whites and Blacks ranged from 6.1 to 12.0. In Puerto Ricans, the relative risks were similarly elevated, but based on smaller numbers.

Autopsy Report (Table 6.10) The presence of an autopsy report was associated with a higher rate of major malformations among White and Black children, giving a relative risk of 1.4.

Table **6.5**

Race-Specific Distribution of Children with Major Malformations by Mother's Age at Registration

	Mother's Age	No. of Children	Children with Major Malformations		Relative Risk
			No.	Rate/1,000	
White	≤14	25	1	40	1.2
	15–19	4,049	99	24	0.7
	20–24	9,012	293	33	1.0*
	25–29	5,208	162	31	0.9
	30–34	2,726	113	41	1.2
	35–39	1,405	57	41	1.2
	40–44	369	22	60	1.8
	≥45	17	1	59	1.8
Black	≤14	394	7	18	0.9
	15–19	6,584	146	22	1.0
	20–24	8,109	173	21	1.0*
	25–29	4,638	99	21	1.0
	30–34	2,610	66	25	1.2
	35–39	1,343	34	25	1.2
	40–44	339	24	71	3.4
	≥45	13	2	154	7.3
Puerto Rican	≤14	10	1	100	4.2
	15–19	842	18	21	0.9
	20–24	1,354	33	24	1.0*
	25–29	746	24	32	1.3
	30–34	319	11	34	1.4
	35–39	136	4	29	1.2
	40–44	34	3	88	3.6
	≥45	0	0	—	—

*Reference category

Table **6.6**

Distribution of Children with Major Malformations by Mother's Prepregnant Weight and Height

		No. of Children	Children with Major Malformations		Relative Risk
			No.	Rate/1,000	
Weight (kg)	≤39	372	13	35	1.3
	40–79	46,164	1,249	27	1.0*
	≥80	2,718	91	33	1.2
	Unknown	1,028	40	39	1.4
Height (cm)	≤149	2,947	84	29	1.1
	150–169	39,483	1,073	27	1.0*
	170–189	5,525	148	27	1.0
	Unknown	2,327	88	38	1.4

*Reference category

Table **6.7**

Race-Specific Distribution of Children with Major Malformations by Child's Birthweight

	Birthweight (grams)	No. of Children	Children with Major Malformations		Relative Risk
			No.	Rate/1,000	
White	≤1,499	357	44	123	4.4
	1,500–1,999	288	33	114	4.1
	2,000–2,499	1,201	77	64	2.3
	≥2,500	20,965	594	28	1.0*
Black	≤1,499	602	42	70	3.9
	1,500–1,999	606	39	64	3.6
	2,000–2,499	2,259	98	43	2.4
	≥2,500	20,563	372	18	1.0*
Puerto Rican	≤1,499	57	4	70	3.3
	1,500–1,999	66	9	136	6.5
	2,000–2,499	244	15	61	2.9
	≥2,500	3,074	66	21	1.0

*Reference category

Table **6.8**

Race-Specific Distribution of Children with Major Malformations by Sex of Child

		No. of Children	Children with Major Malformations		Relative Risk
			No.	Rate/1,000	
White	Male	11,763	426	36	1.2
	Female	11,048	322	29	1.0*
Black	Male	12,038	295	25	1.2
	Female	11,992	256	21	1.0*
Puerto Rican	Male	1,741	45	26	0.9
	Female	1,700	49	29	1.0*

*Reference category

This association was not apparent in Puerto Rican children.

Reproductive History of the Mother

History of Prior Pregnancies (Table 6.11) There was an increase in the rate of major malformations among the offspring of White and Black mothers who had five or more prior pregnancies. For those who had five or six prior pregnan-cies, the relative risks were 1.3 (White) and 1.2 (Black). For mothers who had at least seven prior pregnancies, the relative risks were 1.4 and 1.3. For Puerto Rican mothers who had at least seven prior pregnancies, the relative risk was 1.5.

History of Prior Prematures (Table 6.12) An increased rate of major malformations was found in children whose

Table **6.9**

Race-Specific Distribution of Children with Major Malformations by Survival of the Child

	Survival of Child	No. of Children	Children with Major Malformations		Relative Risk
			No.	Rate/1,000	
White	Stillbirth	327	52	159	6.1
	Neonatal death	302	77	255	9.8
	Infant death	130	34	262	10.1
	Childhood death	91	22	242	9.3
	Survived	21,961	563	26	1.0*
Black	Stillbirth	407	40	98	6.1
	Neonatal death	450	72	160	10.0
	Infant death	229	44	192	12.0
	Childhood death	134	23	172	10.8
	Survived	22,810	372	16	1.0*
Puerto Rican	Stillbirth	64	6	94	5.2
	Neonatal death	54	14	259	14.4
	Infant death	25	8	320	17.8
	Childhood death	14	6	429	23.8
	Survived	3,284	60	18	1.0*

*Reference category

Table **6.10**

Race-Specific Distribution of Dead Children with Major Malformations by Presence of Autopsy Report

	Autopsy Report	No. of Children	Dead Children with Major Malformations		Relative Risk
			No.	Rate/1,000	
White	Present	674	156	232	1.4
	Absent	176	29	165	1.0*
Black	Present	1,008	157	156	1.4
	Absent	213	23	108	1.0*
Puerto Rican	Present	128	27	211	0.9
	Absent	29	7	241	1.0*

*Reference category

Table **6.11**

Race-Specific Distribution of Children with Major Malformations by History of Prior Pregnancies

	No. of Prior Pregnancies[1]	No. of Children	Children with Major Malformations		Relative Risk
			No.	Rate/1,000	
White	None	6,936	228	33	1.1
	1–2	8,866	261	29	1.0*
	3–4	4,224	153	36	1.2
	5–6	1,798	67	37	1.3
	≥7	987	39	40	1.4
Black	None	6,291	136	22	1.0
	1–2	8,347	194	23	1.0*
	3–4	4,913	96	20	0.9
	5–6	2,535	69	27	1.2
	≥7	1,944	56	29	1.3
Puerto Rican	None	941	22	23	0.8
	1–2	1,416	41	29	1.0*
	3–4	665	19	29	1.0
	5–6	281	6	21	0.7
	≥7	138	6	43	1.5

*Reference category
[1]Includes abortions

Table **6.12**

Distribution of Children with Major Malformations by History of Prior Premature Births

No. of Prior Premature Births	No. of Children	Children with Major Malformations		Relative Risk
		No.	Rate/1,000	
None	26,707[1]	719	27	1.0*
1	5,443	160	29	1.1
2	1,677	47	28	1.0
3 or more	901	31	34	1.3
No prior liveborn	15,554	436	28	1.0

*Reference category
[1]Includes unknowns

mothers had had at least 3 prior premature births, giving a relative risk of 1.3.

History of Prior Fetal Loss (Table 6.13) The relative risk for major malformations in children whose mothers had had prior stillbirths or neonatal deaths, was 1.3.

Characteristics and Complications of the Pregnancy

Duration of Pregnancy (Table 6.14) The rate of major malformations was higher in pregnancies which were less than 9 or more than 10 lunar months in duration. Among the three ethnic groups, relative risks ranged from 2.0 to 2.8 for pregnancies of 7 to 8 months duration, and from 2.4 to 4.6 (based on 3 malformed Puerto Rican children) for pregnancies of 5 to 6 months duration. For pregnancies of at least 11 lunar months duration, the relative risks ranged from 1.5 to 2.8.

Placental Weight (Table 6.15) Substantial increases in the rate of major malformations were present when the placenta weighed less than 300 gm, giving relative risks of 2.2 for a placental weight of between 200 and 299 gm, and 3.4 for a placental weight of less than 200 gm.

Single Umbilical Artery (Table 6.16) There was a large increase in the rate of major malformations in children who had only one umbilical artery, giving a relative risk of 5.7.

Signs of Toxemia (Tables 6.17, 6.18) Overall, as seen in Table 6.17, the risk of major malformations was not increased when the mother had generalized edema, a non-specific sign of toxemia. However, when the mother had more severe symptoms of toxemia, the rate of major malformations was increased. The relative risk for proteinuria was 1.2. Relative risks for the various categories of hypertension ranged from 1.1 to 2.4. Based on very small numbers, the relative risk for eclampsia was 3.4.

In Table 6.18, the race-specific rates for combined categories of toxemia are given. The rate of major malformations was elevated among White and Puerto Rican children whose mothers had proteinuria, giving relative risks of 1.7 and 1.9, respectively. The rates were increased for all three ethnic groups when hypertension was present, with relative risks ranging from 1.5 to 2.4.

Hydramnios (Table 6.19) The rate of major malformations was substantially increased in children whose mothers had hydramnios, giving a relative risk of 4.1.

Placental Factors (Table 6.20) The various placental factors were all associated with an increase in the risk of a major malformation; the relative risks for marginal sinus rupture, abruptio placentae, placenta previa, and placental infarct of 3 cm or more ranged from 1.4 to 1.9.

Weight Change during Pregnancy (Table 6.21) There was a slight increase in the risk of major malformations when the mother gained less than 7.5 kg during pregnancy; relative risks were 1.2 among White and Puerto Rican children, and 1.3 among Black children. Among White children whose mothers lost, or did not gain weight, the relative risk was 1.8. When the mother's weight change was unknown, relative risks ranged from 1.3 to 1.6.

Maternal Diabetes (Table 6.22) There was an increase in the rate of major malformations when the mother had treated diabetes for less than 5 years, or more than 5 years, with relative risks of 3.5 and 6.8, respectively.

Other Diseases of the Mother (Table 6.23) The following maternal illnesses were associated with an increase in the risk of a major malformation: functional cardiovascular disorders (relative risk, 1.5), hyperthyroidism (2.0), other endocrine diseases (1.4), urinary tract infection (1.3), hematuria (1.3), bacterial infection after the fourth lunar month (1.6), a convulsive disorder or convulsions during pregnancy (2.5), hemorrhagic shock (3.6), the vena cava syndrome (2.3), and coagulation defects (3.9).

Table **6.13**

Distribution of Children with Major Malformations by History of Prior Fetal or Neonatal Loss

	No. of Children	Children with Major Malformations		Relative Risk
		No.	Rate/1,000	
Prior abortion	9,135	280	31	1.1
No prior abortion[1]	26,979	727	27	1.0*
No prior pregnancy	14,168	386	27	1.0
Prior stillbirth	2,837	100	35	1.3
No prior stillbirth[1]	32,280	873	27	1.0*
No prior pregnancies 20 weeks or over	15,165	420	28	1.0
Prior neonatal death	2,174	79	36	1.3
No prior neonatal death[1]	32,554	878	27	1.0*
No prior liveborn	15,554	436	28	1.0

*Reference category
[1]Includes unknowns

Table **6.14**

Race-Specific Distribution of Children with Major Malformations by Duration of Pregnancy

	Length of Gestation (lunar months)	No. of Children	Children with Major Malformations		Relative Risk
			No.	Rate/1,000	
White	5–6	178	13	73	2.4
	7–8	896	74	83	2.8
	9–10	21,293	638	30	1.0*
	≥11	444	23	52	1.7
Black	5–6	354	21	59	2.9
	7–8	2,147	85	40	2.0
	9–10	21,068	431	20	1.0*
	≥11	461	14	30	1.5
Puerto Rican	5–6	27	3	111	4.6
	7–8	249	12	48	2.0
	9–10	3,075	73	24	1.0*
	≥11	90	6	67	2.8

*Reference category

73

Table **6.15**

Distribution of Children with Major Malformations by Placental Weight

Placental Weight (grams)	No. of Children	Children with Major Malformations		Relative Risk
		No.	Rate/1,000	
≤199	388	34	88	3.4
200–299	2,095	119	57	2.2
≥300	41,385	1,060	26	1.0*
Unknown	6,414	180	28	1.1

*Reference category

Table **6.16**

Distribution of Children with Major Malformations by Number of Umbilical Arteries

No. of Umbilical Arteries	No. of Children	Children with Major Malformations		Relative Risk
		No.	Rate/1,000	
One	341	53	155	5.7
Two or unknown	49,941	1,340	27	1.0*

*Reference category

Table **6.17**

Distribution of Children with Major Malformations by Signs of Toxemia[1]

	No. of Children	Children with Major Malformations		Relative Risk
		No.	Rate/1,000	
Eclampsia	22	2	91	3.4
Uncontrolled chronic hypertension (BP ≥ 160/110 after LM 6)	283	18	64	2.4
Controlled chronic hypertension (without BP ≥ 160/110 after LM 6)	386	12	31	1.1
Acute hypertension (BP ≥ 160/110 after LM 6)	930	45	48	1.8
Proteinuria	1,213	39	32	1.2
Generalized edema	11,425	291	25	0.9
None	36,023	986	27	1.0*

*Reference category
[1]This classification is hierarchical and based on severity—for example, a pregnancy complicated by uncontrolled chronic hypertension is classified as such, even though proteinuria and edema may also be present.

Table **6.18**

Race-Specific Distribution of Children with Major Malformations by Signs of Toxemia[1]

| | | No. of Children | Children with Major Malformations | | Relative Risk |
			No.	Rate/1,000	
White	Eclampsia	3	0	—	—
	High blood pressure and/or chronic hypertension	591	29	49	1.5
	Proteinuria	421	23	55	1.7
	None/generalized edema only	21,796	696	32	1.0*
Black	Eclampsia	19	2	105	4.8
	High blood pressure and/or chronic hypertension	960	43	45	2.0
	Proteinuria	712	12	17	0.8
	None/generalized edema only	22,339	494	22	1.0*
Puerto Rican	Eclampsia	0	0	—	—
	High blood pressure and/or chronic hypertension	48	3	63	2.4
	Proteinuria	80	4	50	1.9
	None/generalized edema only	3,313	87	26	1.0*

*Reference category
[1]The classification in this table is hierarchical. See Table 6.17.

Table **6.19**

Distribution of Children with Major Malformations by Hydramnios

| | No. of Children | Children with Major Malformations | | Relative Risk |
		No.	Rate/1,000	
Hydramnios	694	76	110	4.1
No hydramnios	49,588	1,317	27	1.0*

*Reference category

Table **6.20**

Distribution of Children with Major Malformations by Placental Factors

	No. of Children	Children with Major Malformations		Relative Risk*
		No.	Rate/1,000	
Marginal sinus rupture	639	32	50	1.9
Abruptio placentae	1,030	52	50	1.9
Placenta previa	317	16	50	1.8
Placental infarct ≥ 3 cm diameter	1,501	59	39	1.4

*For each factor, the reference category consists of those without that factor.

Table **6.21**

Race-Specific Distribution of Children with Major Malformations by Weight Change During Pregnancy

	Weight Change (kg)	No. of Children	Children with Major Malformations		Relative Risk
			No.	Rate/1,000	
White	Lost/no change	305	17	56	1.8
	Gained ≤ 7.4	4,707	176	37	1.2
	Gained ≥ 7.5	17,124	527	31	1.0*
	Unknown	675	28	41	1.3
Black	Lost/no change	509	12	24	1.1
	Gained ≤ 7.4	6,334	168	27	1.3
	Gained ≥ 7.5	16,298	343	21	1.0*
	Unknown	889	28	31	1.5
Puerto Rican	Lost/no change	106	3	28	1.1
	Gained ≤ 7.4	933	27	29	1.2
	Gained ≥ 7.5	2,099	52	25	1.0*
	Unknown	303	12	40	1.6

*Reference category

Environmental Factors

Maternal Cigarette Smoking (Table 6.24) Only among Black children whose mothers smoked at least 30 cigarettes per day was the rate of major malformations elevated, and then only slightly, giving a relative risk of 1.2. All other relative risks were at or below unity.

Pelvic or Abdominal X-Ray Exposure (Table 6.25) The rate of major malfor-mations was increased when the mother had had an antenatal X-ray examination of the abdomen (relative risk, 1.3)

Genetic Factors

History of Maternal or Paternal Malfor-mation (Table 6.26) The rate of major malformations was elevated if the child's father had a congenital malformation, giving a relative risk of 1.6. There was no

Table **6.22**

Distribution of Children with Major Malformations by Maternal Diabetes Mellitus

	No. of Children	Children with Major Malformations		Relative Risk
		No.	Rate/1,000	
Treated diabetes for more than 5 years	98	18	184	6.8
Treated diabetes for less than 5 years	96	9	94	3.5
Untreated diabetes or keto-acidosis	142	4	28	1.0
No diabetes	49,946	1,362	27	1.0*

*Reference category

Table **6.23**

Distribution of Children with Major Malformations by Selected Diseases of the Mother and Complications of Pregnancy

	No. of Children	Children with Major Malformations		Relative Risk*
		No.	Rate/1,000	
Functional cardiovascular disorders	314	13	41	1.5
Hyperthyroidism	87	5	57	2.0
Endocrine disease other than diabetes, hypothyroidism, or hyperthyroidism	1,537	60	39	1.4
Urinary tract infection (fever ≥100.4°F)	709	25	35	1.3
Hematuria (≥15 RBC/HPF)	1,059	39	37	1.3
Bacterial infection (after 4th lunar month)	899	39	43	1.6
Convulsive disorder	294	20	68	2.5
Convulsions during pregnancy	131	9	69	2.5
Hemorrhagic shock	99	10	101	3.6
Vena cava syndrome	144	9	63	2.3
Coagulation defects	55	6	109	3.9

*For each disease, the reference category consists of those without that disease.

Table **6.24**

Race-Specific Distribution of Children with Major Malformations by Maternal Cigarette Smoking

| | Cigarette Smoking (no./day) | No. of Children | Children with Major Malformations | | Relative Risk |
			No.	Rate/1,000	
White	Never/Ex/Uncertain	11,334	383	34	1.0*
	≤14	5,100	168	33	1.0
	15–29	4,951	161	33	1.0
	≥30	1,426	36	25	0.7
Black	Never/Ex/Uncertain	14,776	356	24	1.0*
	≤14	7,026	147	21	0.9
	15–29	1,913	39	20	0.8
	≥30	315	9	29	1.2
Puerto Rican	Never/Ex/Uncertain	2,487	76	31	1.0*
	≤14	698	13	19	0.6
	15–29	212	5	24	0.8
	≥30	44	0	—	—

*Reference category

Table **6.25**

Distribution of Children with Major Malformations by Pelvic and/or Abdominal X-Ray Exposure During Pregnancy

| Pelvic and/ or Abdominal X-Ray Exposure | No. of Children | Children with Major Malformations | | Relative Risk |
		No.	Rate/1,000	
Present	11,400	377	33	1.3
Absent	38,882	1,016	26	1.0*

*Reference category

such association with malformations in the mother.

History of Prior Malformed Siblings (Table 6.27) There was a monotonic relationship between the rate of major malformations and the number of prior malformed siblings, giving relative risks of 1.4, and 2.2, respectively, for one and two or more prior malformed siblings.

Rh and ABO Incompatibility and Erythroblastosis (Table 6.28) There was no association with Rh or ABO incompatibility or with ABO erythroblastosis, but there was an increase in the rate of major malformations if there was Rh erythroblastosis (relative risk, 1.6).

Multivariate Analysis

Based on the preceding comparisons, 32 risk factors were selected for multivariate analysis and scaled as binary or ordinal variables; after linear discrimin-

Table **6.26**

Distribution of Children with Major Malformations by History of Maternal or Paternal Malformation

	No. of Children	Children with Major Malformations		Relative Risk*
		No.	Rate/1,000	
Congenital malformation in child's mother	1,168	36	31	1.1
Congenital malformation in child's father	664	29	44	1.6

*For each of the above, the reference category consists of those with a negative parental history.

Table **6.27**

Distribution of Children with Major Malformations by History of Malformation in Prior Siblings

	No. of Children	Children with Major Malformations		Relative Risk
		No.	Rate/1,000	
Congenital malformation in one prior sibling	3,319	123	37	1.4
Congenital malformation in two or more prior siblings	394	23	58	2.2
Prior siblings normal	31,393	827	26	1.0*
Firstborn child	15,166	420	28	1.1

*Reference category

Table **6.28**

Distribution of Major Malformations by Rh and ABO Incompatibility and Erythroblastosis

		No. of Children	Children with Major Malformations		Relative Risk
			No.	Rate/1,000	
Rh incompatibility	Present	3,286	98	30	1.1
	Absent/unknown	46,996	1,295	28	1.0*
ABO incompatibility	Present	9,729	245	25	0.9
	Absent/unknown	40,553	1,148	28	1.0*
Erythroblastosis	Present (Rh)	266	12	45	1.6
	Present (ABO)	162	4	25	0.9
	Absent/unknown	49,854	1,377	28	1.0*

*Reference category

ant function analysis, 24 variables remained. Factors which were excluded because of low coefficients included: prior stillbirths, prior premature births, weight change during pregnancy, functional cardiovascular disorders, urinary tract infections, hematuria, abruptio placentae, and placenta previa. The results of the multiple logistic regression analysis for the remaining factors are presented in Table 6.29.

The following variables had a relative risk of 3.0 or greater: single umbilical artery (4.9), low birthweight (3.9), hydramnios (3.4), and maternal diabetes (3.0); each of these associations with major malformations was statistically significant. A relative risk between 2.0 and 3.0 was seen for convulsive disorder (2.3) and for vena cava syndrome (2.1); these associations also were statistically significant. The remaining variables had a relative risk less than 2.0, of which the following were statistically significant: long pregnancy (1.9), mother aged 40 or greater (1.6), White ethnic group (1.6), two or more prior malformed siblings (1.6), severe signs of toxemia (1.6), bacterial infection during late pregnancy (1.4), other endocrine disorders (1.4), Puerto Rican ethnic group (1.4), male sex (1.3), and smoking during pregnancy (0.8).

Table **6.29**

Factors Related to the Risk of Major Malformations Based Upon Multiple Logistic Risk Function Analysis

	Estimated Risk Function Coefficient	Standard Error of Coefficient	Estimated Standardized Relative Risk
Single umbilical artery	1.58	0.16	4.9
Birthweight < 2,000 grams	1.36	0.10	3.9
Hydramnios	1.22	0.14	3.4
Maternal diabetes	1.11	0.28	3.0
Convulsive disorder	0.82	0.24	2.3
Vena cava syndrome	0.72	0.36	2.1
Pregnancy duration > 11 lunar months	0.66	0.16	1.9
Coagulation defect	0.53	0.46	1.7
Mother aged ≥40	0.49	0.11	1.6
White ethnic group	0.49	0.06	1.6
Two or more prior malformed siblings	0.46	0.14	1.6
Severe signs of toxemia	0.46	0.17	1.6
Hemorrhagic shock	0.43	0.38	1.5
Bacterial infection	0.36	0.17	1.4
Prepregnant weight ≥ 100 kg	0.35	0.25	1.4
Other endocrine disorders[1]	0.33	0.13	1.4
Puerto Rican ethnic group	0.31	0.12	1.4
Male	0.24	0.06	1.3
Placental infarcts ≥ 3 cm in diameter	0.20	0.14	1.2
Marginal sinus rupture	0.16	0.19	1.2
Placental weight < 300 grams	0.13	0.11	1.1
Less than 5 antenatal visits	0.13	0.07	1.1
Antenatal x-ray exposure	0.09	0.06	1.1
Smoking during pregnancy	−0.24	0.06	0.8

[1]Endocrine disease other than hypo- or hyperthyroidism or diabetes mellitus

Table *6.30*

Distribution of Observed and Expected Numbers of Children with Major Malformations by Multiple Logistic Risk Function Scores

Risk Score Percentile[1]	Observed Number of Children with Major Malformations	Expected Number of Children with Major Malformations
99–100	159	152.0
97–98	78	79.6
95–96	63	63.7
93–94	48	54.3
91–92	43	48.2
Subtotal (91–100)	391	397.8
81–90	193	190.7
71–80	155	151.4
61–70	127	128.2
51–60	115	116.9
41–50	98	101.9
31–40	85	93.6
21–30	85	82.2
11–20	74	72.8
1–10	70	57.5
Total	1,393	1,393.0

[1]Each decile contains 5,025 pregnancies, except the lowest which contains 5,057 pregnancies.

As seen in Table 6.30, there was good agreement between the observed number of children with major malformations and the expected number, based on stratification according to the multiple logistic risk function score. The ratio of the numbers of children in the highest decile of risk to the numbers in the lowest decile is over 5, indicating that the model is successful in discriminating among degrees of risk.

CHAPTER 7

Minor
Malformations

Eight hundred and ninety-eight children (17.9 per 1,000) had a total of 957 minor malformations. As shown in Table 7.1, Blacks had a higher rate of minor malformations (23.3 per 1,000) than Whites (13.2 per 1,000) and Puerto Ricans (10.5 per 1,000). Polydactyly was overwhelmingly a Black malformation. It is apparent that the excess of minor malformations in Blacks was due to their high rate of polydactyly. Hypospadias had a more uniform ethnic distribution but was exclusively a male malformation. The remaining minor malformations showed reasonably similar rates by ethnic group and sex of child. Within this group, the individual components showed similar risk factors. Therefore, in the analyses, the three groups, having quite different risk factors, were kept separate and made mutually exclusive. Six individuals having polydactyly jointly with other minor malformations were placed in the Black polydactyly group (330 children); one individual having hypospadias jointly with other minor malformations was placed in the hypospadias group (187 children); the Black polydactyly and hypospadias groups did not intersect. Black polydactyly and hypospadias are discussed in detail in Chapters 10 and 13, respectively. The remainder of this chapter is devoted to the 381 children with minor malformations exclusive of Blacks with polydactyly and males with hypospadias. When the term "minor malformation" is used

Table **7.1**

Minor Malformations According to Ethnic Group (Rates per Thousand)

	White (n=22,811)		Black (n=24,030)		Puerto Rican (n=3,441)		Total (n=50,282)	
	No.	Rate	No.	Rate	No.	Rate	No.	Rate
Any minor malformation	302	13.2	560	23.3	36	10.5	898	17.9
Minor malformations exclusive of polydactyly in Blacks and hypospadias	208	9.1	146	6.1	27	7.8	381	7.6
Hypospadias	95	4.2	84	3.5	9	2.6	188	3.7
Polydactyly	35	1.5	330	13.7	5	1.5	370	7.4

here, it shall refer to these 381 children, unless otherwise stated.

Risk Factors for Minor Malformations

Administrative Data

Number of Antenatal Visits (Table 7.2) There was an increased rate of minor malformations in children whose mothers had fewer than five antenatal visits, giving a relative risk of 1.3.

Personal Characteristics of the Mother

Mother's Age at Registration (Table 7.3) The rates of minor malformations were higher in offspring of mothers older than 24 years than in offspring of younger mothers, giving relative risks of 1.4 for Whites and Blacks and 1.2 for Puerto Ricans.

Mother's Marital Status (Table 7.4) The rate of minor malformations was elevated among children whose mothers were separated, giving a relative risk of 1.3.

Characteristics and Survival of the Offspring

Birthweight (Table 7.5) Low birthweight children were at higher risk of minor malformations. The relative risk was 9.0 for children weighing less than 1,500 gm and 2.4 for children weighing from 1,500 gm to 2,499 gm.

Birth Order (Table 7.6) Higher minor malformation rates were found in Blacks whose birth order was 2 or 3, or greater than 3 (relative risks, 1.6 and 1.7, respectively), and in Whites whose birth order was greater than 3 (relative risk, 1.4). The rate of minor malformations in Puerto Ricans was negligibly affected by birth order.

Reproductive History of the Mother

Prior Premature Births (Table 7.7) The number of prior premature births was associated with an increasing rate of minor malformations. Thus, the relative risks for one, two, and three or more prior premature births were 0.9, 1.4, and 2.0, respectively.

Prior Fetal Loss (Table 7.8) The rate of minor malformations was elevated in children whose mothers had had prior abortions or stillbirths. The relative risk was 1.4 in each category.

Prior Neonatal Deaths (Table 7.9) Higher minor malformation rates were observed in children whose mothers had a history of prior neonatal death, particularly two or more such deaths. For the latter category, the relative risk was 3.3.

Characteristics and Complications of the Pregnancy

Duration of Gestation (Table 7.10) Minor malformations were present

Table **7.2**

Distribution of Children with Minor Malformations Excluding Black Polydactyly and Hypospadias by Number of Antenatal Visits

No. of Antenatal Visits	No. of Children	Children with Minor Malformations		Relative Risk
		No.	Rate/1,000	
1-4	8,624	81	9.4	1.3
≥5	41,658	300	7.2	1.0*

*Reference category

Table **7.3**

Race-Specific Distribution of Children with Minor Malformations Excluding Black Polydactyly and Hypospadias by Mother's Age at Registration

	Mother's Age	No. of Children	Children with Minor Malformations		Relative Risk
			No.	Rate/1,000	
White	<25	13,086	103	7.9	1.0*
	≥25	9,725	105	10.8	1.4
Black	<25	15,087	80	5.3	1.0*
	≥25	8,943	66	7.4	1.4
Puerto Rican	<25	2,206	16	7.3	1.0*
	≥25	1,235	11	8.9	1.2

*Reference category

Table **7.4**

Distribution of Children with Minor Malformations Excluding Black Polydactyly and Hypospadias by Mother's Marital Status

Marital Status	No. of Children	Children with Minor Malformations		Relative Risk
		No.	Rate/1,000	
Separated	3,326	33	9.9	1.3
Other	46,956	348	7.4	1.0*

*Reference category

Table **7.5**

Distribution of Children with Minor Malformations Excluding Black Polydactyly and Hypospadias by Child's Birthweight

Birthweight (grams)	No. of Children	Children with Minor Malformations		Relative Risk
		No.	Rate/1,000	
≤ 1,499	1,016	54	53.1	9.0
1,500 – 2,499	4,664	65	13.9	2.4
≥ 2,500	44,602	262	5.9	1.0*

*Reference category

Table **7.6**

Race-Specific Distribution of Children with Minor Malformations Excluding Black Polydactyly and Hypospadias by Birth Order of Child

	Birth Order[1]	No. of Children	Children with Minor Malformations		Relative Risk
			No.	Rate/1,000	
White	1	7,388	64	8.7	1.0*
	2–3	9,430	69	7.3	0.8
	≥4	5,993	75	12.5	1.4
Black	1	6,740	28	4.2	1.0*
	2–3	8,805	59	6.7	1.6
	≥4	8,485	59	7.0	1.7
Puerto Rican	1	1,038	9	8.7	1.0*
	2–3	1,494	9	6.0	0.7
	≥4	909	9	9.9	1.1

*Reference category
[1]Determined by number of prior liveborn and stillborn siblings

Table **7.7**

Distribution of Children with Minor Malformations Excluding Black Polydactyly and Hypospadias by History of Prior Premature Births

No. of Prior Premature Births	No. of Children	Children with Minor Malformations		Relative Risk
		No.	Rate/1,000	
Prior births not premature	26,707[1]	204	7.6	1.0*
1	5,443	39	7.2	0.9
2	1,677	18	10.7	1.4
≥3	901	14	15.5	2.0
No prior liveborn	15,554	106	6.8	0.9

*Reference category
[1]Includes 952 unknowns

Table **7.8**

Distribution of Children with Minor Malformations Excluding Black Polydactyly and Hypospadias by History of Prior Fetal Loss

	No. of Children	Children with Minor Malformations		Relative Risk
		No.	Rate/1,000	
Prior abortion	9,135	92	10.1	1.4
No prior abortion[1]	26,979	197	7.3	1.0*
No prior pregnancy	14,168	92	6.5	0.9
Prior stillbirth	2,837	30	10.6	1.4
No prior stillbirth[2]	32,280	250	7.7	1.0*
No prior pregnancies 20 weeks or over	15,165	101	6.7	0.9

*Reference category
[1]Includes 108 unknowns
[2]Includes 179 unknowns

Table **7.9**

Distribution of Children with Minor Malformations Excluding Black Polydactyly and Hypospadias by History of Prior Neonatal Deaths

Prior Neonatal Deaths	No. of Children	Children with Minor Malformations		Relative Risk
		No.	Rate/1,000	
None/no prior liveborn/unknown	48,108	357	7.4	1.0*
1	1,884	17	9.0	1.2
≥2	290	7	24.1	3.3

*Reference category

Table **7.10**

Distribution of Children with Minor Malformations Excluding Black Polydactyly and Hypospadias by Duration of Pregnancy

Length of Gestation (lunar months)	No. of Children	Children with Minor Malformations		Relative Risk
		No.	Rate/1,000	
5–7	1,341	47	35.0	5.4
8	2,510	35	13.9	2.2
≥9	46,431	299	6.4	1.0*

*Reference category

in offspring of short duration pregnancies (5-7 LM) at a rate nearly six times that in offspring of normal duration (≥ 9 LM) pregnancies (relative risk, 5.4). The rate for offspring of pregnancies lasting 8 lunar months was intermediate between the two (relative risk, 2.2).

Placental Weight (Table 7.11) Decreasing placental weight was associated with a monotonic increase in the rate of minor malformations. For those whose placentae weighed between 200 and 299 gm, the relative risk was 2.3; for those whose

placentae weighed less than 200 gm, the relative risk was 6.4

Various Complications of Pregnancy (Table 7.12) Vaginal bleeding in the second trimester (relative risk, 2.1), hyperemesis gravidarum (1.6), signs of toxemia (from proteinuria to more serious signs) (1.6), incompetent cervix (4.5), hydramnios (5.1), and hemorrhagic shock (7.1) were all associated with higher rates of minor malformations.

Placental Factors (Table 7.13) Those children who had a single umbilical

Table **7.11**

Distribution of Children with Minor Malformations Excluding Black Polydactyly and Hypospadias by Placental Weight

Placental Weight (grams)	No. of Children	Children with Minor Malformations		Relative Risk
		No.	Rate/1,000	
≤199	388	17	43.8	6.4
200–299	2,095	33	15.8	2.3
≥300	41,385	282	6.8	1.0*
Unknown	6,414	49	7.6	1.1

*Reference category

Table **7.12**

Distribution of Children with Minor Malformations Excluding Black Polydactyly and Hypospadias by Various Complications of Pregnancy

	No. of Children	Children with Minor Malformations		Relative Risk*
		No.	Rate/1,000	
Vaginal bleeding in 2nd trimester	2,546	39	15.3	2.1
Hyperemesis gravidarum	540	7	13.0	1.6
Toxemia signs (proteinuria and/or hypertension and/or eclampsia)	2,834	34	12.0	1.6
Incompetent cervix	184	6	32.6	4.5
Hydramnios	694	25	36.0	5.1
Hemorrhagic shock	99	5	50.5	7.1

*For each condition, the reference category consists of those without that condition.

Table *7.13*

Distribution of Children with Minor Malformations Excluding Black Polydactyly and Hypospadias by Placental Factors

	No. of Children	Children with Minor Malformations		Relative Risk*
		No.	Rate/1,000	
Single umbilical artery	341	23	67.4	9.6
Abruptio placentae	1,030	31	30.1	1.8
Marginal sinus rupture	639	9	14.1	1.9
Placenta previa	318	4	12.6	1.8
Placental infarcts ⩾3 cm	1,501	17	11.3	1.5

*For each condition, the reference category consists of those without that condition.

artery had a relative risk of 9.6. Those whose mothers had abruptio placentae, marginal sinus rupture, placenta previa, or large placental infarcts, were also at increased risk of minor malformations. Relative risks for these factors ranged from 1.5 to 1.9.

Weight Change During Pregnancy (Table 7.14) Women who gained weight during their pregnancies had children with higher rates of minor malformations than women whose weight was unchanged (relative risk, 1.4).

Selected Diseases of the Mother (Table 7.15) The presence of endocrine diseases other than diabetes, hypothyroidism, or hyperthyroidism was associated with a lower minor malformation rate (relative risk, 0.5). All of the remaining listed conditions were associated with higher rates. The increased risk was greatest for offspring of mothers with abnormal fibrinogen (relative risk, 10.9, based on three malformed children). For children of mothers with syphilis, urinary tract infection, hematuria, or diabetes, relative risks varied from 1.4 to 3.2.

Environmental Factors

Maternal Cigarette Smoking (Table 7.16) The rate of minor malformations was increased in children whose mothers smoked 15 to 29, or 30 or more cigarettes per day, with relative risks of 1.2 and 1.6, respectively. No association was apparent in children of light smokers.

Exposure to Pelvic or Abdominal X-Rays and to Rubella Infection (Table 7.17) The rates of minor malformations were elevated in children of mothers who had been exposed to pelvic and/or abdominal

Table *7.14*

Distribution of Children with Minor Malformations Excluding Black Polydactyly and Hypospadias by Weight Change During Pregnancy

Weight Change	No. of Children	Children with Minor Malformations		Relative Risk
		No.	Rate/1,000	
Lost/no change	920	5	5.4	1.0*
Gained	49,362	376	7.6	1.4

*Reference category

Table **7.15**

Distribution of Children with Minor Malformations Excluding Black Polydactyly and Hypospadias by Selected Diseases of the Mother During Pregnancy

	No. of Children	Children with Minor Malformations		Relative Risk*
		No.	Rate/1,000	
Endocrine disease other than diabetes, hypothyroidism, or hyperthyroidism	1,537	6	3.9	0.5
Abnormal fibrinogen	40	3	75.0	10.9
Syphilis	918	11	12.0	1.9
Urinary tract infection (fever ≥100.4°F)	709	12	16.9	2.4
Hematuria (≥15 RBC/HPF)	1,059	11	10.4	1.4
Diabetes	336	8	23.8	3.2

*For each disease, the reference category consists of those without that disease.

Table **7.16**

Race-Specific Distribution of Children with Minor Malformations Excluding Black Polydactyly and Hypospadias by Maternal Cigarette Smoking

Cigarette Smoking (no./day)	No. of Children	Children with Minor Malformations		Relative Risk
		No.	Rate/1,000	
Never/Ex/Uncertain	28,597	211	7.4	1.0*
≤14	12,824	87	6.8	0.9
15-29	7,076	62	8.8	1.2
≥30	1,785	21	11.8	1.6

*Reference category

Table **7.17**

Distribution of Children with Minor Malformations Excluding Black Polydactyly and Hypospadias by Exposure to Pelvic and/or Abdominal X-Rays and to Rubella Infection During Pregnancy

	No. of Children	Children with Minor Malformations		Relative Risk*
		No.	Rate/1,000	
Pelvic and/or abdominal X-ray exposure	11,400	111	9.7	1.4
Exposure to rubella infection in 1st or 2nd trimester	1,404	16	11.4	1.5

*For each exposure, the reference category consists of those without that exposure.

Table **7.18**

Distribution of Children with Minor Malformations Excluding Black Polydactyly and Hypospadias by History of Malformation in Mother and Prior Siblings of Child

	No. of Children	Children with Minor Malformations		Relative Risk*
		No.	Rate/1,000	
Congenital malformation in mother	1,225	15	12.2	1.6
Congenital malformation in one or more prior siblings	3,723	48	12.9	1.8

*For each category, the reference category consists of those with a negative family history.

Table **7.19**

Factors Related to the Risk of Minor Malformations Excluding Black Polydactyly and Hypospadias Based upon Multiple Logistic Risk Function Analysis

	Estimated Risk Function Coefficient	Standard Error of Coefficient	Estimated Standardized Relative Risk
Birthweight < 1,500 gm	1.98	0.17	7.3
Single umbilical artery	1.90	0.24	6.7
Hydramnios	1.33	0.23	3.8
White	0.74	0.21	2.1
Puerto Rican	0.69	0.28	2.0
Abruptio placentae	0.66	0.21	1.9
Urinary tract infection (fever ≥ 100.4°F)	0.64	0.31	1.9
Rubella exposure in 1st or 2nd trimester	0.63	0.36	1.9
Syphilis	0.62	0.32	1.9
Abnormal fibrinogen	0.59	0.65	1.8
Hyperemesis gravidarum	0.51	0.39	1.7
Maternal diabetes	0.50	0.39	1.7
Birth order in Blacks ≥ 2	0.49	0.21	1.6
Signs of toxemia (proteinuria and more severe signs)	0.42	0.19	1.5
Congenital malformation in mother	0.42	0.27	1.5
Prior neonatal deaths ≥ 2	0.41	0.41	1.5
Hemorrhagic shock	0.40	0.53	1.5
Congenital malformation in prior siblings	0.35	0.16	1.4
Birth order in Whites/Puerto Ricans ≥ 4	0.30	0.14	1.3
Vaginal bleeding in 2nd trimester	0.27	0.19	1.3
Incompetent cervix	0.16	0.45	1.2
No weight gain	−0.64	0.46	0.5
Endocrine disease other than diabetes, hyperthyroidism, or hypothyroidism	−0.73	0.42	0.5

X-rays during pregnancy (relative risk, 1.4) or to rubella virus during the first or second trimester (relative risk, 1.5).

Genetic Factors

Family History of Malformations (Table 7.18) History of congenital malformation in the mothers or prior siblings of a child was associated with an increase in the minor malformation rate, giving relative risks of 1.6 and 1.8, respectively.

Multivariate Analysis

Based on the foregoing comparisons, 36 risk factors were selected for multivariate analysis, and scaled as binary or ordinal variables. After linear discriminant function analysis, the following 13 factors were eliminated because of low coefficients: low number of antenatal visits, high maternal age, separated marital status, prior abortions, prior stillbirths, prior premature births, short duration of pregnancy, low placental weight, marginal sinus rupture, large placental infarct, hematuria, heavy cigarette smoking, and exposure to X-rays. The results of the multiple logistic regression analysis for the remaining 23 factors are given in Table 7.19.

Factors with relative risks greater than three were birthweight under 1,500 gm (7.3), single umbilical artery (6.7), and hydramnios (3.8); all were statistically significant. There were two factors with relative risks between two and three, both of which were statistically significant: White (2.1) and Puerto Rican (2.0) ethnic groups. Other factors which had statistically significant relative risks included the following: abruptio placentae (1.9), urinary tract infection (1.9), Black with birth order at least 2 (1.6), proteinuria or more severe signs of toxemia

Table 7.20

Distribution of Observed and Expected Numbers of Children with Minor Malformations Excluding Black Polydactyly and Hypospadias by Multiple Logistic Risk Function Scores

Risk Score Percentile[1]	Observed Number of Children with Minor Malformations	Expected Number of Children with Minor Malformations
99–100	67	69.0
97–98	33	26.2
95–96	18	16.7
93–94	9	13.3
91–92	12	11.0
Total (91–100)	139	136.2
81–90	47	45.8
71–80	44	37.1
61–70	29	30.4
51–60	19	27.1
41–50	28	27.1
31–40	25	24.0
21–30	22	21.2
11–20	17	19.7
1–10	11	12.4
Total	381	381.0

[1]Each decile contains 5,025 pregnancies, except the lowest which contains 5,057 pregnancies.

(1.5), congenital malformation in prior siblings (1.4), and White or Puerto Rican, with birth order at least 4 (1.3).

Table 7.20 shows the 381 mother-child pairs according to percentiles of risk score for minor malformations excluding Black polydactyly and hypospadias. Agreement between observed and predicted numbers within each of the strata was quite satisfactory; the ratio of numbers of children with malformations predicted in the highest decile or risk compared to the lowest was greater than ten, indicating adequate separation by the model in terms of risk.

Table 7.21 shows 898 mother-child pairs according to percentiles of risk score for *any* minor malformation. These were derived by using three separate models to calculate three risk scores for each mother-child pair: one for minor malformations exclusive of Black polydactyly and hypospadias, one for Black polydactyly, and one for hypospadias (see Chapters 10 and 13). The three scores were summed to obtain a single score for risk of *any* minor malformation. The agreement between observed and predicted numbers was satisfactory; once again, the ratio of the numbers predicted in the highest decile of risk compared to those predicted in the lowest was 10.

Table **7.21**

Distribution of Observed and Expected Numbers of Children with *Any* Minor Malformations by Multiple Logistic Risk Function Scores

Risk Score Percentile[1]	Observed Number of Children with Minor Malformations	Expected Number of Children with Minor Malformations
99–100	104	107.6
97–98	59	53.5
95–96	52	39.6
93–94	31	33.4
91–92	33	29.7
Total (91–100)	279	263.8
81–90	108	125.7
71–80	110	103.3
61–70	84	89.3
51–60	95	79.2
41–50	55	68.9
31–40	54	59.9
21–30	54	48.6
11–20	33	33.0
1–10	26	26.3
Total	898	898.0

[1]Each decile contains 5,025 pregnancies, except the lowest which contains 5,057 pregnancies.

CHAPTER **8**

Malformations of the Central Nervous System

Among the 50,282 children, there were 266 children with a total of 365 malformations of the central nervous system (CNS) (5.3 per 1,000). The specific defects in this malformation class are shown in Tables 8.1 and 8.2. The former table lists the more common, and the latter, the less common of the CNS malformations. Table 8.1 shows that microcephaly and hydrocephaly were recorded in 77 (29%) and 75 (28%), respectively, of the 266 affected children. Meningomyelocele was about half as common (36 children, 14%), and anencephaly and craniosynostosis each accounted for approximately 1 in 10 affected children. All other central nervous system malformations were rare: of the 16 different defects listed in Table 8.2, none occurred with a rate exceeding 0.4 per 1,000. Although the 16 rare malformations together accounted for 36% of the affected children, no specific defect accounted for more than 7% of the total. All CNS malformations were classified as major, except for miscellaneous malformations of the sinus tract, which occurred in 10 children.

Apart from anencephaly and craniosynostosis (which were less common in Blacks), and hydrocephaly (which was somewhat more common in Puerto Ricans), there were no striking differences in individual CNS malformation rates among the three ethnic groups (Table 8.1). However, overall, CNS malformations were most common in Puerto

Table **8.1**

Central Nervous System Malformation Rates Classified by Ethnic Group (Rates per Thousand)

Malformation	White (n=22,811)		Black (n=24,030)		Puerto Rican (n=3,441)		Total (n=50,282)	
	No.	Rate	No.	Rate	No.	Rate	No.	Rate
Microcephaly	32	1.40	41	1.71	4	1.16	77	1.53
Hydrocephaly	33	1.45	33	1.37	9	2.62	75	1.49
Meningomyelocele	16	0.70	16	0.67	4	1.16	36	0.72
Anencephaly	19	0.83	4	0.17	3	0.87	26	0.52
Craniosynostosis	15	0.66	6	0.25	5	1.45	26	0.52
Other central nervous system malformations[1]	52	2.28	36	1.50	8	2.32	96	1.91
Any central nervous system malformation	131	5.74	109	4.54	26	7.56	266	5.29

[1]See Table 8.2 for details of this category.

Table **8.2**

Rare Central Nervous System Malformation Rates Classified by Ethnic Group (Rates per Thousand)

Malformation	White (n=22,811)		Black (n=24,030)		Puerto Rican (n=3,441)		Total (n=50,282)	
	No.	Rate	No.	Rate	No.	Rate	No.	Rate
Macrocephaly	12	0.53	5	0.21	1	0.29	18	0.36
Partial hypoplasia of brain	5	0.22	6	0.25	0	—	11	0.22
Hypoplasia/atrophy of brain	5	0.22	5	0.21	0	—	10	0.20
Miscellaneous sinus tract defects	5	0.22	4	0.17	1	0.29	10	0.20
Spina bifida with meningo-myelocele	5	0.22	2	0.08	2	0.58	9	0.18
Miscellaneous brain abnormalities	5	0.22	2	0.08	1	0.29	8	0.16
Rachischisis/cranioschisis	6	0.26	1	0.04	1	0.29	8	0.16
Arnold Chiari/Dandy Walker	3	0.13	4	0.17	1	0.29	8	0.16
Atrophy/hypoplasia optic nerve	4	0.18	3	0.13	0	—	7	0.14
Anomalies of pituitary	4	0.18	3	0.13	0	—	7	0.14
Spina bifida without central nervous system involvement	5	0.22	2	0.08	0	—	7	0.14
Absence olfactory nerve/arhinencephaly	4	0.18	2	0.08	0	—	6	0.12
Encephalocele	2	0.09	3	0.13	0	—	5	0.10
Absent corpus callosum	2	0.09	2	0.08	0	—	4	0.08
Porencephaly/hydrancephaly	0	—	4	0.17	0	—	4	0.08
Malformed medulla	1	0.04	1	0.04	1	0.29	3	0.06

Ricans (7.6 per 1,000), least common in Blacks (4.5 per 1,000), and intermediate in Whites (5.7 per 1,000).

Of the 266 malformed children, 241 had anomalies which affected the brain (91%); cranio-spinal fusion defects were present in 69 (26%); spinal malformations were present in 58 (22%); and cranial nerve anomalies were detected in 10 (4%).

Certain patterns of joint occurrence of malformations within the CNS were apparent: 31 of 75 children with hydrocephaly (41%), 26 of 36 children with meningomyelocele (72%), and 14 of 26 children with anencephaly (54%) had multiple CNS malformations. By contrast, although microcephaly was the most common CNS malformation, affecting 77 children, only 9 children had other CNS malformations as well (12%). The most common associations were between hydrocephaly and spinal fusion defects, and between anencephaly and spinal fusion defects: 22 of the 31 hydrocephalic children had meningomyelocele (71%), in five instances, together with spina bifida; and meningomyelocele or spina bifida occurred in 5 of the 14 children with anencephaly (36%). Other less frequent associations occurred between hydrocephaly and obstructive lesions in the fourth ventricle (5/31:16%, Arnold-Chiari or Dandy-Walker anomalies) and between anencephaly and rachischisis or cranioschisis (5/14:36%).

Table 8.3 provides data on the joint occurrence of malformations in other classes with CNS malformations that occurred in at least 20 children. Of the 266 children with CNS malformations, 36.5% had malformations affecting other systems. For the more common CNS malformation categories, the lowest proportion of malformations occurring elsewhere was in 26 children with craniosynostosis (23.1%). However, the outstanding association was found with anencephaly: fully 21 out of 26 affected children had associated syndromes (81%). In 20, the specific defect was

Table **8.3**

Joint Occurrence of Malformations in Classes Other Than the Central Nervous System (CNS) in Children with Common CNS Malformations

	No. of Children	Cardio-vascular		Musculo-skeletal		Respi-ratory		Gastro-intestinal		Genito-urinary		Eyes/Ears		Syndromes		Tumors		Any Non-CNS Malfor-mation	
		No.	%	No.	%	No.	%	No.	%	No.	%	No.	%	No.	%	No.	%	No.	%
Microcephaly	77	4	5.2	8	10.4	5	6.5	6	7.8	3	3.9	5	6.5	9	11.7	0	—	24	31.2
Hydrocephaly	75	6	8.0	9	12.0	8	10.7	2	2.7	8	10.7	2	2.7	3	4.0	5	6.7	26	34.7
Meningomyelocele	36	3	8.3	9	25.0	8	22.2	6	16.7	9	25.0	0	—	2	5.6	0	—	17	47.2
Anencephaly	26	3	11.5	2	7.7	11	42.3	4	15.4	6	23.1	1	3.8	21	80.8	0	—	22	84.6
Craniosynostosis	26	2	7.7	1	3.8	1	3.8	0	—	1	3.8	1	3.8	2	7.7	1	3.8	6	23.1
Other central nervous system malformations	96	12	12.5	14	14.6	19	19.8	17	17.7	19	19.8	4	4.2	14	14.6	3	3.1	43	44.8
Any central nervous system malformation	266	22	8.3	28	10.5	30	11.3	25	9.4	28	10.5	10	3.8	37	13.9	7	2.6	97	36.5

absence or hypoplasia of the adrenal gland (together with absence of the thyroid gland in one case). Respiratory malformations were also prominent in anencephalic children (42%): among 11 affected children, the specific defect was hypoplasia or agenesis of the lung in five. Apart from anencephaly, the proportion was also rather high in 36 children who had meningomyelocele (47.2%) while the proportions for the remaining common CNS defects were all close to the overall proportion of 36.5%.

Risk Factors for
CNS Malformations

Administrative Data

Duration of Pregnancy at Registration (Table 8.4) The relative risks for CNS malformations, given registration before the third or after the eighth lunar month of pregnancy, were 1.4 and 1.2, respectively.

Number of Antenatal Visits (Table 8.5) The relative risk for mothers who attended for antenatal care fewer than five times during their pregnancies was 2.1. The relative risk was also modestly increased for mothers who attended more than nine times (1.2).

Personal Characteristics of the Mother

Maternal Age at Registration (Table 8.6) For ages up to 39 years, the CNS malformations rates were relatively stable. Among mothers aged 40 years or more, the relative risk was 1.7.

Socioeconomic Status (Table 8.7) Only in Puerto Ricans was there a suggestion

Table *8.4*

Distribution of Children with Central Nervous System (CNS) Malformations by Duration of Pregnancy at Registration

Duration of Pregnancy at Registration (lunar months)	No. of Children	Children with CNS Malformations		Relative Risk
		No.	Rate/1,000	
1-2	1,091	8	7.3	1.4
3-8	41,956	215	5.1	1.0*
≥9	7,235	43	5.9	1.2

*Reference category

Table *8.5*

Distribution of Children with Central Nervous System (CNS) Malformations by Number of Antenatal Visits

No. of Antenatal Visits	No. of Children	Children with CNS Malformations		Relative Risk
		No.	Rate/1,000	
1–4	8,624	76	8.8	2.1
5–9	20,964	88	4.2	1.0*
≥10	20,694	102	4.9	1.2

*Reference category

Table **8.6**

Distribution of Children with Central Nervous System (CNS) Malformations by Mother's Age at Registration

Mother's Age	No. of Children	Children with CNS Malformations		Relative Risk
		No.	Rate/1,000	
≤14	429	2	4.7	0.9
15–19	11,475	57	5.0	0.9
20–24	18,475	97	5.3	1.0*
25–29	10,592	53	5.0	0.9
30–34	5,655	40	7.1	1.3
35–39	2,884	10	3.5	0.7
≥40	772	7	9.1	1.7

*Reference category

Table **8.7**

Race-Specific Distribution of Children with Central Nervous System (CNS) Malformations by Socioeconomic Status (SES)

	SES (Scale of 0–10)	No. of Children	Children with CNS Malformations		Relative Risk
			No.	Rate/1,000	
White	≤3.9	5,042	24	4.8	0.8
	≥4.0	17,304	102	5.9	1.0*
	Unknown	465	5	10.8	1.8
Black	≤3.9	12,718	61	4.8	1.1
	≥4.0	10,957	46	4.2	1.0*
	Unknown	355	2	5.6	1.3
Puerto Rican	≤3.9	1,860	17	9.1	1.6
	≥4.0	1,546	9	5.8	1.0*
	Unknown	35	0	—	—

*Reference category

of a relationship between low socio-economic status and CNS malformations (relative risk, 1.6). Unknown socioeconomic status in Whites and Blacks was associated with elevated relative risks (1.8 and 1.3, respectively). However, these findings were based on small numbers.

Characteristics and Survival of the Offspring

Birthweight (Table 8.8) Decreasing birthweight in all three ethnic groups showed a striking monotonic relationship to the CNS malformation rate. The relative risks ranged from 6.5 to 12.0 for children weighing less than 2 kg, and

97

Table 8.8

Race-Specific Distribution of Children with Central Nervous System (CNS) Malformations by Child's Birthweight

	Birthweight (grams)	No. of Children	Children with CNS Malformations		Relative Risk
			No.	Rate/1,000	
White	≤1,999	645	27	41.9	12.0
	2,000–2,999	5,664	47	8.3	2.4
	≥3,000	16,502	57	3.5	1.0*
Black	≤1,999	1,208	22	18.2	6.5
	2,000–2,999	9,283	49	5.3	1.9
	≥3,000	13,539	38	2.8	1.0*
Puerto Rican	≤1,999	123	6	48.8	10.6
	2,000–2,999	1,156	10	8.7	1.9
	≥3,000	2,162	10	4.6	1.0*

*Reference category

from 1.9 to 2.4 for those weighing 2 to 2.9 kg.

Sex of the Child (Table 8.9) The race-specific CNS malformation rates in male and female children were similar.

Birth Order (Table 8.10) The relative risk among children whose birth order was fourth or higher was 1.4.

Survival of the Child (Table 8.11) CNS malformations were frequently lethal. Fully 14% of the affected children were stillborn; 12% died during the neonatal period; and 21% died thereafter; only half of the children survived the early years of life. The relative risks varied among the three ethnic groups: for stillbirth, the

Table 8.9

Race-Specific Distribution of Children with Central Nervous System (CNS) Malformations by Sex of Child

		No. of Children	Children with CNS Malformations		Relative Risk
			No.	Rate/1,000	
White	Male	11,763	65	5.5	1.0*
	Female	11,048	66	6.0	1.1
Black	Male	12,038	53	4.4	1.0*
	Female	11,992	56	4.7	1.1
Puerto Rican	Male	1,741	15	8.6	1.0*
	Female	1,700	11	6.5	0.8

*Reference category

Table **8.10**

Distribution of Children with Central Nervous System (CNS) Malformations by Birth Order of Child

| Birth Order[1] | No. of Children | Children with CNS Malformations | | Relative Risk |
		No.	Rate/1,000	
1–3	34,895	164	4.7	1.0*
≥4	15,387	102	6.6	1.4

*Reference category
[1]Determined by number of prior liveborn and stillborn siblings

Table **8.11**

Race-Specific Distribution of Children with Central Nervous System (CNS) Malformations by Survival of the Child

| | Survival of Child | No. of Children | Children with CNS Malformations | | Relative Risk |
			No.	Rate/1,000	
White	Stillbirth	327	21	64.2	19.5
	Neonatal death	302	18	59.6	18.1
	Infant death	130	9	69.2	21.0
	Childhood death	91	10	109.9	33.3
	Survived	21,961	73	3.3	1.0*
Black	Stillbirth	407	14	34.4	13.8
	Neonatal death	450	10	22.2	8.9
	Infant death	229	13	56.8	22.7
	Childhood death	134	14	104.5	41.8
	Survived	22,810	58	2.5	1.0*
Puerto Rican	Stillbirth	64	2	31.3	10.4
	Neonatal death	54	4	74.1	24.7
	Infant death	25	5	200.0	66.7
	Childhood death	14	5	357.1	119.0
	Survived	3,284	10	3.0	1.0*

*Reference category

range was 10.4 to 19.5; for neonatal death, 8.9 to 24.7; for infant death, 21.0 to 66.7; and for childhood death, 33.3 to 119.0.

Autopsy Report (Table 8.12) In contrast to many other malformations, the relative risk for CNS malformations was somewhat lower among children who were autopsied (0.7).

Reproductive History of the Mother

Prior Premature Births (Table 8.13) The relative risk for CNS malformations among mothers who had previously given birth to one or more premature children was 1.6.

Prior Fetal or Neonatal Loss (Table 8.14) There was no evidence that prior

Table *8.12*

Distribution of Dead Children with Central Nervous System (CNS) Malformations by Presence of Autopsy Report

Autopsy Report	No. of Children	Dead Children with CNS Malformations		Relative Risk
		No.	Rate/1,000	
Present	1,810	93	51	0.7
Absent	418	32	77	1.0*

*Reference category

Table *8.13*

Distribution of Children with Nervous System (CNS) Malformations by History of Prior Premature Births

	No. of Children	Children with CNS Malformations		Relative Risk
		No.	Rate/1,000	
Prior premature births	8,021	61	7.6	1.6
Prior births not premature	26,707[1]	131	4.9	1.0*
No prior liveborn	15,554	74	4.8	1.0

*Reference category
[1]Includes 952 unknowns

abortion or prior stillbirth increased the risk of CNS malformations. For prior neonatal death, however, the relative risk was 1.6.

Characteristics and Complications of the Pregnancy

Duration of Pregnancy (Table 8.15) The race-specific CNS malformation rates according to the duration of pregnancy are shown. For each ethnic group, the rates were considerably increased for pregnancies lasting less than eight lunar months (relative risks, 4.8 to 6.9); and the rates decreased monotonically as the duration of pregnancy approached nine or more lunar months.

Placental Weight (Table 8.16) There was a monotonic relationship between decreasing placental weight and CNS malformation rates. The relative risks for children with placentae weighing less than 300 gm and 300 to 499 gm were, respectively, 6.0 and 1.9. The relative risk was also increased (1.8) in children whose placental weight was unknown.

Single Umbilical Artery (Table 8.17) The relative risk for CNS malformations in children with single umbilical artery was 8.2.

Signs of Toxemia (Table 8.18) The data suggest that mild manifestations of the toxemia syndrome (edema or proteinuria without hypertension) were not related to CNS defects. For two of the three categories which include hypertension, the relative risks were 2.2 and 2.6.

Vaginal Bleeding (Table 8.19) The

Table 8.14

Distribution of Children with Central Nervous System (CNS) Malformations by History of Prior Fetal or Neonatal Loss

	No. of Children	Children with CNS Malformations		Relative Risk
		No.	Rate/1,000	
Prior abortion	9,135	49	5.4	0.9
No prior abortion[1]	26,979	153	5.7	1.0*
No prior pregnancy	14,168	64	4.5	0.8
Prior stillbirth	2,837	18	6.3	1.1
No prior stillbirth[2]	32,280	178	5.5	1.0*
No prior pregnancies 20 weeks or over	15,165	70	4.6	0.8
Prior neonatal death	2,174	18	8.3	1.6
No prior neonatal death[3]	32,554	174	5.3	1.0*
No prior liveborn	15,554	74	4.8	0.9

*Reference category
[1]Includes 108 unknowns
[2]Includes 179 unknowns
[3]Includes 947 unknowns

Table 8.15

Race-Specific Distribution of Children with Central Nervous System (CNS) Malformations by Duration of Pregnancy

	Length of Gestation (Lunar months)	No. of Children	Children with CNS Malformation		Relative Risk
			No.	Rate/1,000	
White	5–7	375	13	34.7	6.9
	8	699	10	14.3	2.9
	≥9	21,737	108	5.0	1.0*
Black	5–7	885	16	18.1	4.8
	8	1,616	12	7.4	1.9
	≥9	21,529	81	3.8	1.0*
Puerto Rican	5–7	81	3	37.0	5.6
	8	195	2	10.3	1.6
	≥9	3,165	21	6.6	1.0*

*Reference category

Table 8.16

Distribution of Children with Central Nervous System (CNS) Malformations by Placental Weight

Placental Weight (grams)	No. of Children	Children with CNS Malformations		Relative Risk
		No.	Rate/1,000	
≤299	2,483	42	16.9	6.0
300–499	30,964	163	5.3	1.9
≥500	10,421	29	2.8	1.0*
Unknown	6,414	32	5.0	1.8

*Reference category

Table 8.17

Distribution of Children with Central Nervous System (CNS) Malformations by Number of Umbilical Arteries

No. of Umbilical Arteries	No. of Children	Children with CNS Malformations		Relative Risk
		No.	Rate/1,000	
One	341	14	41.1	8.2
Two	44,851	224	5.0	1.0*
Unknown	5,090	28	5.5	1.1

*Reference category

Table 8.18

Distribution of Children with Central Nervous System (CNS) Malformations by Signs of Toxemia[1]

	No. of Children	Children with CNS Malformations		Relative Risk
		No.	Rate/1,000	
Eclampsia	22	0	—	—
Chronic hypertension	669	8	12.0	2.2
Acute hypertension (BP ≥ 160/110 after LM 6)	930	13	14.0	2.6
Proteinuria	1,213	7	5.8	1.1
Generalized edema	11,425	45	3.9	0.7
None	36,023	193	5.4	1.0*

*Reference category
[1]This classification is hierarchical and based on severity—for example, a pregnancy complicated by chronic hypertension is classified as such, even though proteinuria and edema may also be present.

Table **8.19**

Distribution of Children with Central Nervous System (CNS) Malformations According to Vaginal Bleeding During Pregnancy

| Vaginal Bleeding | No. of Children | Children with CNS Malformations | | Relative Risk |
		No.	Rate/1,000	
1st trimester	3,668	17	4.6	0.9
2nd trimester	2,546	18	7.0	1.3
3rd trimester	6,980	37	5.3	1.0
None	37,088	194	5.2	1.0*

*Reference category

relative risk for CNS malformations among mothers who bled during the second trimester was 1.3. Bleeding at other times during pregnancy did not appear to be related to this outcome.

Other Complications of Pregnancy (Table 8.20) In pregnancies complicated by hyperemesis gravidarum, the relative risk was 2.1. Vomiting during pregnancy was not related to central nervous malformations. For pregnancies complicated by hydramnios, the relative risk was 9.0. Hydramnios was thus a strong risk factor for central nervous malformations. The relative risks for hemorrhagic shock and vena cava syndrome were 5.8 and 2.6, respectively. These estimates were based on small numbers.

Placental Factors (Table 8.21) Apart

from marginal sinus rupture, all conditions listed in the table were associated with a higher risk of having a child with a CNS malformation. The relative risks for abruptio placentae, placenta previa, and large placental infarct were 2.7, 2.4, and 1.4, respectively.

Weight Change During Pregnancy (Table 8.22) The table gives the race-specific CNS malformation rates according to four categories of weight change. Among White and Black mothers, there was a relationship between low weight gain and the CNS malformation rate; this was not evident in Puerto Ricans. For White and Black children born to mothers whose weight gain during pregnancy was less than 7.5 kg, the relative risks were, with one exception, at least 1.5. The relative

Table **8.20**

Distribution of Children with Central Nervous System (CNS) Malformations by Various Complications of Pregnancy

| | No. of Children | Children with CNS Malformations | | Relative Risk* |
		No.	Rate/1,000	
Hyperemesis gravidarum	540	6	11.1	2.1
Hydramnios	694	30	43.2	9.0
Hemorrhagic shock	99	3	30.0	5.8
Vena cava syndrome	144	2	13.9	2.6

*For each condition, the reference category consists of those without that condition.

Table **8.21**

Distribution of Children with Central Nervous System (CNS) Malformations According to Placental Factors

	No. of Children	Children with CNS Malformations		Relative Risk*
		No.	Rate/1,000	
Marginal sinus rupture	639	3	4.7	0.9
Abruptio placentae	1,030	14	13.6	2.7
Placenta previa	317	4	12.6	2.4
Placental infarct ≥3 cm diameter	1,501	11	7.3	1.4

*For each condition, the reference category consists of those without that condition.

Table **8.22**

Distribution of Children with Central Nervous System (CNS) Malformations by Weight Change During Pregnancy

	Weight Change (kg)	No. of Children	Children with CNS Malformations		Relative Risk
			No.	Rate/1,000	
White	Lost/no change	305	5	16.4	3.3
	Gained ≤7.4	4,707	36	7.6	1.5
	Gained ≥7.5	17,124	86	5.0	1.0*
	Unknown	675	4	5.9	1.2
Black	Lost/no change	509	0	—	—
	Gained ≤7.4	6,334	37	5.8	1.5
	Gained ≥7.5	16,298	63	3.9	1.0*
	Unknown	889	9	10.1	2.6
Puerto Rican	Lost/no change	106	0	—	—
	Gained ≤7.4	933	6	6.4	0.9
	Gained ≥7.5	2,099	15	7.1	1.0*
	Unknown	303	5	16.5	2.3

*Reference category

risk was also elevated in all three races (1.2 to 2.6) when the amount of weight change was unknown.

Diabetes Mellitus (Table 8.23) Among mothers who had diabetes for at least five years, the relative risk was 9.8. No children with CNS malformations were born to mothers with diabetes of shorter duration.

Other Diseases of the Mother (Table 8.24) The relative risk for hyperthyroidism, based on a numerator of only two children, was 4.4. Among children born to mothers in whom some disturbance of endocrine function other than diabetes, hypothyroidism, or hyperthyroidism was recorded, the relative risk was 1.6. The relative risks among chil-

Table **8.23**

Distribution of Children with Central Nervous System (CNS) Malformations by Maternal Diabetes Mellitus

| | No. of Children | Children with CNS Malformations | | Relative Risk |
		No.	Rate/1,000	
Treated diabetes ≥5 years	98	5	51.0	9.8
Treated diabetes <5 years	96	0	—	—
Untreated diabetes or keto-acidosis	142	0	—	—
No diabetes	49,946	261	5.2	1.0*

*Reference category

Table **8.24**

Distribution of Children with Central Nervous System (CNS) Malformations by Selected Diseases of the Mother During Pregnancy

| | No. of Children | Children with CNS Malformations | | Relative Risk* |
		No.	Rate/1,000	
Hyperthyroidism	87	2	23.0	4.4
Endocrine disease other than diabetes, hypothyroidism, or hyperthyroidism	1,537	13	8.5	1.6
Urinary tract infection (fever ≥100.4°F)	709	7	9.9	1.9
Hematuria (≥15 RBC/HPF)	1,059	9	8.5	1.6
Convulsive disorder	294	6	20.4	3.9

*For each disease, the reference category consists of those without that disease

dren whose mothers had a urinary tract infection, hematuria, or epilepsy were 1.9, 1.6, and 3.9, respectively.

Environmental Factors

Cigarette Smoking (Table 8.25) Among women who smoked 15 to 29 cigarettes per day, and 30 or more cigarettes per day, the relative risks were 1.5 and 1.3, respectively. The CNS malformation rates were not increased in the offspring of light smokers or non-smokers.

Pelvic or Abdominal X-Ray Exposure During Pregnancy (Table 8.26) There was virtually no evidence of exposure to pelvic or abdominal X-rays being related to the risk of CNS malformations (relative risk, 1.1).

Genetic Factors

Family History of Malformations (Table 8.27) Malformations in either of the parents showed no evidence of association with CNS malformations. For children with prior siblings who had malformations affecting the head or spine,

105

Table **8.25**

Distribution of Children with Central Nervous System (CNS) Malformations by Maternal Cigarette Smoking

Cigarette Smoking (no./day)	No. of Children	Children with CNS Malformations		Relative Risk
		No.	Rate/1,000	
Never/Ex/Uncertain	28,597	147	5.1	1.0*
≤14	12,824	51	4.0	0.8
15–29	7,076	56	7.9	1.5
≥30	1,785	12	6.7	1.3

*Reference category

Table **8.26**

Distribution of Children with Central Nervous System (CNS) Malformations by Pelvic and/or Abdominal X-Ray Exposure During Pregnancy

Pelvic and/or Abdominal X-Ray Exposure	No. of Children	Children with CNS Malformations		Relative Risk
		No.	Rate/1,000	
Present	11,400	63	5.5	1.1
Absent	38,882	203	5.2	1.0*

*Reference category

Table **8.27**

Distribution of Children with Central Nervous System (CNS) Malformations by History of Selected Malformations in Prior Siblings

	No. of Children	Children with CNS Malformations		Relative Risk
		No.	Rate/1,000	
Prior siblings with malformations of the head or spine	466	7	15.0	2.7
Prior siblings with miscellaneous malformations[1]	1,301	14	10.8	1.9
Prior siblings not malformed	30,613	170	5.6	1.0*
No prior liveborn	15,166	70	4.6	0.8

*Reference category
[1]Excludes siblings with cleft palate, clubfoot, deformities of the fingers or toes, or congenital heart disease

the relative risk was 2.7. On the other hand, a history of prior siblings with cleft palate, clubfoot, deformities of the fingers or toes, or congenital heart disease was not associated with an increased risk of CNS malformations. For those children whose siblings had miscellaneous malformations other than those listed, the relative risk was 1.9.

Multivariate Analysis

Based on the foregoing comparisons, a total of 22 risk factors were selected for multivariate analysis and scaled as binary or ordinal variables; after linear discriminant function analysis, this number was reduced to 18. The four factors eliminated because of low coefficients were prior neonatal death, short duration of pregnancy, abruptio placentae, and large

placental infarct. The results of the multiple logistic regression analysis for the 18 factors that were retained are given in Table 8.28.

Factors with a relative risk greater than 3 included hydramnios (8.5), single umbilical artery (4.9), and convulsive disorder (3.5); all were statistically significant. Factors with a relative risk between 2 and 3 were Puerto Rican ethnic group (2.2), birthweight under 2,000 gm (2.2), head and/or spine malformations in siblings (2.1), hyperemesis gravidarum (2.1), and chronic hypertension and/or eclampsia (2.0). Only the result for hyperemesis was not statistically significant. Only three of the remaining risk factors were statistically significant: fewer than five antenatal visits (1.5), White ethnic group (1.5), and placental weight under 300 gm (1.2).

Table **8.28**

Factors Related to the Risk of Malformations of the Central Nervous System (CNS) Based Upon Multiple Logistic Risk Function Analysis

	Estimated Risk Function Coefficient	Standard Error of Coefficient	Estimated Standardized Relative Risk
Hydramnios	2.14	0.21	8.5
Single umbilical artery	1.59	0.30	4.9
Convulsive disorder	1.25	0.43	3.5
Puerto Rican ethnic group	0.77	0.22	2.2
Birth weight < 2,000 gm	0.77	0.11	2.2
Head and/or spine malformations in siblings	0.75	0.40	2.1
Hyperemesis gravidarum	0.73	0.42	2.1
Chronic hypertension and/or eclampsia	0.70	0.24	2.0
Treated maternal diabetes, duration ≥ 5 years	0.59	0.53	1.8
Miscellaneous malformations in prior siblings[1]	0.48	0.29	1.6
Urinary tract infection and/or hematuria during pregnancy	0.47	0.27	1.6
Less than five antenatal visits	0.43	0.14	1.5
White ethnic group	0.38	0.14	1.5
Endocrine disorder other than hypothyroidism or diabetes	0.37	0.29	1.4
Hemorrhagic shock during pregnancy	0.28	0.69	1.3
Cigarette smoking in excess of 15 per day during pregnancy	0.27	0.15	1.3
Birth order ≥ 4	0.24	0.13	1.3
Placental weight ≤ 300 gm	0.19	0.08	1.2

[1]Malformations other than cleft lip and/or palate, clubfoot, malformations of fingers and/or toes, malformations of the heart, malformations of the head and/or spine

Table **8.29**

Distribution of Observed and Expected Numbers of Children with Central Nervous System (CNS) Malformations by Multiple Logistic Risk Function Scores

Risk Score Percentile[1]	Observed Number of Children with CNS Malformations	Expected Number of Children with CNS Malformations
99–100	51	50.5
97–98	22	19.6
95–96	13	14.7
93–94	15	11.9
91–92	5	10.1
Subtotal (91–100)	106	106.8
81–90	35	38.0
71–80	28	27.6
61–70	24	21.4
51–60	16	17.6
41–50	14	14.8
31–40	13	12.4
21–30	9	10.9
11–20	9	9.2
1–10	12	7.3
Total	266	266.0

[1]Each decile contains 5,025 pregnancies, except the lowest which contains 5,057 pregnancies.

As seen in Table 8.29, stratification of the 266 children with CNS malformations showed good agreement between observed and expected numbers of malformations. In addition, the ratio of the numbers of children in the top decile of risk to the numbers in the lowest decile is over 8. This indicates that the model is satisfactory in discriminating between degrees of risk.

CHAPTER **9**

Malformations of the Cardiovascular System

A full description of the cardiovascular anomalies in this cohort and their determinants has been published elsewhere.[1] As pointed out in Chapter 2, cardiovascular malformations were ascertained using methods somewhat different from those used to identify other malformations, the net effect of which was to insure more complete and accurate results. Classification of cardiovascular anomalies also presents a problem because of their complexity. Therefore, the presentation in this chapter differs somewhat in its format from that of other chapters.

Among the 50,282 children, 404 had cardiovascular malformations (8.0 per 1,000). The array of anomalies that together constituted this group was large and markedly heterogeneous. In addition, 26% of cardiovascular malformations were multiple. Table 9.1 gives a broad classification based on embryological considerations. Isolated ventricular septal defect, considered together with isolated single ventricle (one case), was the most common malformation, occurring in 110 children (27.2%). Defects of the conus arteriosus (principally transposition of the great arteries and Fallot's tetralogy) were found in 44 children (10.9%); endocardial cushion defects and isolated secundum atrial septal defects occurred in 34 (8.4%) and 28 children (6.9%), respectively.

Table 9.2 lists certain common isolated cardiovascular lesions, as well as

Table **9.1**

Major Developmental Defects of the Cardiovascular System in 50,282 Children

	No. of Children	Rate/1,000
Isolated ventricular septal defect and single ventricle	110	2.19
Conus arteriosus syndrome[1]	44	0.87
Endocardial cushion defect[2]	34	0.68
Isolated atrial septal defect (secundum)	28	0.56
Hypoplastic left heart syndrome[3]	24	0.48
Other defects	164	3.26
Total	404	8.04

[1]Tetralogy of Fallot, Eisenmenger, transposition of great arteries, truncus arteriosus, double outlet right ventricle
[2]Atrial septal defect (primum), atrioventricular canal, cleft mitral valve
[3]Aortic and mitral valve atresia, hypoplastic left heart

Table **9.2**

Cardiovascular System Malformations Classified by Ethnic Group (Rates per Thousand)

	White (n=22,811)		Black (n=24,030)		Puerto Rican (n=3,441)		Total (n=50,282)	
	No.	Rate	No.	Rate	No.	Rate	No.	Rate
Ventricular septal defect[1]	48	2.10	52	2.16	9	2.62	109	2.17
Atrial septal defect[1]	17	0.74	16	0.67	4	1.16	37	0.73
Pulmonic stenosis[1]	15	0.66	17	0.71	2	0.58	34	0.68
Patent ductus arteriosus[1]	8	0.35	18	0.75	3	0.87	29	0.58
Coarctation of aorta[1]	10	0.44	9	0.37	0	—	19	0.38
Tetralogy of Fallot[1]	9	0.39	3	0.12	1	0.29	13	0.26
Ventricular septal defect and pulmonic stenosis[1]	2	0.09	7	0.29	1	0.29	10	0.20
Atrioventricular canal[1]	9	0.39	2	0.08	1	0.29	12	0.24
Aortic and mitral valve atresia[1]	4	0.18	7	0.29	1	0.29	12	0.24
Aortic stenosis[1]	6	0.26	5	0.21	0	—	11	0.22
Endocardial fibroelastosis[1]	3	0.13	7	0.29	1	0.29	11	0.22
Other isolated cardiovascular malformations[2]	26	1.14	12	0.50	0	—	38	0.76
Other multiple cardiovascular malformations[3]	40	1.75	25	1.04	4	1.16	69	1.37
Any cardiovascular malformation	197	8.64	180	7.49	27	7.85	404	8.03

[1]No other cardiovascular anomalies
[2]See Table 9.3
[3]See text

combinations, by ethnic group. Apart from more common syndromes, such as tetralogy, ventricular septal defect and pulmonary stenosis, atrioventricular canal, and atresia of the aortic and mitral valve, a heterogeneous group of multiple cardiovascular malformations affected 69 children (17.1%). It is worth noting that

110

there were only 13 children with tetralogy of Fallot without other cardiovascular anomalies (3.2% of the 404 children). Since this lesion can be surgically corrected, it usually accounts for a considerably greater proportion of cardiac malformations when cases of congenital heart disease are referred to cardiac centers. Table 9.3 lists numerous rare, isolated cardiovascular lesions, none occurring in more than four children.

All cardiovascular malformations were classified as major, except for those judged to be of minor severity: hypoplasia cordis (occurring in 19 children), left vena cava (7), anomalous right subclavian artery (5), Wolff-Parkinson-White syn-

drome (3), hypoplasia pulmonary artery (2), and certain rare single malformations (6).

Overall, cardiovascular malformation rates were similar among the three ethnic groups, being 8.6, 7.5, and 7.9 per 1,000 in Whites, Blacks, and Puerto Ricans respectively (Table 9.2).

Table 9.4 provides data on the joint occurrence of malformations in other classes with cardiovascular malformations classified on an embryological basis. Of the 404 children with cardiovascular malformations, 28.7% had malformations affecting other systems. It is particularly noteworthy that 71% of children with endocardial cushion defect had

Table **9.3**

Rare Isolated Cardiovascular System Malformations Classified by Ethnic Group (Rates per Thousand)

	White (n=22,811)		Black (n=24,030)		Total (n=50,282)[1]	
	No.	**Rate**	**No.**	**Rate**	**No.**	**Rate**
Right subclavian artery	3	0.13	1	0.04	4	0.08
Vascular ring	1	0.04	2	0.08	3	0.06
Anomalous coronary artery	2	0.09	1	0.04	3	0.06
Wolff-Parkinson-White syndrome	3	0.13	0	—	3	0.06
Mitral insufficiency	1	0.04	1	0.04	2	0.04
Truncus arteriosus	2	0.09	0	—	2	0.04
Double outlet right ventricle	0	—	2	0.08	2	0.04
Endomyocardial fibrosis	1	0.04	1	0.04	2	0.04
Aortic insufficiency	2	0.09	0	—	2	0.04
Absent mitral valve	1	0.04	0	—	1	0.02
Ebstein's anomaly	1	0.04	0	—	1	0.02
Tricuspid valve atresia	0	—	1	0.04	1	0.02
Pulmonary atresia	1	0.04	0	—	1	0.02
Hypoplastic pulmonary artery	0	—	1	0.04	1	0.02
Single pulmonary artery and vein	1	0.04	0	—	1	0.02
Absent pulmonary vein	1	0.04	0	—	1	0.02
Transposition of great arteries	1	0.04	0	—	1	0.02
Single ventricle	1	0.04	0	—	1	0.02
Hypoplastic heart	0	—	1	0.04	1	0.02
Hypoplastic left atrium	1	0.04	0	—	1	0.02
Anomalous renal artery and vein	1	0.04	0	—	1	0.02
Anomalous origin of renal artery	0	—	1	0.04	1	0.02
Vena azygos	1	0.04	0	—	1	0.02
Stenosis ductus venosus	1	0.04	0	—	1	0.02
Total	26	1.14	12	0.50	38	0.76

[1]None of these anomalies occurred in 3,441 Puerto Ricans

Table 9.4

Joint Occurrence of Malformations in Classes Other Than the Cardiovascular System (CVS) in Children with Common CVS Malformations

	No. of Children	Central Nervous		Musculo-skeletal		Respiratory		Gastro-intestinal		Genito-urinary		Eye/Ear		Syndromes		Tumors		Any Non-CVS Malformation	
		No.	%	No.	%	No.	%	No.	%	No.	%	No.	%	No.	%	No.	%	No.	%
Isolated ventricular septal defect and single ventricle	110	3	2.7	5	4.5	3	2.7	3	2.7	0	0.0	1	0.9	7	6.4	1	0.9	17	15.4
Conus arteriosus syndrome	44	4	9.1	2	4.5	5	11.4	9	20.4	3	6.8	2	4.5	5	11.4	1	2.3	12	27.3
Endocardial cushion defect	34	4	11.8	7	20.6	8	23.5	8	23.5	8	23.5	2	5.9	15	44.1	0	—	24	70.6
Isolated atrial septal defect (secundum)	28	0	—	2	7.1	0	—	2	7.1	1	3.6	0	—	1	3.6	0	—	3	10.7
Hypoplastic left heart syndrome	24	2	8.3	2	8.3	4	16.7	5	20.8	5	20.8	0	—	2	8.3	0	—	9	37.5
Any other cardiovascular malformation	164	9	5.5	8	4.9	12	7.3	15	9.1	17	10.4	5	3.0	18	11.0	2	1.2	51	31.1
Any cardiovascular malformation	404	22	5.4	26	6.4	32	7.9	42	10.4	34	8.4	10	2.5	48	11.9	4	1.0	116	28.7

widespread malformations. It is also worth noting that the proportion of children with cardiovascular malformations who also had syndromes was higher than the proportion with other malformations classes. This is because of the well-known fact that Down syndrome is frequently associated with cardiovascular anomalies.

Risk Factors for Cardiovascular Malformations

Administrative Data

Ordinal Number of Entry (Table 9.5) Congenital heart disease was more common in children born to women with a first, or only, pregnancy registered into the study (relative risk, 1.4).

Duration of Pregnancy at Registration *(Table 9.6)* In children born to mothers who registered during the first two lunar months of pregnancy, the rate of cardiovascular malformations was lower than in those whose mothers registered later, giving a relative risk of 0.3. However, this observation is based on small numbers.

Number of Antenatal Visits (Table 9.7) Cardiovascular defects were slightly more common when the mother attended for fewer than 10 antenatal visits, giving a relative risk of 1.2.

Personal Characteristics of the Mother

Mother's Age at Registration (Table 9.8) Maternal age was a strong determinant of cardiovascular malformations. In Whites and Blacks, the relative risk increased monotonically with age, reaching

Table **9.5**

Distribution of Children with Cardiovascular System (CVS) Malformations by Mother's Ordinal Number of Entry to the Study

Ordinal Number of Entry	No. of Children	Children with CVS Malformations		Relative Risk
		No.	Rate/1,000	
1	41,796	352	8.4	1.4
≥2	8,486	52	6.1	1.0*

*Reference category

Table *9.6*

Distribution of Children with Cardiovascular System (CVS) Malformations by Duration of Pregnancy at Registration

Duration of Pregnancy at Registration (lunar months)	No. of Children	Children with CVS Malformations		Relative Risk
		No.	Rate/1,000	
1–2	1,091	3	2.7	0.3
≥3	49,191	401	8.2	1.0*

*Reference category

Table **9.7**

Distribution of Children with Cardiovascular System (CVS) Malformations by Number of Antenatal Visits

| No. of Antenatal Visits | No. of Children | Children with CVS Malformations | | Relative Risk |
		No.	Rate/1,000	
1–9	29,588	254	8.6	1.2
≥10	20,694	150	7.3	1.0*

*Reference category

Table **9.8**

Race-Specific Distribution of Children with Cardiovascular System (CVS) Malformations by Mother's Age at Registration

| | Mother's Age | No. of Children | Children with CVS Malformations | | Relative Risk |
			No.	Rate/1,000	
White	≤19	4,074	22	5.4	1.0*
	20–29	14,220	110	7.7	1.4
	30–39	4,131	54	13.1	2.4
	≥40	386	11	28.5	5.3
Black	≤19	6,978	45	6.5	1.0*
	20–29	12,747	97	7.6	1.2
	30–39	3,953	32	8.1	1.3
	≥40	352	6	17.1	2.6
Puerto Rican	≤19	852	6	7.0	1.0*
	20–29	2,100	18	8.6	1.2
	30–39	455	3	6.6	0.9
	≥40	34	0	—	—

*Reference category

values of 5.3 and 2.6, respectively. Based on small numbers, there did not appear to be a similar relationship in Puerto Ricans.

Mother's Marital Status (Table 9.9) There were 34 affected children born to mothers who were separated, giving a relative risk of 1.3.

Mother's Religion (Table 9.10) The rate of cardiovascular malformations was elevated in the offspring of White mothers whose religion was recorded as "other" (mostly Jewish), giving a relative risk of 1.6. In Blacks and Puerto Ricans, no association between religion and cardiovascular defects was noted.

Ponderal Index (Table 9.11) The rate of cardiovascular defects was elevated in children born to mothers with a ponderal index of 3.0 or over, giving a relative risk of 1.5. The malformation rate was also increased when the ponderal index was unknown (relative risk, 1.6).

114

Table **9.9**

Distribution of Children with Cardiovascular System (CVS) Malformations by
Mother's Marital Status

| Marital Status | No. of Children | Children with CVS Malformations | | Relative Risk |
		No.	Rate/1,000	
Separated	3,326	34	10.2	1.3
Other	46,956	370	7.9	1.0*

*Reference category

Table **9.10**

Race-Specific Distribution of Children with Cardiovascular System (CVS) Malformations by
Mother's Religion

| | | No. of Children | Children with CVS Malformations | | Relative Risk |
			No.	Rate/1,000	
White	Protestant	9,031	72	8.0	1.0*
	Roman Catholic	11,943	103	8.6	1.1
	Other	1,441	18	12.5	1.6
	Unknown	396	4	10.1	1.3
Black	Protestant	20,620	155	7.5	1.0*
	Roman Catholic	2,833	23	8.1	1.1
	Other	366	2	5.5	0.7
	Unknown	211	0	—	—
Puerto Rican	Protestant	279	0	—	—
	Roman Catholic	3,136	27	8.6	—
	Other	6	0	—	—
	Unknown	20	0	—	—

*Reference category

Table **9.11**

Distribution of Children with Cardiovascular System (CVS) Malformations According to the
Prepregnant Ponderal Index of the Mother

| Ponderal Index (weight × 1,000)/(height)^2 | No. of Children | Children with CVS Malformations | | Relative Risk |
		No.	Rate/1,000	
≤3.0	44,381	335	7.6	1.0*
≥3.0	3,106	36	11.6	1.5
Unknown	2,795	33	11.8	1.6

*Reference category

Characteristics and Survival
of the Child

Birthweight (Table 9.12) In each ethnic group, there was an increase in the frequency of cardiovascular malformations with decreasing birthweight. For birthweights between 2,500 and 2,999 gm, relative risks ranged from 1.4 to 1.9. For birthweights under 2,500 gm, relative risks ranged from 3.5 to 4.8.

Birth Order (Table 9.13) The car-

diovascular malformation rates were elevated for children of birth order four to seven (relative risk, 1.3), and for children ranking eighth or higher (relative risk, 2.2).

Survival of the Child (Table 9.14) Of the 404 children with cardiovascular malformations, 164 (41%) were either stillborn or died during the four- to seven-year follow-up period. The cardiovascular malformation rate was in-

Table *9.12*

Race-Specific Distribution of Children with Cardiovascular System (CVS) Malformations by Birthweight

	Birthweight (grams)	No. of Children	Children with CVS Malformations		Relative Risk
			No.	Rate/1,000	
White	≤2,499	1,846	48	26.0	4.4
	2,500–2,999	4,463	51	11.4	1.9
	≥3,000	16,502	98	5.9	1.0*
Black	≤2,499	3,467	62	17.9	3.5
	2,500–2,999	7,024	49	7.0	1.4
	≥3,000	13,539	69	5.1	1.0*
Puerto Rican	≤2,499	367	9	24.5	4.8
	2,500–2,999	912	7	7.7	1.5
	≥3,000	2,162	11	5.1	1.0*

*Reference category

Table *9.13*

Distribution of Children with Cardiovascular System (CVS) Malformations by Birth Order of Child

Birth Order[1]	No. of Children	Children with CVS Malformations		Relative Risk
		No.	Rate/1,000	
1	15,166	110	7.3	1.0*
2–3	19,729	137	6.9	0.9
4–7	13,294	124	9.3	1.3
≥8	2,093	33	15.8	2.2

*Reference category
[1]Determined by number of prior liveborn and stillborn siblings

116

Table **9.14**

Race-Specific Distribution of Children with Cardiovascular System (CVS) Malformations by Survival of the Child

	Survival of Child	No. of Children	Children with CVS Malformations		Relative Risk
			No.	Rate/1,000	
White	Stillbirth	327	20	61.2	11.9
	Neonatal death	302	36	119.2	23.2
	Infant death	130	18	138.5	26.9
	Childhood death	91	10	109.9	21.4
	Survived	21,961	113	5.2	1.0*
Black	Stillbirth	407	10	24.6	5.0
	Neonatal death	450	30	66.7	13.6
	Infant death	229	19	83.0	16.9
	Childhood death	134	9	67.2	13.7
	Survived	22,810	112	4.9	1.0*
Puerto Rican	Stillbirth	64	4	62.5	13.7
	Neonatal death	54	6	111.1	24.3
	Infant death	25	2	80.0	17.5
	Childhood death	14	0	—	—
	Survived	3,284	15	4.6	1.0*

*Reference category

creased about 15-fold in non-survivors. Relative risks varied among the three ethnic groups: for stillbirth, the range was 5.0 to 13.7; for neonatal death, 13.6 to 24.3; for infant death, 16.9 to 26.9; and for childhood death, 13.7 to 21.4 (in this category there were 14 Puerto Rican children, none of whom had cardiovascular malformations).

Autopsy Report (Table 9.15) The presence of an autopsy report was associated with a higher rate of cardiovascular malformations among those who died, giving a relative risk of 2.5.

Reproductive History of the Mother

Prior Fetal or Neonatal Loss (Table 9.16) A history of prior abortion was associated with an increased cardiovascular malformation rate. This increase was only

Table **9.15**

Distribution of Dead Children with Cardiovascular System (CVS) Malformations by Presence of Autopsy Report

Autopsy Report	No. of Children	Dead Children with CVS Malformations		Relative Risk
		No.	Rate/1,000	
Present	1,810	151	83.4	2.5
Absent	418	14	33.5	1.0*

*Reference category

Table **9.16**

Distribution of Children with Cardiovascular System (CVS) Malformations by History of Prior Fetal or Neonatal Loss

	No. of Children	Children with CVS Malformations		Relative Risk
		No.	Rate/1,000	
Two or more prior abortions	2,504	33	13.2	1.7
One prior abortion	6,631	60	9.1	1.2
No prior abortion[1]	26,979	212	7.9	1.0*
No prior pregnancy	14,168	99	7.0	0.9
Prior stillbirth	2,837	33	11.6	1.4
No prior stillbirth[2]	32,280	261	8.1	1.0*
No prior pregnancies 20 weeks or over	15,165	110	7.3	0.9
Prior neonatal death	2,174	28	12.9	1.6
No prior neonatal death[3]	32,554	262	8.1	1.0*
No prior liveborn	15,554	114	7.3	0.9

*Reference category
[1]Includes 108 unknowns
[2]Includes 179 unknowns
[3]Includes 947 unknowns

slight when there was one prior abortion (relative risk, 1.2) and larger when there had been repeated abortions (relative risk, 1.7). Histories of prior stillbirth (relative risk, 1.4) and prior siblings who died within 28 days of birth (relative risk, 1.6) were also associated with cardiovascular malformations.

Characteristics and Complications of the Pregnancy

Duration of Pregnancy (Table 9.17) The cardiovascular malformation rates, in each ethnic group, were increased with the pregnancies lasted less than 9 lunar months, or longer than 10 lunar months. For pregnancies of 7 to 8 months duration, the relative risks ranged from 1.7 to 3.0. Pregnancies of 5 to 6 months duration were only associated with an increased malformation rate in Whites (relative risk, 2.2). For pregnancies of 11 months duration, the relative risks ranged from 2.6 to 3.1 (the latter, for Puerto Ricans, based on two malformed children).

Placental Weight (Table 9.18) Low placental weight was associated with cardiovascular malformations. In White children, the rate began to rise as the placental weight dropped below 400 gm (relative risk, 1.8), while in Black and Puerto Rican children, a trend only became evident at placental weights of less than 300 gm (relative risk, 1.6). The relative risk for Whites in the latter category was 3.6.

Signs of Toxemia (Table 9.19) With the exception of eclampsia, in which there were only 22 pregnancies, there was a steady monotonic decrease in the relative risk estimates from 3.0 to 0.8, corresponding with decreasing degrees of severity, until proteinuria without hypertension and generalized edema (without other features of toxemia) gave no evidence of being a risk factor for cardiovascular malformations.

Various Complications of Pregnancy (Table 9.20) The table lists seven further complications of pregnancy that were found to be related to increased rates of

Table **9.17**

Race-Specific Distribution of Children with Cardiovascular System (CVS) Malformations by Duration of Pregnancy

	Length of Gestation (lunar months)	No. of Children	Children with CVS Malformations		Relative Risk
			No.	Rate/1,000	
White	5–6	178	3	16.9	2.2
	7–8	896	21	23.4	3.0
	9–10	21,293	164	7.7	1.0*
	≥11	444	9	20.3	2.6
Black	5–6	354	2	5.7	0.9
	7–8	2,147	30	14.0	2.1
	9–10	21,068	140	6.7	1.0*
	≥11	461	8	17.4	2.6
Puerto Rican	5–6	27	0	—	—
	7–8	249	3	12.1	1.7
	9–10	3,075	22	7.2	1.0*
	≥11	90	2	22.2	3.1

*Reference category

Table **9.18**

Race-Specific Distribution of Children with Cardiovascular System (CVS) Malformations by Placental Weight

	Placental Weight (grams)	No. of Children	Children with CVS Malformations		Relative Risk
			No.	Rate/1,000	
White	≤299	864	21	24.3	3.6
	300–399	5,377	65	12.1	1.8
	≥400[1]	16,570	111	6.7	1.0*
Black and Puerto Rican	≤299	1,619	20	12.4	1.6
	300–399	7,738	49	6.3	0.8
	≥400[2]	18,114	138	7.6	1.0*

*Reference category
[1]Includes 2,644 unknowns
[2]Includes 3,770 unknowns

Table **9.19**

Distribution of Children with Cardiovascular System (CVS) Malformations by Signs of Toxemia[1]

	No. of Children	Children with CVS Malformations		Relative Risk
		No.	Rate/1,000	
Eclampsia	22	0	—	—
Uncontrolled chronic hypertension (BP ≥ 160/110 after LM 6)	283	7	24.7	3.0
Controlled chronic hypertension (without BP 160/110 after LM 6)	386	7	18.1	2.2
Acute hypertension (BP ≥ 160/110 after LM 6)	930	11	11.8	1.4
Proteinuria	1,213	10	8.2	1.0
Generalized edema	11,425	74	6.5	0.8
None	36,023	295	8.2	1.0*

*Reference category
[1]This classification is hierarchical and based on severity—for example, a pregnancy complicated by uncontrolled chronic hypertension is classified as such, even though proteinuria and edema may also be present.

Table **9.20**

Distribution of Children with Cardiovascular System (CVS) Malformations by Various Complications of Pregnancy

	No. of Children	Children with CVS Malformations		Relative Risk*
		No.	Rate/1,000	
Single umbilical artery	341	19	55.7	7.2
Hemorrhagic shock	99	4	40.4	5.1
Placenta previa	131	4	30.5	3.8
Hydramnios	694	18	25.9	3.3
Vena cava syndrome	144	3	20.8	2.6
Abruptio placentae	1,030	12	11.7	1.5

*For each condition, the reference category consists of those without that condition.

cardiovascular malformations in this study. For single umbilical artery the relationship is well known. However, a point estimate of relative risk of 7.2 is noteworthy. There were 99 pregnancies complicated by hemorrhagic shock (due to placenta previa and/or abruptio placentae in two-thirds, and other causes in the remainder). There were four children with cardiovascular malformations born to this group, giving a relative risk of 5.1. For placenta previa, the relative risk was 3.8. Other complications associated with congenital heart disease were: hydramnios, vena cava syndrome, and abruptio placentae; relative risks were 3.3, 2.6, and 1.5, respectively.

Weight Change During Pregnancy (Table 9.21) The rate of cardiovascular malformations was doubled in children whose

Table **9.21**

Distribution of Children with Cardiovascular System (CVS) Malformations by Weight Change During Pregnancy

| | No. of Children | Children with CVS Malformations | | Relative Risk |
		No.	Rate/1,000	
Lost weight	753	12	15.9	2.0
Other[1]	49,529	392	7.9	1.0*

*Reference category
[1]Includes 1,867 unknowns

mothers lost weight during their pregnancies, compared with those whose mothers did not. Thus, the relative risk was 2.0.

Maternal Diabetes (Table 9.22) The cardiovascular malformation rates were considerably elevated in the offspring of diabetic mothers. The data showed a monotonic trend: for treated diabetes of at least five years duration, the relative risk was 7.8; for diabetes treated with insulin and/or oral antidiabetic drugs for less than five years, the relative risk was 4.0.

Selected Diseases of the Mother (Table 9.23) The relative risk for cardiovascular malformations among children of mothers who had thrombophlebitis was 3.5. For endocrine disorder other than diabetes or malfunction of the thyroid gland, urinary tract infection, hematuria, or bacterial infection during the second or third trimester, the relative risks ranged from 1.3 to 2.0. Clinically diagnosed anemia was negatively associated with cardiovascular malformations (relative risk, 0.8).

Environmental Factors

Pelvic or Abdominal X-Ray Exposure During Pregnancy (Table 9.24) The cardiovascular malformation rate was increased among children of mothers exposed to pelvic and/or abdominal X-rays, giving a relative risk of 1.3.

Rubella Exposure (Table 9.25) Among children whose mothers were exposed to rubella during the first two trimesters of

Table **9.22**

Distribution of Children with Cardiovascular System (CVS) Malformations by Maternal Diabetes Mellitus

| | No. of Children | Children with CVS Malformations | | Relative Risk |
		No.	Rate/1,000	
Treated diabetes ≥ 5 years	98	6	61.2	7.8
Treated diabetes < 5 years	96	3	31.3	4.0
Untreated diabetes or ketoacidosis	142	1	7.1	0.9
No diabetes	49,946	394	7.9	1.0*

*Reference category

Table **9.23**

Distribution of Children with Cardiovascular System (CVS) Malformations by Selected Diseases of the Mother During Pregnancy

	No. of Children	Children with CVS Malformations		Relative Risk*
		No.	Rate/1,000	
Thrombophlebitis	144	4	27.8	3.5
Endocrine disorder other than diabetes, hypothyroidism, or hyperthyroidism	1,537	16	10.4	1.3
Urinary tract infection (fever ≥ 100.4°F)	709	9	12.7	1.6
Hematuria (≥15 RBC/HPF)	1,059	15	14.2	1.8
Bacterial infection during 2nd and/or 3rd trimester	899	14	15.6	2.0
Anemia	11,761	82	7.0	0.8

*For each disease, the reference category consists of those without that disease.

Table **9.24**

Distribution of Children with Cardiovascular System (CVS) Malformations by Pelvic and/or Abdominal X-Ray Exposure During Pregnancy

Pelvic and/or Abdominal X-Ray Exposure	No. of Children	Children with CVS Malformations		Relative Risk
		No.	Rate/1,000	
Present	11,400	111	9.7	1.3
Absent	38,882	293	7.5	1.0*

*Reference category

Table **9.25**

Distribution of Children with Cardiovascular System (CVS) Malformations by Maternal Exposure to Rubella Infection During Pregnancy

Rubella Exposure	No. of Children	Children with CVS Malformations		Relative Risk
		No.	Rate/1,000	
1st and/or 2nd trimester	1,404	17	12.1	1.5
3rd trimester	583	2	3.4	0.4
None	48,295	385	8.0	1.0*

*Reference category

pregnancy, the relative risk for cardiovascular malformations was 1.5. There was no evidence of an effect in late pregnancy.

Genetic Factors

Family History of Malformation (Table 9.26) There was some increase in the cardiovascular malformation rate in offspring of fathers recorded as having a physical birth defect (relative risk, 1.6). There was essentially no increase in risk among the offspring of malformed mothers. A variety of malformations in prior siblings were related to a high cardiovascular malformation rate. They included: congenital heart disease (relative risk, 2.9), malformations affecting the head and/or spine (2.8), and malformations of the fingers and/or toes (2.1). The less accurately defined category of prior siblings with other miscellaneous malformations also appeared to be associated with an increased risk (relative risk, 1.6).

Multivariate Analysis

Fifteen of the 39 factors initially selected and scaled as binary or ordinal variables for multivariate analysis were eliminated after linear discriminant function analysis: low number of antenatal visits, ethnic group, separated marital status, high ponderal index, history of abortion, stillbirth or neonatal death, short gestation, abruptio placentae, anemia, "other" endocrine disorders, urinary tract infection, pelvic or abdominal X-ray exposure, parental history of malformations, and history of miscellaneous birth defects in siblings. The results of the multiple logistic regression analysis for the remaining 24 variables are given in Table 9.27.

Factors with a relative risk greater than three included single umbilical artery (5.1), low birthweight (3.6), maternal diabetes (3.3), and thrombophlebitis (3.1). All were statistically significant. Factors with a relative risk between two and three included vena cava syndrome (2.7), hydramnios (2.4), congenital heart disease in a prior sibling (2.2), malformations of the fingers and/or toes in a prior sibling (2.0), and malformations of the head and/or spine in a prior sibling (2.0).

Table **9.26**

Distribution of Children with Cardiovascular System (CVS) Malformations by Family History of Malformation

	No. of Children	Children with CVS Malformations		Relative Risk*
		No.	Rate/1,000	
Congenital malformation in child's father	690	9	13.0	1.6
Congenital malformation in child's mother	1,225	11	9.0	1.1
Congenital heart disease in a prior sibling	662	15	22.7	2.9
Malformation of head and/or spine in a prior sibling	597	13	21.8	2.8
Malformation of finger and/or toe in a prior sibling	474	8	16.9	2.1
Miscellaneous other malformations in a prior sibling	1,797	22	12.2	1.6

*For each of the above, the reference category consists of those with a negative family history.

Table **9.27**

Factors Related to the Risk of Cardiovascular System (CVS) Malformations Based Upon Multiple Logistic Risk Function Analysis

	Estimated Risk Function Coefficient	Standard Error of Coefficient	Estimated Standardized Relative Risk
Single umbilical artery	1.63	0.25	5.1
Birthweight < 2,500 gm	1.29	0.13	3.6
Maternal diabetes, duration ≥ 5 years	1.19	0.44	3.3
Thrombophlebitis during pregnancy	1.14	0.52	3.1
Vena cava syndrome (positional shock)	0.01	0.60	2.7
Hydramnios	0.86	0.26	2.4
Congenital heart disease in prior sibling	0.81	0.27	2.2
Malformation of finger and/or toe in prior sibling	0.71	0.36	2.0
Malformation of head and/or spine in prior sibling	0.71	0.30	2.0
Bacterial infection in 2nd and/or 3rd trimester	0.57	0.28	1.8
Hematuria (≥ 15 RBC/HPF) during pregnancy	0.55	0.27	1.7
White and religion other than Protestant or Roman Catholic	0.54	0.25	1.7
Age of mother 40 years or greater	0.53	0.21	1.7
Hemorrhagic shock during pregnancy	0.53	0.58	1.7
Placenta previa	0.50	0.55	1.7
Chronic hypertension and/or eclampsia	0.46	0.27	1.6
Weight loss (without weight gain) during pregnancy	0.43	0.30	1.5
First entry to the study	0.43	0.15	1.5
Birth order 8th or higher	0.40	0.19	1.5
Exposure to rubella in 1st and/or 2nd trimester	0.39	0.25	1.5
White and placental weight less than 400 gm	0.38	0.13	1.5
Duration of gestation 11 lunar months or more	0.11	0.02	1.1
Entry to the study during the first two lunar months	−0.11	0.06	0.9
Black or Puerto Rican and placental weight less than 300 gm	−0.29	0.25	0.8

All were statistically significant except for vena cava syndrome and malformations of fingers and/or toes. Of the remaining factors, the following were statistically significant: bacterial infection in the second or third trimester (1.8), hematuria (1.7), religion other than Roman Catholic or Protestant in Whites (1.7), maternal age at least 40 years (1.7), first entry to the study (1.5), birth order eighth or higher (1.5), placental weight less than 400 gm in Whites (1.5), and length of gestation at least 11 lunar months (1.1).

Table 9.28 evaluates the adequacy of the model as fitted to the data. The observed and expected numbers of malformed children within each decile of risk are similar. In addition, the separation between the highest and lowest decile of risk (a ratio greater than 14) suggests that the model is satisfactory in separating high and low risk groups.

124

Table **9.28**

Distribution of Observed and Expected Numbers of Children with Cardiovascular System (CVS) Malformations by Multiple Logistic Risk Function Scores

Risk Score Percentile[1]	Observed Number of Children with CVS Malformations	Expected Number of Children with CVS Malformations
99–100	60	55.4
97–98	22	26.4
95–96	18	21.0
93–94	17	18.0
91–92	16	15.7
Subtotal (91–100)	133	136.5
81–90	64	61.3
71–80	37	42.9
61–70	42	33.8
51–60	28	29.3
41–50	28	25.6
31–40	19	21.9
21–30	23	20.8
11–20	21	17.9
1–10	9	14.0
Total	404	404.0

[1]Each decile contains 5,025 mother-child pairs, except the lowest which contains 5,057 mother-child pairs.

CHAPTER 10

Malformations of the Musculo-skeletal System

Among the 50,282 children, there were 717 with malformations of the musculo-skeletal system (MS) (14.3 per 1,000). The more common specific defects affecting at least 20 children are shown in Table 10.1. Of the affected children, 370 had polydactyly (53%); syndactyly was also common, being present in 125 children (18%). Dislocation of the hip occurred in 92 (9%), and the corresponding numbers for hypoplasia of a limb (or part thereof) and absence of a limb (or part thereof) were 51 (7%) and 32 (5%), respectively. Micrognathia affected 21 of the malformed children (2%).

The less common malformations are listed in Table 10.2: none of them accounted for more than 3% of the children with MS malformations. It is of particular interest that true hemimelia or phocomelia was rare, affecting only 7 children (1.0% of those with MS deformities). Absence, atrophy, or hypoplasia of various muscle groups was also uncommon: the combined category of muscular anomalies of this type comprised 17 children (2.4%). As a combined group, all of the less common malformations together accounted for 14% of the 717 affected children.

It should be noted that clubfoot and some rare anomalies affecting the hands or fingers are not considered in this chapter; data concerning these malformations are presented in Chapter 17, which deals with those malformations that showed

Table **10.1**

Musculoskeletal Malformation Rates Classified by Race (Rates per Thousand)

Malformation	White (n=22,811) No.	Rate	Black (n=24,030) No.	Rate	Puerto Rican (n=3,441) No.	Rate	Total (n=50,282) No.	Rate
Polydactyly	35	1.53	330	13.73	5	1.45	370	7.36
Syndactyly	93	4.08	26	1.08	6	1.74	125	2.49
Dislocation of hip	72	3.16	13	0.54	7	2.03	92	1.83
Hypoplasia of limb or part	25	1.10	23	0.96	3	0.87	51	1.01
Absence of limb or part	16	0.70	13	0.54	3	0.87	32	0.64
Micrognathia/hypoplastic jaw	16	0.70	3	0.12	2	0.58	21	0.42
Other musculoskeletal malformations[1]	54	2.37	40	1.66	7	2.03	101	2.01
Any musculoskeletal malformation	268	11.75	418	17.39	31	9.01	717	14.26

[1]See Table 10.2 for details of this category.
Note: Clubfoot and abnormalities of hands/fingers are not included; they are presented in Chapter 17.

Table **10.2**

Rare Musculoskeletal Malformation Rates Classified by Race (Rates per Thousand)

Malformation	White (n=22,811) No.	Rate	Black (n=24,030) No.	Rate	Puerto Rican (n=3,441) No.	Rate	Total (n=50,282) No.	Rate
Anomalies of rib and sternum	9	0.39	5	0.21	2	0.58	16	0.32
Hemivertebrae	9	0.39	3	0.12	1	0.29	13	0.26
Webbed neck	7	0.31	2	0.08	1	0.29	10	0.20
Other vertebral anomalies	8	0.35	5	0.21	0	—	13	0.26
Deformed and/or abnormally implanted toes	5	0.22	7	0.29	0	—	12	0.24
Other miscellaneous anomalies of foot	7	0.31	3	0.12	0	—	10	0.20
Hemimelia/phocomelia	5	0.22	2	0.08	0	—	7	0.14
Absence/atrophy/hypoplasia of pectoral muscles	5	0.22	4	0.17	1	0.29	10	0.20
Absence/atrophy/hypoplasia of rectus abdominis	0	—	4	0.17	0	—	4	0.08
Absence/atrophy/hypoplasia of other muscles	0	—	2	0.08	1	0.29	3	0.06
Arthrogryposis	3	0.13	3	0.12	0	—	6	0.12
Abnormal face and/or skull	4	0.18	1	0.04	0	—	5	0.10
Other miscellaneous musculoskeletal malformations	4	0.18	5	0.21	1	0.29	10	0.20

gross variability in their hospital distributions.

There were some striking differences in the rates of specific malformations by ethnic group (Table 10.1). The most common malformation, polydactyly, was nine times more common among Blacks (13.7 per 1,000) than among Whites (1.5 per 1,000) or Puerto Ricans (1.5 per 1,000). Conversely, syndactyly was about four times more common among Whites (4.1 per 1,000) than among Blacks (1.1 per 1,000). Syndactyly was uncommon among Puerto Rican children (1.7 per 1,000).

The overwhelming preponderance of polydactyly in Black children was responsible for their high overall MS malformation rate of 17.4 per 1,000, as against 11.7 per 1,000 among White children and 9.0 per 1,000 among Puerto Ricans. Apart from polydactyly, however, MS malformations tended to be appreciably more common in White and Puerto Rican children.

Polydactyly was judged, on clinical grounds, to be of minor severity; certain anomalies of the chest wall (16 children), anomalies of the vertebrae (13), deformed or abnormally implanted toes (10), abnormalities of the foot (10), and webbed neck (10) were also designated as minor. Thus, over half of the MS malformations were minor, but only a small proportion of the MS anomalies other than polydactyly were of minor severity.

Of the 717 children with MS malformations, 62 had more than one malformation affecting the MS system. However, there was considerable variability in the proportion of multiple malformations according to which malformation was considered as the referent. Thus, 4.1% of the 370 children with polydactyly had more than one MS anomaly. Similarly, 5.4% of 92 children with congenital dislocation of the hip were thus affected. By contrast, 22 of 32 children who were born with an absent limb had multiple MS anomalies (69%), and for 51 children with hypo-

plasia of a limb, the corresponding number was 27 (53%). Syndactyly was intermediate: 27 of 125 affected children (22%) had multiple MS anomalies. Of the 62 children with multiple MS anomalies, 39 had two MS anomalies (63%), 14 had three (23%), and the remainder had more than three.

Table 10.3 summarizes the occurrence of MS malformations overall, and MS malformations affecting at least 20 children, in relation to the occurrence of malformations in other classes. Polydactyly (4.9%), congenital dislocation of the hip (6.5%), and syndactyly (8.8%) tended to be class-specific. All other MS malformations, including the more common categories of hypoplastic or absent limbs and micrognathia or absent jaws, tended to be commonly associated with malformations affecting other systems, with rates varying from 27.5% to 47.6%.

The low overall association between MS malformations, in general, and anomalies in other classes, is due to disproportionate weighting by polydactyly, syndactyly, and congenital dislocation of the hip. More detailed inspection of Table 10.3 does not reveal any striking association between the class of MS malformations or its components and any other malformation class. The only relationships that are perhaps noteworthy are between micrognathia and two malformation classes, respiratory malformations (29%) and syndromes (38%), and between the combined category of uncommon MS malformations, each individual one affecting fewer than 20 children, and genitourinary malformations (25%).

As is well known, polydactyly has a large genetic component and occurs principally in Blacks. In the cohort under study, children with this condition comprise a substantial fraction (53%) of those affected by MS malformations, particularly among Blacks (79%). Moreover, in these data, the set of risk factors for polydactyly differs appreciably from the set for other MS malformations.

Table 10.3

Joint Occurrence of Malformations in Classes Other Than the Musculoskeletal System (MS) in Children with Common MS Malformations

	No. of Children	Central Nervous		Cardio-vascular		Respiratory		Gastro-intestinal		Genito-urinary		Eyes/Ears		Syndromes		Tumors		Any Malformation Other Than MS	
		No.	%	No.	%	No.	%	No.	%	No.	%	No.	%	No.	%	No.	%	No.	%
Polydactyly	370	4	1.1	7	1.9	10	2.7	4	1.1	3	0.8	5	1.4	3	0.8	1	0.3	18	4.9
Syndactyly	125	3	2.4	1	0.8	4	3.2	3	2.4	2	1.6	1	0.8	4	3.2	0	—	11	8.8
Congenital dislocation of hip	92	2	2.2	1	1.1	1	1.1	2	2.2	1	1.1	0	—	1	1.1	0	—	6	6.5
Hypoplasia of limb or part thereof	51	4	7.8	6	11.8	3	5.9	4	7.8	2	3.9	0	—	7	13.8	1	2.0	14	27.5
Absence of limb or part thereof	32	2	6.3	3	9.4	4	12.5	6	18.7	3	9.4	2	6.3	3	9.4	1	3.1	10	31.3
Micrognathia or hypoplastic jaw	21	2	9.5	2	9.5	6	28.6	1	4.8	2	9.5	0	—	8	38.1	0	—	10	47.6
Any other musculoskeletal malformation	101	22	21.8	16	15.8	19	18.8	15	14.9	25	24.8	4	4.0	14	13.9	4	4.0	48	47.5
Any musculoskeletal malformation	717	28	3.9	26	3.6	37	5.2	26	3.5	30	4.2	10	1.4	25	3.5	6	0.8	88	12.3

Because ethnic group was such a strong determinant, it seemed reasonable analytic strategy to treat polydactyly as a separate outcome among the Black members of the cohort. Black children whose only MS malformation was polydactyly were consequently no longer considered to be affected by a MS malformation when the relation between drugs and this class was analyzed, and will be dealt with separately in a later section.

Syndactyly has, *mutatis mutandis,* some of the same features as polydactyly, but less prominently. In particular, syndactyly is not as large a component of the MS malformation class and is less race-specific. Furthermore, the set of risk factors for syndactyly proved to be much the same as that for MS malformations other than polydactyly or syndactyly. It was decided on these grounds to retain syndactyly in the MS malformation class. Note, therefore, that in the next two sections, the term "musculoskeletal (MS) malformations" will be used to refer to this malformation class after the exclusion of polydactyly in Black children.

Risk Factors for Musculoskeletal Malformations Other Than Polydactyly in Blacks

Administrative Data
Number of Antenatal Visits (Table 10.4)
Compared to the group of mothers who attended fewer than 10 times for antenatal care, the relative risk of a MS malformation for the group attending 10 to 14 times was 1.4, and it was 2.0 in the group attending at least 15 times.

Personal Characteristics of the Mother
Ethnic Group (Table 10.5) As mentioned in the introduction to this chapter, the rate of MS malformations other than polydactyly was considerably higher in White children and Puerto Rican children than in Black children, giving relative risks of 2.9 and 2.3, respectively.

Mother's Age at Registration (Table 10.6) Apart from the handful of malformed children born to very young mothers, the relative risks for MS malformations rose monotonically with increasing maternal age, from 0.6 in children of mothers aged 15 to 19 years to 2.1 in children of mothers over 40 years old.

Characteristics and Survival
of the Offspring
Birthweight (Table 10.7) Among all three ethnic groups, the MS malformation rate was about 3 times greater among infants weighing under 2 kg at birth than among infants weighing at least 2.5 kg at birth, with relative risks ranging from 2.8 to 3.2. Children whose birthweight was in the range of 2 to 2.5 kg had relative risks ranging from 1.1 to 1.5.

Survival of the Child (Table 10.8) MS

Table **10.4**

Distribution of Children with Musculoskeletal (MS) Malformations by Number of Antenatal Visits

No. of Antenatal Visits	No. of Children	Children with MS Malformations		Relative Risk
		No.	Rate/1,000	
1–4	8,624	57	6.6	1.0
5–9	20,964	136	6.5	1.0*
10–14	16,994	154	9.1	1.4
≥15	3,700	48	13.0	2.0

*Reference category

Table **10.5**

Distribution of Children with Musculoskeletal (MS) Malformations by Ethnic Group

	No. of Children	Children with MS Malformations		Relative Risk
		No.	Rate/1,000	
White	22,811	268	11.7	2.9
Black	24,030	96	4.0	1.0*
Puerto Rican	3,441	31	9.0	2.3

*Reference category

Table **10.6**

Distribution of Children with Musculoskeletal (MS) Malformations by Mother's Age at Registration

Mother's Age	No. of Children	Children with MS Malformations		Relative Risk
		No.	Rate/1,000	
≤14	429	3	7.0	0.9
15–19	11,475	58	5.1	0.6
20–24	18,475	146	7.9	1.0*
25–29	10,592	89	8.4	1.1
30–34	5,655	55	9.7	1.2
35–39	2,884	31	10.7	1.4
≥40	772	13	16.8	2.1

*Reference category

malformations were frequently associated with fetal or later death, particularly among Blacks: 26% of affected Black children died before 4 years of age, compared to 13% of the Whites and 16% of the Puerto Ricans. The relative risks of MS malformations associated with death at various stages ranged from 3.1 to 5.0 in Whites, 2.4 to 8.6 in Blacks, and 2.0 to 18.0 in Puerto Ricans. The findings for Puerto Ricans were based on small numbers.

Reproductive History of the Mother

Prior Fetal or Neonatal Loss (Table 10.9) There was no evidence that a history of prior stillbirths or of one prior abortion was associated with an increased rate of MS malformations. The rate was somewhat higher in children of mothers who had experienced prior neonatal death (relative risk, 1.2) or who had had at least two prior abortions (relative risk, 1.5).

Characteristics and Complications of the Pregnancy

Duration of Pregnancy (Table 10.10) Compared to children born after at least 9 lunar months, the relative risks of MS malformations in children born at 7 lunar months or less were 1.9, 2.4, and 3.0 in Whites, Blacks, and Puerto Ricans,

131

Table **10.7**

Race-Specific Distributions of Children with Musculoskeletal (MS) Malformations by Child's Birthweight

	Birthweight (grams)	No. of Children	Children with MS Malformations		Relative Risk
			No.	Rate/1,000	
White	≤1,999	645	20	31.0	2.8
	2,000–2,499	1,201	20	16.7	1.5
	≥2,500	20,965	228	10.9	1.0*
Black	≤1,999	1,208	14	11.6	3.2
	2,000–2,499	2,259	9	4.0	1.1
	≥2,500	20,563	73	3.6	1.0*
Puerto Rican	≤1,999	123	3	24.4	3.0
	2,000–2,499	244	3	12.3	1.5
	≥2,500	3,074	25	8.1	1.0*

*Reference category

Table **10.8**

Race-Specific Distributions of Children with Musculoskeletal (MS) Malformations by Survival of the Child

	Survival of Child	No. of Children	Children with MS Malformations		Relative Risk
			No.	Rate/1,000	
White	Stillbirth	327	11	33.6	3.2
	Neonatal death	302	16	53.0	5.0
	Infant death	130	5	38.5	3.6
	Childhood death	91	3	33.0	3.1
	Survived	21,961	233	10.6	1.0*
Black	Stillbirth	407	7	17.2	5.5
	Neonatal death	450	12	26.7	8.6
	Infant death	229	5	21.8	7.0
	Childhood death	134	1	7.5	2.4
	Survived	22,810	71	3.1	1.0*
Puerto Rican	Stillbirth	64	1	15.6	2.0
	Neonatal death	54	1	18.5	2.3
	Infant death	25	1	40.0	5.1
	Childhood death	14	2	142.9	18.0
	Survived	3,284	26	7.9	1.0*

*Reference category

Table **10.9**

Distribution of Children with Musculoskeletal (MS) Malformations by History of Prior Fetal or Neonatal Loss

	No. of Children	Children with MS Malformations		Relative Risk
		No.	Rate/1,000	
One prior abortion	6,631	50	7.5	1.0
At least two prior abortions	2,504	27	10.8	1.5
No prior abortion[1]	26,979	195	7.2	1.0*
No prior pregnancy	14,168	123	8.7	1.2
Prior stillbirth	2,837	21	7.4	1.0
No prior stillbirth[2]	32,280	245	7.6	1.0*
No prior pregnancies 20 weeks or over	15,165	129	8.5	1.1
Prior neonatal death	2,174	19	8.7	1.2
No prior neonatal death[3]	32,554	242	7.4	1.0*
No prior liveborn	15,554	134	8.6	1.2

*Reference category
[1]Includes 108 unknowns
[2]Includes 179 unknowns
[3]Includes 947 unknowns

Table **10.10**

Race-Specific Distribution of Children with Musculoskeletal (MS) Malformations by Duration of Pregnancy

	Length of Gestation (lunar months)	No. of Children	Children with MS Malformations		Relative Risk
			No.	Rate/1,000	
White	5–7	375	8	21.3	1.9
	8	699	13	18.6	1.6
	≥9	21,737	247	11.4	1.0*
Black	5–7	885	8	9.0	2.4
	8	1,616	6	3.7	1.0
	≥9	21,529	82	3.8	1.0*
Puerto Rican	5–7	81	2	24.7	3.0
	8	195	3	15.4	1.9
	≥9	3,165	26	8.2	1.0*

*Reference category

respectively. In Whites and Puerto Ricans, the intermediate category of children showed intermediate rates (relative risks, 1.6, 1.9), but in Blacks the rate in this category was similar to the rate among longer-term infants.

Placental Weight (Table 10.11) The relative risk of MS malformations among children with placentae weighing less than 300 gm was 2.1.

Single Umbilical Artery (Table 10.12) The MS malformation rate was increased more than eight-fold when only one umbilical artery was present, giving a relative risk of 8.5.

Signs of Toxemia (Table 10.13) In children of mothers whose most severe toxemia sign was proteinuria, the relative risk for MS malformations was 1.6. However, toxemia signs which included

hypertension (but not eclampsia) were associated with only a modest increase in risk (1.3 for children whose mothers had high blood pressure after LM 6). The relative risk of 6.0 for eclampsia was based on only one malformed child.

Vaginal Bleeding (Table 10.14) The relative risk for MS malformations in children whose mothers bled during the first or second trimester was 1.3. Bleeding during the third trimester did not appear to be related to this outcome.

Marginal Sinus Rupture (Table 10.15) An association with MS malformations was evident only among Blacks (relative risk, 4.1) and Puerto Ricans (relative risk, 8.7, based on one case among 13 affected mothers).

Other Placental Factors and Hydramnios (Table 10.16) Both placental conditions

Table **10.11**

Distribution of Children with Musculoskeletal (MS) Malformations by Placental Weight

Placental Weight (grams)	No. of Children	Children with MS Malformations		Relative Risk
		No.	Rate/1,000	
≤299	2,483	40	16.1	2.1
≥300	41,385	314	7.6	1.0*
Unknown	6,414	41	6.4	0.8

*Reference category

Table **10.12**

Distribution of Children with Musculoskeletal (MS) Malformations by Number of Umbilical Arteries

No. of Umbilical Arteries	No. of Children	Children with MS Malformations		Relative Risk
		No.	Rate/1,000	
One	341	22	64.5	8.5
Two	44,851	340	7.6	1.0*
Unknown	5,090	33	6.5	0.9

*Reference category

Table **10.13**

Distribution of Children with Musculoskeletal (MS) Malformations by Signs of Toxemia[1]

| | No. of Children | Children with MS Malformations | | Relative Risk |
		No.	Rate/1,000	
Eclampsia	22	1	45.5	6.0
Chronic hypertension	669	5	7.5	1.0
Acute hypertension (BP ≥ 160/110 after LM 6)	930	9	9.7	1.3
Proteinuria	1,213	15	12.4	1.6
Generalized edema	11,425	93	8.1	1.1
None	36,023	272	7.6	1.0*

*Reference category
[1]The classification is hierarchical and based on severity—for example, a pregnancy complicated by chronic hypertension is classified as such even though proteinuria and edema may also be present.

Table **10.14**

Distribution of Children with Musculoskeletal (MS) Malformations According to Vaginal Bleeding During Pregnancy

| Vaginal Bleeding | No. of Children | Children with MS Malformations | | Relative Risk |
		No.	Rate/1,000	
1st trimester	3,668	35	9.5	1.3
2nd trimester	2,546	26	10.2	1.3
3rd trimester	6,980	51	7.3	1.0
None	37,088	283	7.6	1.0*

*Reference category

listed in the table were associated with a higher risk of having a child with a MS malformation. The relative risks for abruptio placentae and placenta previa were 1.4 and 1.6, respectively. Fifteen children whose mothers had hydramnios also had MS malformations, giving a relative risk of 2.8.

Weight Change During Pregnancy (Table 10.17) Among children born to mothers whose weight gain during pregnancy was 15.0 kg or more, the relative risk for MS malformations was 1.5. The risk was also increased when the amount of weight change was unknown (relative risk, 1.4).

Anemia (Table 10.18) The children of anemic Black and Puerto Rican mothers experienced a lower rate of MS malformations than did the children of mothers without this diagnosis (relative risks, 0.6 and 0.3, respectively). This association was not apparent in Whites.

Selected Diseases of the Mother (Table 10.19) The relative risk for MS malformations among children of mothers with a urinary tract infection was 1.7. Mothers who had diabetes for at least five years or

135

Table **10.15**

Race-Specific Distribution of Children with Musculoskeletal (MS) Malformations by Marginal Sinus Rupture

	Marginal Sinus Rupture	No. of Children	Children with MS Malformations		Relative Risk
			No.	Rate/1,000	
White	Present	303	4	13.2	1.1
	Absent	22,508	264	11.7	1.0*
Black	Present	323	5	15.5	4.1
	Absent	23,707	91	3.8	1.0*
Puerto Rican	Present	13	1	76.9	8.7
	Absent	3,428	30	8.8	1.0*

*Reference category

Table **10.16**

Distribution of Children with Musculoskeletal (MS) Malformations by Placental Factors and Hydramnios

	No. of Children	Children with MS Malformations		Relative Risk*
		No.	Rate/1,000	
Abruptio placentae	1,030	11	10.7	1.4
Placenta previa	318	4	12.6	1.6
Hydramnios	694	15	21.6	2.8

*For each condition, the reference category consists of those without that condition.

Table **10.17**

Distribution of Children with Musculoskeletal (MS) Malformations by Weight Change During Pregnancy

Weight Change (kg)	No. of Children	Children with MS Malformations		Relative Risk
		No.	Rate/1,000	
Lost/no change	920	4	4.3	0.6
0.1–7.4	11,974	99	8.3	1.2
7.5–14.9	29,135	207	7.1	1.0*
≥15.0	6,386	66	10.3	1.5
Unknown	1,867	19	10.2	1.4

*Reference category

Table **10.18**

Race-Specific Distribution of Children with Musculoskeletal (MS) Malformations by Mother's Anemia During Pregnancy

| | Anemia | No. of Children | Children with MS Malformations | | Relative Risk |
			No.	Rate/1,000	
White	Present	2,213	25	11.3	1.0
	Absent	20,598	243	11.8	1.0*
Black	Present	8,299	24	2.9	0.6
	Absent	15,731	72	4.6	1.0*
Puerto Rican	Present	1,249	4	3.2	0.3
	Absent	2,192	27	12.3	1.0*

*Reference category

Table **10.19**

Distribution of Children with Musculoskeletal (MS) Malformations by Selected Diseases of the Mother During Pregnancy

| | No. of Children | Children with MS Malformations | | Relative Risk* |
		No.	Rate/1,000	
Urinary tract infection (fever ≥ 100.4°F)	709	9	12.7	1.7
Treated and long-term (≥ 5 years) diabetes	194	7	36.1	4.7

*For each disease, the reference category consists of those without that disease.

treated diabetes of shorter duration also had an increased risk of giving birth to children with MS malformations (relative risk, 4.7).

Environmental Factors

Pelvic or Abdominal X-Ray Exposure During Pregnancy (Table 10.20). There was some evidence that exposure to pelvic or abdominal X-rays was associated with MS malformations: the relative risk for 11,400 exposed mother-child pairs was 1.4.

Exposure to Rubella Infection During Pregnancy (Table 10.21) Among the gravidas with reported exposure to rubella infection in the first and second trimesters, the relative risks for MS malformations were, respectively, 2.4 and 1.5. Exposure during the third trimester did not appear to be associated with an increased risk.

Genetic Factors

Parental History of Malformations (Table 10.22) Malformations in the mothers

Table **10.20**

Distribution of Children with Musculoskeletal (MS) Malformations by Pelvic and/or Abdominal X-Ray Exposure During Pregnancy

Pelvic and/or Abdominal X-Ray Exposure	No. of Children	Children with MS Malformations		Relative Risk
		No.	Rate/1,000	
Present	11,400	115	10.1	1.4
Absent	38,882	280	7.2	1.0*

*Reference category

Table **10.21**

Distribution of Children with Musculoskeletal (MS) Malformations by Maternal Exposure to Rubella Infection During Pregnancy

Rubella Exposure	No. of Children	Children with MS Malformations		Relative Risk
		No.	Rate/1,000	
1st trimester	535	10	18.7	2.4
2nd trimester	869	10	11.5	1.5
3rd trimester	583	4	6.9	0.9
None	48,295	371	7.7	1.0*

*Reference category

Table **10.22**

Distribution of Children with Musculoskeletal (MS) Malformations by a History of Maternal or Paternal Malformation

	No. of Children	Children with MS Malformations		Relative Risk*
		No.	Rate/1,000	
Congenital malformation in child's mother	1,168	10	8.6	1.1
Congenital malformation in child's father	664	9	13.6	1.7

*For each of the above, the reference category consists of those with a negative parental history.

showed no evidence of association with MS malformations, while malformations in the fathers were associated with a relative risk of 1.7.

History of Selected Malformations in Prior Siblings (Table 10.23) For children with prior siblings who had malformations affecting the fingers or toes and for children with prior siblings with cleft anomalies, the relative risk was 4.2. A history of prior siblings with clubfoot was associated with a relative risk of 3.5.

Multivariate Analysis

Twenty-four of the factors described above were scaled as binary or ordinal variables and subjected to linear discriminant function analysis. Seven were eliminated by this procedure, their coefficients having been reduced to low values by the presence of the other covariates. The omitted factors were histories of prior abortion and neonatal death, short pregnancy, signs of toxemia, abruptio placentae, placenta previa, and vaginal bleeding. The results of the multiple logistic regression analysis for the remaining 17 factors are given in Table 10.24.

Factors with relative risks greater than 3 were single umbilical artery (6.2), clubfoot and various other malformations in prior siblings (3.7), and marginal sinus rupture in Blacks and Puerto Ricans (3.5). All were statistically significant. Factors with relative risks between 2 and 3 included maternal diabetes (treated and/or duration of at least five years) (2.8), Puerto Rican ethnic group (2.7), White ethnic group (2.5), and birthweight under 2,000 gm (2.1). Again, all were statistically significant. Of the remaining factors, the following were statistically significant: hydramnios (1.9), maternal exposure to rubella in the first or second trimester (1.8), mother's age at least 40 years (1.7), placental weight under 300 gm (1.6), weight gain during pregnancy at least 15 kg (1.6), at least 15 antenatal visits (1.5), and anemia in Blacks and Puerto Ricans (0.5).

Table 10.25 shows the results of stratification of the 395 children with MS malformations according to risk score. Comparison of the observed and expected numbers within each stratum of risk shows reasonable agreement. In addition, the ratio of the numbers of children in the top decile of risk to the numbers in

Table 10.23

Distribution of Children with Musculoskeletal (MS) Malformations by History of Selected Malformations in Prior Siblings

	No. of Children	Children with MS Malformations		Relative Risk
		No.	Rate/1,000	
Cleft palate and/or lip	106	3	28.3	4.2
Clubfoot	291	7	24.1	3.5
Malformations of fingers/toes	453	13	28.7	4.2
Prior siblings not malformed	30,613	208	6.8	1.0*
No prior liveborn	15,166	129	8.5	1.3

*Reference category

Table **10.24**

Factors Related to the Risk of Musculoskeletal (MS) Malformations Based on Multiple Logistic Risk Function Analysis

	Estimated Risk Function Coefficient	Standard Error of Coefficient	Estimated Standardized Relative Risk
Single umbilical artery	1.83	0.23	6.2
Clubfoot, cleft palate/lip, or malformations of fingers/toes in prior siblings	1.31	0.22	3.7
Marginal sinus rupture in Blacks and Puerto Ricans	1.25	0.43	3.5
Maternal diabetes, treated and/or duration ≥ 5 years	1.02	0.42	2.8
Puerto Rican ethnic group	0.98	0.21	2.7
White ethnic group	0.94	0.13	2.5
Birthweight < 2,000 gm	0.76	0.21	2.1
Hydramnios	0.62	0.28	1.9
Maternal exposure to rubella in first or second trimester	0.58	0.23	1.8
Mother's age ≥ 40 years	0.53	0.20	1.7
Urinary tract infection during pregnancy	0.48	0.35	1.6
Placental weight < 300 gm	0.47	0.21	1.6
Weight gain ≥ 15 kg during pregnancy	0.45	0.14	1.6
At least 15 antenatal visits	0.40	0.16	1.5
Malformation in father	0.29	0.34	1.3
Exposure to pelvic and/or abdominal X-rays during pregnancy	0.11	0.11	1.1
Anemia in Blacks and Puerto Ricans	−0.60	0.22	0.5

the lowest decile is over 13, indicating that the model is satisfactory in discriminating between degrees of risk.

Risk Factors for Polydactyly in Black Children

Administrative Data

Institution (Table 10.26) In comparison to the Boston hospitals and the New York Medical Center, all other medical institutions participating in the study had relatively high rates of Black polydactyly, giving a relative risk of 1.7.

Number of Antenatal Visits (Table 10.27) The number of antenatal visits was not associated with great variations in the rate of polydactyly. All relative risks were at or near unity, with the exception of a relative risk of 0.4 for at least 15 visits.

Personal Characteristics of the Mother

Mother's Age at Registration (Table 10.28) In general, children born to mothers aged 15 or more had a lower risk of polydactyly than that observed in the group of 394 mothers who were younger, for whom the relative risk was 1.5. There was one child with polydactyly born to a mother older than 44 years (relative risk, 5.0).

Characteristics and Survival of the Offspring

Birthweight (Table 10.29) Polydactyly among Black children occurred more frequently as birthweight increased. Thus, for children in the lower birthweight categories, the relative risk was 0.7.

Birth Order (Table 10.30) As a child's order of birth increased within the family, it appeared that the risk of polydactyly

Table **10.25**

Distribution of Observed and Expected Numbers of Children with Musculoskeletal (MS) Malformations by Multiple Logistic Risk Function Scores

Risk Score Percentile*	Observed Number of Children with MS Malformations	Expected Number of Children with MS Malformations
99–100	49	50.8
97–98	23	23.1
95–96	17	17.9
93–94	16	15.5
91–92	15	14.2
Subtotal (91–100)	120	121.5
81–90	50	58.9
71–80	59	48.2
61–70	43	42.1
51–60	34	35.9
41–50	40	30.9
31–40	14	20.6
21–30	15	15.5
11–20	11	13.1
1–10	9	8.3
Total	395	395.0

*Each decile contains 5,025 pregnancies, except the lowest which contains 5,057 pregnancies.

Table **10.26**

Distribution of Black Children with Polydactyly by Institution

Location of Institution	No. of Children	Black Children with Polydactyly		Relative Risk
		No.	Rate/1,000	
Boston, MA or New York, NY (N.Y. Medical)	2,613	22	8.4	1.0*
Other locations	21,417	308	14.4	1.7

*Reference category

141

Table **10.27**

Distribution of Black Children with Polydactyly by Number of Antenatal Visits

No. of Antenatal Visits	No. of Children	Black Children with Polydactyly		Relative Risk
		No.	Rate/1,000	
1–4	5,140	86	16.7	1.1
5–9	11,585	140	12.1	0.8
10–14	6,459	99	15.3	1.0*
≥15	846	5	5.9	0.4

*Reference category

Table **10.28**

Distribution of Black Children with Polydactyly by Mother's Age at Registration

Mother's Age	No. of Children	Black Children with Polydactyly		Relative Risk
		No.	Rate/1,000	
≤14	394	9	22.8	1.5
15–19	6,584	87	13.2	0.9
20–24	8,109	126	15.5	1.0*
25–29	4,638	63	13.6	0.9
30–34	2,610	24	9.2	0.6
35–39	1,343	16	11.9	0.8
40–44	339	4	11.8	0.8
≥45	13	1	76.9	5.0

*Reference category

Table **10.29**

Distribution of Black Children with Polydactyly by Child's Birthweight

Birthweight (grams)	No. of Children	Black Children with Polydactyly		Relative Risk
		No.	Rate/1,000	
≤1,999	1,208	12	9.9	0.7
2,000–2,499	2,259	23	10.2	0.7
≥2,500	20,563	295	14.3	1.0*

*Reference category

Table **10.30**

Distribution of Black Children with Polydactyly by Birth Order of Child

Birth Order[1]	No. of Children	Black Children with Polydactyly		Relative Risk
		No.	Rate/1,000	
1	6,740	96	14.2	1.0
2–3	8,805	130	14.8	1.0*
4–5	4,798	60	12.5	0.8
6–7	2,254	29	12.9	0.9
8–9	931	11	11.8	0.8
≥10	502	4	8.0	0.5

*Reference category
[1]Determined by number of prior liveborn and stillborn siblings

decreased. Thus, the relative risks for children whose birth order was between 4 and 9 were all slightly below unity, while the relative risk for children of birth order 10 or above was 0.5.

Survival of the Child (Table 10.31) The frequency of polydactyly among Black children did not appear to be strongly related to the survival status of the children. Relative risks varied from 0.4 for stillbirth to 1.3 for infant death. All were based on small numbers of exposed and malformed children.

Reproductive History of the Mother

Prior Neonatal Loss (Table 10.32) The malformation rate in children born to mothers having a history of prior neonatal death was 18.8 per 1,000, giving a relative risk of 1.4.

Characteristics and Complications of the Pregnancy

Duration of Pregnancy (Table 10.33) As the length of gestation increased, there was a corresponding increase in the rate of polydactyly. Thus, among mothers whose pregnancies lasted 5 to 6 lunar months, the relative risk was 0.6, while for those whose pregnancies lasted 7 to 8 months, the relative risk was 0.8.

Single Umbilical Artery (Table 10.34) The relative risk for polydactyly in

Table **10.31**

Distribution of Black Children with Polydactyly by Survival of the Child

Survival of Child	No. of Children	Black Children with Polydactyly		Relative Risk
		No.	Rate/1,000	
Stillbirth	407	2	4.9	0.4
Neonatal death	450	5	11.1	0.8
Infant death	229	4	17.5	1.3
Childhood death	134	1	7.5	0.5
Survived	22,810	318	13.9	1.0*

*Reference category

Table **10.32**

Distribution of Black Children with Polydactyly by History of Prior Neonatal Loss

	No. of Children	Black Children with Polydactyly		Relative Risk
		No.	Rate/1,000	
Prior neonatal death	1,226	23	18.8	1.4
No prior neonatal deaths[1]	15,866	209	13.2	1.0*
No prior liveborn	6,938	98	14.1	1.1

*Reference category
[1]Includes 490 unknowns

Table **10.33**

Distribution of Black Children with Polydactyly by Duration of Pregnancy

Length of Gestation (lunar months)	No. of Children	Black Children with Polydactyly		Relative Risk
		No.	Rate/1,000	
5–6	354	3	8.5	0.6
7–8	2,147	24	11.2	0.8
9–10	21,068	296	14.0	1.0*
≥11	461	7	15.2	1.1

*Reference category

Table **10.34**

Distribution of Black Children with Polydactyly by Number of Umbilical Arteries

No. of Umbilical Arteries	No. of Children	Black Children with Polydactyly		Relative Risk
		No.	Rate/1,000	
One	107	4	37.4	2.8
Two	21,399	285	13.3	1.0*
Unknown	2,524	41	16.2	1.2

*Reference category

144

Black children with one umbilical artery was 2.8.

Signs of Toxemia (Table 10.35) An increased rate of polydactyly was present among children born to mothers who had chronic hypertension without either eclampsia or elevated blood pressure late in pregnancy (relative risk, 1.8). In addition, 1 of the 19 Black children whose mothers had eclampsia during pregnancy had polydactyly (relative risk, 3.8).

Umbilical Cord Knot (Table 10.36) The relative risk for polydactyly in children who had an umbilical cord knot (tight or loose) was 1.4.

Selected Diseases of the Mother (Table 10.37) Of 172 mothers who had a functional cardiovascular disorder, 7 gave birth to children with polydactyly (relative risk, 3.0). The relative risk for polydactyly in children whose mothers had syphilis (mostly inactive) during pregnancy was 1.4. Among children whose mothers had hematuria, the relative risk for polydactyly was 1.5.

Table **10.35**

Distribution of Black Children with Polydactyly by Signs of Toxemia[1]

	No. of Children	Black Children with Polydactyly		Relative Risk
		No.	Rate/1,000	
Eclampsia	19	1	52.6	3.8
Uncontrolled chronic hypertension (BP ≥ 160/110 after LM 6)	213	2	9.4	0.7
Controlled chronic hypertension (without BP ≥ 160/110 after LM 6)	312	8	25.6	1.8
Acute hypertension (BP ≥ 160/110 after LM 6)	435	4	9.2	0.7
Proteinuria	712	5	7.0	0.5
Generalized edema	3,898	54	13.9	1.0
None	18,441	256	13.9	1.0*

*Reference category
[1]This classification is hierarchical and based on severity—for example, a pregnancy complicated by uncontrolled chronic hypertension is classified as such even though proteinuria and edema may also be present.

Table **10.36**

Distribution of Black Children with Polydactyly by Umbilical Cord Knot

Cord Knot	No. of Children	Black Children with Polydactyly		Relative Risk
		No.	Rate/1,000	
Yes	207	4	19.3	1.4
No[1]	23,823	326	13.7	1.0*

*Reference category
[1]Includes 552 unknowns

145

Table **10.37**

Distribution of Black Children with Polydactyly by Selected Diseases of the Mother During Pregnancy

	No. of Children	Black Children with Polydactyly		Relative Risk*
		No.	Rate/1,000	
Functional cardiovascular disorders	172	7	40.7	3.0
Syphilis	747	14	18.7	1.4
Hematuria (≥15 RBC/HPF)	692	14	20.2	1.5

*For each disease, the reference category consists of those without that disease.

Genetic Factors

Family History of Malformations (Table 10.38) Malformations in the child's parents were related to an increased frequency of polydactyly. Among children whose mothers had congenital malformations, the relative risk was 4.6. Among children whose fathers had a malformation, the relative risk was 5.9.

History of Malformations of the Fingers or Toes in Prior Siblings (Table 10.39) Among children with prior siblings with anomalies of the fingers or toes, the relative risk for polydactyly was 8.0.

Mother-Child ABO Incompatibility (Table 10.40) There were 1,750 mothers who had blood type O and gave birth to children with blood type A (a strong in-compatibility). Among these mother-child pairs, the relative risk for polydac-tyly was 1.5.

Multivariate Analysis

Seventeen of the above factors were initially selected for multivariate analysis and scaled as dichotomous variables. Discriminant function analysis elimi-nated 2 factors from further consideration because of low coefficients: duration of pregnancy and the presence of an umbili-cal cord knot. Results of the multiple logistic regression analysis of the remain-ing 15 variables are shown in Table 10.41.

Factors with relative risks greater than 3 included the following, all of which

Table **10.38**

Distribution of Black Children with Polydactyly by History of Maternal or Paternal Malformation

	No. of Children	Black Children with Polydactyly		Relative Risk*
		No.	Rate/1,000	
Congenital malformation in child's mother	406	24	59.1	4.6
Congenital malformation in child's father	167	13	77.8	5.9

*For each of the above, the reference category consists of those with a negative parental history.

Table **10.39**

Distribution of Black Children with Polydactyly by History of Malformations of the Fingers or Toes in Prior Siblings

Malformation of Fingers/Toes	No. of Children	Black Children with Polydactyly		Relative Risk
		No.	Rate/1,000	
Yes	298	30	100.7	8.0
No	23,732	300	12.6	1.0*

*Reference category

Table **10.40**

Distribution of Black Children with Polydactyly by ABO Incompatibility

	No. of Children	Black Children with Polydactyly		Relative Risk
		No.	Rate/1,000	
Mother O, child A	1,750	37	21.1	1.5
Other than above	20,110	276	13.7	1.0*
Unknown	2,170	17	7.8	0.6

*Reference category

Table **10.41**

Factors Related to the Risk of Occurrence of Polydactyly in Black Children Based Upon Multiple Logistic Risk Function Analysis

	Estimated Risk Function Coefficient	Standard Error of Coefficient	Estimated Standardized Relative Risk
Prior sibling with malformation of fingers/toes	1.95	0.22	7.0
Paternal congenital malformation	1.37	0.31	3.9
Maternal congenital malformation	1.26	0.23	3.5
Single umbilical artery	1.25	0.52	3.5
Functional cardiovascular disease	1.13	0.40	3.1
Fewer than 15 antenatal vists	0.92	0.45	2.5
Maternal age at registration < 15 yrs	0.53	0.35	1.7
ABO incompatibility (mother O, offspring A)	0.51	0.18	1.7
Hospitals other than in Boston and New York (N.Y. Medical)	0.50	0.22	1.6
Birthweight ≥ 2,500 gm	0.45	0.18	1.6
Hematuria (≥ 15 RBC/HPF)	0.45	0.28	1.6
Chronic hypertension or eclampsia	0.45	0.32	1.6
Any prior neonatal death	0.38	0.23	1.5
Maternal syphilis	0.38	0.28	1.5
Birth order < 4	0.35	0.15	1.4

Table **10.42**

Distribution of Observed and Expected Numbers of Black Children with Polydactyly by Multiple Logistic Risk Function Scores

Risk Score Percentile[1]	Observed Number of Black Children with Polydactyly	Expected Number of Black Children with Polydactyly
99–100	45	42.3
97–98	20	18.3
95–96	9	11.6
93–94	12	10.3
91–92	9	10.1
Total (91–100)	95	92.6
81–90	39	37.5
71–80	28	31.1
61–70	33	31.1
51–60	34	31.1
41–50	23	29.2
31–40	23	22.1
21–30	17	22.1
11–20	18	19.6
1–10	20	13.6
Total	330	330.0

[1]Each decile contains 2,400 pregnancies, except the lowest which contains 1,950 pregnancies.

were statistically significant: prior sibling with malformation of fingers/toes (7.0), paternal congenital malformation (3.9), maternal congenital malformation (3.5), single umbilical artery (3.5), and functional cardiovascular disease of the mother (3.1). The only factor with a relative risk between 2 and 3 was fewer than 15 antenatal visits (2.5), which achieved marginal statistical significance. Of the factors with relative risks below 2, the following were statistically significant: ABO incompatibility (1.7), hospitals other than at Boston and New York (New York Medical Center) (1.6), birthweight at least 2,500 gm (1.6), and birth order less than fourth (1.4).

An indication of the adequacy of the logistic model in describing the risk of polydactyly observed among Black children is given in Table 10.42. In this table, each decile lists the numbers of Black polydactyly observed and expected based on the logistic regression model. The fit is quite acceptable. The ratio between the observed numbers in the uppermost decile and the numbers in the lowest decile (about 5) shows that the model has achieved adequate classification of the higher and lower risk children.

CHAPTER 11

Malformations of the Respiratory Tract

Pectus excavatum and cleft gum are not considered here because of their uneven distribution in the participating hospitals (see Chapter 17). Apart from these anomalies, there were 218 (4.3 per 1,000) children with observed respiratory tract (RT) malformations in the cohort of 50,282 mother-child pairs. Among these 218 children, there were 240 RT malformations. The specific RT malformation distributions by ethnic group are given in Tables 11.1 and 11.2. As in previous chapters, the initial table describes the rates observed for the more common malformations, whereas the latter table is concerned with the less common malformations. There was no single malformation entity in the respiratory tract which was recorded significantly more often than others. As shown in Table 11.1, the most common malformation was hypoplasia/agenesis of the lung, occurring in 32 of the 218 affected children (15%); anomalies of the lung were observed in 26 of the malformed children (12%).

Aside from isolated cleft gum all other cleft anomalies amounted to 36% of the 240 RT defects (79 malformed children). Isolated cleft palate (31 children) represented 14% of the total. Isolated cleft lip was observed as often as was co-existent cleft lip and palate (11%). Among the less common RT malformations (occurring with a rate of less than 4 per 1,000), anomalies of the teeth occurred in 19

Table 11.1

Respiratory Malformation Rates Classified by Ethnic Group (Rates per Thousand)

Malformation	White (n=22,811) No.	Rate	Black (n=24,030) No.	Rate	Puerto Rican (n=3,441) No.	Rate	Total (n=50,282) No.	Rate
Hypoplasia/agenesis lung	21	0.92	8	0.33	3	0.87	32	0.64
Cleft palate only	16	0.70	12	0.50	3	0.87	31	0.62
Malformed lung	13	0.57	11	0.46	2	0.58	26	0.52
Cleft lip only	18	0.79	5	0.21	1	0.29	24	0.48
Co-existent cleft lip and palate	13	0.57	11	0.46	0	—	24	0.48
Other respiratory malformation[1]	47	2.06	45	1.87	5	1.45	97	1.93
Any respiratory malformation	117	5.13	87	3.62	14	4.07	218	4.34

[1]See Table 11.2 for details of this category.
Note: Pectus excavatum and cleft gum are not included; they are presented in Chapter 17.

Table 11.2

Rare Respiratory Malformations Classified by Ethnic Group (Rates per Thousand)

Malformation	White (n=22,811) No.	Rate	Black (n=24,030) No.	Rate	Puerto Rican (n=3,441) No.	Rate	Total (n=50,282) No.	Rate
Anomalies of the teeth	5	0.22	12	0.50	2	0.58	19	0.38
Malformations of the thoracic wall	11	0.48	6	0.25	1	0.29	18	0.36
Bilobed lung	7	0.31	6	0.25	1	0.29	14	0.28
Diaphragmatic hernia	8	0.35	4	0.17	1	0.29	13	0.26
Malformations of the diaphragm	6	0.26	5	0.21	0	—	11	0.22
Hiatal hernia	3	0.13	4	0.17	1	0.29	8	0.16
Laryngeal/tracheal malacia	0	—	4	0.17	0	—	4	0.08
Choanal atresia	3	0.13	0	—	0	—	3	0.06
Other miscellaneous respiratory malformations	3	0.13	2	0.08	0	—	5	0.10
Some epiglottis/bronchi malformations	4	0.18	4	0.17	0	—	8	0.16

children (9%), and 18 children (8%) had malformations of the thoracic wall (Table 11.2). Seventy-two or 30% of all RT anomalies involved the lung. Malformed lung, bilobed lung, and anomalies of the teeth and gum were judged to be of minor severity. All other RT malformations were considered to be major.

In general, there was no consistent racial pattern among the RT group of mal-formations. Blacks did have lower rates among the more commonly reported anomalies; however, this ranking did not obtain for the more rare defects. Overall, the rates per thousand were 5.1 for Whites, 3.6 for Blacks, and 4.1 for Puerto Ricans (Table 11.1).

Of the 218 children with observed RT malformations, 30 (14%) had more than one RT malformation. Among these 30 children, 19 (63%) had defects affecting other classes. There were 18 children with at least two or more RT malformations; of these, 11 had hypoplasia/agenesis of the lung. Among these 11 children, 8 had malformations of the diaphragm. There were 5 children who had isolated cleft gum along with other RT malformations; 4 of these children had hypoplasia/agenesis of the lung or malformations of the diaphragm. All other instances of a joint occurrence of RT defects consisted of a single case.

Table 11.3 presents the joint occurrence of malformations in other systems for those RT malformations affecting at least 20 children. The two RT malformation categories that had the highest proportion of joint occurrence with other malformation classes were hypoplasia/agenesis of the lung (88%) and other malformations of the lung (62%). In both categories, approximately 31% of the involved children also had a gastrointestinal malformation. Furthermore, among the 32 children with hypoplasia/agenesis of the lung, 15 (47%) also had recorded anomalies of the genitourinary tract. In the latter group of 15 children, 6 had joint RT defects involving the genitalia only, 7 had joint RT defects involving the urinary tract only, and 2 had joint RT defects with both genital and urinary tract involvement. In addition, among the 32 children with hypoplasia/agenesis of the lung, 12 (38%) had cardiovascular defects, 10 (31%) had musculoskeletal defects, 10 had gastrointestinal defects, and 10 had syndromes.

Risk Factors for Respiratory Tract Malformations

Administrative Data

Duration of Pregnancy at Registration (Table 11.4) There was an increased risk of RT malformations among the offspring of mothers who registered early in their pregnancies (relative risk, 1.7).

Number of Antenatal Visits (Table 11.5) In general, there was an inverse monotonic relationship between the number of antenatal visits and the risk of RT malformations. Among the 3,700 mothers who visited the study clinics 15 times or more, the relative risk was less than half (0.7) that observed for the 8,624 mothers who attended the clinics 4 times or less (1.6).

Personal Characteristics of the Mother

Maternal Age at Registration (Table 11.6) Mothers whose age at registration was 40 years or more were at greatest risk of bearing a child with an RT malformation (relative risk, 3.0).

Mother's Religion (Table 11.7) Roman Catholic mothers had a relative risk of 1.3 in comparison to all other religions combined.

Characteristics and Survival of the Offspring

Birthweight (Table 11.8) In general, there was a marked monotonic association between decreasing birthweight and the frequency of RT malformations. For White mother-child pairs, the relative risks ranged from 3.4 for children with birthweights between 2,000 and 2,499 gm to 18.8 for children whose birthweights were less than 1,500 gm. Among Black mother-child pairs, the corresponding range was 2.0 to 6.9. In Puerto Ricans, the highest relative risk was 13.3, for birthweight between 1,500 and 1,999 gm.

Sex of the Child (Table 11.9) Male children had slightly higher rates of RT malformations than did female children, giving a relative risk of 1.2.

Birth Order (Table 11.10) As birth order increased, the risk of RT anomalies also increased. For the 13,294 children who ranked between fourth- and seventh-born in the family, the relative risk was 1.2, as compared with a relative risk of 1.3 for those with a ranking greater than seventh-born.

Survival of the Child (Table 11.11) Survival status of the child was strongly

Table 11.3

Joint Occurrence of Malformations in Classes Other Than the Respiratory Tract (RT) in Children with Common RT Malformations

	No. of Children	Central Nervous		Cardio-vascular		Musculo-skeletal		Gastro-intestinal		Genito-urinary		Eyes/Ears		Syndromes		Tumors		Any Non-RT Malformation	
		No.	%	No.	%	No.	%	No.	%	No.	%	No.	%	No.	%	No.	%	No.	%
Hypoplasia/agenesis lung	32	9	28.1	12	37.5	10	31.3	10	31.3	15	46.9	1	3.1	10	31.3	0	—	28	87.5
Cleft palate only	31	6	19.4	3	9.7	9	29.0	2	6.5	3	9.7	1	3.2	7	22.6	0	—	13	41.9
Malformed lung	26	4	15.4	6	23.1	6	23.1	8	30.8	6	23.1	0	—	5	19.2	1	3.8	16	61.5
Cleft lip only	24	0	—	0	—	2	8.3	0	—	4	16.7	0	—	0	—	0	—	6	25.0
Co-existent cleft lip and palate	24	4	16.7	2	8.3	4	16.7	3	12.5	2	8.3	3	12.5	3	12.5	0	—	9	37.5
Other respiratory tract malformations	97	13	13.4	15	15.5	11	11.3	19	19.6	14	14.4	2	2.1	8	8.2	2	2.1	34	35.1
Any respiratory tract malformation	218	30	13.8	32	14.7	37	17.0	33	15.1	36	16.5	5	2.3	29	13.3	3	1.4	91	41.7

Table **11.4**

Distribution of Children with Respiratory Tract (RT) Malformations by Duration of Pregnancy at Registration

Duration of Pregnancy at Registration (lunar months)	No. of Children	Children with RT Malformations		Relative Risk
		No.	Rate/1,000	
1–2	1,091	8	7.3	1.7
3–8	41,956	185	4.4	1.0*
≥9	7,235	25	3.4	0.8

*Reference category

Table **11.5**

Distribution of Children with Respiratory Tract (RT) Malformations by Number of Antenatal Visits

No. of Antenatal Visits	No. of Children	Children with RT Malformations		Relative Risk
		No.	Rate/1,000	
1–4	8,624	56	6.5	1.6
5–14	37,958	151	4.0	1.0*
≥15	3,700	11	3.0	0.7

*Reference category

Table **11.6**

Distribution of Children with Respiratory Tract (RT) Malformations by Mother's Age at Registration

Mother's Age	No. of Children	Children with RT Malformations		Relative Risk
		No.	Rate/1,000	
≤19	11,904	45	3.8	0.9
20–39	37,606	163	4.3	1.0*
≥40	772	10	13.0	3.0

*Reference category

Table **11.7**

Distribution of Children with Respiratory Tract (RT) Malformations by Mother's Religion

	No. of Children	Children with RT Malformations		Relative Risk
		No.	Rate/1,000	
Roman Catholic	17,912	93	5.2	1.3
Other	32,370	125	3.9	1.0*

*Reference category

Table **11.8**

Race-Specific Distribution of Children with Respiratory Tract (RT) Malformations by Child's Birthweight

	Birthweight (grams)	No. of Children	Children with RT Malformations		Relative Risk
			No.	Rate/1,000	
White	≤1,499	357	23	64.4	18.8
	1,500–1,999	288	8	27.8	8.1
	2,000–2,499	1,201	14	11.7	3.4
	≥2,500	20,965	72	3.4	1.0*
Black	≤1,499	602	11	18.3	6.9
	1,500–1,999	606	10	16.5	6.3
	2,000–2,499	2,259	12	5.3	2.0
	≥2,500	20,563	54	2.6	1.0*
Puerto Rican	≤1,499	57	1	17.5	7.7
	1,500–1,999	66	2	30.3	13.3
	2,000–2,499	244	4	16.4	7.2
	≥2,500	3,074	7	2.3	1.0*

*Reference category

Table **11.9**

Distribution of Children with Respiratory Tract (RT) Malformations by Sex of Child

	No. of Children	Children with RT Malformations		Relative Risk
		No.	Rate/1,000	
Male	25,542	119	4.7	1.2
Female	24,740	99	4.0	1.0*

*Reference category

Table **11.10**

Distribution of Children with Respiratory Tract (RT) Malformations by Birth Order

Birth Order[1]	No. of Children	Children with RT Malformations		Relative Risk
		No.	Rate/1,000	
≤3	34,895	143	4.1	1.0*
4–7	13,294	64	4.8	1.2
≥8	2,093	11	5.3	1.3

*Reference category
[1]Determined by number of prior liveborn and stillborn siblings

Table **11.11**

Race-Specific Distribution of Children with Respiratory Tract (RT) Malformations by Survival of the Child

	Survival of Child	No. of Children	Children with RT Malformations		Relative Risk
			No.	Rate/1,000	
White	Stillbirth	327	24	73.4	25.2
	Neonatal death	302	23	76.2	26.2
	Infant death	130	5	38.5	13.2
	Childhood death	91	1	11.0	3.8
	Survived	21,961	64	2.9	1.0*
Black	Stillbirth	407	17	41.8	19.0
	Neonatal death	450	16	35.6	16.2
	Infant death	229	4	17.5	8.0
	Childhood death	134	0	—	—
	Survived	22,810	50	2.2	1.0*
Puerto Rican	Stillbirth	64	3	46.9	25.7
	Neonatal death	54	5	92.6	50.7
	Infant death	25	0	—	—
	Childhood death	14	0	—	—
	Survived	3,284	6	1.8	1.0*

*Reference category

related to the reported frequency of RT malformations, where the lowest relative risk was 3.8 for White childhood deaths. The highest relative risks were seen among the stillbirths, with a range of 19.0 to 25.7, and neonatal deaths, with a range of 16.2 to 50.7. It should be noted that the relative risks for Puerto Ricans were based on small numbers.

Reproductive History of the Mother
Prior Stillbirth (Table 11.12) Neonatal deaths in prior siblings did not markedly elevate rates of RT malformations.

*Table **11.12***

Distribution of Children with Respiratory Tract (RT) Malformations by History of Prior Stillbirth

	No. of Children	Children with RT Malformations		Relative Risk
		No.	Rate/1,000	
Prior stillbirth	2,837	19	6.7	1.6
No prior stillbirth[1]	32,280	138	4.3	1.0*
No prior pregnancies 20 weeks or over	15,165	61	4.0	0.9

*Reference category
[1]Includes 179 unknowns

However, this was not the case for prior stillbirths, where the relative risk was 1.6.

Characteristics and Complications of the Pregnancy

Duration of Pregnancy (Table 11.13) The relative risks for those mother-child pairs whose length of gestation was 5 to 6 lunar months, or 7 to 8 lunar months were 7.4 and 3.9, respectively. The relative risk was also elevated for mothers with gestation lasting more than 10 lunar months (2.1).

Placental Weight (Table 11.14) Among the mother-child pairs where the information was known, there was a monotonic association between increasing placental weight and decreasing rates of RT anomalies. Thus, the highest relative risk was observed in the category of placental weights below 200 gm (4.7). For placental weights between 200 and 299 gm, the relative risk was 2.6.

Number of Umbilical Arteries (Table 11.15) The relative risk for the 341 children with a single umbilical artery was 13.2.

Signs of Toxemia and Eclampsia (Table 11.16) The two categories with elevated risks for the development of an RT malformation were those children whose mothers had hypertension (relative risk, 1.5), and those whose mothers had proteinuria (relative risk, 1.2).

Vaginal Bleeding (Table 11.17) The relative risk for vaginal bleeding during the second trimester was 2.0.

Other Complications of Pregnancy (Table 11.18) Among the factors selected for display in this table, hydramnios is particularly marked as a risk factor for the

*Table **11.13***

Distribution of Children with Respiratory Tract (RT) Malformations by Duration of Pregnancy

Length of Gestation (lunar months)	No. of Children	Children with RT Malformations		Relative Risk
		No.	Rate/1,000	
5–6	559	14	25.0	7.4
7–8	3,292	43	13.1	3.9
9–10	45,436	154	3.4	1.0*
≥11	995	7	7.0	2.1

*Reference category

156

Table **11.14**

Distribution of Children with Respiratory Tract (RT) Malformations by Placental Weight

Placental Weight (grams)	No. of Children	Children with RT Malformations		Relative Risk
		No.	Rate/1,000	
≤199	388	8	20.6	4.7
200–299	2,095	24	11.5	2.6
300–399	13,115	58	4.4	1.0*
≥400	28,270	95	3.4	0.8
Unknown	6,414	33	5.1	1.2

*Reference category

Table **11.15**

Distribution of Children with Respiratory Tract (RT) Malformations by Number of Umbilical Arteries

No. of Umbilical Arteries	No. of Children	Children with RT Malformations		Relative Risk
		No.	Rate/1,000	
One	341	18	52.8	13.2
Two or unknown	49,941	200	4.0	1.0*

*Reference category

Table **11.16**

Distribution of Children with Respiratory Tract (RT) Malformations by Signs of Toxemia[1]

	No. of Children	Children with RT Malformations		Relative Risk
		No.	Rate/1,000	
Eclampsia	22	0	—	—
Hypertension	1,599	10	6.3	1.5
Proteinuria	1,213	6	4.9	1.2
Generalized edema	11,425	51	4.5	1.1
None	36,023	151	4.2	1.0*

*Reference category
[1]This classification is hierarchical and based on severity—for example, a pregnancy complicated by hypertension is classified as such, even though proteinuria and edema may also be present.

157

Table **11.17**

Distribution of Children with Respiratory Tract (RT) Malformations by Vaginal Bleeding During Pregnancy

| Vaginal Bleeding | No. of Children | Children with RT Malformations | | Relative Risk |
		No.	Rate/1,000	
1st trimester	3,668	17	4.6	1.2
2nd trimester	2,546	20	7.9	2.0
3rd trimester	6,980	33	4.7	1.2
None	37,088	148	4.0	1.0*

*Reference category

Table **11.18**

Distribution of Children with Respiratory Tract (RT) Malformations by Selected Complications of Pregnancy

| | No. of Children | Children with RT Malformations | | Relative Risk* |
		No.	Rate/1,000	
Hydramnios	694	27	38.9	10.1
Coagulation defect	46	2	43.5	10.1
Hemorrhagic shock	99	3	30.3	7.1

*For each condition, the reference category consists of those without that condition.

development of RT malformations. Of the 694 mothers with this condition, 27 had children who were eventually diagnosed as having an RT malformation, giving a relative risk of 10.1. Based on smaller numbers, maternal coagulation defects and hemorrhagic shock were also related to increased malformation rates, having relative risks of 10.1 and 7.1, respectively.

Placental Factors (Table 11.19) Mothers with the placental factors displayed in this table delivered children who were at increased risk of having an RT malformation. For marginal sinus rupture, abruptio placentae, and placenta previa, the relative risks were 3.0, 2.3, and 2.2, respectively.

Diabetes Mellitus (Table 11.20) Among diabetics there was a monotonically increasing risk of bearing a child with RT malformations as the duration of the disease increased. The relative risk for untreated, short-term maternal diabetes was 3.4; for treated diabetes of short duration, it was 5.0; for long-term diabetes, 9.7.

Other Maternal Diseases During Pregnancy (Table 11.21) If the mother had anemia or urinary tract infection during pregnancy, the child was at greater risk for developing an RT malformation; the relative risks associated with each disease were 1.2 and 3.4, respectively.

Genetic Factors

Family History of Malformations (Table 11.22) Children whose fathers had any

158

Table **11.19**

Distribution of Children with Respiratory Tract (RT) Malformations by Placental Factors

	No. of Children	Children with RT Malformations		Relative Risk*
		No.	Rate/1,000	
Marginal sinus rupture	639	8	12.5	3.0
Abruptio placentae	1,030	10	9.7	2.3
Placenta previa	317	3	9.5	2.2

*For each condition, the reference category consists of those without that condition.

Table **11.20**

Distribution of Children with Respiratory Tract (RT) Malformations by Maternal Diabetes Mellitus

	No. of Children	Children with RT Malformations		Relative Risk
		No.	Rate/1,000	
Treated diabetes $\geq$ 5 years	98	4	40.8	9.7
Treated diabetes $<$ 5 years	96	2	20.8	5.0
Untreated diabetes or keto-acidosis	142	2	14.1	3.4
No diabetes	49,946	210	4.2	1.0*

*Reference category

Table **11.21**

Distribution of Children with Respiratory Tract (RT) Malformations by Selected Diseases of the Mother During Pregnancy

	No. of Children	Children with RT Malformations		Relative Risk*
		No.	Rate/1,000	
Anemia	11,761	57	4.9	1.2
Urinary tract infection (fever $\geq$ 100.4°F)	709	10	14.1	3.4

*For each disease, the reference category consists of those without that disease.

Table **11.22**

Distribution of Children with Respiratory Tract (RT) Malformations by Family History of Malformation

	No. of Children	Children with RT Malformations		Relative Risk*
		No.	Rate/1,000	
Congenital malformation in child's father	664	9	13.6	3.2
Congenital malformation in prior sibling(s)	3,723	24	6.4	1.5
Prior sibling with cleft lip/palate	106	4	37.7	8.9

*For each of the above, the reference category consists of those with a negative family history.

Table **11.23**

Distribution of Children with Respiratory Tract (RT) Malformations by ABO Incompatibility

ABO Incompatibility	No. of Children	Children with RT Malformations		Relative Risk
		No.	Rate/1,000	
Mother O, child A	4,492	21	4.7	1.5
Other than above	41,562	129	3.1	1.0*
Unknown	4,228	68	16.1	5.2

*Reference category

congenital malformation (including RT) had an increased risk of RT malformations in comparison with children whose fathers had a negative history (relative risk, 3.2). This was also true for children whose siblings had a history of congenital malformations in general (relative risk, 1.5), and, in particular, for those children whose prior siblings had a history of a cleft lip and/or palate (relative risk, 8.9).

ABO Incompatibility and Erythroblastosis (Table 11.23) There was an increase in the rate of RT anomalies among children when the mother was type O and the child was type A, giving a relative risk of 1.5. When the blood type of the mother or child was unknown, the relative risk was 5.2.

Multivariate Analysis

Based on the foregoing comparisons, a total of 28 risk factors was selected for multivariate analysis, and scaled as binary or ordinal variables. After linear discriminant function analysis, the following 9 factors were eliminated because of low coefficients: high birth order, prior stillbirths, short duration of pregnancy, low placental weight, signs of toxemia, vaginal bleeding during pregnancy, abruptio placentae, placenta previa, and prior malformed siblings. The results of the multiple logistic regression analysis

160

for the 19 factors that were retained are given in Table 11.24.

Factors with a relative risk greater than three included single umbilical artery (8.2), prior malformed siblings with cleft lip and/or palate (7.3), hydramnios (7.0), birthweight under 2,000 gm (5.2), and malformed father (3.6); all were statistically significant. Factors with relative risks between 2 and 3 included unknown ABO group (2.7, statistically significant), coagulation defect (2.7), urinary tract infection (2.6, statistically significant), maternal diabetes of at least 5 years duration (2.4, statistically significant), and

maternal age of at least 40 years (2.2). Among the remaining factors, only the association with White ethnic group (1.4) was statistically significant.

As seen in Table 11.25, stratification of the 218 children with RT malformations showed satisfactory agreement between observed and expected numbers of malformations, particularly in the highest and lowest deciles of computed risk. The ratio of the numbers of children in the highest decile to the numbers in the lowest decile is large (about 16), indicating that the model is adequate in discriminating between degrees of risk.

Table **11.24**

Factors Related to the Risk of Occurrence of Respiratory Tract (RT) Malformations Based Upon Multiple Logistic Risk Function Analysis

	Estimated Risk Function Coefficient	Standard Error of Coefficient	Estimated Standardized Relative Risk
Single umbilical artery	2.10	0.28	8.2
Prior malformed sibling with cleft lip/palate	1.99	0.54	7.3
Hydramnios	1.94	0.23	7.0
Birthweight < 2,000 gm	1.65	0.20	5.2
Malformed father	1.28	0.35	3.6
Unknown ABO group	1.01	0.17	2.7
Coagulation defect	0.99	0.65	2.7
Urinary tract infection	0.95	0.34	2.6
Maternal diabetes ≥ 5 years	0.88	0.52	2.4
Maternal age ≥ 40 years	0.79	0.34	2.2
Lunar months 1–2 at registration	0.55	0.38	1.7
ABO incompatibility (mother O, child A)	0.44	0.24	1.6
Number of prenatal visits ≤ 4	0.37	0.28	1.5
White ethnic group	0.36	0.15	1.4
Marginal sinus rupture	0.29	0.38	1.3
Anemia	0.26	0.16	1.3
Male infant	0.22	0.14	1.2
Roman Catholic	0.21	0.15	1.2
Hemorrhagic shock	−0.30	0.75	0.7

Table **11.25**

Distribution of Observed and Expected Numbers of Children with Respiratory Tract (RT) Malformations by Multiple Logistic Risk Function Scores

Risk Score Percentile[1]	Observed Number of Children with RT Malformations	Expected Number of Children with RT Malformations
99–100	52	56.8
97–98	24	18.8
95–96	17	12.2
93–94	12	9.2
91–92	2	7.6
Total (91–100)	107	104.6
81–90	17	26.0
71–80	25	17.5
61–70	9	14.0
51–60	16	11.8
41–50	9	11.0
31–40	12	9.8
21–30	11	8.8
11–20	6	7.9
1–10	6	6.6
Total	218	218

[1]Each decile contains 5,025 pregnancies, except the lowest which contains 5,057 pregnancies.

CHAPTER 12

Malformations of the Gastro-intestinal Tract

Among the 50,282 children, there were 301 children with malformations of the gastrointestinal tract (GIT) (6.0 per 1,000), with a total of 346 GIT malformations. The specific defects are listed in Tables 12.1 and 12.2. As shown in Table 12.1, the most common malformations were pyloric stenosis, which occurred in 95 children (32% of 301 with GIT malformations), and umbilical hernia, which occurred in 51 children (17%). Among the less common malformations listed in Table 12.2, Hirschsprung's disease affected 13 children (4.3%), tracheo-esophageal fistula affected 11 (3.7%), and various types of atresia each accounted for about 2% to 3% of GIT malformations. All other GIT malformations were extremely rare. Inguinal hernia, which affected 683 children, is considered separately in Chapter 17.

The only specific GIT malformation which had a strong association with ethnic group was pyloric stenosis, which occurred four times more commonly in Whites than in Blacks, and also more commonly in Whites than in Puerto Ricans (Table 12.1). Overall, the rate (per 1,000) of GIT malformations was 7.4 in Whites, 5.0 in Blacks, and 3.8 in Puerto Ricans.

A number of GIT malformations were considered minor; among the more common are umbilical hernia (51 malformed children), malrotation (25), accessory spleen (23), and Meckel's

163

Table 12.1

Gastrointestinal Tract Malformation Rates Classified by Ethnic Group (Rates per Thousand)

Malformation	White (n=22,811) No.	Rate	Black (n=24,030) No.	Rate	Puerto Rican (n=3,441) No.	Rate	Total (n=50,282) No.	Rate
Pyloric stenosis	73	3.20	20	0.83	2	0.58	95	1.89
Umbilical hernia	18	0.79	32	1.33	1	0.29	51	1.01
Anal atresia	14	0.61	12	0.50	0	—	26	0.52
Malrotation	11	0.48	12	0.50	2	0.58	25	0.50
Accessory spleen	11	0.48	12	0.50	0	—	23	0.46
Omphalocele	8	0.35	14	0.58	0	—	22	0.44
Meckel's diverticulum	13	0.57	5	0.21	3	0.87	21	0.42
Other gastrointestinal malformations[1]	35	1.53	30	1.25	8	2.32	73	1.45
Any gastrointestinal malformation	168	7.36	120	4.99	13	3.78	301	5.99

[1]See Table 12.2 for details of this category.
Note: Inguinal hernia is not included; it is presented in Chapter 17.

Table 12.2

Rare Gastrointestinal Tract Malformation Rates Classified by Ethnic Group (Rates per Thousand)

Malformation	White (n=22,811) No.	Rate	Black (n=24,030) No.	Rate	Puerto Rican (n=3,441) No.	Rate	Total (n=50,282) No.	Rate
Hirschsprung's disease	8	0.35	4	0.17	1	0.29	13	0.26
TE fistula	3	0.13	5	0.21	3	0.87	11	0.22
Biliary atresia	5	0.22	3	0.12	0	—	8	0.16
Atresia/hypoplasia small intestine	5	0.22	1	0.04	1	0.29	7	0.14
Duodenal atresia	2	0.09	4	0.17	1	0.29	7	0.14
Anomalies of pancreas	2	0.09	3	0.12	1	0.29	6	0.12
Hernia other than umbilical	2	0.09	3	0.12	0	—	5	0.10
Anomalies of gallbladder	3	0.13	2	0.08	0	—	5	0.10
Anomalous shaped/lobation of liver	2	0.09	3	0.12	0	—	5	0.10
Anomalies of liver	3	0.13	0	—	0	—	3	0.06
Asplenia	1	0.04	1	0.04	1	0.29	3	0.06
Atresia/agenesis of colon	3	0.13	0	—	0	—	3	0.06
Other gastrointestinal malformations	3	0.13	3	0.12	1	0.29	7	0.14

diverticulum (21). Altogether, 29.8% of the GIT malformations, affecting 130 children, were classified as minor; the rest were considered major.

As shown in Table 12.3, 28.9% of the children with a GIT malformation also had a malformation of another organ system. With the exception of pyloric stenosis, the overall rate of other malformations among children with specific GIT malformations was at least 3 times that of the total cohort.

Table 12.3

Joint Occurrence of Gastrointestinal Tract (GIT) Malformations with Other Classes of Malformations

	No. of Children	Central Nervous		Cardio-vascular		Musculo-skeletal		Respi-ratory		Genito-urinary		Eyes/Ears		Syndromes		Tumors		Any Non-GIT Malfor-mation	
		No.	%	No.	%	No.	%	No.	%	No.	%	No.	%	No.	%	No.	%	No.	%
Pyloric stenosis	95	2	2.1	0	—	0	—	1	1.1	1	1.1	1	1.1	1	1.1	1	1.1	5	5.3
Umbilical hernia	51	2	3.9	0	—	2	3.9	3	5.9	1	2.0	0	—	2	3.9	2	3.9	7	13.7
Anal atresia	26	6	23.1	1	3.8	5	19.2	8	30.8	13	50.0	1	3.8	6	23.1	1	3.8	17	65.4
Malrotation	25	7	28.0	0	—	9	36.0	9	36.0	7	28.0	0	—	6	24.0	6	24.0	17	68.0
None of the above	129	18	14.0	4	3.1	27	20.9	33	25.6	28	21.7	1	0.8	20	15.5	15	11.6	61	47.3
All gastrointestinal malformations	301	26	8.6	4	1.3	33	11.0	42	14.0	39	13.0	2	0.7	25	8.3	19	6.3	87	28.9

Risk Factors for Gastrointestinal Tract Malformations

Administrative Data

Duration of Pregnancy at Registration (Table 12.4) The rate of GIT malformations in children whose mothers registered for prenatal care in the first or second lunar month of pregnancy was almost twice as high as the rate in children of other mothers, giving a relative risk of 1.9.

Personal Characteristics of the Mother

Maternal Age at Registration (Table 12.5) The rate of GIT malformations was lowest in children born to young mothers and increased about 50% in children born to mothers aged 40 and above, giving relative risks of 0.6 and 1.6, respectively.

Mother's Socioeconomic Status (Table 12.6) There was no consistent association between socioeconomic status and the rate of GIT malformations. All relative risks were near unity, with one exception: among Puerto Ricans of the lowest socioeconomic grouping, the relative risk was 0.5.

Characteristics and Survival of the Offspring

Birthweight (Table 12.7) A large increase in the rate of GIT malformations was observed in children of low birthweight, for all ethnic groups. For birthweights under 1.5 kg, relative risks

Table **12.4**

Distribution of Children with Gastrointestinal Tract (GIT) Malformations by Duration of Pregnancy at Registration

Duration of Pregnancy at Registration (lunar months)	No. of Children	Children with GIT Malformations		Relative Risk
		No.	Rate/1,000	
1–2	1,091	12	11.0	1.9
3–8	41,956	242	5.8	1.0*
≥9	7,235	47	6.5	1.1

*Reference category

Table **12.5**

Distribution of Children with Gastrointestinal Tract (GIT) Malformations by Mother's Age at Registration

Mother's Age	No. of Children	Children with GIT Malformations		Relative Risk
		No.	Rate/1,000	
≤19	11,904	47	3.9	0.6
20–39	37,606	246	6.5	1.0*
≥40	772	8	10.4	1.6

*Reference category

Table **12.6**

Race-Specific Distribution of Children with Gastrointestinal Tract (GIT) Malformations by Mother's Socioeconomic Status (SES)

	SES (scale of 0–10)	No. of Children	Children with GIT Malformations		Relative Risk
			No.	Rate/1,000	
White	≤3.9	5,042	29	5.8	0.8
	4.0–7.9	13,172	98	7.4	1.0*
	≥8.0	4,132	38	9.2	1.2
	Unknown	465	3	6.5	0.9
Black	≤3.9	12,718	60	4.7	0.9
	4.0–7.9	10,512	56	5.3	1.0*
	≥8.0	445	2	4.5	0.8
	Unknown	355	2	5.6	1.1
Puerto Rican	≤3.9	1,860	5	2.7	0.5
	4.0–7.9	1,513	8	5.3	1.0*
	≥8.0	33	0	—	—
	Unknown	35	0	—	—

*Reference category

Table **12.7**

Race-Specific Distribution of Children with Gastrointestinal Tract (GIT) Malformations by Child's Birthweight

	Birthweight (grams)	No. of Children	Children with GIT Malformations		Relative Risk
			No.	Rate/1,000	
White	≤1,499	357	14	39.2	6.4
	1,500–1,999	288	10	34.7	5.7
	2,000–2,499	1,201	16	13.3	2.2
	≥2,500	20,965	128	6.1	1.0*
Black	≤1,499	602	15	24.9	6.9
	1,500–1,999	606	10	16.5	4.6
	2,000–2,499	2,259	20	8.9	2.5
	≥2,500	20,563	75	3.6	1.0*
Puerto Rican	≤1,499	57	1	17.5	6.0
	1,500–1,999	66	1	15.2	5.2
	2,000–2,499	244	2	8.2	2.8
	≥2,500	3,074	9	2.9	1.0*

*Reference category

ranged from 6.0 to 6.9; for those between 1.5 and 1.99 kg, the range was 4.6 to 5.7; for those between 2.0 and 2.49 kg, the range was 2.2 to 2.8.

Sex of Child (Table 12.8) The rate of GIT malformations was about 50% higher in boys.

Survival of the Child (Table 12.9) For stillbirth, relative risks were 11.6 and 11.9 among Whites and Blacks, respectively. For neonatal death, they were 11.9 and 16.9; for infant death, 14.6 and 24.1; and for childhood death, 5.2 and 6.2. It should be noted that the extremely high relative risks among Puerto Ricans were based on small numbers.

Table *12.8*

Distribution of Children with Gastrointestinal Tract (GIT) Malformations by Sex of Child

	No. of Children	Children with GIT Malformations		Relative Risk
		No.	Rate/1,000	
Male	25,542	184	7.2	1.5
Female	24,740	117	4.7	1.0*

*Reference category

Table *12.9*

Race-Specific Distribution of Children with Gastrointestinal Tract (GIT) Malformations by Survival of the Child

	Survival of Child	No. of Children	Children with GIT Malformations		Relative Risk
			No.	Rate/1,000	
White	Stillbirth	327	20	61.2	11.6
	Neonatal death	302	19	62.9	11.9
	Infant death	130	10	76.9	14.6
	Childhood death	91	3	33.0	6.2
	Survived	21,961	116	5.3	1.0*
Black	Stillbirth	407	14	34.4	11.9
	Neonatal death	450	22	48.9	16.9
	Infant death	229	16	69.9	24.1
	Childhood death	134	2	14.9	5.2
	Survived	22,810	66	2.9	1.0*
Puerto Rican	Stillbirth	64	3	46.9	30.8
	Neonatal death	54	5	92.6	61.7
	Infant death	25	0	—	—
	Childhood death	14	0	—	—
	Survived	3,284	5	1.5	1.0*

*Reference category

Reproductive History of the Mother

History of Prior Prematures (Table 12.10) The relative risk for women who had had two or more premature births was 1.4.

Prior Fetal or Neonatal Loss (Table 12.11) The relative risk for GIT malformations was increased in children born to mothers who had had a prior stillborn child (1.8) or a child who died within one month of birth (1.5).

Characteristics and Complications of the Pregnancy

Duration of Pregnancy (Table 12.12) The relative risk for GIT malformations increased as duration of pregnancy decreased. For a pregnancy of 7 to 8 lunar months gestation, the relative risk was 3.0; for 5 to 6 lunar months, it was 3.5. For a pregnancy which lasted 11 months or longer, the relative risk was also elevated (1.6).

Table **12.10**

Distribution of Children with Gastrointestinal Tract (GIT) Malformations by History of Prior Premature Births

No. of Prior Premature Births	No. of Children	Children with GIT Malformations		Relative Risk
		No.	Rate/1,000	
None[1]	26,707	158	5.9	1.0*
1	5,443	24	4.4	0.7
≥2	2,578	21	8.1	1.4
No prior liveborn	15,554	98	6.3	1.1

*Reference category
[1]Includes 952 unknowns

Table **12.11**

Distribution of Children with Gastrointestinal Tract (GIT) Malformations by History of Prior Fetal or Neonatal Loss

	No. of Children	Children with GIT Malformations		Relative Risk
		No.	Rate/1,000	
Prior stillbirth	2,837	28	9.9	1.8
No prior stillbirth[1]	32,280	178	5.5	1.0*
No prior pregnancies 20 weeks or over	15,165	95	6.3	1.1
Prior neonatal death	2,174	18	8.3	1.5
No prior neonatal death[2]	32,554	185	5.7	1.0*
No prior liveborn	15,554	98	6.3	1.1

*Reference category
[1]Includes 179 unknowns
[2]Includes 947 unknowns

Table **12.12**

Distribution of Children with Gastrointestinal Tract (GIT) Malformations by Duration of Pregnancy

Length of Gestation (lunar months)	No. of Children	Children with GIT Malformations		Relative Risk
		No.	Rate/1,000	
5–6	559	10	17.9	3.5
7–8	3,292	50	15.2	3.0
9–10	45,436	233	5.1	1.0*
≥11	995	8	8.0	1.6

*Reference category

Placental Weight (Table 12.13) There was evidence of a monotonic relationship between decreasing placental weight and GIT malformation rates. The relative risks for placental weights of less than 200 gm and 200 to 299 gm were 6.2 and 2.5, respectively.

Number of Umbilical Arteries (Table 12.14) The relative risk for GIT malformations in children with single umbilical artery was 12.1.

Signs of Toxemia (Table 12.15) Among a total of 1,621 pregnancies complicated by hypertension, there were 15 children with GIT malformations (relative risk, 1.5). One of these was born to an eclamptic mother.

Various Complications of Pregnancy (Table 12.16) The relative risk for vaginal bleeding during the first and second trimesters was 1.5. Substantially elevated relative risks were seen for hydramnios (6.5) and hemorrhagic shock (10.3).

Placental Factors (Table 12.17) All of the factors listed in the table had elevated relative risks. They included marginal sinus rupture (2.1), abruptio placentae (4.0), placenta previa (3.8), and large placental infarct (1.8).

Maternal Diabetes (Table 12.18) The rate of GIT malformations was increased for both treated (relative risk, 5.2) and untreated maternal diabetes (relative risk, 2.4 — based on 2 malformed children).

Other Diseases of the Mother (Table 12.19) Syphilis, mostly inactive (relative risk, 1.5), urinary tract infection with

Table **12.13**

Distribution of Children with Gastrointestinal Tract (GIT) Malformations by Placental Weight

Placental Weight (grams)	No. of Children	Children with GIT Malformations		Relative Risk
		No.	Rate/1,000	
≤199	388	13	33.5	6.2
200–299	2,095	28	13.4	2.5
≥300	41,385	225	5.4	1.0*
Unknown	6,414	35	5.5	1.0

*Reference category

Table **12.14**

Distribution of Children with Gastrointestinal Tract (GIT) Malformations by Number of Umbilical Arteries

No. of Umbilical Arteries	No. of Children	Children with GIT Malformations		Relative Risk
		No.	Rate/1,000	
One	341	23	67.4	12.1
Two or unknown	49,941	278	5.6	1.0*

*Reference category

Table **12.15**

Distribution of Children with Gastrointestinal Tract (GIT) Malformations by Signs of Toxemia[1]

	No. of Children	Children with GIT Malformations		Relative Risk
		No.	Rate/1,000	
Eclampsia and/or any hypertension	1,621	15	9.3	1.5
Proteinuria	1,213	6	4.9	0.8
Generalized edema	11,425	65	5.7	1.0
None	36,023	215	6.0	1.0*

*Reference category
[1]This classification is hierarchical and based on severity—for example, a pregnancy complicated by hypertension is classified as such, even though proteinuria and edema may also be present.

Table **12.16**

Distribution of Children with Gastrointestinal Tract (GIT) Malformations by Various Complications of Pregnancy

	No. of Children	Children with GIT Malformations		Relative Risk*
		No.	Rate/1,000	
Vaginal Bleeding				
1st trimester	3,668	31	8.5	1.5
2nd trimester	2,546	21	8.3	1.5
3rd trimester	6,980	42	6.0	1.1
Hydramnios	694	25	36.0	6.5
Hemorrhagic shock	99	6	60.6	10.3

*For each condition, the reference category consists of those without that condition.

171

Table **12.17**

Distribution of Children with Gastrointestinal Tract (GIT) Malformations by Placental Factors

| | No. of Children | Children with GIT Malformations | | Relative Risk* |
		No.	Rate/1,000	
Marginal sinus rupture	639	8	12.5	2.1
Abruptio placentae	1,030	23	22.3	4.0
Placenta previa	317	7	22.1	3.8
Placental infarct				
≥ 3 cm diameter	1,501	16	10.7	1.8

*For each condition, the reference category consists of those without that condition.

Table **12.18**

Distribution of Children with Gastrointestinal Tract (GIT) Malformations Classified by Maternal Diabetes Mellitus

| | No. of Children | Children with GIT Malformations | | Relative Risk |
		No.	Rate/1,000	
Treated diabetes	194	6	30.9	5.2
Untreated diabetes				
or keto-acidosis	142	2	14.1	2.4
No diabetes	49,946	293	5.9	1.0*

*Reference category

Table **12.19**

Distribution of Children with Gastrointestinal Tract (GIT) Malformations by Selected Diseases of the Mother During Pregnancy

| | No. of Children | Children with GIT Malformations | | Relative Risk* |
		No.	Rate/1,000	
Syphilis	918	8	8.7	1.5
Urinary tract infection				
(fever ≥ 100.4°F)	709	9	12.7	2.2
Convulsive disorder	294	5	17.0	2.9

*For each disease, the reference category consists of those without that disease.

fever (2.2), and convulsive disorder (2.9) were all positively associated with GIT malformations.

Environmental Factors

Pelvic or Abdominal X-Ray Exposure During Pregnancy (Table 12.20) GIT malformations were somewhat more common in children who were exposed *in utero* to radiation of the mother's pelvis or abdomen (relative risk, 1.3).

Genetic Factors

Family History of Malformation (Table 12.21) A family history of congenital malformation was positively associated with GIT malformations. The relative risks, given malformations in the child's father or mother and cardiovascular malformations in prior siblings, were 1.9, 1.5, and 3.1, respectively. Other malformations in prior siblings were not related to GIT malformations.

Rh and ABO Incompatibility and Erythroblastosis (Table 12.22) Elevated relative risks were seen for erythroblastosis (Rh — 2.5, ABO — 2.1) and Rh incompatibility (2.1). The relative risks were also elevated for erythroblastosis (6.3) and exchange transfusion (2.2) in prior siblings. However, only the relative risk for Rh incompatibility was based on substantial numbers of exposed and malformed children.

Table **12.20**

Distribution of Children with Gastrointestinal Tract (GIT) Malformations by Pelvic and/or Abdominal X-Ray Exposure During Pregnancy

Pelvic and/or Abdominal X-Ray Exposure	No. of Children	Children with GIT Malformations		Relative Risk
		No.	Rate/1,000	
Present	11,400	81	7.1	1.3
Absent	38,882	220	5.7	1.0*

*Reference category

Table **12.21**

Distribution of Children with Gastrointestinal Tract (GIT) Malformations by Family History of Malformation

	No. of Children	Children with GIT Malformations		Relative Risk*
		No.	Rate/1,000	
Congenital malformation in child's mother	1,168	13	11.1	1.9
Congenital malformation in child's father	664	6	9.0	1.5
Cardiovascular malformation in a prior sibling	329	6	18.2	3.1

*For each of the above, the reference category consists of those with a negative family history.

Table **12.22**

Distribution of Children with Gastrointestinal Tract (GIT) Malformations Classified by Rh and ABO Incompatibility and Erythroblastosis

		No. of Children	Children with GIT Malformations		Relative Risk
			No.	Rate/1,000	
Erythroblastosis	Present (Rh)	266	4	15.0	2.5
	Present (ABO)[1]	162	2	12.4	2.1
	Absent/unknown	49,854	295	5.9	1.0*
Rh incompatibility	Present	3,286	39	11.9	2.1
	Absent/unknown	46,996	262	5.6	1.0*
Prior erythroblastosis	Present	53	2	37.7	6.3
	Absent/unknown	50,229	299	6.0	1.0*
Prior exchange transfusion	Present	232	3	12.9	2.2
	Absent/unknown	50,050	298	6.0	1.0*

*Reference category
[1]Includes seven cases of varieties of erythroblastosis other than Rh or ABO.

Table **12.23**

Factors Related to the Risk of Malformations of the Gastrointestinal Tract (GIT) Based Upon Multiple Logistic Risk Function Analysis

	Estimated Risk Function Coefficient	Standard Error of Coefficient	Estimated Standardized Relative Risk
Single umbilical artery	2.19	0.24	8.8
Birthweight < 1,500 gm	1.63	0.24	5.4
Hydramnios	1.55	0.23	4.7
Hemorrhagic shock	1.00	0.52	2.6
Convulsive disorder	0.94	0.46	2.5
Rh incompatibility	0.74	0.18	2.2
Maternal age ≥ 40	0.68	0.29	2.0
Malformation in parent; heart malformation in prior sibling	0.64	0.21	1.9
Abruptio placentae	0.57	0.24	1.8
Urinary tract infection (fever ≥ 100.4°F)	0.56	0.35	1.8
Syphilis	0.53	0.37	1.7
Duration of pregnancy ≥ 11 lunar months	0.47	0.36	1.6
Diabetes	0.47	0.41	1.6
Gestational age at registration < 3 lunar months	0.46	0.30	1.6
Male sex	0.44	0.12	1.6
White ethnic group	0.33	0.12	1.4
Placenta previa	0.33	0.44	1.4
Placental infarcts ≥ 3 cm	0.33	0.27	1.4
Toxemia (hypertension, eclampsia)	0.22	0.27	1.2
Placental weight < 200 gm	0.15	0.34	1.2

Multivariate Analysis

Based on the preceding comparisons, 27 risk factors were selected and scaled as binary or ordinal variables. A linear discriminant function analysis was applied to evaluate them jointly. The following variables were eliminated from further consideration because of low coefficients: socioeconomic status, prior fetal loss, prior premature children, vaginal bleeding during pregnancy, marginal sinus rupture, prenatal X-ray exposure, and exchange transfusion in a prior sibling.

The relation of the remaining 20 factors to GIT malformations is presented in Table 12.23. Variables with a relative risk greater than 3 were single umbilical artery (8.8), birthweight under 1,500 gm (5.4), and hydramnios (4.7). The association of each of these variables with GIT malformations was statistically significant. Variables with a relative risk between 2 and 3 were hemorrhagic shock (2.6), convulsive disorder (2.5), Rh incompatibility (2.2), and maternal age of 40 or above (2.0). The last three in this category were statistically significant. Of the remaining variables, malformation in a family member (1.9), abruptio placentae (1.8), male sex (1.6), and White ethnic group (1.4) were statistically significant.

As seen in Table 12.24, stratification of the 301 children with a GIT malformation according to the percentile of risk score showed good agreement between the observed and expected numbers of children with malformations. The ratio of numbers in the top decile of risk to the numbers in the lowest decile is over 19, indicating that the model is satisfactory in discriminating between degrees of risk.

Table *12.24*

Distribution of Observed and Expected Numbers of Children with Gastrointestinal Tract (GIT) Malformations by Multiple Logistic Risk Function Scores

Risk Score Percentile[1]	Observed Number of Children with GIT Malformations	Expected Number of Children with GIT Malformations
99–100	46	55.3
97–98	26	21.0
95–96	22	14.8
93–94	10	11.6
91–92	14	10.5
Subtotal (91–100)	118	113.2
81–90	31	38.6
71–80	36	28.1
61–70	27	26.2
51–60	22	20.2
41–50	18	19.4
31–40	19	17.4
21–30	11	14.8
11–20	13	12.5
1–10	6	10.6
Total	301	301.0

[1]Each decile contains 5,025 pregnancies, except the lowest which contains 5,057 pregnancies.

CHAPTER **13**

Malformations of the Genitourinary System

Among the 50,282 children, 366 were diagnosed as having at least one malformation of the genitourinary system (GUS) other than urethral obstruction for a total of 463 GUS malformations. In Table 13.1 the more common specific defects are listed together with a broad categorization of the less common malformations; the latter are presented in more detail in Table 13.2. From Table 13.1 it is clear that by far the most common specific defect was hypospadias, occurring in 188 of the affected children (51.4%), followed by polycystic kidney (33 children, 9.0%), stenotic ureter (26 children, 7.1%), hydronephrosis (23 children, 6.3%), and hydroureter (21 children, 5.7%). Of the affected children, 65 had some other malformation of the urinary tract (17.8%); 37 had a malformation of the male genitalia other than hypospadias (10.1%); and 43 had malformations of the female genitalia (11.7%). A large number of genitourinary malformations affected less than 20 children (Table 13.2). Urethral obstruction, which affected 68 children, is considered separately in Chapter 17.

Hypospadias, hydrocele, and sundry other malformations of the genitalia — for instance, chordee (3 cases) among male infants, and vaginal tag (7 cases) and labial adhesions (10 cases) among females — were classified as minor (a total of 226 cases, 61.7% of all children with GUS malformations other than urethral obstruction). The rest were classified as

176

Table **13.1**

Genitourinary Malformation Rates Classified by Ethnic Group (Rates per Thousand)

Malformation	White (n=22,811)		Black (n=24,030)		Puerto Rican (n=3,441)		Total (n=50,282)	
	No.	Rate	No.	Rate	No.	Rate	No.	Rate
Hypospadias	95	4.16	83	3.50	9	2.62	188	3.74
Polycystic kidney	13	0.57	20	0.83	0	—	33	0.66
Stenotic ureter	15	0.66	11	0.46	0	—	26	0.52
Hydronephrosis	12	0.53	11	0.46	0	—	23	0.46
Hydroureter	12	0.53	9	0.37	0	—	21	0.42
Other malformations of the urinary system[1]	30	1.32	32	1.33	3	0.87	65	1.29
Other malformations of male genitalia[1]	22	0.96	12	0.50	3	0.87	37	0.74
Minor malformations of female genitalia	16	0.70	5	0.21	1	0.29	22	0.44
Other malformations of female genitalia[1]	15	0.66	6	0.25	0	—	21	0.42
Any genitourinary malformation	189	8.29	161	6.70	16	4.65	366	7.28

[1]See Table 13.2 for details of these categories.
Note: Urethral obstruction is not included; it is presented in Chapter 17.

Table **13.2**

Rare Genitourinary Malformation Rates Classified by Ethnic Group (Rates per Thousand)

Malformation	White (n=22,811)		Black (n=24,030)		Puerto Rican (n=3,441)		Total (n=50,282)	
	No.	Rate	No.	Rate	No.	Rate	No.	Rate
Hypoplastic kidney	6	0.26	9	0.37	0	—	15	0.30
Malformations of bladder/ureter	6	0.26	6	0.25	1	0.29	13	0.26
Absence of one or both kidneys	6	0.26	5	0.21	2	0.58	13	0.26
Undescended testes	9	0.39	3	0.12	0	—	12	0.24
Double collecting system	4	0.18	6	0.25	1	0.29	11	0.22
Absent ureter	3	0.13	5	0.21	2	0.58	10	0.20
Hydrocele	2	0.09	6	0.25	2	0.58	10	0.20
Horseshoe kidney	6	0.26	2	0.08	0	—	8	0.16
Abnormal ovary	6	0.26	2	0.08	0	—	8	0.16
Recto-fistula	4	0.18	3	0.12	0	—	7	0.14
Some miscellaneous uterine malformations	3	0.13	4	0.17	0	—	7	0.14
Major malformations of the female external genitalia	3	0.13	3	0.12	0	—	6	0.12
Minor malformations of the male genitalia	5	0.22	1	0.04	0	—	6	0.12
Malposition/ectopic kidney	2	0.09	3	0.12	0	—	5	0.10
Ambiguous genitalia	4	0.18	0	—	1	0.29	5	0.10
Hypoplasia of penis	3	0.13	1	0.04	0	—	4	0.08
Mullerian malfusion	4	0.18	0	—	0	—	4	0.08
Other testicular malformations	2	0.09	1	0.04	0	—	3	0.06
Other kidney malformations	2	0.09	0	—	0	—	2	0.04

major (147 children, 7 having both a major and a minor defect).

GUS malformations were somewhat less common in Blacks than in Whites (6.7 per 1,000 against 8.3 per 1,000; and still less common in Puerto Ricans (4.6 per 1,000). The difference in rates between Whites and Blacks was mainly due to the higher frequency of malformations of the genitalia among the former, particularly defects other than hypospadias (2.3 per 1,000 in Whites, 1.0 per 1,000 in Blacks).

Minor GUS malformations tended to occur in isolation (i.e., without concomitant malformations of either the genitourinary system or any other). Only five children with hypospadias had another GUS malformation, four of which were some malformation of the male genitalia. Two of six children with minor malformations of the male genitalia other than hydrocele or hypospadias had a urinary malformation as well, but all the minor anomalies of the female genitalia occurred singly except in one case where a respiratory system malformation was also present.

On the other hand, many of the children with major GUS malformations were multiply afflicted, both with other GUS defects and with anomalies in other classes. With respect to the joint occurrence of more than one malformation within the genitourinary system, it was generally true that at least half of the children with a specific major GUS malformation or subgroup of such malformations had at least one other major GUS malformation. There were two exceptions: none of the 8 children with horseshoe kidney and only 1 of the 11 children with a double collecting system had an additional GUS malformation.

As shown in Table 13.3, malformations of the GUS were commonly associated with malformations elsewhere. Two exceptions were hypospadias and minor malformations of the female genitalia. Of the remainder, at least 40% of the affected children had malformations affecting

other systems. For major malformations of the female genitalia, this proportion was 81%. In general, with the exceptions noted above, genitourinary anomalies were prominent indicators of widespread congenital malformations.

Hypospadias is overwhelmingly a condition affecting male infants (although there was one diagnosis of hypospadias in a female) and, as pointed out above, tends to occur in isolation. Therefore we decided to examine the effect of drugs on hypospadias only in those pregnancies resulting in a male birth and to consider GUS malformations other than hypospadias, together with the one female case of hypospadias, as a separate outcome. As noted earlier, the overlap is only five cases. We were strengthened in our decision by the observation that hypospadias had a different set of risk factors than the remaining GUS malformations. Therefore, the expression "GUS malformations" will, in the next two sections, refer to genitourinary malformations other than hypospadias and urethral obstruction; hypospadias will be treated separately in later sections of this chapter.

Risk Factors for GUS Malformations Other Than Hypospadias

Administrative Data

Duration of Pregnancy at Registration (Table 13.4) The GUS malformation rate was elevated in pregnancies registered in the first two lunar months, giving a relative risk of 2.2.

Number of Antenatal Visits (Table 13.5) The relative risk for mothers who attended for antenatal care fewer than five times during their pregnancies was 1.7.

Personal Characteristics of the Mother

Ethnic Group (Table 13.6) The GUS malformation rates were somewhat higher in Whites (relative risk, 1.3), and

Table 13.3

Joint Occurrence of Malformations in Classes Other Than the Genitourinary System (GUS) in Children with Common GUS Malformations

	No. of Children	Central Nervous		Cardio-vascular		Musculo-skeletal		Respiratory		Gastro-intestinal		Eye/Ear		Syndromes		Tumors		Any Non-GUS Malformation	
		No.	%	No.	%	No.	%	No.	%	No.	%	No.	%	No.	%	No.	%	No.	%
Hypospadias	188	2	1.1	2	1.1	2	1.1	3	1.6	0	—	1	0.5	1	0.5	1	0.5	11	5.9
Polycystic kidney	33	6	18.2	7	21.2	10	30.3	12	36.4	9	27.3	3	9.1	5	15.2	1	3.0	22	66.7
Stenotic ureter	26	5	19.2	6	23.1	5	19.2	4	15.4	5	19.2	0	—	1	3.8	0	—	11	42.3
Hydronephrosis	23	7	30.4	6	26.1	6	26.1	6	26.1	8	34.8	0	—	6	26.1	1	4.3	17	73.9
Minor malformations of female genitalia	22	0	—	0	—	0	—	1	4.5	0	—	0	—	0	—	0	—	1	4.5
Hydroureter	21	6	28.6	4	19.0	4	19.0	5	23.8	6	28.6	0	—	5	23.8	2	9.5	16	76.2
Other malformations of the urinary system	65	10	15.4	14	21.5	14	21.5	13	20.0	21	32.3	3	4.6	4	6.2	3	4.6	38	58.5
Other malformations of male genitalia	37	6	16.2	4	10.8	5	13.5	7	18.9	5	13.5	0	—	2	5.4	0	—	15	40.5
Major malformations of female genitalia	21	6	28.6	8	38.1	7	33.3	10	47.6	9	42.9	2	9.5	8	38.1	1	4.8	17	81.0
Any genitourinary malformation	366	28	7.7	34	9.3	30	8.2	36	9.8	39	10.7	6	1.6	21	5.7	6	1.6	97	26.5

179

Table **13.4**

Distribution of Children with Genitourinary System (GUS) Malformations Other Than Hypospadias by Duration of Pregnancy at Registration

Duration of Pregnancy at Registration (lunar months)	No. of Children	Children with GUS Malformations		Relative Risk
		No.	Rate/1,000	
1–2	1,091	9	8.2	2.2
3–8	41,956	154	3.7	1.0*
≥9	7,235	21	2.9	0.8

*Reference category

Table **13.5**

Distribution of Children with Genitourinary System (GUS) Malformations Other Than Hypospadias by Number of Antenatal Visits

No. of Antenatal Visits	No. of Children	Children with GUS Malformations		Relative Risk
		No.	Rate/1,000	
1–4	8,624	49	5.7	1.7
5–9	20,964	70	3.3	1.0*
≥10	20,694	65	3.1	0.9

*Reference category

Table **13.6**

Distribution of Children with Genitourinary System (GUS) Malformations Other Than Hypospadias by Ethnic Group

	No. of Children	Children with GUS Malformations		Relative Risk
		No.	Rate/1,000	
White	22,811	98	4.3	1.3
Black	24,030	79	3.3	1.0*
Puerto Rican	3,441	7	2.0	0.6

*Reference category

somewhat lower in Puerto Ricans (relative risk, 0.6), than they were in Blacks.

Mother's Age at Registration (Table 13.7) For ages up to 39 years, the GUS malformation rates were relatively stable, and it was only beyond that age that there was an increase. Among mothers aged 40 years or more, there were seven children with GUS malformations, giving a relative risk of 2.3.

Characteristics and Survival of the Offspring

Birthweight (Table 13.8) Decreasing birthweight in all three ethnic groups showed a striking monotonic relationship to the GUS malformation rate. The relative risks ranged from 9.1 to 14.4 for children weighing less than 2 kg, and from 2.0 to 7.7 for those weighing 2 to 2.5 kg.

Table **13.7**

Distribution of Children with Genitourinary System (GUS) Malformations Other Than Hypospadias by Mother's Age at Registration

Mother's Age	No. of Children	Children with GUS Malformations		Relative Risk
		No.	Rate/1,000	
≤14	429	0	—	—
15–19	11,475	40	3.5	0.9
20–24	18,475	73	4.0	1.0*
25–29	10,592	32	3.0	0.8
30–34	5,655	20	3.5	0.9
35–39	2,884	12	4.2	1.1
≥40	772	7	9.1	2.3

*Reference category

Table **13.8**

Race-Specific Distribution of Children with Genitourinary System (GUS) Malformations Other Than Hypospadias by Child's Birthweight

	Birthweight (grams)	No. of Children	Children with GUS Malformations		Relative Risk
			No.	Rate/1,000	
White	≤1,999	645	23	35.7	14.4
	2,000–2,499	1,201	23	19.2	7.7
	≥2,500	20,965	52	2.5	1.0*
Black	≤1,999	1,208	24	19.9	9.1
	2,000–2,499	2,259	10	4.4	2.0
	≥2,500	20,563	45	2.2	1.0*
Puerto Rican	≤1,999	123	2	16.3	12.5
	2,000–2,499	244	1	4.1	3.1
	≥2,500	3,074	4	1.3	1.0*

*Reference category

Birth Order (Table 13.9) For Whites, the relative risk for GUS malformations was 1.5 among firstborn children. No such association was noted in Blacks or Puerto Ricans. The rates in both major ethnic groups were somewhat elevated among children with birth order greater than five (relative risks, 1.4 for Whites, 1.3 for Blacks).

Survival of the Child (Table 13.10) GUS malformations other than hypospadias were frequently associated with the death of the child. Fully 20% of the affected children were stillborn; 27% died during the neonatal period, and an additional 8% died thereafter; less than half the children (45%) survived the early years of life. The relative risks among the three ethnic groups given stillbirth, neonatal death, infant death, and childhood death ranged from 12.8 to 30.7, 15.2 to 40.9, 16.1 to 32.8, and 5.5 to 10.1, respectively. The associations with childhood death were all based on at most two malformed children, while all the findings for Puerto Ricans were based on one malformed child.

Reproductive History of the Mother

Prior Premature Births (Table 13.11) The GUS malformation rate was elevated in children of White mothers who had previously given birth to premature children, giving a relative risk of 2.4. No association was evident in the other two ethnic groups.

Prior Fetal Loss (Table 13.12) The relative risks for GUS malformations among the offspring of mothers with a history of prior abortion or stillbirth were 1.5 and 1.8, respectively.

Prior Neonatal Death (Table 13.13) The GUS malformation rate was elevated among offspring of White mothers with a history of prior neonatal death (relative risk, 4.9); this was not the case in the other ethnic groups. Among White women delivering their first liveborn child, the relative risk was 1.8.

Characteristics and Complications of the Pregnancy

Duration of Pregnancy (Table 13.14) For both Whites and Blacks, the rates

Table **13.9**

Race-Specific Distribution of Children with Genitourinary System (GUS) Malformations Other Than Hypospadias by Birth Order of Child

	Birth Order[1]	No. of Children	Children with GUS Malformations		Relative Risk
			No.	Rate/1,000	
White	1	7,388	40	5.4	1.5
	2–5	13,446	48	3.6	1.0*
	⩾6	1,977	10	5.1	1.4
Black	1	6,740	20	3.0	0.9
	2–5	13,603	44	3.2	1.0*
	⩾6	3,687	15	4.1	1.3
Puerto Rican	1	1,038	2	1.9	0.8
	2–5	2,095	5	2.4	1.0*
	⩾6	308	0	0.0	—

*Reference category
[1]Determined by number of prior liveborn and stillborn siblings

182

Table **13.10**

Race-Specific Distribution of Children with Genitourinary System (GUS) Malformations Other Than Hypospadias by Survival of the Child

	Survival of Child	No. of Children	Children with GUS Malformations		Relative Risk
			No.	Rate/1,000	
White	Stillbirth	327	19	58.1	26.6
	Neonatal death	302	23	76.2	34.8
	Infant death	130	6	46.2	21.1
	Childhood death	91	2	22.0	10.1
	Survived	21,961	48	2.2	1.0*
Black	Stillbirth	407	17	41.8	30.7
	Neonatal death	450	25	55.6	40.9
	Infant death	229	5	21.8	16.1
	Childhood death	134	1	7.5	5.5
	Survived	22,810	31	1.4	1.0*
Puerto Rican	Stillbirth	64	1	15.6	12.8
	Neonatal death	54	1	18.5	15.2
	Infant death	25	1	40.0	32.8
	Childhood death	14	0	—	—
	Survived	3,284	4	1.2	1.0*

*Reference category

Table **13.11**

Race-Specific Distributions of Children with Genitourinary System (GUS) Malformations Other Than Hypospadias by History of Prior Premature Births

		No. of Children	Children with GUS Malformations		Relative Risk
			No.	Rate/1,000	
White	Prior prematures	2,547	18	7.1	2.4
	Prior births not premature[1]	12,715	38	3.0	1.0*
	No prior liveborn	7,549	42	5.6	1.9
Black	Prior prematures	4,930	17	3.4	1.0
	Prior births not premature[2]	12,162	41	3.4	1.0*
	No prior liveborn	6,938	21	3.0	0.9
Puerto Rican	Prior prematures	544	1	1.8	0.8
	Prior births not premature[3]	1,830	4	2.2	1.0*
	No prior liveborn	1,067	2	1.9	0.9

*Reference category
[1]Includes 439 unknowns
[2]Includes 491 unknowns
[3]Includes 22 unknowns

Table **13.12**

Distribution of Children with Genitourinary System (GUS) Malformations Other Than Hypospadias by History of Prior Fetal Loss

	No. of Children	Children with GUS Malformations		Relative Risk
		No.	Rate/1,000	
Prior abortion	9,135	43	4.7	1.5
No prior abortion[1]	26,979	86	3.2	1.0*
No prior pregnancy	14,168	55	3.9	1.2
Prior stillbirth	2,837	17	6.0	1.8
No prior stillbirth[2]	32,280	105	3.3	1.0*
No prior pregnancies 20 weeks or over	15,165	62	4.1	1.3

*Reference category
[1]Includes 108 unknowns
[2]Includes 179 unknowns

were considerably increased for pregnancies lasting less than eight lunar months, giving relative risks of 6.2 and 4.2, respectively.

Placental Weight (Table 13.15) The table shows that there was a monotonic relationship between decreasing placental weight and GUS malformation rates.

The relative risks for children with placentae weighing less than 200 gm and 200 to 399 gm were, respectively, 13.8 and 2.0.

Single Umbilical Artery (Table 13.16) The relative risk for GUS malformations in children with single umbilical artery was 18.8.

Table **13.13**

Race-Specific Distribution of Children with Genitourinary System (GUS) Malformations Other Than Hypospadias by History of Prior Neonatal Loss

		No. of Children	Children with GUS Malformations		Relative Risk
			No.	Rate/1,000	
White	Prior neonatal death	805	12	14.9	4.9
	No prior neonatal death[1]	14,457	44	3.0	1.0*
	No prior liveborn	7,549	42	5.6	1.8
Black	Prior neonatal death	1,226	5	4.1	1.2
	No prior neonatal death[2]	15,866	53	3.3	1.0*
	No prior liveborn	6,938	21	3.0	0.9
Puerto Rican	Prior neonatal death	143	0	—	—
	No prior neonatal death[3]	2,231	5	2.2	1.0*
	No prior liveborn	1,067	2	1.9	0.8

*Reference category
[1]Includes 437 unknowns
[2]Includes 490 unknowns
[3]Includes 20 unknowns

Table **13.14**

Race-Specific Distribution of Children with Genitourinary System (GUS) Malformations Other Than Hypospadias by Duration of Pregnancy

	Length of Gestation (lunar months)	No. of Children	Children with GUS Malformations		Relative Risk
			No.	Rate/1,000	
White	5–8	1,074	23	21.4	6.2
	≥9	21,737	75	3.5	1.0*
Black	5–8	2,501	26	10.4	4.2
	≥9	21,529	53	2.5	1.0*
Puerto Rican	5–8	276	0	—	—
	≥9	3,165	7	2.2	1.0*

*Reference category

Table **13.15**

Distribution of Children with Genitourinary System (GUS) Malformations Other Than Hypospadias by Placental Weight

Placental Weight (grams)	No. of Children	Children with GUS Malformations		Relative Risk
		No.	Rate/1,000	
≤199	388	14	36.1	13.8
200–399	15,210	78	5.1	2.0
≥400	28,270	74	2.6	1.0*
Unknown	6,414	18	2.8	1.1

*Reference category

Table **13.16**

Distribution of Children with Genitourinary System (GUS) Malformations Other Than Hypospadias by Number of Umbilical Arteries

No. of Umbilical Arteries	No. of Children	Children with GUS Malformations		Relative Risk
		No.	Rate/1,000	
One	341	21	61.6	18.8
Two	44,851	147	3.3	1.0*
Unknown	5,090	16	3.1	1.0

*Reference category

Signs of Toxemia (Table 13.17) In the table the GUS malformation rates for each of the categories forming this syndrome are displayed. The data suggest that symptoms not including hypertension were only weak risk factors (relative risk, 1.2). For two hypertensive categories (excluding eclampsia) the relative risks were 2.2 and 1.8.

Various Complications of Pregnancy (Table 13.18) Nineteen children whose mothers had hydramnios had GUS malformations, giving a relative risk of 8.2. Four children whose mothers had hemorrhagic shock while pregnant had GUS

malformations, giving a relative risk of 11.3.

Placental Factors (Table 13.19) All conditions listed in the table were associated to some degree with a higher risk of having a child with a GUS malformation. The relative risks for marginal sinus rupture, abruptio placentae, placenta previa, and large placental infarct were 3.5, 2.7, 3.5, and 1.7, respectively.

Weight Change During Pregnancy (Table 13.20) The relative risk for GUS malformations among the children of mothers who gained less than 7.5 kg during pregnancy was 1.6. The relative risk was also

Table **13.17**

Distribution of Children with Genitourinary System (GUS) Malformations Other Than Hypospadias by Signs of Toxemia[1]

	No. of Children	Children with GUS Malformations		Relative Risk
		No.	Rate/1,000	
Eclampsia	22	0	—	—
Chronic hypertension	669	4	6.0	1.8
Acute hypertension (BP $\geq$ 160/110 after LM 6)	930	7	7.5	2.2
Proteinuria	1,213	5	4.1	1.2
Generalized edema	11,425	47	4.1	1.2
None	36,023	121	3.4	1.0*

*Reference category
[1]This classification is hierarchical and based on severity—for example, a pregnancy complicated by chronic hypertension is classified as such, even though proteinuria and edema may also be present.

Table **13.18**

Distribution of Children with Genitourinary System (GUS) Malformations Other Than Hypospadias by Various Complications of Pregnancy

	No. of Children	Children with GUS Malformations		Relative Risk*
		No.	Rate/1,000	
Hydramnios	694	19	27.4	8.2
Hemorrhagic shock	99	4	40.4	11.3

*For each condition, the reference category consists of those without that condition.

186

Table **13.19**

Distribution of Children with Genitourinary System (GUS) Malformations Other Than
Hypospadias by Placental Factors

| | No. of Children | Children with GUS Malformations | | Relative Risk* |
		No.	Rate/1,000	
Marginal sinus rupture	639	8	12.5	3.5
Abruptio placentae	1,030	10	9.7	2.7
Placenta previa	318	4	12.6	3.5
Placental infarct ≥ 3 cm diameter	1,501	9	6.0	1.7

*For each condition, the reference category consists of those without that condition.

Table **13.20**

Distribution of Children with Genitourinary System (GUS) Malformations Other Than
Hypospadias by Weight Change During Pregnancy

| Weight Change (kg) | No. of Children | Children with GUS Malformations | | Relative Risk |
		No.	Rate/1,000	
Gained ≤ 7.4	12,894	64	5.0	1.6
Gained ≥ 7.5	35,521	109	3.1	1.0*
Unknown	1,867	11	5.9	1.9

*Reference category

higher in the group with unknown values for this factor (1.9).

Anemia (Table 13.21) The GUS malformation rate was slightly increased in children of White and Puerto Rican anemic mothers (relative risk, 1.3). By contrast, the rate was decreased among children of Black women with anemia (relative risk, 0.4).

Selected Diseases of the Mother (Table 13.22) Eight mothers who had treated diabetes gave birth to children with GUS malformations (relative risk, 11.7). Only one child with a GUS malformation was born to a mother with untreated diabetes of short duration. The relative risks for GUS malformations were elevated among children whose mothers had urinary tract infections (2.0) or bacterial infections in the second or third trimester (1.9).

Environmental Factors

Pelvic or Abdominal X-Ray Exposure During Pregnancy (Table 13.23) Exposure to pelvic or abdominal X-rays was related to the risk of GUS malformations (relative risk, 1.5).

Genetic Factors

Family History of Malformations (Table 13.24) Malformations in either of the parents showed no evidence of association with GUS malformations. The rate was somewhat higher among children with at least one sibling affected by congenital heart disease (relative risk, 1.8)

Table **13.21**

Race-Specific Distribution of Children with Genitourinary System (GUS) Malformations Other Than Hypospadias by Mother's Anemia During Pregnancy

	Anemia	No. of Children	Children with GUS Malformations		Relative Risk
			No.	Rate/1,000	
White	Present	2,213	12	5.4	1.3
	Absent	20,598	86	4.2	1.0*
Black	Present	8,299	14	1.7	0.4
	Absent	15,731	65	4.1	1.0*
Puerto Rican	Present	1,249	3	2.4	1.3
	Absent	2,192	4	1.8	1.0*

*Reference category

Table **13.22**

Distribution of Children with Genitourinary System (GUS) Malformations Other Than Hypospadias by Selected Diseases of the Mother During Pregnancy

	No. of Children	Children with GUS Malformations		Relative Risk*
		No.	Rate/1,000	
Treated diabetes	194	8	41.2	11.7
Urinary tract infection (fever ≥ 100.4°F)	709	5	7.1	2.0
Bacterial infection in 2nd and/or 3rd trimester	899	6	6.7	1.9

*For each disease, the reference category consists of those without that disease.

Table **13.23**

Distribution of Children with Genitourinary System (GUS) Malformations Other Than Hypospadias by Pelvic and/or Abdominal X-Ray Exposure During Pregnancy

Pelvic and/or Abdominal X-Ray Exposure	No. of Children	Children with GUS Malformations		Relative Risk
		No.	Rate/1,000	
Present	11,400	56	4.9	1.5
Absent	38,882	128	3.3	1.0*

*Reference category

188

Table **13.24**

Distribution of Children with Genitourinary System (GUS) Malformations Other Than Hypospadias by History of Selected Malformations in Prior Siblings

	No. of Children	Children with GUS Malformations		Relative Risk
		No.	Rate/1,000	
Prior sibling(s) with congenital heart disease[1]	662	4	6.0	1.8
Prior sibling(s) with other miscellaneous malformations[1]	1,797	10	5.6	1.6
Prior sibling(s) not malformed[2]	31,393	106	3.4	1.0*
First born	15,166	62	4.1	1.2

*Reference category
[1]Includes children whose sibling malformation histories are uncertain
[2]Includes 780 unknowns

and among those with at least one sibling recorded as having one of a miscellaneous set of malformations which includes GUS malformations (relative risk, 1.6).

Multivariate Analysis

Twenty-seven of the factors described above were scaled as binary or ordinal variables and were subjected to linear discriminant function analysis. Eleven were eliminated by this procedure, their coefficients having been reduced to low values by the presence of the other covariates. The omitted factors were ethnic group, low number of antenatal visits, histories of prior abortion, stillbirth, or premature births, signs of toxemia, abruptio placentae, large placental infarcts, small weight change, and histories of siblings with heart or other malformations. The remaining factors are listed in Table 13.25.

Factors with relative risks greater than 3 included the following, all of which were statistically significant: single umbilical artery (10.8), low birthweight (9.9), hydramnios (5.0), and diabetes mellitus in its more serious forms (4.5). Hemorrhagic shock during pregnancy (2.5), prior neonatal death (among Whites only) (2.2), and early registration (2.0) had rela-

tive risks between 2 and 3. Only the finding for prior neonatal death was statistically significant. Of the remaining factors, only White firstborn child (1.8), and anemia in Blacks (0.5) had statistically significant relative risks.

The mother-child pairs were ordered according to risk score for GUS malformations; Table 13.26 shows the resulting distribution. Comparing observed and expected numbers of affected children within the strata shows agreement to be good. The ratio of the numbers in the top decile of risk to the numbers in the lowest decile is over 15, suggesting that the model leads to good discrimination between degrees of risk.

Risk Factors for Hypospadias

Administrative Data

Hospital (Table 13.27) The hypospadias rate among children of Black mothers at Johns Hopkins University, Medical College of Virginia, and University of Tennessee was considerably lower than the rate for the remaining institutions, giving a relative risk of 0.3. This pattern did not hold true for Whites, and there was only one Puerto Rican child at the above three institutions.

189

Table **13.25**

Factors Related to the Risk of Genitourinary System (GUS) Malformations Other Than Hypospadias Based on Multiple Logistic Risk Function Analysis

	Estimated Risk Function Coefficient	Standard Error of Coefficient	Estimated Standardized Relative Risk
Single umbilical artery	2.38	0.27	10.8
Birthweight < 2,000 gm	2.29	0.28	9.9
Hydramnios	1.60	0.28	5.0
Treated maternal diabetes	1.49	0.43	4.5
Hemorrhagic shock during pregnancy	0.93	0.62	2.5
At least one prior neonatal death (Whites only)	0.77	0.33	2.2
Duration of pregnancy at registration < 3 lunar months	0.69	0.35	2.0
Placental weight < 200 gm	0.64	0.34	1.9
Mother's age ≥ 40 years	0.63	0.40	1.9
Firstborn child (White only)	0.56	0.19	1.8
Marginal sinus rupture	0.44	0.39	1.5
Bacterial infection in 2nd or 3rd trimester of pregnancy	0.34	0.44	1.4
Urinary tract infection (fever ≥ 100.4°F)	0.30	0.48	1.4
Pelvic and/or abdominal X-ray exposure during pregnancy	0.18	0.17	1.2
Duration of pregnancy ≤ 8 lunar months	−0.34	0.26	0.7
Anemia (Blacks only)	−0.75	0.29	0.5

Duration of Pregnancy at Registration (Table 13.28) The relative risk for hypospadias in pregnancies registered in the first two lunar months was 0.2. Among pregnancies registered between three and four lunar months, the relative risk was 0.7.

Number of Antenatal Visits (Table 13.29) The relative risk for children of mothers who attended for antenatal care at least 15 times during their pregnancies was 0.5.

Personal Characteristics of the Mother

Ethnic Group (Table 13.30) The rate of hypospadias was highest among White children and lowest among Puerto Rican children.

Marital Status (Table 13.31) The relative risk for hypospadias among the sons of widowed and divorced women was 2.2.

Ponderal Index (Table 13.32) In children of mothers whose ponderal index was less than 1.9, the relative risk for hypospadias was 1.5.

Characteristics and Survival of the Offspring

Birthweight (Table 13.33) Decreasing birthweight in Whites and Puerto Ricans showed a monotonic relationship to the hypospadias rate. The trend was less clear in Blacks. The relative risks ranged from 2.3 to 11.0 for children weighing less than 2 kg, and from 1.9 to 5.3 for those weighing 2 to 2.5 kg. The findings for Puerto Ricans were based on small numbers.

Birth Order (Table 13.34) The hypospadias rate among firstborn children was elevated compared with the rate among children whose birth order was two or more, giving a relative risk of 1.2.

Survival of the Child (Table 13.35) Hypospadias was not very strongly associated with early death, if at all. Some 3% of the affected children were stillborn (relative risk, 2.0); 1% died

Table **13.26**

Distribution of Observed and Expected Numbers of Children with Genitourinary System (GUS) Malformations (Other Than Hypospadias) by Multiple Logistic Risk Function Scores

Risk Score Percentile[1]	Observed Number of Children with GUS Malformations	Expected Number of Children with GUS Malformations
99–100	47	49.1
97–98	16	16.7
95–96	15	11.2
93–94	11	7.6
91–92	5	6.4
Subtotal (91–100)	94	91.0
81–90	19	20.5
71–80	12	14.8
61–70	13	11.1
51–60	10	10.1
41–50	6	9.0
31–40	6	8.3
21–30	11	8.3
11–20	7	6.9
1–10	6	4.0
Total	184	184.0

[1]Each decile contains 5,025 pregnancies, except the lowest which contains 5,057 pregnancies.

Table **13.27**

Race-Specific Distribution of Male Children with Hypospadias by Institution

	Location of Institution	No. of Children	Male Children with Hypospadias		Relative Risk
			No.	Rate/1,000	
White	Baltimore, MD Richmond, VA Memphis, TN	799	6	7.5	0.9
	All others	10,964	89	8.1	1.0*
Black	Baltimore, MD Richmond, VA Memphis, TN	4,152	13	3.1	0.3
	All others	7,886	70	8.9	1.0*
Puerto Rican	Baltimore, MD Richmond, VA Memphis, TN	1	0	—	—
	All others	1,740	9	5.2	1.0*

*Reference category

191

Table **13.28**

Distribution of Male Children with Hypospadias by Duration of Pregnancy at Registration

Duration of Pregnancy at Registration (lunar months)	No. of Children	Male Children with Hypospadias		Relative Risk
		No.	Rate/1,000	
1–2	535	1	1.9	0.2
3–4	6,226	36	5.8	0.7
≥5	18,781	150	8.0	1.0*

*Reference category

Table **13.29**

Distribution of Male Children with Hypospadias by Number of Antenatal Visits

No. of Antenatal Visits	No. of Children	Male Children with Hypospadias		Relative Risk
		No.	Rate/1,000	
1–4	4,403	34	7.7	1.0
5–14	19,246	146	7.6	1.0*
≥15	1,893	7	3.7	0.5

*Reference category

Table **13.30**

Distribution of Male Children with Hypospadias by Ethnic Group

	No. of Children	Male Children with Hypospadias		Relative Risk
		No.	Rate/1,000	
White	11,763	95	8.1	1.0*
Black	12,038	83	6.9	0.9
Puerto Rican	1,741	9	5.2	0.6

*Reference category

Table **13.31**

Distribution of Male Children with Hypospadias by Mother's Marital Status

Marital Status	No. of Children	Male Children with Hypospadias		Relative Risk
		No.	Rate/1,000	
Single	3,782	27	7.1	1.0
Married[1]	19,702	143	7.3	1.0*
Separated	1,629	10	6.1	0.8
Widowed or Divorced	429	7	16.3	2.2

*Reference category
[1]Includes common-law marriages

Table **13.32**

Distribution of Male Children with Hypospadias According to the Prepregnant Ponderal Index of the Mother

Ponderal Index (weight × 1,000)/(height)^2	No. of Children	Male Children with Hypospadias		Relative Risk
		No.	Rate/1,000	
≤1.9	1,837	20	10.9	1.5
≥2.0	22,356	161	7.2	1.0*
Unknown	1,349	6	4.4	0.6

*Reference category

Table **13.33**

Race-Specific Distribution of Male Children with Hypospadias by Child's Birthweight

	Birthweight (grams)	No. of Children	Male Children with Hypospadias		Relative Risk
			No.	Rate/1,000	
White	<2,000	326	9	27.6	3.8
	2,000–2,499	498	7	14.1	1.9
	≥2,500	10,939	79	7.2	1.0*
Black	<2,000	600	8	13.3	2.3
	2,000–2,499	965	13	13.5	2.3
	≥2,500	10,473	62	5.9	1.0*
Puerto Rican	<2,000	57	2	35.1	11.0
	2,000–2,499	118	2	16.9	5.3
	≥2,500	1,566	5	3.2	1.0*

*Reference category

Table **13.34**

Distribution of Male Children with Hypospadias by Birth Order of Child

		Male Children with Hypospadias		
Birth Order[1]	No. of Children	No.	Rate/1,000	Relative Risk
1	7,733	65	8.4	1.2
≥2	17,809	122	6.9	1.0*

*Reference category
[1]Determined by number of prior liveborn and stillborn siblings

Table **13.35**

Distribution of Male Children with Hypospadias by Survival of the Child

		Male Children with Hypospadias		
Survival of Child	No. of Children	No.	Rate/1,000	Relative Risk
Stillbirth	414	6	14.5	2.0
Neonatal death	453	2	4.4	0.6
Infant death	234	4	17.1	2.6
Childhood death	137	1	7.3	1.0
Survived	24,304	174	7.2	1.0*

*Reference category

during the neonatal period (relative risk, 0.6); a further 2% died as infants (relative risk, 2.6).

Reproductive History of the Mother

Prior Fetal or Neonatal Loss (Table 13.36) There was no evidence that prior stillbirth increased the risk of hypospadias. For prior neonatal death, however, the relative risk was 1.9, while for prior abortion it was 1.3.

Characteristics and Complications of the Pregnancy

Duration of Pregnancy (Table 13.37) For pregnancies lasting 8 lunar months, relative risks were 1.8 (Whites) and 1.4 (Blacks). For those of 5 to 7 months duration, relative risks were 2.6 (Whites) and 1.7 (Blacks). In Puerto Ricans, the relative risk for pregnancies of 8 lunar months duration was 8.7 (based on 3 children with hypospadias). For pregnancies lasting 11 lunar months or more, the rates were again somewhat higher in both Whites and Blacks (relative risks, 1.2 and 2.0, respectively).

Placental Weight (Table 13.38) The relative risk for hypospadias in children whose placental weight was below 300 gm was 1.8.

Vaginal Bleeding (Table 13.39) The hypospadias rate was increased in children of mothers who bled during the third trimester (relative risk, 1.6).Bleeding at other times during pregnancy did not appear to be related to this outcome.

Placental Factors (Table 13.40) Of the

Table **13.36**

Distribution of Male Children with Hypospadias by History of Prior Fetal or Neonatal Loss

	No. of Children	Male Children with Hypospadias		Relative Risk
		No.	Rate/1,000	
Prior abortion	4,626	39	8.4	1.3
No prior abortion[1]	13,695	89	6.5	1.0*
No prior pregnancy	7,221	59	8.2	1.3
Prior stillbirth	1,408	10	7.1	1.0
No prior stillbirth[2]	16,402	112	6.8	1.0*
No prior pregnancies 20 weeks or over	7,732	65	8.4	1.2
Prior neonatal death	134	14	12.3	1.9
No prior neonatal death[3]	16,494	106	6.4	1.0*
No prior liveborn	7,914	67	8.5	1.3

*Reference category
[1]Includes 48 unknowns
[2]Includes 81 unknowns
[3]Includes 470 unknowns

Table **13.37**

Race-Specific Distribution of Male Children with Hypospadias by Duration of Pregnancy

	Length of Gestation (lunar months)	No. of Children	Male Children with Hypospadias		Relative Risk
			No.	Rate/1,000	
White	5–7	200	4	20.0	2.6
	8	355	5	14.1	1.8
	9–10	10,986	84	7.6	1.0*
	≥11	222	2	9.0	1.2
Black	5–7	461	5	10.8	1.7
	8	771	7	9.1	1.4
	9–10	10,576	68	6.4	1.0*
	≥11	230	3	13.0	2.0
Puerto Rican	5–7	34	0	—	—
	8	91	3	33.0	8.7
	9–10	1,574	6	3.8	1.0*
	≥11	42	0	—	—

*Reference category

Table **13.38**

Distribution of Male Children with Hypospadias by Placental Weight

| Placental Weight (grams) | No. of Children | Male Children with Hypospadias | | Relative Risk |
		No.	Rate/1,000	
≤299	1,205	15	12.4	1.8
≥300	21,094	147	7.0	1.0*
Unknown	3,243	25	7.7	1.1

*Reference category

Table **13.39**

Distribution of Male Children with Hypospadias by Vaginal Bleeding During Pregnancy

| Vaginal Bleeding | No. of Children | Male Children with Hypospadias | | Relative Risk |
		No.	Rate/1,000	
1st trimester	1,866	13	7.0	1.0
2nd trimester	1,292	6	4.6	0.7
3rd trimester	3,579	39	10.9	1.6
None	18,805	129	6.9	1.0*

*Reference category

Table **13.40**

Distribution of Male Children with Hypospadias by Placental Factors

| | No. of Children | Male Children with Hypospadias | | Relative Risk* |
		No.	Rate/1,000	
Marginal sinus rupture	362	1	2.8	0.4
Abruptio placentae	540	9	16.7	2.3
Placenta previa	153	1	6.5	0.9
Placental infarcts ≥ 3 cm in diameter	829	8	9.7	1.3

*For each condition, the reference category consists of those without that condition.

factors listed in the table, only abruptio placentae and large placental infarcts were associated with a higher risk of having a child with hypospadias, with relative risks of 2.3 and 1.3, respectively.

Environmental Factors

Cigarette Smoking (Table 13.41) Hypospadias was not related to light or moderate smoking in pregnancy. However, there was evidence of association in women who smoked 30 or more cigarettes per day. Among these heavy smokers, the relative risk was 2.0.

Rubella Exposure (Table 13.42) The relative risk for hypospadias among the offspring of mothers exposed to rubella in the third trimester was 2.8; among those whose mothers were exposed during the second trimester, it was 1.3.

Genetic Factors

Family History of Malformations (Table 13.43) Malformations in the mothers were associated with a slightly increased hypospadias rate (relative risk, 1.6). Among children with at least one malformed sibling, the relative risk was slightly elevated (1.2).

Multivariate Analysis

Based on the foregoing comparisons, 18 factors were selected for multivariate analysis and scaled as binary or ordinal variables. After linear discriminant

Table **13.41**

Distribution of Male Children with Hypospadias by Maternal Cigarette Smoking

Cigarette Smoking (no./day)	No. of Children	Male Children with Hypospadias		Relative Risk
		No.	Rate/1,000	
Never/Ex/Uncertain	14,515	108	7.4	1.0*
≤14	6,495	38	5.9	0.8
15–29	3,603	27	7.5	1.0
≥30	929	14	15.1	2.0

*Reference category

Table **13.42**

Distribution of Male Children with Hypospadias by Maternal Exposure to Rubella Infection During Pregnancy

Rubella Exposure	No. of Children	Male Children with Hypospadias		Relative Risk
		No.	Rate/1,000	
1st trimester	273	0	—	—
2nd trimester	427	4	9.4	1.3
3rd trimester	297	6	20.2	2.8
None	24,545	177	7.2	1.0*

*Reference category

Table **13.43**

Distribution of Male Children with Hypospadias by History of Malformations in the Mother or Prior Siblings

| | No. of Children | Male Children with Hypospadias | | Relative Risk* |
		No.	Rate/1,000	
Malformation in mother	608	7	11.5	1.6
Malformation in at least one prior sibling	1,881	16	8.5	1.2

*For each of the above, the reference category consists of those with a negative family history.

function analysis, 3 factors were eliminated because of low coefficients: low placental weight, large placental infarcts, and family history of malformations. The results of the multiple logistic regression analysis for the remaining 15 variables are listed in Table 13.44.

The only factor with a relative risk greater than 3 was low birth weight (3.8); this result was statistically significant. Relative risks between 2 and 3 were found for exposure to rubella in the third trimester of pregnancy (2.9) and mother widowed or divorced (2.0); the former result was statistically significant. Relative risks for the following factors were also statistically significant: vaginal bleeding in the third trimester of pregnancy (1.5), firstborn child (1.4), and Black born at certain hospitals (0.3).*

*Hypospadias was considered with the uniform malformations because by the $\chi^2_{(22)}$ = test, its occurrence by ethnic group and hospital did not vary significantly.

Table **13.44**

Factors Related to the Risk of Hypospadias Based Upon Multiple Logistic Risk Function Analysis

	Estimated Risk Function Coefficient	Standard Error of Coefficient	Estimated Standardized Relative Risk
Birthweight < 2,000 gm	1.33	0.33	3.8
Exposure to rubella in 3rd trimester of pregnancy	1.07	0.42	2.9
Mother widowed or divorced	0.67	0.40	2.0
Fewer than 15 antenatal visits	0.60	0.40	1.8
Cigarette smoking ≥ 30 per day during pregnancy	0.55	0.28	1.7
At least one prior neonatal death	0.53	0.29	1.7
Duration of pregnancy ≥ 11 lunar months	0.43	0.46	1.5
Vaginal bleeding in 3rd trimester of pregnancy	0.42	0.18	1.5
Gestational age at registration > 4 lunar months	0.36	0.19	1.4
Abruptio placentae	0.36	0.37	1.4
Ponderal index < 2.0	0.32	0.24	1.4
Firstborn child	0.32	0.16	1.4
Duration of pregnancy < 9 lunar months	−0.34	0.33	0.7
Puerto Rican	−0.45	0.35	0.6
Black born at Baltimore, MD, Richmond, VA, Memphis, TN	−1.10	0.29	0.3

The mother-child pairs were ordered according to risk score for hypospadias. Table 13.45 shows the resulting distribution. Comparison of the observed and expected numbers within each stratum of risk indicates that there is reasonable agreement between the numbers of children with hypospadias predicted on the basis of the summed risks for the pregnancies constituting the strata and the numbers of cases actually observed. In addition, the ratio of the numbers in the top decile of risk to the numbers in the lowest decile is over 8, indicating that the model is satisfactory in discriminating between degrees of risk.

Table **13.45**

Distribution of Observed and Expected Numbers of Male Children with Hypospadias by Multiple Logistic Risk Function Scores

Risk Score Percentile[1]	Observed Number of Male Children with Hypospadias	Expected Number of Male Children with Hypospadias
99–100	15	17.3
97–98	14	10.5
95–96	9	8.5
93–94	10	7.3
91–92	4	6.4
Subtotal (91–100)	52	50.0
81–90	29	26.5
71–80	18	21.8
61–70	18	18.6
51–60	11	15.8
41–50	20	15.8
31–40	11	14.1
21–30	12	10.8
11–20	10	8.3
1–10	6	5.3
Total	187	187.0

[1]Each decile contains 2,550 pregnancies, except the lowest which contains 2,592 pregnancies.

CHAPTER 14

Malformations of the Eye and Ear

Congenital malformations of the eye and ear were observed in 121 children in the study cohort of 50,282 (2.4 per 1,000). In all, the 121 children had 137 anomalies affecting the eye and ear systems, 4% of the 3,291 malformations reported. Table 14.1 lists the race-specific distributions of the malformation entities involving these systems. By far the most commonly observed eye and ear defects were cataracts, which affected 44 children (36.4%), and pre-auricular skin tags, found in 38 children (31.4%). In terms of frequency of occurrence, these defects were followed by coloboma (10.7%), anophthalmia/microphthalmia (9.1%), glaucoma/buphthalmos (8.3%), absent or abnormal external meatus (7.4%), corneal opacity (6.6%), and other eye malformations (3.3%).

Although there were only 12 (9.9%) Puerto Rican children out of the 121 who had an eye or ear malformation, the rates for this ethnic group were the highest in each of the three malformation categories in which they occurred. In general, eye and ear malformations were more commonly recorded in Puerto Ricans (3.5 per 1,000), while Whites and Blacks had similar overall rates (2.4 per 1,000 and 2.3 per 1,000, respectively).

There were 47 children who had malformations involving the auditory system. None of these children had an anomaly of the eye. Of the 121 children with eye or ear malformations, 70 (57.8%)

Table **14.1**

Eye and Ear Malformation Rates Classified by Ethnic Group (Rates per Thousand)

Malformation	White (n=22,811)		Black (n=24,030)		Puerto Rican (n=3,441)		Total (n=50,282)	
	No.	Rate	No.	Rate	No.	Rate	No.	Rate
Cataract	23	1.01	17	0.71	4	1.16	44	0.88
Pre-auricular skin tag	11	0.48	20	0.83	7	2.03	38	0.76
Coloboma	8	0.35	5	0.21	0	—	13	0.26
Anophthalmia/microphthalmia	3	0.13	6	0.25	2	0.58	11	0.22
Glaucoma/buphthalmos	4	0.18	6	0.25	0	—	10	0.20
Absent/abnormal external meatus	5	0.22	4	0.17	0	—	9	0.18
Corneal opacity	5	0.22	3	0.12	0	—	8	0.16
Other eye malformations	2	0.09	2	0.08	0	—	4	0.08
Any eye and/or ear malformation	54	2.37	55	2.29	12	3.49	121	2.41

had defects considered to be major, 7 (5.8%) had both major and minor defects, and 44 (36.4%) had minor malformations only. All defects except pre-auricular skin tag and coloboma were classified as major.

There were 13 (10.7%) children who had multiple eye malformations; none of the 47 children who had an ear anomaly (absent/abnormal external meatus or pre-auricular skin tag) had multiple defects affecting this system. Table 14.2 gives the joint distribution of the more common eye and ear malformations in relation to the other classes of malformations. In the group of children with cataracts (44), 31.8% had anomalies affecting systems other than the eye and ear; of these, 8 (18.2%) involved the cardiovascular system. There were 13 cases of coloboma, 6 (46.2%) of which occurred in children with a variety of other malformations. This was also true in the case of 7 (63.6%) of the 11 offspring with anophthalmia/microphthalmia. Altogether, 31 (25.6%) of the 121 children had both eye or ear malformations and other anomalies. In marked contrast to defects involving the eye, there were only 2 children with malformations of both the ear and other anatomical systems.

Risk Factors for Eye and Ear Malformations

Administrative Data

Ordinal Number of Entry (Table 14.3) Among the offspring of 8,486 mothers who entered the study more than twice, there were 30 eye or ear malformations, resulting in a relative risk of 1.6.

Duration of Pregnancy at Registration (Table 14.4) For White mother-child pairs entering the study before the seventh month of pregnancy, the risk of an eye or ear malformation was increased, giving relative risks of 1.2 for those five to six months pregnant and 1.5 for those less than five months pregnant. Among Black and Puerto Rican mothers, however, the risk was less if they entered the study before the seventh month.

Number of Antenatal Visits (Table 14.5) The relative risk for eye and ear malformations in children whose mothers visited the prenatal clinics fewer than five times during pregnancy was 1.3.

Personal Characteristics of the Mother

Religion (Table 14.6) The rates of eye and ear malformations were higher for Roman Catholics in all three ethnic groups; in Whites, the observed relative risk was 1.6, and in Blacks, it was 1.7. In

Table *14.2*

Joint Occurrence of Malformations in Classes Other Than the Eye and Ear (E/E) in Children with Common E/E Malformations

	No. of Children	Central Nervous		Cardio-vascular		Musculo-skeletal		Respi-ratory		Gastro-intestinal		Genito-urinary		Syndromes		Tumors		Any Non-E/E Malfor-mation	
		No.	%	No.	%	No.	%	No.	%	No.	%	No.	%	No.	%	No.	%	No.	%
Cataract	44	2	4.5	8	18.2	4	9.1	2	4.5	3	6.8	2	4.5	3	6.8	1	2.3	14	31.8
Pre-auricular skin tag	38	0	—	0	—	2	5.3	0	—	0	—	0	—	0	—	0	—	2	5.3
Coloboma	13	2	15.4	3	23.1	3	23.1	3	23.1	3	23.1	3	23.1	2	15.4	0	—	6	46.2
Anophthalmia/microphthalmia	11	4	36.4	3	27.3	4	36.4	3	27.3	2	18.2	1	9.1	2	18.2	0	—	7	63.6
Glaucoma/buphthalmos	10	2	20.0	1	10.0	1	10.0	0	—	0	—	0	—	1	10.0	0	—	3	30.0
Other eye and ear malformations	21	2	9.5	2	9.5	1	4.8	2	9.5	1	4.8	3	14.3	1	4.8	2	9.5	7	33.3
Any eye and ear malformations	121	10	8.3	10	8.3	10	8.3	5	4.1	4	3.3	6	5.0	6	5.0	3	2.5	31	25.6

Table **14.3**

Distribution of Children with Eye/Ear (E/E) Malformations by Ordinal Number of Entry into the Study

Ordinal Number of Entry	No. of Children	Children with E/E Malformations		Relative Risk
		No.	Rate/1,000	
1	41,796	91	2.2	1.0*
≥2	8,486	30	3.5	1.6

*Reference category

Table **14.4**

Race-Specific Distribution of Children with Eye/Ear (E/E) Malformations by Duration of Pregnancy at Registration

	Duration of Pregnancy at Registration (lunar months)	No. of Children	Children with E/E Malformations		Relative Risk
			No.	Rate/1,000	
White	1–4	8,400	24	2.9	1.5
	5–6	6,526	15	2.3	1.2
	≥7	7,885	15	1.9	1.0*
Black	1–4	4,269	8	1.9	0.7
	5–6	8,557	19	2.2	0.9
	≥7	11,204	28	2.5	1.0*
Puerto Rican	1–4	766	1	1.3	0.2
	5–6	1,286	2	1.6	0.2
	≥7	1,389	9	6.5	1.0*

*Reference category

Table **14.5**

Distribution of Children with Eye/Ear (E/E) Malformations by Number of Antenatal Vists

No. of Antenatal Visits	No. of Children	Children with E/E Malformations		Relative Risk
		No.	Rate/1,000	
1–4	8,624	26	3.0	1.3
5–9	20,964	48	2.3	1.0*
≥10	20,694	47	2.3	1.0

*Reference category

Table **14.6**

Race-Specific Distribution of Children with Eye/Ear (E/E) Malformations by Mother's Religion

		No. of Children	Children with E/E Malformations		Relative Risk
			No.	Rate/1,000	
White	Roman Catholic	11,943	34	2.8	1.6
	Other[1]	10,868	20	1.8	1.0*
Black	Roman Catholic	2,833	10	3.5	1.7
	Other[2]	21,197	45	2.1	1.0*
Puerto Rican	Roman Catholic	3,136	11	3.5	1.1
	Other[3]	305	1	3.3	1.0*

*Reference category
[1]Includes 396 unknowns
[2]Includes 211 unknowns
[3]Includes 20 unknowns

Puerto Ricans the increased risk was negligible.

Characteristics and Survival of the Offspring

Birthweight (Table 14.7) For Whites, Blacks, and Puerto Ricans, the rate of eye and ear malformations increased as the child's birthweight decreased. The relative risks in the lowest birthweight category ranged from 2.9 to 7.2. The relative risks for birthweight between 2,000 and 2,999 gm ranged from 1.2 to 3.3.

Birth Order (Table 14.8) Among the 35,116 children whose birth ranking was second or more, there were 95 with eye or

Table **14.7**

Race-Specific Distribution of Children with Eye/Ear (E/E) Malformations by Child's Birthweight

	Birthweight (grams)	No. of Children	Children with E/E Malformations		Relative Risk
			No.	Rate/1,000	
White	≤1,999	645	4	6.2	2.9
	2,000–2,999	5,664	15	2.6	1.2
	≥3,000	16,502	35	2.1	1.0*
Black	≤1,999	1,208	9	7.5	7.2
	2,000–2,999	9,283	32	3.4	3.3
	≥3,000	13,539	14	1.0	1.0*
Puerto Rican	≤1,999	123	1	8.1	2.9
	2,000–2,999	1,156	5	4.3	1.6
	≥3,000	2,162	6	2.8	1.0*

*Reference category

Table **14.8**

Distribution of Children with Eye/Ear (E/E) Malformations by Birth Order

Birth Order[1]	No. of Children	Children with E/E Malformations		Relative Risk
		No.	Rate/1,000	
1	15,166	26	1.7	1.0*
≥2	35,116	95	2.7	1.6

*Reference category
[1]Determined by number of prior liveborn and stillborn siblings

ear malformations, with a relative risk of 1.6.

Reproductive History of the Mother
Prior Premature Births (Table 14.9) There was an increased risk of eye and ear malformations as the number of prior premature births increased. The relative risk of malformation for those whose mothers had a history of two or more such births was 1.9; for those whose mothers had a single prior premature birth, the relative risk was 1.2.

Characteristics and Complications of the Pregnancy
Duration of Pregnancy (Table 14.10) The relative risk for eye and ear malformations among offspring of mothers whose pregnancy lasted between five and eight lunar months was 2.6.

Placental Weight (Table 14.11) Children whose placental weight was less than 300 gm had a relative risk of 2.6, while those whose placental weight was between 300 and 399 gm had a relative risk of 1.5.

Signs of Toxemia (Table 14.12) In general, there was an increased risk of eye and ear malformations in offspring of mothers who had signs of toxemia during pregnancy. With the exceptions of proteinuria and eclampsia, the relative risks for all the conditions in the table were elevated, ranging from 1.2 to 3.1. It should be noted that the results for conditions which included chronic hypertension were based on small numbers of malformed children.

Various Complications of Pregnancy (Table 14.13) The relative risks for vomiting during pregnancy, hyperemesis

Table **14.9**

Distribution of Children with Eye/Ear (E/E) Malformations by History of Prior Premature Births

No. of Prior Premature Births	No. of Children	Children with E/E Malformations		Relative Risk
		No.	Rate/1,000	
None[1]	26,707	66	2.5	1.0*
1	5,443	16	2.9	1.2
≥2	2,578	12	4.7	1.9*
No Prior Liveborn	15,554	27	1.7	0.7

*Reference category
[1]Includes 952 unknowns

Table **14.10**

Distribution of Children with Eye/Ear (E/E) Malformations by Duration of Pregnancy

Length of Gestation (lunar months)	No. of Children	Children with E/E Malformations		Relative Risk
		No.	Rate/1,000	
5–8	3,851	23	6.0	2.6
9	22,603	53	2.3	1.0*
≥10	23,828	45	1.9	0.8

*Reference category

Table **14.11**

Distribution of Children with Eye/Ear (E/E) Malformations by Placental Weight

Placental Weight (grams)	No. of Children	Children with E/E Malformations		Relative Risk
		No.	Rate/1,000	
≤299	2,483	13	5.2	2.6
300–399	13,115	40	3.0	1.5
≥400	34,684	68	2.0	1.0*

*Reference category

Table **14.12**

Distribution of Children with Eye/Ear (E/E) Malformations by Signs of Toxemia[1]

	No. of Children	Children with E/E Malformations		Relative Risk
		No.	Rate/1,000	
Eclampsia	22	0	—	—
Uncontrolled chronic hypertension (BP ≥ 160/110 after LM 6)	283	2	7.1	3.1
Controlled chronic hypertension (without BP ≥ 160/110 after LM 6)	386	1	2.6	1.2
Acute hypertension (BP ≥ 160/110 after LM 6)	930	5	5.4	2.4
Proteinuria	1,213	2	1.6	0.7
Generalized edema	11,425	30	2.6	1.2
None	36,023	81	2.2	1.0*

*Reference category
[1]This classification is hierarchical and based on severity—for example, a pregnancy complicated by uncontrolled chronic hypertension is classified as such, even though proteinuria and edema may also be present.

Table **14.13**

Distribution of Children with Eye/Ear (E/E) Malformations by Various Complications of Pregnancy

	No. of Children	Children with E/E Malformations		Relative Risk*
		No.	Rate/1,000	
Vomiting during pregnancy	33,341	86	2.6	1.2
Hyperemesis gravidarum	540	5	9.3	4.0
Vaginal bleeding				
1st trimester	3,668	12	3.3	1.4
2nd trimester	2,546	8	3.1	1.4
3rd trimester	6,980	15	2.2	0.9
Hydramnios	694	4	5.8	2.5

*For each condition, the reference category consists of those without that condition.

gravidarum, vaginal bleeding during the first and second trimesters, and hydramnios were 1.2, 4.0, 1.4, and 2.5, respectively.

Environmental Factors

Cigarette Smoking (Table 14.14) Eye and ear malformations were generally related to the smoking of cigarettes by the mother during pregnancy, but there was no consistent pattern of association. Except for the offspring of Blacks who smoked fewer than 15 cigarettes per day, the relative risk of the malformations was at least 1.3, and ranged as high as 2.1.

Pelvic or Abdominal X-Ray Exposure During Pregnancy (Table 14.15) There were 35 children with eye or ear malformations among the 11,400 who were exposed *in utero* to X-rays, giving a relative risk of 1.4.

Genetic Factors

History of Maternal or Paternal Malformations (Table 14.16) There was an increased risk of eye and ear malformations in children whose mothers had a congenital malformation (relative risk, 1.8), as well as in children whose fathers had a malformation (relative risk, 1.3 — based on two malformed children).

History of Malformations in Prior Siblings (Table 14.17) If the child had prior siblings with congenital malformations, the relative risk was 1.4.

Multivariate Analysis

Based on the foregoing comparisons, 19 variables were selected for multivariate analysis, and scaled as binary or ordinal variables. After linear discriminant function analysis, 8 variables were eliminated: duration of pregnancy at registration, low number of antenatal visits, history of prior premature births, low placental weight, vaginal bleeding, maternal cigarette smoking, maternal exposure to X-rays, and prior malformed siblings. The results of the multiple logistic regression analysis for the remaining 11 factors are given in Table 14.18.

Two factors had relative risks greater than 3: hyperemesis gravidarum (4.0) and birthweight under 2,500 gm (3.2). Both were statistically significant. Hydramnios had a relative risk of 2.3, but this finding was not statistically significant. Among the remaining factors, only the relative risk of 1.5 for Roman Catholic religion was statistically significant.

Table 14.19 gives the distribution of

Table **14.14**

Race-Specific Distribution of Children with Eye/Ear (E/E) Malformations by Maternal Cigarette Smoking

	Cigarette Smoking (no./day)	No. of Children	Children with E/E Malformations		Relative Risk
			No.	Rate/1,000	
White	Never/Ex/Uncertain	11,334	20	1.8	1.0*
	≤14	5,100	19	3.7	2.1
	≥15	6,377	15	2.4	1.3
Black	Never/Ex/Uncertain	14,776	34	2.3	1.0*
	≤14	7,026	13	1.9	0.8
	≥15	2,228	8	3.6	1.6
Puerto Rican	Never/Ex/Uncertain	2,487	7	2.8	1.0*
	≤14	698	4	5.7	2.0
	≥15	256	1	3.9	1.4

*Reference category

Table **14.15**

Distribution of Children with Eye/Ear (E/E) Malformations by Pelvic and/or Abdominal X-Ray Exposure During Pregnancy

Pelvic and/or Abdominal X-Ray Exposure	No. of Children	Children with E/E Malformations		Relative Risk
		No.	Rate/1,000	
Present	11,400	35	3.1	1.4
Absent	38,882	86	2.2	1.0*

*Reference category

Table **14.16**

Distribution of Children with Eye/Ear (E/E) Malformations by History of Maternal or Paternal Malformation

	No. of Children	Children with E/E Malformations		Relative Risk*
		No.	Rate/1,000	
Congenital malformation of child's mother	1,168	5	4.3	1.8
Congenital malformation of child's father	664	2	3.0	1.3

*For each of the above, the reference category consists of those with a negative parental history.

Table **14.17**

Distribution of Children with Eye/Ear (E/E) Malformations by History of Malformation in Prior Siblings

	No. of Children	Children with E/E Malformations		Relative Risk
		No.	Rate/1,000	
Congenital malformation in prior sibling(s)	3,723	14	3.8	1.4
Firstborn child	15,166	26	1.7	0.7
Prior siblings not malformed	30,613	80	2.6	1.0*

*Reference category

Table **14.18**

Factors Related to the Risk of Malformations of the Eye or Ear Based Upon Multiple Logistic Risk Function Analysis

	Estimated Risk Function Coefficient	Standard Error of Coefficient	Estimated Standardized Relative Risk
Hyperemesis gravidarum	1.39	0.46	4.0
Birthweight < 2,500 gm	1.15	0.27	3.2
Hydramnios	0.82	0.51	2.3
Hypertension or eclampsia	0.63	0.37	1.9
Parental malformations	0.51	0.39	1.7
Roman Catholic religion	0.41	0.19	1.5
Birth order > 1	0.41	0.23	1.5
More than one entry into study	0.38	0.22	1.5
Duration of pregnancy < 9 lunar months	0.33	0.28	1.4
White ethnic group	0.29	0.32	1.3
Vomiting during pregnancy	0.26	0.20	1.3

the 121 cases of eye or ear malformations in percentiles of risk estimated by multivariate techniques. There is generally good agreement between observed and expected numbers of malformations. Furthermore, the ratio (sixfold) between the numbers in the highest risk decile and those in the lowest risk decile shows that the model was successful in discriminating between those children who were at greatest risk of an eye or ear malformation and those who were at lowest risk.

*Table **14.19***

Distribution of Observed and Expected Numbers of Children with Eye/Ear (E/E) Malformations by Multiple Logistic Risk Function Scores

Risk Score Percentile[1]	Observed Number of Children with E/E Malformations	Expected Number of Children with E/E Malformations
99–100	11	12.3
97–98	11	7.6
95–96	6	6.1
93–94	6	5.4
91–92	2	4.7
Total (91–100)	36	36.1
81–90	14	18.6
71–80	20	13.9
61–70	10	11.3
51–60	11	9.9
41–50	5	8.2
31–40	9	6.9
21–30	7	6.6
11–20	3	5.3
1–10	6	4.2
Total	121	121.0

[1]Each decile contains 5,025 pregnancies, except the lowest which contains 5,057 pregnancies.

CHAPTER 15

Syndromes

Among the 50,282 children, there were 176 with syndrome malformations (3.5 per 1,000) with a total of 182 specific syndromes. The specific defects of this group are shown in Tables 15.1 and 15.2. One-third of the children with syndromes had Down syndrome and one-quarter had abnormalities of the adrenal gland. Each of the other syndromes was rare, with fewer than 17 children affected. As indicated in Table 15.1, the overall rates of syndromes were 4.0 per 1,000 in Whites, 3.1 per 1,000 in Blacks, and 2.9 per 1,000 in Puerto Ricans. Most of this difference was due to syndromes other than Down syndrome. The rates of Down syndrome among Whites and Blacks were 1.3 and 1.2 per 1,000, respectively. Only two Puerto Rican children were affected.

As shown in Table 15.3, children with syndromes frequently had malformations of other systems: 27% had malformations of the cardiovascular system, while 21% had malformations of the central nervous system; tumors and eye/ear malformations were the least common other malformations, occurring in approximately 3% of those with syndromes.

Of the children with adrenal atrophy or hypoplasia, 92% had a malformation of another system, primarily of the central nervous system (85%). Of the children with other chromosomal abnormalities, 89% had a musculoskeletal malformation. The only syndrome group in which fewer than 25% of the children had a

Table **15.1**

Syndrome Rates Classified by Ethnic Group (Rates per Thousand)

Syndrome	White (n=22,811)		Black (n=24,030)		Puerto Rican (n=3,441)		Total (n=50,282)	
	No.	Rate	No.	Rate	No.	Rate	No.	Rate
Down syndrome	30	1.32	29	1.21	2	0.58	61	1.21
Hypoplasia/atrophy adrenal	17	0.75	7	0.29	2	0.58	26	0.52
Other syndromes[1]	46	2.02	38	1.58	6	1.74	90	1.79
Any syndrome	92	4.03	74	3.08	10	2.91	176	3.50

[1]See Table 15.2 for details of this category.

Table **15.2**

Rare Syndrome Rates Classified by Ethnic Group (Rates per Thousand)

Syndrome	White (n=22,811)		Black (n=24,030)		Puerto Rican (n=3,441)		Total (n=50,282)	
	No.	Rate	No.	Rate	No.	Rate	No.	Rate
Situs inversus/dextrocardia	5	0.22	6	0.25	1	0.29	12	0.24
Inborn errors metabolism	0	—	7	0.29	2	0.58	9	0.18
Anomalies of thyroid	3	0.13	3	0.12	1	0.29	7	0.14
Caffey's	1	0.04	5	0.21	0	—	6	0.12
Albinism	1	0.04	3	0.12	1	0.29	5	0.10
Hypertrophy/enlarged adrenal	5	0.22	0	—	0	—	5	0.10
Miscellaneous other adrenal	12	0.53	4	0.17	0	—	16	0.32
Adrenogenital	2	0.09	1	0.04	1	0.29	4	0.08
Achondroplasia	2	0.09	2	0.08	0	—	4	0.08
Pierre Robin	2	0.09	1	0.04	0	—	3	0.06
Turner's	3	0.13	0	—	0	—	3	0.06
Other trisomies	4	0.18	1	0.04	0	—	5	0.10
Klinefelter's syndrome	1	0.04	0	—	0	—	1	0.02
Other miscellaneous syndromes	10	0.44	5	0.21	0	—	15	0.30

malformation of another system was inborn errors of metabolism, where only 2 of the 9 children (22%) had another malformation.

Since the risk factors for Down syndrome were quite different from those for the other syndromes, these two groups will be described separately. In the next two sections, the term "syndromes" will refer to syndromes excluding Down syndrome, found in 115 children.

Risk Factors for Syndromes Other Than Down Syndrome

Administrative Data

Number of Antenatal Visits (Table 15.4) The rate of syndromes was 40% higher in children whose mothers had fewer than five antenatal visits, giving a relative risk of 1.4.

Characteristics of the Mother

Ethnic Group (Table 15.5) The relative risks for syndromes excluding Down

Table **15.3**

Joint Occurrence of Malformations Other Than Syndromes in Children with Syndromes

	No. of Children	Central Nervous		Cardio-vascular		Musculo-skeletal		Respiratory		Gastro-intestinal		Genito-urinary		Eyes/Ears		Tumors		Any Malformations Other Than Syndromes	
		No.	%	No.	%	No.	%	No.	%	No.	%	No.	%	No.	%	No.	%	No.	%
Down syndrome	61	8	13.1	25	41.0	3	4.9	2	3.3	4	6.6	0	—	0	—	0	—	34	55.7
Adrenal atrophy/hypoplasia	26	22	84.6	3	11.5	1	3.9	10	38.5	5	19.2	3	11.5	1	3.9	1	3.9	24	92.3
Other adrenal	19	2	10.5	6	31.6	2	10.5	5	26.3	4	21.1	5	26.3	1	5.3	1	5.3	11	57.9
Situs inversus/dextrocardia	12	0	—	8	66.7	1	8.3	3	25.0	4	33.3	0	—	0	—	1	8.3	9	75.0
Inborn errors of metabolism	9	0	—	0	—	0	—	0	—	0	—	1	11.1	1	11.1	0	—	2	22.2
Other chromosomal abnormalities	9	1	11.1	6	66.7	8	88.9	5	55.5	2	22.2	3	33.3	2	22.2	0	—	8	88.9
Thyroid abnormalities	7	1	14.3	1	14.3	0	—	0	—	3	42.9	0	—	0	—	0	—	3	42.9
Other syndromes	37	4	10.8	1	2.7	11	29.7	6	16.2	1	2.7	5	13.5	2	5.4	2	5.4	18	48.7
All syndromes	176	37	21.0	48	27.3	25	14.2	29	16.5	19	10.8	21	11.9	6	3.4	5	2.8	105	59.7

Table **15.4**

Distribution of Children with Syndromes Excluding Down Syndrome by Number of Antenatal Visits

No. of Antenatal Visits	No. of Children	Children with Syndromes		Relative Risk
		No.	Rate/1,000	
1–4	8,624	26	3.0	1.4
5–9	20,964	43	2.1	1.0*
≥10	20,694	46	2.2	1.1

*Reference category

Table **15.5**

Distribution of Children with Syndromes Excluding Down Syndrome by Ethnic Group

	No. of Children	Children with Syndromes		Relative Risk
		No.	Rate/1,000	
White	22,811	62	2.7	1.4
Black	24,030	45	1.9	1.0*
Puerto Rican	3,441	8	2.3	1.2

*Reference category

syndrome were elevated for Whites (1.4) and Puerto Ricans (1.2).

Maternal Age at Registration (Table 15.6) The rate of syndromes was increased in children born to White mothers aged 30 and over, giving a relative risk of 1.5.

Religion (Table 15.7) The syndrome rate was higher in children born to White or Black mothers of the Catholic faith, giving relative risks of 1.6 and 1.5, respectively, but was not increased in Puerto Rican children whose mothers were Catholic. The relative risk was also increased for Blacks of other religions (2.1).

Characteristics of the Offspring

Birthweight (Table 15.8) There was a strong association of syndromes with low birthweight. This association was stronger in Whites, with relative risks ranging from 5.4 for 2,000 to 2,499 gm, to 14.8 for less than 1,500 gm. In Blacks and Puerto Ricans, the range was 1.3 to 7.6.

Survival of the Child (Table 15.9) Death of the child was strongly associated with the risk of having a syndrome. Relative risks for the various categories of death ranged from 40.8 to 77.2 in Whites, and from 9.6 to 25.1 in Blacks and Puerto Ricans.

Reproductive History of the Mother

Prior Premature Births (Table 15.10) There was an increase in the rate of syndromes in children whose mothers had given birth to a premature child (relative risk, 1.6).

Prior Fetal or Neonatal Loss (Table 15.11) The risk of having a child with a

214

Table **15.6**

Race-Specific Distribution of Children with Syndromes Excluding Down Syndrome by Mother's Age at Registration

	Age	No. of Children	Children with Syndromes		Relative Risk
			No.	Rate/1,000	
White	<20	4,074	12	2.9	1.2
	20–29	14,220	34	2.4	1.0*
	≥30	4,517	16	3.5	1.5
Black and	<20	7,830	15	1.9	1.0
Puerto Rican	20–29	14,847	28	1.9	1.0*
	≥30	4,794	10	2.1	1.1

*Reference category

Table **15.7**

Race-Specific Distribution of Children with Syndromes Excluding Down Syndrome by Mother's Religion

		No. of Children	Children with Syndromes		Relative Risk
			No.	Rate/1,000	
White	Protestant	9,031	19	2.1	1.0*
	Catholic	11,943	39	3.3	1.6
	Other/none	1,837	4	2.2	1.1
Black	Protestant	20,620	36	1.7	1.0*
	Catholic	2,833	7	2.5	1.5
	Other/none	577	2	3.5	2.1
Puerto Rican	Protestant	279	2	7.2	1.0*
	Catholic	3,136	6	1.9	0.3
	Other/none	26	0	—	—

*Reference category

syndrome was almost three times higher in mothers who had given birth to a child who died during the neonatal period (relative risk, 2.8). Also, there was a slight increase in the rate among children born to mothers who had had a prior abortion or stillbirth, giving relative risks of 1.4 and 1.3, respectively.

Characteristics and Complications of the Pregnancy

Duration of Pregnancy (Table 15.12) The rate of syndromes was increased over three times when the pregnancy was less than 9 or greater than 10 lunar months in duration, giving relative risks of 3.4 for 7 to 8 lunar months, 4.9 for 5 to

215

Table **15.8**

Race-Specific Distribution of Children with Syndromes Excluding Down Syndrome by Child's Birthweight

	Birthweight (grams)	No. of Children	Children with Syndromes		Relative Risk
			No.	Rate/1,000	
White	≤1,499	357	9	25.2	14.8
	1,500–1,999	288	6	20.8	12.2
	2,000–2,499	1,201	11	9.2	5.4
	≥2,500	20,965	36	1.7	1.0*
Black and	≤1,499	659	8	12.1	7.6
Puerto Rican	1,500–1,999	672	2	3.0	1.9
	2,000–2,499	2,503	5	2.0	1.3
	≥2,500	23,637	38	1.6	1.0*

*Reference category

Table **15.9**

Race-Specific Distribution of Children with Syndromes Excluding Down Syndrome by Survival of the Child

	Survival of Child	No. of Children	Children with Syndromes		Relative Risk
			No.	Rate/1,000	
White	Stillbirth	327	12	36.7	40.8
	Neonatal death	302	21	69.5	77.2
	Infant death	130	5	38.5	42.8
	Childhood death	91	5	54.9	61.0
	Survived	21,961	19	0.9	1.0*
Black and	Stillbirth	471	5	10.6	9.6
Puerto Rican	Neonatal death	504	12	23.8	21.6
	Infant death	254	7	27.6	25.1
	Childhood death	148	0	—	—
	Survived	26,094	29	1.1	1.0*

*Reference category

Table **15.10**

Distribution of Children with Syndromes Excluding Down Syndrome by History of Prior Premature Births

Prior Premature Births	No. of Children	Children with Syndromes		Relative Risk
		No.	Rate/1,000	
No	26,707[1]	52	1.9	1.0*
Yes	8,021	25	3.1	1.6
No prior liveborn	15,554	38	2.4	1.3

*Reference category
[1]Includes 952 unknowns

Table **15.11**

Distribution of Children with Syndromes Excluding Down Syndrome by History of Prior Fetal or Neonatal Loss

	No. of Children	Children with Syndromes		Relative Risk
		No.	Rate/1,000	
Prior abortion	9,135	26	2.8	1.4
No prior abortion[1]	26,979	56	2.1	1.0*
No prior pregnancy	14,168	33	2.3	1.1
Prior stillbirth	2,837	8	2.8	1.3
No prior stillbirth[2]	32,280	70	2.2	1.0*
No prior pregnancies 20 weeks or over	15,165	37	2.4	1.1
Prior neonatal death	2,174	12	5.5	2.8
No prior neonatal death[3]	32,554	65	2.0	1.0*
No prior liveborn	15,554	38	2.4	1.2

*Reference category
[1]Includes 108 unknowns
[2]Includes 179 unknowns
[3]Includes 947 unknowns

6 lunar months, and 3.9 for at least 11 lunar months duration.

Placental Weight (Table 15.13) Low placental weight was associated with an increased risk of having a syndrome (relative risk, 3.6). The risk was also increased when the placenta weighed at least 600 gm (relative risk, 1.8).

Number of Umbilical Arteries (Table 15.14) There was a strong association between single umbilical artery and syndromes, with a relative risk of 10.5.

Signs of Toxemia (Table 15.15) Both eclampsia and/or hypertension and proteinuria were associated with increased syndrome rates, giving relative risks of 1.9 and 3.6, respectively.

Selected Complications of Pregnancy

Table **15.12**

Distribution of Children with Syndromes Excluding Down Syndrome by Duration of Pregnancy

Length of Gestation (lunar months)	No. of Children	Children with Syndromes		Relative Risk
		No.	Rate/1,000	
5–6	559	5	8.9	4.9
7–8	3,292	20	6.1	3.4
9–10	45,436	83	1.8	1.0*
≥11	995	7	7.0	3.9

*Reference category

Table **15.13**

Distribution of Children with Syndromes Excluding Down Syndrome by Placental Weight

Placental Weight (grams)	No. of Children	Children with Syndromes		Relative Risk
		No.	Rate/1,000	
≤299	2,483	18	7.2	3.6
300–599	38,886	78	2.0	1.0*
≥600	2,499	9	3.6	1.8
Unknown	6,414	10	1.6	0.8

*Reference category

Table **15.14**

Distribution of Children with Syndromes Excluding Down Syndrome by Number of Umbilical Arteries

No. of Umbilical Arteries	No. of Children	Children with Syndromes		Relative Risk
		No.	Rate/1,000	
One	341	8	23.5	10.5
Two	44,851	100	2.2	1.0*
Unknown	5,090	7	1.4	0.6

*Reference category

Table **15.15**

Distribution of Children with Syndromes Excluding Down Syndrome by Signs of Toxemia[1]

	No. of Children	Children with Syndromes		Relative Risk
		No.	Rate/1,000	
Eclampsia and/or hypertension	1,621	7	4.3	1.9
Proteinuria	1,213	10	8.2	3.6
Generalized edema	11,425	16	1.4	0.6
None	36,023	82	2.3	1.0*

*Reference category
[1]This classification is hierarchical and based on severity—for example, a pregnancy complicated by hypertension is classified as such, even though proteinuria and edema may also be present.

(Table 15.16) The relative risks for hyperemesis gravidarum and hydramnios were, respectively, 2.4 and 15.2.

Placental Factors (Table 15.17) Marginal sinus rupture (relative risk, 2.9), abruptio placentae (2.2), and large placental infarct (1.5) were all associated with increased syndrome rates.

Weight Change during Pregnancy (Table 15.18) Unusually low and unusually high weight gain were both associated with increased rates of syndromes, giving relative risks of 1.4 and 1.7, respectively. The relative risk was also elevated among those children whose mothers' weight gains were unknown (1.7).

Selected Diseases of the Mother (Table 15.19) Elevated relative risks were found for hyperthyroidism (10.0), other endocrine disease (2.1), urinary tract infection (1.8), and bacterial infection (2.0).

The finding for hyperthyroidism was based on small numbers of exposed and malformed children.

Environmental Factors

Maternal Cigarette Smoking (Table 15.20) The rate of syndromes was higher in children whose mothers smoked 30 or more cigarettes per day (relative risk, 1.7).

Pelvic or Abdominal X-Ray Exposure During Pregnancy (Table 15.21) Children whose mothers were exposed to an abdominal or pelvic X-ray during pregnancy had an increased risk of having syndromes (relative risk, 1.6).

Genetic Factors

History of Malformations in Prior Siblings (Table 15.22) The rate of syndromes was twice as high in children who had a

Table **15.16**

Distribution of Children with Syndromes Excluding Down Syndrome by Various Complications of Pregnancy

	No. of Children	Children with Syndromes		Relative Risk*
		No.	Rate/1,000	
Hyperemesis gravidarum	540	3	5.6	2.4
Hydramnios	694	20	28.8	15.2

*For each condition, the reference category consists of those without that condition.

Table **15.17**

Distribution of Children with Syndromes Excluding Down Syndrome by Placental Factors

	No. of Children	Children with Syndromes		Relative Risk*
		No.	Rate/1,000	
Marginal sinus rupture	639	4	6.3	2.9
Abruptio placentae	1,030	5	4.9	2.2
Placental infarct ⩾ 3 cm	1,501	5	3.3	1.5

*For each condition, the reference category consists of those without that condition.

Table **15.18**

Distribution of Children with Syndromes Excluding Down Syndrome by Weight Change During Pregnancy

Weight Change (kg)	No. of Children	Children with Syndromes		Relative Risk
		No.	Rate/1,000	
⩽7.4	12,894	34	2.6	1.4
7.5–14.9	29,135	55	1.9	1.0*
⩾15.0	6,386	20	3.1	1.7
Unknown	1,867	6	3.2	1.7

*Reference category

Table **15.19**

Distribution of Children with Syndromes Excluding Down Syndrome by Selected Diseases of the Mother During Pregnancy

	No. of Children	Children with Syndromes		Relative Risk*
		No.	Rate/1,000	
Hyperthyroidism	87	2	23.0	10.0
Endocrine disease other than diabetes or malfunction of the thyroid gland	1,537	7	4.6	2.1
Urinary tract infection (fever ⩾ 100.4°F)	709	3	4.2	1.8
Bacterial infection	899	4	4.4	2.0

*For each disease, the reference category consists of those without that disease.

Table **15.20**

Distribution of Children with Syndromes Excluding Down Syndrome by Maternal Cigarette Smoking

Cigarette Smoking (no./day)	No. of Children	Children with Syndromes		Relative Risk
		No.	Rate/1,000	
None/uncertain	28,597	74	2.6	1.0*
≤29	19,900	33	1.7	0.7
≥30	1,785	8	4.5	1.7

*Reference category

Table **15.21**

Distribution of Children with Syndromes Excluding Down Syndrome by Pelvic and/or Abdominal X-Ray Exposure During Pregnancy

Pelvic and/or Abdominal X-Ray Exposure	No. of Children	Children with Syndromes		Relative Risk
		No.	Rate/1,000	
Present	11,400	36	3.2	1.6
Absent	38,882	79	2.0	1.0*

*Reference category

Table **15.22**

Distribution of Children with Syndromes Excluding Down Syndrome by History of Malformation in Prior Siblings

	No. of Children	Children with Syndromes		Relative Risk
		No.	Rate/1,000	
Congenital malformations in prior sibling(s)	3,723	15	4.0	2.0
None[1]	31,393	63	2.0	1.0*
First born child	15,166	37	2.4	1.2

*Reference category
[1]Includes 780 unknowns

prior sibling with a malformation as in children who did not, giving a relative risk of 2.0.

Multivariate Analysis

Based on the above data, 28 factors were selected for discriminant function analysis and scaled as binary or ordinal variables. The following variables were eliminated from further consideration because of low coefficients: low number of antenatal visits, high age of mother, prior abortions, stillbirths or premature births, pregnancy of less than 9 lunar months in duration, abruptio placentae, placental infarcts, weight gain of less than 7.5 kg, urinary tract infection, and ethnic group. The results of the multiple logistic regression analysis for the remaining 17 factors are presented in Table 15.23.

The following factors had a relative risk greater than 3: hydramnios (11.2), single umbilical artery (6.0), birthweight less than 2,000 gm (5.3), and gestation greater than 10 lunar months (3.9). Each of these associations was statistically significant. The following factors had a relative risk between 2 and 3: signs of toxemia (2.2), hyperemesis gravidarum (2.2), hyperthyroidism and endocrine diseases other than diabetes or hypothyroidism (2.1), and placental weight less than 300 gm (2.0). All of these associations were statistically significant, except for that with hyperemesis gravidarum. Among the remaining variables, only the following associations were statistically significant: weight gain of 15 kg or more during pregnancy (1.7), and Catholic religion among Whites (1.6).

In Table 15.24, the 115 children with syndromes other than Down syndrome are stratified on the basis of the multivariate risk score. There is good agreement between the observed and expected numbers of children with syndromes. In addition, the ratio of the numbers in the

Table *15.23*

Factors Related to the Risks of Syndromes Other Than Down Syndrome Based Upon Multiple Logistic Risk Function Analysis

	Estimated Risk Function Coefficient	Standard Error of Coefficient	Estimated Standardized Relative Risk
Hydramnios	2.42	0.26	11.2
Single umbilical artery	1.79	0.40	6.0
Birthweight < 2,000 gm	1.67	0.34	5.3
Gestation ⩾ 11 lunar months	1.36	0.40	3.9
Signs of toxemia (proteinuria, hypertension, eclampsia)	0.78	0.24	2.2
Hyperemesis gravidarum	0.77	0.61	2.2
Hyperthyroidism and other endocrine diseases[1]	0.75	0.36	2.1
Placental weight < 300 gm	0.70	0.32	2.0
Bacterial infection second or third trimester	0.53	0.52	1.7
Weight gain ⩾ 15 kg	0.53	0.25	1.7
Placental weight ⩾ 600 gm	0.49	0.37	1.6
Catholic religion among Whites	0.46	0.21	1.6
Smoking ⩾ 30 cig./day	0.44	0.38	1.6
Prior malformed siblings	0.40	0.29	1.5
Prior neonatal death	0.38	0.33	1.5
Marginal sinus rupture	0.36	0.53	1.4
Prenatal X-ray exposure	0.11	0.21	1.1

[1]Excluding diabetes, hypothyroidism

Table *15.24*

Distribution of Observed and Expected Numbers of Children with Syndromes Other Than Down Syndrome by Multiple Logistic Risk Function Scores

Risk Score Percentile[1]	Observed Number of Children with Syndromes	Expected Number of Children with Syndromes
99–100	29	29.8
97–98	12	9.2
95–96	10	6.2
93–94	0	4.6
91–92	2	3.9
Total (91–100)	53	53.7
81–90	13	13.9
71–80	9	9.8
61–70	11	8.1
51–60	6	6.4
41–50	5	5.9
31–40	7	5.4
21–30	4	4.2
11–20	6	3.8
1–10	1	3.8
Total	115	115.0

[1]Each decile contains 5,025 pregnancies, except the lowest which contains 5,057 pregnancies.

top decile of risk to the numbers in the lowest decile is large, indicating that the model is satisfactory in discriminating between degrees of risk.

Risk Factors for Down Syndrome

Personal Characteristics of the Mother

Mother's Age at Registration (Table 15.25) The age and race-specific rates of Down syndrome are given in this table. There was a general increase in the risk of Down syndrome as the mother's age increased. Thus, relative risks ranged from 2.4 to 11.5 with increasing age in Whites; in Blacks and Puerto Ricans, the range was 1.2 to 45.2.

Mother's Marital Status (Table 15.26) The relative risk for Down syndrome in children born to mothers who were not single, married, or divorced was 2.2.

Mother's Religion (Table 15.27) Among the children whose mother's religion was other than Protestant, the relative risk for Down syndrome was 1.6.

Maternal Ponderal Index (Table 15.28) The rate of syndromes was increased in Black and Puerto Rican children when the mother's ponderal index was between 2.5 and 2.9, or at least 3.0, giving relative risks of 1.5 and 3.4, respectively. The rate was also elevated among both Whites and others when the mother's ponderal index was unknown, with relative risks of 2.6 and 2.3, respectively.

Characteristics and Survival of the Offspring

Birthweight (Table 15.29) There was an increased risk of Down syndrome as the child's birthweight decreased. Thus, among children who had a birthweight below 2,500 gm, the relative risk was 9.3. For birthweights between 2,500 and 2,999 gm, and for those between 3,000 and

Table **15.25**

Race-Specific Distribution of Children with Down Syndrome by Mother's Age at Registration

	Mother's Age	No. of Children	Children with Down Syndrome		Relative Risk
			No.	Rate/1,000	
White	≤29	18,294	16	0.9	1.0*
	30–34	2,726	6	2.2	2.4
	35–39	1,405	4	2.8	3.1
	≥40	386	4	10.4	11.5
Black and Puerto Rican	≤29	22,677	13	0.6	1.0*
	30–34	2,929	2	0.7	1.2
	35–39	1,479	6	4.1	7.1
	≥40	386	10	25.9	45.2

*Reference category

Table **15.26**

Distribution of Children with Down Syndrome by Mother's Marital Status

Marital Status	No. of Children	Children with Down Syndrome		Relative Risk
		No.	Rate/1,000	
Single, married, or divorced	46,093	51	1.1	1.0*
Other	4,189	10	2.4	2.2

*Reference category

Table **15.27**

Distribution of Children with Down Syndrome by Mother's Religion

	No. of Children	Children with Down Syndrome		Relative Risk
		No.	Rate/1,000	
Protestant	29,930	29	1.0	1.0*
Other	20,352	32	1.6	1.6

*Reference category

Table **15.28**

Race-Specific Distribution of Children with Down Syndrome According to Prepregnant Ponderal Index of Mother

	Ponderal Index (weight × 1000)/(height)²	No. of Children	Children with Down Syndrome		Relative Risk
			No.	Rate/1,000	
White	≤2.4	17,319	22	1.3	1.0*
	2.5–2.9	2,668	2	0.7	0.5
	≥3.0	1,037	0	—	—
	Unknown	1,787	6	3.4	2.6
Black and Puerto Rican	≤2.4	19,827	17	0.9	1.0*
	2.5–2.9	4,567	6	1.3	1.5
	≥3.0	2,069	6	2.9	3.4
	Unknown	1,008	2	2.0	2.3

*Reference category

Table **15.29**

Distribution of Children with Down Syndrome by Child's Birthweight

Birthweight (grams)	No. of Children	Children with Down Syndrome		Relative Risk
		No.	Rate/1,000	
≤2,499	5,680	16	2.8	9.3
2,500–2,999	12,399	19	1.5	5.0
3,000–3,499	19,608	22	1.1	3.7
≥3,500	12,595	4	0.3	1.0*

*Reference category

3,499 gm, the relative risks were 5.0 and 3.7, respectively.

Sex of the Child (Table 15.30) The relative risk for Down syndrome in male children was 1.3.

Birth Order (Table 15.31) In all three ethnic groups, the risk of Down syndrome increased as the birth order increased. For White children of birth order 2 to 7, the relative risk was 3.0; for those of birth order 8 or more, it was 10.6. Similarly, among Black children and Puerto Rican children of birth order 2 to 7, the relative risk was 2.0 while for those with 7 or more prior siblings, it was 10.2.

Survival of the Child (Table 15.32) In general, the rates of Down syndrome were higher in stillborn children and in those children who died during the neonatal, infant, or childhood periods. The relative risks shown in this table were highest in the category infant deaths, for both Whites (30.8) and Blacks and Puerto Ricans (41.1).

Table **15.30**

Distribution of Children with Down Syndrome by Sex of Child

| | No. of Children | Children with Down Syndrome | | Relative Risk |
		No.	Rate/1,000	
Male	25,542	35	1.4	1.3
Female	24,740	26	1.1	1.0*

*Reference category

Table **15.31**

Race-Specific Distribution of Children with Down Syndrome by Birth Order of Child

| | Birth Order[1] | No. of Children | Children with Down Syndrome | | Relative Risk |
			No.	Rate/1,000	
White	1	7,388	4	0.5	1.0*
	2–7	14,856	23	1.5	3.0
	≥8	567	3	5.3	10.6
Black and	1	7,778	4	0.5	1.0*
Puerto Rican	2–7	18,167	19	1.0	2.0
	≥8	1,526	8	5.2	10.2

*Reference category
[1]Determined by number of prior liveborn and stillborn siblings

Reproductive History of the Mother

Prior Fetal or Neonatal Loss (Table 15.33) Children born to mothers who had more than one prior abortion had an observed rate of Down syndrome of 4.0 per 1,000 (relative risk, 2.8). (For those whose mothers had one prior abortion, however, the relative risk was 0.5.) Similarly, the corresponding rates of the syndrome were higher in the offspring of mothers who had prior stillbirths and prior neonatal deaths (relative risks, 1.7 and 1.9, respectively).

Characteristics and Complications of the Pregnancy

Placental Weight (Table 15.34) The rates of Down syndrome were increased when the placental weight was less than 400 gm or unknown (relative risks, 2.6 and 2.1, respectively).

Various Complications of Pregnancy (Table 15.35) There were three children with Down syndrome among those whose mothers had hyperemesis gravidarum, giving a relative risk of 4.7. Among the children whose mothers had hydramnios during pregnancy, three had Down syndrome, for a relative risk of 3.6. The relative risk among the children of mothers who suffered from endocrine diseases other than diabetes, hypothyroidism, or hyperthyroidism was 3.5.

Weight Change During Pregnancy (Table 15.36) The offspring of mothers who gained less than 5.0 kg during their preg-

Table **15.32**

Race-Specific Distribution of Children with Down Syndrome by Survival of the Child

	Survival of Child	No. of Children	Children with Down Syndrome		Relative Risk
			No.	Rate/1,000	
White	Stillbirth	327	1	3.1	3.1
	Neonatal death	302	2	6.6	6.6
	Infant death	130	4	30.8	30.8
	Childhood death	91	0	—	—
	Survived	21,961	23	1.0	1.0*
Black and	Stillbirth	471	1	2.1	2.8
Puerto Rican	Neonatal death	504	1	2.0	2.6
	Infant death	254	8	31.5	41.1
	Childhood death	148	1	6.8	8.8
	Survived	26,094	20	0.8	1.0*

*Reference category

Table **15.33**

Distribution of Children with Down Syndrome by History of Prior Fetal or Neonatal Loss

	No. of Children	Children with Down Syndrome		Relative Risk
		No.	Rate/1,000	
1 prior abortion	6,631	5	0.8	0.5
≥ 2 prior abortions	2,504	10	4.0	2.8
No prior abortion	26,871	39	1.5	1.0*
No prior pregnancy	14,168	7	0.5	0.3
Prior stillbirth	2,837	7	2.5	1.7
No prior stillbirth[2]	32,280	46	1.4	1.0*
No prior pregnancies 20 weeks or over	15,165	8	0.5	0.4
Prior neonatal death	2,174	6	2.8	1.9
No prior neonatal death[3]	32,554	47	1.4	1.0*
No prior liveborn	15,554	8	0.5	0.4

*Reference category
[1]Includes 108 unknowns
[2]Includes 179 unknowns
[3]Includes 947 unknowns

Table **15.34**

Distribution of Children with Down Syndrome by Placental Weight

Placental Weight (grams)	No. of Children	Children with Down Syndrome		Relative Risk
		No.	Rate/1,000	
≤399	15,598	30	1.9	2.6
≥400	28,270	21	0.7	1.0*
Unknown	6,414	10	1.6	2.1

*Reference category

Table **15.35**

Distribution of Children with Down Syndrome by Various Complications of Pregnancy

	No. of Children	Children with Down Syndrome		Relative Risk*
		No.	Rate/1,000	
Hyperemesis gravidarum	540	3	5.6	4.7
Hydramnios	694	3	4.3	3.6
Endocrine disease other than diabetes, hypothyroidism, or hyperthyroidism	1,537	6	3.9	3.5

*For each condition, the reference category consists of those without that condition.

Table **15.36**

Distribution of Children with Down Syndrome by Weight Change During Pregnancy

Weight Change (kg)	No. of Children	Children with Down Syndrome		Relative Risk
		No.	Rate/1,000	
Gained ≤ 4.9	5,948	14	2.4	2.1
Gained 5.0–12.4	28,572	32	1.1	1.0*
Gained ≥ 12.5	13,895	10	0.7	0.6
Unknown	1,867	5	2.7	2.5

*Reference category

nancy were at greater risk of Down syndrome than those born of mothers who gained more than 4.9 kg, with a relative risk of 2.1. The relative risk when the mother's weight change was unknown was 2.5.

Environmental Factors

Cigarette Smoking (Table 15.37) There were seven cases of Down syndrome among children whose mothers were former cigarette smokers (relative risk, 3.3). The rate was also elevated among those whose mothers never smoked, compared with those whose mothers were current smokers (relative risk, 1.6).

Genetic Factors

History of Malformed Siblings (Table 15.38) The relative risk for Down syndrome among the children with at least one prior malformed sibling was 1.6. Among those children where the existence of prior malformed siblings was unknown, the relative risk was 3.9.

Multivariate Analysis

Based on the foregoing comparisons, a total of 17 risk factors were selected for multivariate analysis and scaled as binary or ordinal variables; after linear discriminant function analysis, this number

Table **15.37**

Distribution of Children with Down Syndrome by Maternal Cigarette Smoking

| Cigarette Smoking | No. of Children | Children with Down Syndrome | | Relative Risk |
		No.	Rate/1,000	
Never	21,567	31	1.4	1.6
Ex	2,309	7	3.0	3.3
Current	26,406	23	0.9	1.0*

*Reference category

Table **15.38**

Distribution of Children with Down Syndrome by History of Malformation in Prior Siblings

| | No. of Children | Children with Down Syndrome | | Relative Risk |
		No.	Rate/1,000	
Congenital malformation in prior sibling(s)	3,723	8	2.1	1.6
Firstborn child	15,166	8	0.5	0.4
Prior siblings not malformed	30,613	41	1.3	1.0*
Unknown	780	4	5.1	3.9

*Reference category

Table **15.39**

Factors Related to the Risk of Occurrence of Down Syndrome Based Upon Multiple Logistic Risk Function Analysis

	Estimated Risk Function Coefficient	Standard Error of Coefficient	Estimated Standardized Relative Risk
Maternal age ≥ 40 years	2.91	0.35	18.4
Hyperemesis gravidarum	1.33	0.61	3.8
Maternal endocrine disease other than diabetes, hypothyroidism, or hyperthyroidism	1.03	0.44	2.8
Hydramnios	0.84	0.61	2.3
Birthweight < 3,000 gm	0.80	0.29	2.2
Non-smoker (cigarettes)	0.71	0.27	2.0
Number of prior abortions > 1	0.61	0.36	1.8
Marital status (widowed, divorced, or separated)	0.60	0.36	1.8
Religion other than Protestant	0.55	0.26	1.7
Placental weight < 400 gm	0.50	0.28	1.6
Male infant	0.38	0.26	1.5
Weight gain < 5 kg	0.35	0.31	1.4
Prior neonatal death	0.31	0.44	1.4

Table **15.40**

Distribution of Observed and Expected Numbers of Children with Down Syndrome by Multiple Logistic Risk Function Scores

Risk Score Percentile[1]	Observed Number of Children with Down Syndrome	Expected Number of Children with Down Syndrome
99–100	15	17.9
97–98	7	5.3
95–96	5	3.5
93–94	2	2.7
91–92	3	2.3
Total (91–100)	32	31.7
81–90	4	8.0
71–80	9	5.5
61–70	4	4.0
51–60	4	3.3
41–50	5	2.5
31–40	1	2.1
21–30	2	1.7
11–20	0	1.3
1–10	0	0.9
Total	61	61.0

[1]Each decile contains 5,025 pregnancies, except the lowest which contains 5,057 pregnancies.

was reduced to 13. The 4 factors eliminated because of low coefficients were high birth order, prior stillbirth, prior malformed siblings, and high values of ponderal index. The results of the multiple logistic regression analysis for the 18 factors that were retained are given in Table 15.39.

Factors with relative risks greater than 3 included maternal age at least 40 years (18.4) and hyperemesis gravidarum (3.8). Both were statistically significant. Factors with relative risks between 2 and 3 included maternal endocrine disease other than diabetes, hypothyroidism, or hyperthyroidism (2.8), hydramnios (2.8), birthweight under 3,000 gm (2.2), and non-cigarette smoker (2.0). All were statistically significant except the finding for hydramnios. Of the remaining factors, only religion other than Protestant, with a relative risk of 1.7, was statistically significant.

Table 15.40 displays the distribution of the 61 children with Down syndrome according to risk score. The agreement between the numbers expected and observed is acceptable. The ratio of the numbers in the top decile of risk to the numbers in the lowest decile is large, indicating that the model is successful in discriminating between degrees of risk.

CHAPTER 16

Tumors

There were 164 children with tumors (3.3 per 1,000) (Table 16.1). Most of the tumors were benign and were distributed without striking variation among the ethnic groups. Only 24 malignant tumors were identified; none was found in Puerto Rican children, consistent with the small size of the Puerto Rican group. The 2 mixed tumors that occurred are, henceforth, grouped with the 138 benign tumors, in accordance with international classification procedures, giving a total of 140.

Tables 16.2 and 16.3 show the distributions of the individual tumor types by ethnic groups. Cysts, other than dermoid, were the most common benign tumors, occurring in 42 children (26%) (Table 16.2). CNS tumors and leukemias were the most common malignant tumors, each occurring in 8 children (5%) (Table 16.3). There were no striking differences in tumor rates among the ethnic groups. Whites had a somewhat higher overall tumor rate of 3.9 per 1,000, compared with 2.8 per 1,000 in Blacks and 2.9 per 1,000 in Puerto Ricans. This was largely due to their higher rate of cysts other than dermoid (Table 13.2).

Tumor rates rose between 1958 and 1961 and then declined, as shown in Table 16.4. The high rates of malignant tumors in the years 1959 to 1962 relative to the other years are discussed later in relationship to one of the drugs to which the study women were exposed,

Table **16.1**

Malignant, Benign, and Mixed Tumor Rates Classified by Ethnic Group (Rates per Thousand)

	White (n=22,811)		Black (n=24,030)		Puerto Rican (n=3,441)		Total (n=50,282)	
Tumor	No.	Rate	No.	Rate	No.	Rate	No.	Rate
Malignant[1]	14	0.61	10	0.42	0	—	24	0.48
Benign	72	3.16	56	2.33	10	2.91	138	2.74
Mixed	2	0.09	0	—	0	—	2	0.04

[1]Includes 8 children with CNS tumors, 8 with leukemia, 5 with Wilms' tumor and 8 with other malignancies (see Table 16.3).

Table **16.2**

Tumor Rates Classified by Ethnic Group (Rates per Thousand)

	White (n=22,811)		Black (n=24,030)		Puerto Rican (n=3,441)		Total (n=50,282)	
Tumor	No.	Rate	No.	Rate	No.	Rate	No.	Rate
Any cyst (except dermoid)	27	1.18	13	0.54	2	0.58	42	0.84
Hairy nevus	11	0.48	9	0.37	2	0.58	22	0.44
Benign tumors other than cysts, hairy nevus, hemangioma/granuloma, papillomas/polyps, lymphangioma	10	0.44	12	0.50	2	0.58	24	0.48
Other tumors[1]	40	1.75	32	1.33	4	1.16	76	1.51
Any tumors	88	3.86	66	2.75	10	2.91	164	3.26

[1]See Table 16.3 for details of this category.

Table **16.3**

Rare Tumor Rates Classified by Ethnic Group (Rates per Thousand)

	White (n=22,811)		Black (n=24,030)		Puerto Rican (n=3,441)		Total (n=50,282)	
Tumor	No.	Rate	No.	Rate	No.	Rate	No.	Rate
Hemangioma/granuloma	8	0.35	9	0.37	2	0.58	19	0.38
Papillomas/polyps	5	0.22	5	0.21	2	0.58	12	0.24
Dermoid cysts	8	0.35	3	0.12	0	—	11	0.22
Lymphangioma	3	0.13	5	0.21	0	—	8	0.16
CNS tumors	5	0.22	3	0.12	0	—	8	0.16
Leukemias	6	0.26	2	0.08	0	—	8	0.16
Wilms' tumor	2	0.09	3	0.12	0	—	5	0.10
Other malignant tumors	1	0.04	2	0.08	0	—	3	0.06
Mixed tumors (benign/malignant)	2	0.09	0	—	0	—	2	0.04

Table **16.4**

Benign and Malignant Tumor Rates According to Year of Mother's Last Menstrual Period (LMP) (Rates per Thousand)

Year of LMP	No. of Mother-Child Pairs	Benign Tumors		Malignant Tumors		Total	
		No.	Rate	No.	Rate	No.	Rate
1958	1,877	3	1.6	0	—	3	1.6
1959	5,735	16	2.8	5	0.9	21	3.7
1960	7,285	21	2.9	6	0.8	27	3.7
1961	7,441	30	4.0	5	0.7	35	4.7
1962	8,216	31	3.8	6	0.7	37	4.5
1963	7,986	20	2.5	0	—	20	2.5
1964	7,817	14	1.8	1	0.1	15	1.9
1965	3,925	5	1.3	1	0.3	6	1.5
Total	50,282	140	2.8	24	0.5	164	3.3

poliomyelitis vaccine (see Chapter 22). Table 16.5 shows the rates of the individual types of benign tumors by year of the mother's last menstrual period (LMP). No single tumor type was responsible for the peak around 1961; among the chief contributors were cysts other than dermoid, hemangiomas/granulomas, and hairy nevus. Table 16.6 shows the tumor rate by calendar month of the mother's LMP. It can be seen that there were no obvious seasonal trends.

There were no children with more than one morphological type of tumor. Tables 16.7 and 16.8 show the joint occurrence of other malformations with tumors. Benign tumors occurred jointly with other malformation classes less often than did most other malformation groups. For example, 36.5% and 25.6% of those with CNS or eye/ear malformations, respectively, had other malformations, whereas only 12.9% of those with benign tumors had other malformations (Table 16.7). As for malignant tumors, one-third of those afflicted had other malformations in addition (Table 16.8). The three children with CNS tumors had associated malformations that were probably caused by their tumors (e.g., hydrocephaly). The two individuals with Wilms' tumor had, respec-

tively, polycystic kidney, hydronephrosis, hydroureter, and malposition/ectopic kidney among their additional malformations. One child with leukemia had a double ureter, and one with nephroblastic nodules also had a double ureter with hydronephrosis and hydroureter, thus accounting for the four genitourinary malformations listed in Table 16.8. The two cardiovascular malformations occurring jointly with leukemia and Wilms' tumor were an atrial septal defect and a ventricular septal defect, respectively.

Risk Factors for Tumors

Administrative Data

Duration of Pregnancy at Registration (Table 16.9) The relative risk for tumors was 1.5 among those who registered during the first four months of pregnancy. This held true for both malignant and benign tumors.

Personal Characteristics of the Mother
Maternal Age at Registration (Table 16.10) There was no convincing association between maternal age and the rate of benign tumors. However, the rate of

Table **16.5**

Benign Tumors According to Year of Mother's Last Menstrual Period (LMP) (Rates per Thousand)

Year of LMP	No. of Mother-Child Pairs	Papillomas/ Polyps		Dermoid Cysts		Cysts Other Than Dermoid		Hemangioma/ Granuloma		Hairy Nevus		Lymphangioma		Other Benign Tumors	
		No.	Rate	No.	Rate	No.	Rate	No.	Rate	No.	Rate	No.	Rate	No.	Rate
1958	1,877	0	—	0	—	0	—	1	0.53	0	—	1	0.53	1	0.53
1959	5,735	1	0.17	2	0.35	4	0.70	1	0.17	2	0.35	4	0.70	2	0.35
1960	7,285	1	0.14	3	0.41	7	0.96	1	0.14	3	0.41	1	0.14	5	0.69
1961	7,441	3	0.40	3	0.40	9	1.21	5	0.67	4	0.54	1	0.13	5	0.67
1962	8,216	3	0.37	2	0.24	12	1.46	2	0.24	6	0.73	0	—	6	0.73
1963	7,986	1	0.13	1	0.13	4	0.50	5	0.63	4	0.50	1	0.13	4	0.50
1964	7,817	1	0.13	0	—	6	0.77	3	0.38	2	0.26	0	—	2	0.26
1965	3,925	2	0.51	0	—	0	—	1	0.25	1	0.25	0	—	1	0.25
Total	50,282	12	0.24	11	0.22	42	0.84	19	0.38	22	0.44	8	0.16	26	0.52

Table **16.6**

Distribution of Children with Tumors by Month of Mother's Last Menstrual Period (LMP) (Rates per Thousand)

		Children with Tumors	
Month of LMP	No. of Mother-Child Pairs	No.	Rate
January	4,185	11	2.6
February	4,075	8	2.0
March	4,136	18	4.3
April	4,154	14	3.4
May	4,194	18	4.3
June	4,118	12	2.9
July	3,817	9	2.4
August	4,001	13	3.2
September	4,049	14	3.5
October	4,539	12	2.6
November	4,412	20	4.5
December	4,602	15	3.3
Total	50,282	164	3.3

malignant tumors was slightly elevated when the mother was 31 years or older.

Mother's Prepregnant Weight and Height (Table 16.11) The rate of tumors, both benign and malignant, was higher in offspring of mothers whose prepregnant weight was at least 60 kg, compared to those who weighed 59 kg or less, giving a relative risk of 1.4. There was no association between the tumor rate and height of the mother.

Characteristics and Survival of the Offspring

Birthweight (Table 16.12) Low birthweight was associated with increased risk of malignant tumors but not of benign tumors. For those weighing between 1,000 and 1,999 gm, and for those weighing less than 1,000 gm, the relative risks for malignant tumors were 2.8 and 11.0, respectively.

Birth Order (Table 16.13) Benign tumor rates did not vary with birth order. Birth order of four or more was associated with a higher risk of malignant tumors in Whites but not in Blacks (relative risk, 2.5).

Survival of the Child (Table 16.14) Malignant tumors were usually lethal; relative risks among those who died ranged from 25.0 to 418.0. The benign tumor rate was also somewhat higher in those who died than in those who lived.

Reproductive History of the Mother

Prior Fetal or Neonatal Loss (Tables 16.15, 16.16) The relative risks of benign and malignant tumors were slightly higher (1.3 and 2.4, respectively) in offspring of mothers who had previously given birth to a stillborn (Table 16.15). For prior neonatal death, the relative risk of benign tumors was 2.1 for Whites and 1.9 for Blacks, but was not increased for malignant tumors (Table 16.16).

Characteristics and Complications of the Pregnancy

Duration of Pregnancy (Table 16.17) For the offspring of those women whose pregnancies lasted 8 lunar months or

Table **16.7**

Joint Occurrence of Malformations in Classes Other Than Benign Tumors in Children With Benign Tumors

	No. of Children	Cardio-vascular		Central Nervous		Musculo-skeletal		Respi-ratory		Gastro-intestinal		Genito-urinary		Eyes/Ears		Syndromes		Any Malformation Except Tumors	
		No.	%	No.	%	No.	%	No.	%	No.	%	No.	%	No.	%	No.	%	No.	%
Any cyst (except dermoid)	42	1	2.4	1	2.4	0	—	0	—	1	2.4	1	2.4	1	2.4	2	4.8	7	16.7
Hairy nevus	22	0	—	0	—	1	4.5	0	—	0	—	0	—	0	—	0	—	1	4.5
Hemangioma/granuloma	19	1	5.3	0	—	1	5.3	1	5.3	0	—	0	—	1	5.3	0	—	3	15.8
Papillomas/polyps	12	0	—	0	—	1	8.3	0	—	0	—	0	—	0	—	0	—	1	8.3
Dermoid	11	0	—	0	—	1	9.1	0	—	0	—	0	—	0	—	0	—	1	9.1
Lymphangioma	8	0	—	0	—	0	—	0	—	0	—	0	—	0	—	0	—	0	—
Other tumors	26	0	—	3	11.5	1	3.8	2	7.7	0	—	1	3.8	0	—	1	3.8	5	19.2
Any beign tumors	140	2	1.4	4	2.9	5	3.6	3	2.1	1	0.7	2	1.4	2	1.4	4	2.9	18	12.9

237

Table 16.8

Joint Occurrence of Malformations in Classes Other Than Malignant Tumors in Children with Malignant Tumors

	No. of Children	Cardio-vascular		Central Nervous		Musculo-skeletal		Respi-ratory		Gastro-intestinal		Genito-urinary		Eyes/Ears		Syndromes		Any Mal-formation Except Tumors	
		No.	%	No.	%	No.	%	No.	%	No.	%	No.	%	No.	%	No.	%	No.	%
Leukemias	8	1	12.5	0	—	0	—	0	—	0	—	1	12.5	0	—	1	12.5	2	25.0
CNS tumors	8	0	—	3	37.5	0	—	0	—	0	—	0	—	0	—	0	—	3	37.5
Wilms' tumor	5	1	20.0	0	—	1	20.0	0	—	1	20.0	2	40.0	1	20.0	0	—	2	40.0
Other tumors	3	0	—	0	—	0	—	0	—	0	—	1	33.3	0	—	0	—	1	33.3
Any malignant tumors	24	2	8.3	3	12.5	1	4.2	0	—	1	4.2	4	16.7	1	4.2	1	4.2	8	33.3

238

Table 16.9

Distribution of Children with Tumors by Duration of Pregnancy at Registration

Duration of Pregnancy at Registration (lunar months)	No. of Children	Children with Tumors		Relative Risk
		No.	Rate/1,000	
1–4	13,435	59	4.4	1.5
≥5	36,847	105	2.9	1.0*

*Reference category

Table 16.10

Distribution of Children with Malignant Tumors by Mother's Age at Registration

Mother's Age	No. of Children	Children with Malignant Tumors		Relative Risk
		No.	Rate/1,000	
≤19	11,904	4	0.3	0.8
20–24	18,475	8	0.4	1.0*
25–29	10,592	3	0.3	0.8
30–34	5,655	6	1.1	2.8
≥35	3,656	3	0.8	2.0

*Reference category

Table 16.11

Distribution of Children with Tumors by Mother's Prepregnant Weight and Height

		No. of Children	Children with Tumors		Relative Risk
			No.	Rate/1,000	
Weight (kg)	≤59[1]	31,986	91	2.8	1.0*
	≥60	18,296	73	4.0	1.4
Height (cm)	≤149	2,947	10	3.4	1.1
	150–169[2]	41,810	133	3.2	1.0*
	170–189	5,525	21	3.8	1.2

*Reference category
[1]Includes 1,028 unknowns
[2]Includes 2,327 unknowns

Table **16.12**

Distribution of Children with Tumors by Malignancy and by Child's Birthweight

| Tumor | Birthweight (grams) | No. of Children | Children with Tumors | | Relative Risk |
			No.	Rate/1,000	
Malignant	≤999	548	3	5.5	11.0
	1,000–1,999	1,428	2	1.4	2.8
	2,000–2,999	16,103	4	0.3	0.6
	≥3,000	32,203	15	0.5	1.0*
Benign	≤999	548	2	3.7	1.2
	1,000–1,999	1,428	1	0.7	0.2
	2,000–2,999	16,103	38	2.4	0.8
	≥3,000	32,203	99	3.1	1.0*

*Reference category

Table **16.13**

Race-Specific Distribution of Children with Malignant Tumors by Birth Order of Child

| | Birth Order[1] | No. of Children | Children with Malignant Tumors | | Relative Risk |
			No.	Rate/1,000	
White	1	7,388	3	0.4	1.0*
	2–3	9,430	5	0.5	1.2
	≥4	5,993	6	1.0	2.5
Black	1	6,740	3	0.4	1.0*
	2–3	8,805	4	0.5	1.2
	≥4	8,485	3	0.4	1.0

*Reference category
[1]Determined by number of prior liveborn and stillborn siblings

less, the relative risk of malignant or benign tumors was 1.5 in Whites and 2.1 in Blacks. Of the 19 tumors in offspring of the shorter pregnancies, 4 were malignant.

Single Umbilical Artery (Table 16.18) Among those children born with one umbilical artery, two had benign tumors and one had a malignant tumor for a relative risk of 2.7.

Signs of Toxemia (Table 16.19) The risk of tumors increased with severity of toxemia for both malignant and benign tumors. Compared to the reference category, consisting of generalized edema without other signs and those with no signs of toxemia, the relative risks for benign and malignant tumors in those with toxemia ranged from 1.2 to 2.8 and 3.7 to 5.8, respectively.

240

Table **16.14**

Distribution of Children with Tumors by Malignancy and Survival of the Child

	Survival of Child	No. of Children	Children with Tumors		Relative Risk
			No.	Rate/1,000	
Benign	Stillbirth	798	5	6.3	2.3
	Neonatal death	806	2	2.5	0.9
	Infant death	384	3	7.8	2.9
	Childhood death	239	1	4.2	1.6
	Survived	48,055	129	2.7	1.0*
Malignant	Stillbirth	798	2	2.5	25.0
	Neonatal death	806	5	6.2	62.0
	Infant death	384	3	7.8	78.0
	Childhood death	239	10	41.8	418.0
	Survived	48,055	4	0.1	1.0*

*Reference category

Table **16.15**

Distribution of Children with Tumors by Malignancy and History of Prior Stillbirths

	Prior Stillbirths	No. of Children	Children with Tumors		Relative Risk
			No.	Rate/1,000	
Benign	Yes	2,837	10	3.5	1.3
	No	47,445	130	2.7	1.0*
Malignant	Yes	2,837	3	1.1	2.4
	No	47,445	21	0.4	1.0*

*Reference category. Includes no prior pregnancies 20 weeks or over and 179 unknowns.

Table 16.16

Race-Specific Distribution of Children with Benign Tumors by History of Prior Neonatal Deaths

	Prior Neonatal Deaths	No. of Children	Children with Benign Tumors		Relative Risk
			No.	Rate/1,000	
White	Yes	805	5	6.2	2.1
	No[1]	22,006	67	3.0	1.0*
Black	Yes	1,226	5	4.1	1.9
	No[2]	22,804	51	2.2	1.0*
Puerto Rican	Yes	143	0	—	—
	No[3]	3,298	10	3.0	1.0*

*Reference category
[1]Includes no prior liveborns and 437 unknowns
[2]Includes no prior liveborns and 490 unknowns
[3]Includes no prior liveborns and 20 unknowns

Table 16.17

Race-Specific Distribution of Children with Tumors by Duration of Pregnancy

	Length of Gestation (lunar months)	No. of Children	Children with Tumors		Relative Risk
			No.	Rate/1,000	
White	5–8	1,074	6	5.6	1.5
	≥9	21,737	82	3.8	1.0*
Black	5–8	2,501	13	5.2	2.1
	≥9	21,529	53	2.5	1.0*
Puerto Rican	5–8	276	0	—	—
	≥9	3,165	10	3.2	1.0*

*Reference category

Table **16.18**

Distribution of Children with Tumors by Number of Umbilical Arteries

No. of Umbilical Arteries	No. of Children	Children with Tumors		Relative Risk
		No.	Rate/1,000	
One	341	3	8.8	2.7
Two	44,851	148	3.3	1.0*
Unknown	5,090	13	2.6	0.8

*Reference category

Table **16.19**

Distribution of Children with Tumors by Malignancy and by Signs of Toxemia[1]

		No. of Children	Children with Tumors		Relative Risk
			No.	Rate/1,000	
Benign	Eclampsia	22	0	—	—
	Chronic hypertension	669	5	7.5	2.8
	Acute hypertension (BP ≥ 160/110 after LM 6)/ proteinuria	2,143	7	3.3	1.2
	Generalized edema/ none	47,448	128	2.7	1.0*
Malignant	Eclampsia	22	0	—	—
	Chronic hypertension	669	1	1.5	3.7
	Acute hypertension (BP ≥ 160/110 after LM 6)/ proteinuria	2,143	5	2.3	5.8
	Generalized edema/ none	47,448	18	0.4	1.0*

*Reference category
[1]This classification is hierarchical and based on severity—for example, a pregnancy complicated by chronic hypertension is classified as such, even though proteinuria and edema may also be present.

Various Complications of Pregnancy (Table 16.20) The rates of tumors in offspring of individuals with abruptio placentae, hydramnios, hemorrhagic shock, or vena cava syndrome were higher than those in children of individuals without these conditions, giving relative risks of 1.8, 1.8, 3.1, and 4.3, respectively. All of the tumors were benign except for one of the six in children of mothers with abruptio placentae, one of the two in children of mothers with vena cava syndrome, and the one tumor occurring in a child of a mother with hemorrhagic shock.

Placental Infarcts (Table 16.21) The risk of both malignant and benign tumors was almost doubled in those with placental infarcts. Relative risks for Whites, Blacks, and Puerto Ricans were 1.8, 1.5, and 1.8, respectively. Seven of the 48 tumors in those with placental infarcts were malignant.

Weight Change During Pregnancy (Table 16.22) The relative risk of malignant tumors in offspring of those mothers who

Table **16.20**

Distribution of Children with Tumors by Various Complications of Pregnancy

	No. of Children	Children with Tumors		Relative Risk*
		No.	Rate/1,000	
Abruptio placentae	1,030	6	5.8	1.8
Hydramnios	694	4	5.8	1.8
Hemorrhagic shock	99	1	10.1	3.1
Vena cava syndrome	144	2	13.7	4.3

*For each condition, the reference category consists of those without that condition.

Table **16.21**

Race-Specific Distribution of Children with Tumors by Presence of Placental Infarcts

	Placental Infarct	No. of Children	Children with Tumors		Relative Risk
			No.	Rate/1,000	
White	Present	5,876	33	5.6	1.8
	Absent[1]	16,935	55	3.2	1.0*
Black	Present	3,063	12	3.9	1.5
	Absent[2]	20,967	54	2.6	1.0*
Puerto Rican	Present	680	3	4.4	1.8
	Absent[3]	2,761	7	2.5	1.0*

*Reference category
[1]Includes 1,923 unknowns
[2]Includes 2,873 unknowns
[3]Includes 306 unknowns

Table **16.22**

Distribution of Children with Tumors by Malignancy and Weight Change During Pregnancy

		No. of Children	Children with Tumors		Relative Risk
			No.	Rate/1,000	
Benign	Gain ≤ 4.9 kg	5,948	16	2.7	1.0
	Gain ≥ 5.0 kg/unknown[1]	44,334	124	2.8	1.0*
Malignant	Gain ≤ 4.9 kg	5,948	8	1.3	3.7
	Gain ≥ 5.0 kg/unknown[1]	44,334	16	0.4	1.0*

*Reference category
[1]Includes 1,867 unknowns

gained 4.9 kg or less during pregnancy was 3.7. No association was observed for benign tumors.

Selected Diseases of the Mother (Table 16.23) Tumor rates were elevated in offspring of those who had endocrine disorders other than diabetes or malfunction of the thyroid gland, hematuria, or convulsive disorder, giving relative risks of 1.8, 1.8, and 3.2, respectively. Two of the tumors in the other endocrine disorder group and one of those in the convulsive disorder group were malignant.

Environmental Factors

Maternal Cigarette Smoking (Table 16.24) The rate of malignant tumors was elevated in smokers of 15 to 29 cigarettes per day (relative risk, 3.3) and in ex-smokers (relative risk, 5.7). Benign tumor rates in different smoking categories were similar with the exception of ex-smokers, where the relative risk was 1.8.

Pelvic or Abdominal X-Ray Exposure During Pregnancy (Table 16.25) The offspring of those women who were exposed to pelvic or abdominal X-rays dur-

Table **16.23**

Distribution of Children with Tumors by Selected Diseases of the Mother During Pregnancy

	No. of Children	Children with Tumors		Relative Risk*
		No.	Rate/1,000	
Endocrine disease other than diabetes, hypothyroidism, or hyperthyroidism	1,537	9	5.8	1.8
Hematuria (≥ 15 RBC/HPF)	1,059	6	5.7	1.8
Convulsive disorder	294	3	10.3	3.2

*For each disease, the reference category consists of those without that disease.

Table **16.24**

Distribution of Children with Tumors by Malignancy and by Maternal Cigarette Smoking

	Cigarette Smoking (no./day)	No. of Children	Children with Tumors		Relative Risk
			No.	Rate/1,000	
Benign	Never/Uncertain	26,288	69	2.6	1.0*
	Ex-smoker	2,309	11	4.8	1.8
	≤14	12,824	32	2.5	1.0
	15–29	7,076	23	3.3	1.3
	≥30	1,785	5	2.8	1.1
Malignant	Never/Uncertain	26,288	9	0.3	1.0*
	Ex-smoker	2,309	4	1.7	5.7
	≤14	12,824	4	0.3	1.0
	15–29	7,076	7	1.0	3.3
	≥30	1,785	0	—	—

*Reference category

Table **16.25**

Distribution of Children with Tumors by Malignancy and by Pelvic and/or Abdominal X-Ray Exposure During Pregnancy

	Pelvic and/or Abdominal X-Ray Exposure	No. of Children	Children with Tumors		Relative Risk
			No.	Rate/1,000	
Benign	Present	11,400	50	4.4	1.9
	Absent	38,882	90	2.3	1.0*
Malignant	Present	11,400	9	0.8	2.0
	Absent	38,882	15	0.4	1.0*

*Reference category

ing pregnancy had benign and malignant tumor rates about twice those of offspring of non-exposed women, with relative risks of 1.9 and 2.0, respectively.

Genetic Factors

Family History of Malformation (Table 16.26) There was no association be- tween a history of malformation in a prior sibling and malignant tumors. The rate of benign tumors was elevated in children with prior malformed siblings, giving a relative risk of 1.4.

ABO Incompatibility (Table 16.27) The relative risk of malignant tumors in off- spring of pregnancies in which there was

246

Table **16.26**

Distribution of Children with Tumors by Malignancy and by History of Malformations in Prior Siblings

		No. of Children	Children with Tumors		Relative Risk
			No.	Rate/1,000	
Benign	No Prior malformed siblings/no prior pregnancies ≥ 20 weeks/ unknown	46,559	126	2.7	1.0*
	Prior malformed sibling(s)	3,723	14	3.7	1.4
Malignant	No prior malformed siblings/no prior pregnancies ≥ 20 weeks/ unknown	46,559	22	0.5	1.0*
	Prior malformed sibling(s)	3,723	2	0.5	1.0

*Reference category

mother-offspring ABO incompatibility was 3.0. Of the nine for whom ABO incompatibility was present, six had strong incompatibility (mother O, offspring A or mother O, offspring B) and three had mild incompatibility (mother B or A, offspring AB). In addition, there was one child with a malignant tumor in whom ABO erythroblastosis occurred. The relative risk among those where the presence or absence of ABO incompatibility was unknown was also 3.0.

Multivariate Analysis

Seventeen factors were selected for multivariate analysis and were scaled as dichotomous variables. After linear discriminant function analysis, 6 factors were eliminated on the basis of having coefficients that were close to zero. Those

Table **16.27**

Distribution of Children with Malignant Tumors by ABO Incompatibility

ABO Incompatibility	No. of Children	Children with Malignant Tumors		Relative Risk
		No.	Rate/1,000	
Present	9,729	9	0.9	3.0
Absent	36,325	11	0.3	1.0*
Unknown	4,228	4	0.9	3.0

*Reference category

Table **16.28**

Factors Related to the Risk of Tumors Based Upon Multiple Logistic Risk Function Analysis

	Estimated Risk Function Coefficient	Standard Error of Coefficient	Estimated Standardized Relative Risk
Convulsive disorder	1.03	0.59	2.8
Single umbilical artery	0.85	0.59	2.3
Birthweight < 1,000 gm	0.65	0.52	1.9
Pelvic or abdominal X-ray exposure	0.56	0.17	1.8
Toxemia (proteinuria, hypertension, eclampsia)	0.56	0.25	1.8
Hematuria	0.53	0.42	1.7
Placental infarcts	0.51	0.17	1.7
Endocrine disorders other than diabetes, hypothyroidism, or hyperthyroidism	0.51	0.35	1.7
Duration of pregnancy ≤ 8 LM	0.39	0.28	1.5
Length of gestation at registration ≤ 4 LM	0.34	0.16	1.4
Prepregnant weight ≥ 60 kg	0.29	0.16	1.3

Table **16.29**

Distribution of Observed and Expected Numbers of Children with Tumors by Multiple Logistic Risk Function Scores

Risk Score Percentile[1]	Observed Number of Children with Tumors	Expected Number of Children with Tumors
99–100	12	12.9
97–98	6	8.2
95–96	7	6.9
93–94	8	6.5
91–92	10	5.6
Total (91–100)	43	40.1
81–90	23	23.5
71–80	23	19.6
61–70	9	16.1
51–60	13	14.5
41–50	14	12.2
31–40	6	11.3
21–30	15	9.7
11–20	7	8.5
1–10	11	8.5
Total	164	164.0

[1]Each decile contains 5,025 pregnancies, except the lowest which contains 5,057 pregnancies.

eliminated were history of prior stillbirth, history of prior neonatal death, abruptio placentae, hydramnios, low weight gain during pregnancy, and prior malformed siblings. The results of the multiple logistic risk function analysis for the 11 variables that were retained are shown in Table 16.28.

Factors with relative risks greater than 2 included convulsive disorder (2.8) and single umbilical artery (2.3). Neither was statistically significant. Of the remaining factors, pelvic or abdominal X-ray exposure during pregnancy (1.8), toxemia (1.8), placental infarcts (1.7), and length of gestation at registration of at least 4 lunar months (1.4) were all statistically significant.

Table 16.29 shows the 164 children with tumors, classified according to risk score. The top decile of risk contained about one-quarter of the tumors and the ratio of numbers in this decile to those in the lowest decile was about five, showing good discrimination by the model between degrees of risk. Within deciles of risk, agreement between observed and expected numbers of pregnancies resulting in offspring with tumors was satisfactory.

CHAPTER 17

Malformations With Non-Uniform Frequencies in the Hospitals

Race-specific comparisons of malformation rates where numbers were adequate revealed six outcomes that showed considerable variability among the participating institutions; these are hereafter referred to as "non-uniform" malformations and include inguinal hernia, clubfoot, pectus excavatum, urethral obstruction, cleft gum, and miscellaneous abnormalities of the hands and fingers. As explained in Chapter 2, these outcomes have been considered separately in order to simplify the analytical procedures.

Of the six non-uniform malformations, abnormalities of the hands and fingers affected only 10 children. There was clearly no need to analyze this outcome by multivariate analysis. All associations between drug exposure and this outcome are documented in Appendix 4 in terms of relative risk standardized for hospital variability.

There were 110 children with cleft gum and this outcome was evaluated in terms of all of the risk factors selected for analysis. None of them was found to show any appreciable association with cleft gum and it was not possible to utilize multivariate techniques in any meaningful way. Data on associations between drugs and cleft gum are also presented in Appendix 4.

Similar analysis of 68 children recorded as having urethral obstruction again failed to uncover consistent associations with any risk factors. As for abnormalities of the hands and fingers and for cleft gum, data for associations between drugs and urethral obstruction are presented only in Appendix 4.

Table 17.1 presents the race-specific hospital distribution of cleft gum, urethral obstruction, and abnormal hands and fingers. It can be seen that there is considerable inter-hospital variability in the rates of all three malformations.

The remaining three non-uniform malformations, inguinal hernia, clubfoot, and pectus excavatum, are described below. Because of the inter-hospital variability in the rates of these malformations, it would be necessary, in contrast with previous chapters, to present each risk factor stratified not only by ethnic group, but also by institution. This has proved to be unacceptably complicated, and we have therefore elected to omit the univariate tables.

Inguinal Hernia

There were 683 children with inguinal hernia (13.6 per 1,000). Table 17.2 gives the race-specific rates by hospital. It is evident that there was considerable variability, with rates ranging from zero to 16.5 per 1,000, 8.8 to 111.1 per 1,000, and zero to 8.8 per 1,000 in Whites, Blacks and Puerto Ricans, respectively. As shown in Table 17.3, Blacks in six hospitals — in Boston, Buffalo, New York (Columbia), Minnesota, Oregon, and Pennsylvania — had inguinal hernia rates that were higher than those of Blacks at other hospitals or Whites and Puerto Ricans. The overall rates of inguinal hernia in Whites and Puerto Ricans were 12.7 and 8.1 per 1,000, respectively, while Blacks in the hospitals mentioned above had a rate of 19.0 and other Blacks, a rate of 11.9 per 1,000.

Risk Factors for Inguinal Hernia
According to Multivariate Analysis
Selection of risk factors for multivariate analysis was based on univariate comparisons; for each factor, the four race-hospital groups described in Table 17.3 were used. Twenty factors were selected and scaled as binary or ordinal variables. The following factors were eliminated after linear discriminant function analysis: history of prior premature births, low placental weight, cord knot, vena cava syndrome, and bacterial infection. The results of the multiple logistic risk function analysis (allowing for hospital variability) for the remaining 15 factors are given in Table 17.4.

Two factors had relative risks greater than 3: male sex (6.8) and birthweight under 2,000 gm (3.8); both were statistically significant. Two factors had relative risks between 2 and 3, both of which were statistically significant: single umbilical artery (2.7), and maternal diabetes (2.3). Of the remaining factors, the following were statistically significant: height of mother equal to or greater than 170 cm (1.8), exposure to rubella after the third lunar month (1.6), Black born in certain hospitals (1.5), history of prior malformed siblings (1.3), cigarette smoking during pregnancy (1.3), pelvic and/or abdominal X-ray exposure during pregnancy (1.2), and vaginal bleeding during the second or third trimester (1.2).

Table 17.5 shows the 683 children with inguinal hernia stratified by risk score as based on the multiple logistic model. Agreement between observed and expected numbers of inguinal hernias within the strata is quite satisfactory. The ratio of the numbers in the highest risk decile to those in the lowest is large, showing good discrimination among degrees of risk.

Clubfoot

Clubfoot was recorded in 192 children (3.8 per 1,000); 81 of these were White (3.6 per 1,000), 102 were Black (4.2 per 1,000), and 9 were Puerto Rican (2.6 per 1,000). Within ethnic groups, the frequency with which clubfoot was diagnosed varied ap-

251

Table 17.1

Race-Specific Distributions of Cleft Gum, Urethral Obstruction, and Abnormalities of the Hands and Fingers by Institution (Rates per Thousand)

Location of Institution	No. of Mother-Child Pairs			Cleft Gum						Urethral Obstruction						Miscellaneous Abnormalities of Hands and Fingers					
	W	B	PR	W No.	W Rate	B No.	B Rate	PR No.	PR Rate	W No.	W Rate	B No.	B Rate	PR No.	PR Rate	W No.	W Rate	B No.	B Rate	PR No.	PR Rate
Boston, MA	10,207	1,124	25	2	0.20	7	6.23	0	—	5	0.49	0	—	0	—	1	0.10	0	—	0	—
Buffalo, NY	2,225	55	11	4	1.80	0	—	0	—	3	1.35	1	18.18	0	—	3	1.35	0	—	0	—
New Orleans, LA	0	2,507	0	—	—	1	0.40	—	—	—	—	2	0.80	—	—	—	—	1	0.40	—	—
New York, NY (Columbia)	613	848	585	1	1.63	16	18.87	0	—	1	1.63	0	—	1	1.71	0	—	1	1.18	0	—
Baltimore, MD	774	2,622	1	0	—	9	3.43	0	—	0	—	1	0.38	0	—	0	—	0	—	0	—
Richmond, VA	796	2,262	0	3	3.77	28	12.38	0	—	1	1.26	1	0.44	0	—	0	—	0	—	0	—
Minneapolis, MN	2,914	18	2	0	—	0	—	0	—	3	1.03	0	—	0	—	0	—	0	—	0	—
New York, NY (N.Y. Medical)	253	1,489	2,506	0	—	3	2.01	1	0.40	0	—	0	—	2	0.80	0	—	0	—	0	—
Portland, OR	2,417	819	0	0	—	4	4.88	0	—	1	0.47	3	3.66	0	—	0	—	0	—	0	—
Philadelphia, PA	840	8,236	306	0	—	28	3.40	0	—	2	2.38	39	4.74	0	—	0	—	0	—	0	—
Providence, RI	2,022	654	5	0	—	1	1.53	0	—	1	0.50	0	—	0	—	0	—	2	3.06	0	—
Memphis, TN	20	3,396	0	0	—	2	0.59	0	—	0	—	1	0.29	0	—	0	—	2	0.59	0	—

Table **17.2**

Race-Specific Distribution of Inguinal Hernia by Institution (Rates per Thousand)

| | White | | | Black | | | Puerto Rican | | |
| | No. of Children | Children with Inguinal Hernia | | No. of Children | Children with Inguinal Hernia | | No. of Children | Children with Inguinal Hernia | |
Location of Institution		No.	Rate		No.	Rate		No.	Rate
Boston, MA	10,207	124	12.1	1,124	23	20.5	25	0	—
Buffalo, NY	2,225	36	16.2	55	1	18.2	11	0	—
New Orleans, LA	0	—	—	2,507	28	11.2	0	—	—
New York, NY (Columbia)	613	9	14.7	848	18	21.2	585	4	6.8
Baltimore, MD	774	9	11.6	2,622	34	13.0	1	0	—
Richmond, VA	796	7	8.8	2,262	34	15.0	0	—	—
Minneapolis, MN	2,914	48	16.5	18	2	111.1	2	0	—
New York, NY (NY Medical)	253	3	11.9	1,489	21	14.1	2,506	22	8.8
Portland, OR	2,147	27	12.6	819	16	19.5	0	—	—
Philadelphia, PA	840	9	10.7	8,236	151	18.3	306	2	6.5
Providence, RI	2,022	18	8.9	654	7	10.7	5	0	—
Memphis, TN	20	0	—	3,396	30	8.8	0	—	—

Table **17.3**

Distribution of Children with Inguinal Hernia by Ethnic Group

| | No. of Children | Children with Inguinal Hernia | |
		No.	Rate/1,000
White	22,811	290	12.7
Black			
Group 1[1]	11,100	211	19.0
Group 2[2]	12,930	154	11.9
Puerto Rican	3,441	28	8.1

[1]Group 1: Boston, MA, Buffalo, NY, New York, NY (Columbia), Minneapolis, MN, Portland, OR, Philadelphia, PA.
[2]Group 2: New Orleans, LA, Baltimore, MD, Richmond, VA, New York, NY (NY Medical), Providence, RI, Memphis, TN.

Table **17.4**

Factors Related to the Risk of Inguinal Hernia Based Upon Multiple Logistic Risk Function Analysis

	Estimated Risk Function Coefficient	Standard Error of Coefficient	Estimated Standardized Relative Risk
Male Sex	1.91	0.11	6.8
Birthweight < 2,000 gm	1.34	0.16	3.8
Single umbilical artery	1.01	0.28	2.7
Maternal diabetes	0.82	0.40	2.3
Height of mother ≥ 170 cm	0.61	0.18	1.8
Exposure to rubella after LM 3	0.50	0.19	1.6
Black, born at Boston, Buffalo, New York (Columbia), Minnesota, Oregon, Pennsylvania	0.41	0.08	1.5
At least 2 prior stillbirths	0.29	0.23	1.3
Prior malformed sibling(s)	0.28	0.13	1.3
Cigarette smoking during pregnancy	0.25	0.08	1.3
Incompetent cervix	0,23	0.41	1.3
Pelvic/abdominal X-ray exposure during pregnancy	0.20	0.09	1.2
Vaginal bleeding in second or third trimester	0.19	0.09	1.2
Length of gestation ≤ 9 LM	0.10	0.14	1.1

Table **17.5**

Distribution of Observed and Expected Numbers of Children with Inguinal Hernia by Multiple Logistic Risk Function Scores

Risk Score Percentile[1]	Observed Number of Children with Inguinal Hernia	Expected Number of Children with Inguinal Hernia
99–100	83	84.8
97–98	50	51.1
95–96	42	39.8
93–94	28	33.9
91–92	31	30.4
Total (91–100)	234	240.0
81–90	129	121.3
71–80	83	92.7
61–70	78	75.6
51–60	59	60.4
41–50	55	37.7
31–40	19	20.2
21–30	15	14.7
11–20	7	11.6
1–10	4	8.8
Total	683	683.0

[1]Each decile contains 5,025 pregnancies, except the lowest which contains 5,057 pregnancies.

preciably by hospital (Table 17.6). Rates ranged from 1.3 to 8.2, 0.3 to 18.9, and 1.2 to 10.3 per 1,000 in Whites, Blacks, and Puerto Ricans, respectively.

Risk Factors for Clubfoot
According to Multivariate Analysis

Selection of risk factors for multivariate analysis was based on univariate comparisons, using, for each factor, six race-hospital groups. Twenty-one factors were selected and scaled as dichotomous variables.

Three were eliminated after linear discriminant function analysis: short duration of pregnancy at registration, marginal sinus rupture, and one race-hospital variable. The remaining 18 variables were entered into the multiple logistic risk function analysis, the results of which are presented in Table 17.7.

Variables with relative risks greater than three included Blacks at Buffalo or

New York (Columbia) (4.6), single umbilical artery (3.5), Puerto Ricans at New York (Columbia) (3.2), and birthweight under 2,000 gm (3.2); all were statistically significant. Variables with relative risks between 2 and 3 were hydramnios (2.6), maternal syphilis (mostly inactive) (2.1) and Whites at Buffalo, Columbia, or Virginia (2.1). The association with syphilis was not statistically significant. Of the remaining variables, the following were statistically significant: low placental weight (1.9), any signs of toxemia in Blacks (1.7), family history of malformations (1.7), male infant (1.6), first-born child (1.4), and Blacks at Tennessee (0.1).

In Table 17.8, comparisons of the observed and expected numbers within each stratum of computed risk indicate that there is good agreement between the numbers of children with clubfoot predicted on the basis of the summed risks

Table **17.6**

Distribution of Children with Clubfoot by Ethnic Group[1] and Institution (Rates per Thousand)

Location of Institution	White			Black		
	No. of Children	Children with Clubfoot		No. of Children	Children with Clubfoot	
		No.	Rate		No.	Rate
Boston, MA	10,207	30	2.9	1,124	2	1.8
Buffalo, NY	2,225	14	6.3	55	1	18.2
New Orleans, LA	0	—	—	2,507	11	4.4
New York, NY (Columbia)	613	5	8.2	848	16	18.9
Baltimore, MD	774	1	1.3	2,622	8	3.1
Richmond, VA	796	6	7.5	2,262	8	3.5
Minneapolis, MN	2,914	11	3.8	18	0	—
New York, NY (NY Medical)	253	1	4.0	1,489	7	4.7
Portland, OR	2,147	6	2.8	819	2	2.4
Philadelphia, PA	840	2	2.4	8,236	44	5.3
Providence, RI	2,022	5	2.5	654	2	3.1
Memphis, TN	20	0	—	3,396	1	0.3
Total	22,811	81	3.6	24,030	102	4.2

[1]Puerto Ricans: New York, NY (Columbia): 6/585 (10.3 per 1000), New York, NY (NY Medical): 3/2,506 (1.2 per 1000) Total: 9/3,441 (2.6 per 1000).

255

Table **17.7**

Factors Related to the Risk of Clubfoot Based on Multiple Logistic Risk Function Analysis

	Estimated Risk Function Coefficient	Standard Error of Coefficient	Estimated Standardized Relative Risk
Blacks at Buffalo, NY or New York, NY (Columbia)	1.52	0.27	4.6
Single umbilical artery	1.25	0.43	3.5
Puerto Ricans at New York, NY (Columbia)	1.17	0.42	3.2
Birthweight < 2,000 gm	1.15	0.32	3.2
Hydramnios	0.95	0.37	2.6
Syphilis (mostly inactive)	0.76	0.39	2.1
Whites at Buffalo, NY, New York, NY (Columbia), or Richmond, VA	0.75	0.22	2.1
Placental weight < 300 gm	0.65	0.28	1.9
Signs of toxemia in Blacks	0.53	0.20	1.7
Malformations in the mother and/or clubfoot and/or miscellaneous malformations in sibling(s)[1]	0.52	0.26	1.7
Urinary tract infection with fever and/or hematuria during pregnancy	0.51	0.30	1.7
Male infant	0.45	0.15	1.6
Vaginal bleeding in first trimester	0.44	0.23	1.6
Firstborn child	0.33	0.16	1.4
Placental weight ≥ 500 gm	0.31	0.18	1.4
Duration of pregnancy < 8 lunar months	−0.28	0.38	0.8
Puerto Ricans at New York, NY (NY Medical)	−0.93	0.59	0.4
Blacks at Memphis, TN	−2.52	1.00	0.1

[1]Malformations other than cardiac, head/spine, finger/toe, cleft lip/palate, clubfoot.

for the mother-child pairs constituting the strata and the numbers of malformed children actually observed. In addition, the ratio of the numbers in the top decile of risk to the numbers in the lowest decile is large. This high ratio suggests that the model is adequate in discriminating between degrees of risk.

Pectus Excavatum

Pectus excavatum was recorded in 92 children (1.8 per 1,000). Only 9 of these were Black (10%), while 5 were Puerto Rican (5%). The rates among Whites, Blacks, and Puerto Ricans were 3.4, 0.4, and 1.5 per 1,000, respectively.

The distribution of pectus excavatum by ethnic group and hospital is given in Table 17.9. Fully 28 of the 78 White cases were recorded in Buffalo (36%, 12.6 per 1,000), whereas in Minnesota and Ore-

gon, only 3 cases (1.0 per 1,000) and 1 case (0.5 per 1,000), respectively, were recorded. There were no cases recorded in Tennessee. The rates for Whites at the other institutions were in the range 2.4 to 6.5 per 1,000. The rates for Blacks and Puerto Ricans ranged from zero to 1.8 and zero to 5.1 per 1,000, respectively.

Risk Factors for Pectus Excavatum According to Multivariate Analysis

Selection of risk factors for multivariate analysis was based on univariate comparisons, using, for each factor, six race-hospital groups. Nineteen factors were selected and scaled as dichotomous variables.

After linear discriminant function analysis, two factors, small number of antenatal visits and endocrine disorders other than diabetes or malfunction of the thyroid gland in the mother, were elimi-

Table **17.8**

Distribution of Observed and Expected Numbers of Children with Clubfoot by Multiple Logistic Risk Function Scores

Risk Score Percentile[1]	Observed Number of Children with Clubfoot	Expected Number of Children with Clubfoot
99–100	33	26.8
97–98	7	13.3
95–96	9	10.4
93–94	9	8.4
91–92	5	7.4
Total (91–100)	63	66.3
81–90	25	28.6
71–80	21	20.9
61–70	19	17.3
51–60	14	14.9
41–50	12	12.6
31–40	15	11.7
21–30	13	9.4
11–20	6	7.9
1–10	4	2.4
Total	192	192.0

[1]Each decile contains 5,025 pregnancies, except the lowest which contains 5,057 pregnancies.

nated because of low coefficients. The 17 remaining factors are listed in Table 17.10, with their multiple logistic risk function coefficients, the standard errors, and the estimated standardized relative risks derived from these coefficients.

Factors with relative risks greater than 3 were vena cava syndrome (8.0), abruptio placentae at Buffalo (4.0), and convulsive disorder (3.0). The first two were statistically significant. Factors with relative risks between 2 and 3 included male child (2.8), registration at Buffalo (2.6), low socioeconomic status at Buffalo (2.4), family history of malformations (2.2), and birthweight at least 4,000 gm (2.0). The only one of these statistically significant was low socioeconomic status.

Of the remaining factors, the following were statistically significant: vomiting during pregnancy (1.8), first-born child (1.8), history of prior abortions (1.7), White at Minnesota and Oregon (0.3), and Black ethnic group (0.1).

The mother-child pairs were ordered by risk function score for pectus excavatum. The results are shown in Table 17.11; it is clear that the multiple logistic risk function model adequately differentiates among pregnancies with differing degrees of risk, with good agreement between observed and expected numbers of children with pectus excavatum, and with the ratio of the numbers in the highest decile to the numbers in the lowest being very large.

Table **17.9**

Distribution of Pectus Excavatum by Ethnic Group[1] and Institution (Rates per Thousand)

Location of Institution	White			Black		
	No. of Children	Pectus Excavatum		No. of Children	Pectus Excavatum	
		No.	Rate		No.	Rate
Boston, MA	10,207	26	2.5	1,124	2	1.8
Buffalo, NY	2,225	28	12.6	55	0	—
New Orleans, LA	0	—	—	2,507	1	0.4
New York, NY (Columbia)	613	4	6.5	848	0	—
Baltimore, MD	774	2	2.6	2,622	1	0.4
Richmond, VA	796	3	3.8	2,262	0	—
Minneapolis, MN	2,914	3	1.0	18	0	—
New York, NY (NY Medical)	253	1	4.0	1,489	1	0.7
Portland, OR	2,147	1	0.5	819	0	—
Philadelphia, PA	840	2	2.4	8,236	3	0.4
Providence, RI	2,022	8	4.0	654	0	—
Memphis, TN	20	0	—	3,396	1	0.3
Total	22,811	78	3.4	24,030	9	0.4

[1]Puerto Ricans: 3/585 at Columbia (5.1 per 1000), 2/2,506 at New York Medical (0.8 per 1000), 0/306 at Philadelphia, PA. No other institution had more than 25 children. Total: 5/3,441 (1.5 per 1000).

Table **17.10**

Factors Related to the Risk of Pectus Excavatum Based on Multiple Logistic Risk Function Analysis

	Estimated Risk Function Coefficient	Standard Error of Coefficient	Estimated Standardized Relative Risk
Vena cava syndrome	2.08	0.73	8.0
Abruptio placentae at Buffalo, NY	1.39	0.45	4.0
Convulsive disorder	1.11	0.75	3.0
Male child	1.05	0.24	2.8
Children's Hospital of Buffalo, NY	0.95	0.30	2.6
Socioeconomic status < 6.0 at Buffalo, NY	0.86	0.47	2.4
Malformations in mother, father, and/or at least two siblings	0.79	0.33	2.2
Birthweight ≥ 4,000 gm	0.71	0.32	2.0
Vomiting during pregnancy	0.60	0.27	1.8
First-born child	0.60	0.22	1.8
History of prior abortion(s)	0.55	0.25	1.7
Placental infarcts ≥ 3 cm diameter	0.46	0.40	1.6
Duration of pregnancy at registration ≤ 4 lunar months	0.32	0.23	1.4
Non-smoking mother	0.30	0.21	1.3
Puerto Rican ethnic group	−0.60	0.48	0.6
White born in Minnesota and Oregon	−1.34	0.52	0.3
Black ethnic group	−1.91	0.37	0.1

Table *17.11*

Distribution of Observed and Expected Numbers of Children with Pectus Excavatum by Multiple Logistic Risk Function Scores

Risk Score Percentile[1]	Observed Number of Children with Pectus Excavatum	Expected Number of Children with Pectus Excavatum
99–100	27	24.4
97–98	6	9.2
95–96	12	6.8
93–94	2	5.5
91–92	2	4.5
Subtotal (91–100)	49	50.4
81–90	11	15.7
71–80	12	9.1
61–70	9	5.7
51–60	2	3.8
41–50	5	2.7
31–40	2	1.9
21–30	0	1.3
11–20	1	0.9
1–10	1	0.5
Total	92	92.0

[1]Each decile contains 5,025 pregnancies, except the lowest which contains 5,057 pregnancies.

CHAPTER 18

Drug Utilization

Several hundred distinct pharmacological entities were taken by the 50,282 women in the Collaborative Perinatal Project. Before these drugs can be evaluated as possible teratogens, it is necessary to consider patterns of drug utilization. For this reason, the chapter is divided into three parts: a description of the classification used in this study; a description of drug use, both in general and as related to various risk factors for malformations; and a consideration of the problem of under-reporting of drug exposure as it may affect relationships between drugs and malformations.

Classification of Drugs

Since many drugs have widespread and complex actions, no classification can ever be entirely satisfactory. The classification adopted in this study is based on pharmacological considerations, therapeutic indications, and how commonly particular agents were used. Also, agents such as vaccines are included in the classification.

The classification is generically based and does not include brand names or (with a few exceptions, such as oral contraceptives) preparations containing combinations of drugs. For combination drugs, the generic ingredients have been identified and classified accordingly.

As shown in Table 18.1, the drugs taken by the women in the cohort have

Table **18.1**

Broad Classification of Drug Exposure in 50,282 Mother-Child Pairs From the First Day of the Last Menstrual Period to 48 Hours Before Delivery

	Mother-Child Pairs Exposed			
	Lunar Months 1–4		Anytime During Pregnancy	
	No.	%	No.	%
Analgesic and antipyretic drugs	15,909	31.6	33,841	67.3
Nonaddicting analgesics and antipyretics	15,463	30.8	32,856	65.3
Narcotic analgesics	1,564	3.1	6,745	13.4
Antimicrobial and antiparasitic agents	8,088	16.1	17,538	34.9
Antibiotics	4,444	8.8	9,560	19.0
Sulfonamides	1,455	2.9	5,689	11.3
Miscellaneous antimicrobial and antiparasitic agents	981	2.0	3,185	6.3
Antimicrobial drugs used for topical application	2,918	5.8	4,792	9.5
Immunizing agents	9,222	18.3	22,707	45.2
Antinauseants, antihistamines, and phenothiazines	6,194	12.0	14,641	29.1
Antihistamines and antinauseants	5,401	10.4	12,678	25.2
Phenothiazines	1,309	2.6	3,675	7.3
Sedatives, tranquilizers, and antidepressants	3,122	6.2	14,278	28.4
Barbiturates	2,413	4.8	12,639	25.1
Tranquilizers and nonbarbiturate sedatives	946	1.9	3,231	6.4
Antidepressants	59	0.1	152	0.3
Drugs affecting the autonomic nervous system	4,657	9.2	12,502	24.9
Sympathomimetic drugs	3,082	6.1	9,719	19.3
Parasympatholytic drugs	2,323	4.6	5,623	11.2
Parasympathomimetic drugs	30	0.1	44	0.1
Anesthetics, anticonvulsants, muscle relaxants, and stimulants	2,657	5.3	6,990	13.9
Local anesthetics	2,165	4.3	5,703	11.3
General anesthetics and oxygen	218	0.4	492	1.0
Nonbarbiturate anticonvulsants	151	0.3	425	0.9
General nervous system stimulants	60	0.1	228	0.5
Muscle relaxants	83	0.2	266	0.5
Smooth muscle stimulants	57	0.1	196	0.4
Caffeine and other xanthine derivatives	5,773	11.5	13,509	26.9
Diuretics and drugs taken for cardiovascular disorders	392	0.8	15,887	31.6
Diuretics	280	0.6	15,671	31.2
Antihypertensive agents	53	0.1	525	1.0
Vasodilators	39	0.1	129	0.3
Digitalis glycosides	52	0.1	129	0.3

Table **18.1** (Continued)

Table *18.1*   (Continued)

| | Mother-Child Pairs Exposed | | | |
| | Lunar Months 1–4 | | Anytime During Pregnancy | |
	No.	%	No.	%
Cough Medicines	948	1.9	7,941	15.8
Expectorants	864	1.7	6,277	12.5
Antitussives	344	0.7	867	1.7
Unspecified cough medicines	55	0.1	1,789	3.6
Drugs used for gastrointestinal disturbances	440	0.9	1,500	3.0
Hormones, hormone antagonists, and contraceptives	2,327	4.6	3,506	7.0
Progestational agents	866	1.7	1,399	2.8
Estrogenic agents	614	1.2	761	1.5
Thyroid hormones	560	1.1	825	1.6
Corticosteroids and corticotropin	145	0.3	275	5.5
Antidiabetic drugs	139	0.3	234	4.7
Miscellaneous hormones	131	0.3	433	8.6
Thyroid suppressants	25	0.1	38	7.6
Oral contraceptives	278	0.6	309	6.1
Local contraceptives	462	0.9	466	9.3
Inorganic compounds and certain vitamins	2,542	5.1	10,116	20.1
Bromides, fluorides, and iodides	1,526	3.0	5,312	10.6
Calcium, parenteral iron, and vitamins (B_{12} and K)	1,091	2.2	5,598	11.1
Diagnostic aids	108	0.2	313	0.6
Radiopaque media	69	0.1	150	0.3
Intravenous dilution test agents	22	0.0	127	0.3
Radioactive material	21	0.0	50	0.1
Technical aids	431	0.9	1,736	3.4
Local irritants and keratolytics	386	0.8	1,661	3.3
Enzymes	19	0.0	51	0.1
Agents used for wound protection	27	0.1	31	0.1
Rare drugs	300	0.6	777	1.5
Miscellaneous infrequently used drugs	50	0.1	148	0.3
Drugs with unknown ingredients	250	0.5	632	1.3

been divided into 16 broad groups with further subgroups. The complete list of all drugs comprising each of the subgroups is given in Appendix 3. The arrangement of the table shows the principles used in making the classification. For example, division of autonomic drugs into sympathomimetic, parasympatholytic, and parasympathomimetic drugs is in accord with the usual pharmacological classifications. At the other extreme, diuretics and drugs taken for cardiovascular disorders represent a mixed group of drugs consisting of diuretics, antihypertensives, vasodilators, and digitalis glycosides. Their pharmacological actions are not at all comparable, but they are unified by their indication in the

262

treatment of cardiovascular disorders (especially during early pregnancy) or edema. Similarly, some antinauseants, antihistamines, and phenothiazines are not similar in terms of chemical structure or pharmacological action. They are grouped together in this study because the main indication for their use was nausea and vomiting.

It should be kept in mind that iron preparations (when taken by mouth) and antacids were not considered in this study. Vitamins were also disregarded, with the exceptions of vitamin B_{12} and vitamin K, when received by injection.

Patterns of Drug Utilization

This section gives a broad overall description of drug use and an evaluation of drug use in terms of some administrative and pregnancy-related variables.

Overall Drug Utilization

Table 18.2 has been excerpted from Table 18.1 to more easily show rates of exposure to the drug groups as classified in this study. Fully 31.6% of the gravidas took analgesics (mostly aspirin) during early pregnancy, and by the time pregnancy ended, over two-thirds (67.3%)

Table **18.2**

Percentages of Drug Exposure in 50,282 Mother-Child Pairs from the First Day of the Last Menstrual Period to 48 Hours Before Delivery

| | Mother-Child Pairs Exposed | | | | | | | |
| | White (n=22,811) | | Black (n=24,030) | | Puerto Rican (n=3,441) | | Total (n=50,282) | |
	Early[1]	Any-time[2]	Early[1]	Any-time[2]	Early[1]	Any-time[2]	Early[1]	Any-time[2]
Analgesic and antipyretic drugs	31.4	68.4	34.6	69.2	12.6	46.9	31.6	67.3
Antimicrobial and antiparasitic agents	14.5	32.2	18.6	38.0	9.1	30.7	16.1	34.9
Immunizing agents	25.5	56.6	12.0	31.7	15.6	63.8	18.3	45.2
Antinauseants, antihistamines, and phenothiazines	16.7	35.8	8.6	23.6	4.8	15.7	12.0	28.6
Sedatives, tranquilizers, and antidepressants	8.2	32.7	4.9	26.0	1.9	16.5	6.2	28.4
Drugs affecting the autonomic nervous system	12.6	29.1	7.1	22.8	2.3	10.8	9.3	24.9
Anesthetics, anticonvulsants, muscle relaxants, and stimulants	7.5	18.9	3.7	10.5	1.4	4.8	5.3	13.9
Caffeine and other xanthine derivatives	10.4	25.0	13.8	30.6	2.8	13.3	11.5	26.9
Diuretics and drugs taken for cardiovascular disorders	1.0	32.4	0.7	31.7	0.03	25.8	0.8	31.6
Cough medicines	2.0	18.2	2.0	13.8	1.0	14.4	1.9	15.8
Drugs used for gastrointestinal disturbances	0.8	2.5	1.1	3.8	0.1	0.4	0.9	3.0
Hormones, hormone antagonists, and contraceptives	6.2	9.2	3.6	5.5	1.2	2.3	4.6	7.0
Inorganic compounds and certain vitamins	4.9	18.3	5.6	23.3	2.0	10.3	5.1	20.1
Diagnostic aids	0.2	0.6	0.2	0.7	0.1	0.1	0.2	0.6
Technical aids	1.0	3.6	0.8	1.5	0.2	0.6	0.9	2.4
Rare drugs	0.6	1.6	0.7	1.7	0.2	0.6	0.6	1.5

[1]Lunar Months 1–4
[2]Anytime from LMP to 48 hours before onset of labor

263

had used this group of drugs. Similarly, almost one-fifth of the mothers (18.3%) received immunizing agents (principally killed polio virus vaccine) in the first trimester, and 45.2% received such agents before term.

In general, drugs more commonly used in early pregnancy were also more commonly used in late pregnancy, but there were some exceptions. The most striking exception applied to diuretics and drugs taken for cardiovascular disorders: while such drugs were used by only 0.8% of the gravidas during early pregnancy, 31.6% used them before term. This was mostly due to the great increase in the use of diuretics as pregnancy progressed.

With the single exception of immunizing agents, drug exposure rates in Puerto Rican women were either lower than in Black women or (in the case of cough medicines only) similar. The following differences during early pregnancy between Black women and White women are noteworthy: receipt of immunizing agents by White women (25.5%) was almost twice that of Black women (12.0%), and drugs generally used to treat nausea or vomiting (antinauseants, antihistamines, and phenothiazines) were taken by 16.7% of the White women and 8.6% of the Black women; hormones, hormone antagonists, and oral contraceptives were used by 6.2% of the White and 3.6% of the Black women. Other differences were less sharp, but generally drug usage across most of the categories was more common in White women. Table 18.2 also shows that while drug usage rates were substantially higher when the entire pregnancy was taken into account, differences in usage rates between Black women and White women were still present although, for the most part, they were less sharp.

Number of Products
Used by Pregnant Women

In this section, the number of products taken by women in the three ethnic groups is examined, initially in terms of secular trends and hospital distributions, and then in terms of some risk factors for various malformation outcomes.

It should be stressed that here *products*, not *drugs*, are under consideration: many products contain more than one ingredient (e.g., combinations of aspirin, phenacetin, caffeine, and pseudoephedrine). However, if two commercial brands happen to have the identical ingredients, they are counted here as one *product*. It is also worth re-emphasizing that iron or vitamin preparations (particularly multivitamins), taken by mouth, and antacids are not considered.

Secular Trends

In Table 18.3 the mean number of products used throughout pregnancy is given according to the year of the last menstrual period and according to ethnic group. Overall, the mean number of preparations taken by the mothers was 3.8. In 1958, the mean was 2.6 per pregnancy, and there was a steady increase over the years until 1965 when the mean was 4.5. The mean for White mothers was 4.2, and the corresponding values for Blacks and Puerto Ricans were 3.5 and 2.7, respectively. In contrast to Whites and Blacks, there were no discernable trends among Puerto Ricans.

The time-related trend can again be observed in Table 18.4. Overall, in only 5.8% of the gravidas was there no record of drug use, and the proportion of mothers who took no drugs decreased from 9.4% in 1958 to 4.4% in 1965. The proportion also decreased for mothers taking only one product: in 1958, this was 21.3% and by 1965 it had dropped to 12.4%.

Similarly, over the years of the study the proportions of mothers taking 2 to 4 preparations decreased from 55.3% in 1958 to 43.0% in 1965. By contrast, the proportion of gravidas taking 5 to 10 products increased from 13.8% to 33.4%. A relatively small proportion of gravidas

Table **18.3**

Mean Number of Pharmaceutical Products Used in 50,282 Pregnancies Classified by Ethnic Group and Year of Mother's Last Menstrual Period (LMP)

Year of LMP	No. of Mother-Child Pairs	White (n=22,811)	Black (n=24,030)	Puerto Rican (n=3,441)	Total (n=50,282)
1958	1,877	2.6	2.6	2.2	2.6
1959	5,735	3.5	2.6	2.5	3.0
1960	7,285	3.6	2.9	2.6	3.2
1961	7,441	4.1	3.6	2.8	3.8
1962	8,216	4.5	3.9	3.1	4.1
1963	7,986	4.5	3.9	2.8	4.1
1964	7,817	4.7	3.8	2.5	4.1
1965	3,925	5.0	4.2	2.7	4.5
Total	50,282	4.2	3.5	2.7	3.8

Table **18.4**

Percentages of 50,282 Mother-Child Pairs Exposed to Various Numbers of Pharmaceutical Products According to Year of Mother's Last Menstrual Period (LMP)

Year of LMP	No. of Mother-Child Pairs	Number of Pharmaceutical Products				
		None	1	2–4	5–10	≥10
1958	1,877	9.4	21.3	55.3	13.8	0.2
1959	5,735	7.6	19.2	52.1	19.9	1.1
1960	7,258	8.9	19.1	49.1	21.0	1.8
1961	7,441	5.3	15.0	49.4	27.0	3.2
1962	8,216	4.5	12.2	48.2	31.3	3.7
1963	7,986	4.0	12.8	48.3	30.8	4.1
1964	7,817	5.2	13.0	47.2	29.7	4.8
1965	3,925	4.4	12.4	43.0	33.4	6.7
Total	50,282	5.8	14.9	48.7	27.1	3.4

took 10 or more preparations, the overall rate being 3.4%. However, even here there was a striking upward trend over the years, with only 0.2% using over 10 products in 1958 and 6.7% using this number in 1965.

During the years of the study, including the period from 1962 onward when thalidomide was given a great deal of publicity, the evidence points overwhelmingly to a secular increase in drug use by pregnant women. It is clear that publicity directed to avoiding unnecessary use of drugs during pregnancy was a failure.

Hospital Distributions

Table 18.5 presents the mean number of products as used in the 12 hospital centers. There was considerable variability. The highest values for early use (2.9 to 3.0) and for use at any time (6.3 to 7.3) in

Table **18.5**

Mean Number of Products Used in Pregnancy by Ethnic Group and Hospital

Location of Institution	Lunar Months 1–4			Anytime in Pregnancy			No. of Mother-Child Pairs		
	W	B	PR	W	B	PR	W	B	PR
Boston, MA	1.3	1.4	1.8	4.0	4.2	5.3	10,207	1,124	25
Buffalo, NY	3.0	3.1	2.9	6.6	7.3	6.9	2,225	55	11
New Orleans, LA	—	0.9	—	—	3.6	—	—	2,507	—
New York, NY (Columbia)	0.9	0.8	0.8	3.9	4.0	3.7	613	848	585
New York, NY (NY Medical)	0.5	0.6	0.4	2.7	2.7	2.4	253	1,489	2,506
Baltimore, MD	1.0	1.2	0.0	3.5	3.5	0.0	774	2,622	1
Richmond, VA	0.9	1.1	—	4.1	3.8	—	796	2,262	—
Minneapolis, MN	1.2	1.3	0.5	4.1	3.8	1.0	2,914	18	2
Portland, OR	0.9	0.9	—	3.6	3.1	—	2,147	819	—
Philadelphia, PA	0.9	1.1	0.9	3.5	3.6	3.0	840	8,236	306
Providence, RI	1.1	1.1	1.0	4.1	4.0	3.8	2,022	654	5
Memphis, TN	1.2	0.9	—	3.6	3.0	—	20	3,396	—
Total	1.4	1.1	0.5	4.2	3.5	2.7	22,811	24,030	3,441

pregnancy were found in Buffalo. Most of the women in that institution were private or insured patients. The lowest usage rate was in the New York Medical College Metropolitan Hospital (early 0.4 to 0.6; any time, 2.4 to 2.7). Overall, the mean numbers of products taken in early pregnancy by White, Black, and Puerto Rican women, respectively, were 1.4, 1.1, and 0.5; corresponding values for the entire pregnancy were 4.2, 3.5, and 2.7.

Table 18.5 also shows that much of the apparent difference between White women and Black women in the number of products used is accounted for by institutional variability: within institutions, differences were generally slight. However, with the exception of Boston (25 women), Puerto Rican women used fewer products.

As already mentioned, the institutional differences are quite large. There is clearly a possibility that hospital variability could confound further analyses of drug use in relation to factors such as

hydramnios or toxemia. In the following section, two strategies are used to insure that confounding from hospital variability is adequately controlled. First, all the analyses are kept race-specific. From Table 18.5, it is evident that this has the effect of partially controlling institutional variability. Second, in some of the tables, data are also given for subsets of women selected as follows: 10,207 White women from Boston (44.7% of all White women in the cohort); 8,236 Black women from Philadelphia (34.3%), and 2,506 Puerto Rican women from the New York Medical College Metropolitan Hospital (72.8%). For these three subsets, there can be no institutional confounding. To the extent that the data in the subsets agree with the overall data, confounding of any material importance is unlikely.

Drug Use in Relation to Risk Factors for Malformations

In Tables 18.6 through 18.21, the mean number of *products* (some containing more than one drug) used during pregnancy is examined in relation to certain variables, all of which were associated with one or more of the outcomes analyzed in this study.

Number of Antenatal Visits (Table 18.6) The mean number of products

taken in pregnancy was consistently higher among women who attended more frequently for antenatal care.

Age at Registration (Table 18.7) Among Whites and Blacks, drug use in early pregnancy was lowest below

Table **18.6**

Mean Number of Products Used in Pregnancy: Number of Antenatal Visits

No. of Antenatal Visits	Lunar Months 1–4			Anytime in Pregnancy			No. of Gravidas		
	W	B	PR	W	B	PR	W	B	PR
1–9	0.8	0.8	0.3	3.3	3.0	2.3	10,725	16,725	2,138
≥10	1.8	1.4	0.7	5.0	4.6	3.4	12,086	7,305	1,303

Table **18.7**

Mean Number of Products Used in Pregnancy: Mother's Age at Registration[1]

Age (Years)	Lunar Months 1–4			Anytime in Pregnancy			No. of Gravidas		
	W	B	PR	W	B	PR	W	B	PR
<15	1.0	0.7	0.6	3.2	2.8	2.6	25	394	10
	(0.0)	(0.7)	(0.7)	(2.2)	(3.0)	(2.6)	(5)	(98)	(9)
15–19	1.0	0.9	0.4	3.7	3.0	2.4	4,049	6,584	842
	(1.0)	(0.9)	(0.4)	(3.7)	(3.0)	(2.2)	(1,403)	(2,307)	(679)
20–24	1.4	1.1	0.6	4.1	3.5	2.7	9,012	8,109	1,354
	(1.3)	(1.2)	(0.4)	(4.0)	(3.6)	(2.3)	(4,138)	(2,786)	(959)
25–29	1.6	1.2	0.6	4.5	3.9	3.0	5,208	4,638	746
	(1.4)	(1.3)	(0.5)	(4.2)	(3.9)	(2.6)	(2,411)	(1 586)	(534)
30–34	1.5	1.2	0.6	4.4	4.0	2.9	2,726	2,610	319
	(1.3)	(1.3)	(0.4)	(4.2)	(4.0)	(2.5)	(1,349)	(917)	(208)
35–39	1.3	1.1	0.6	4.5	4.0	3.3	1,405	1,343	136
	(1.2)	(1.2)	(0.4)	(4.1)	(4.1)	(2.7)	(696)	(441)	(92)
40–44	1.3	1.1	0.6	4.5	4.2	3.1	369	339	34
	(1.3)	(1.1)	(0.5)	(4.5)	(4.2)	(2.8)	(195)	(96)	(25)
≥45	0.8	0.9	—	5.9	3.7	—	17	13	—
	(0.8)	(0.6)	(—)	(6.8)	(3.2)	(—)	(10)	(5)	(—)

[1] Data in parentheses refer to White women in Boston, Black women in Philadelphia, and Puerto Rican women at the New York Medical College Metropolitan Hospital.

the age of 20 years. It increased from 20 to 24 years, to reach maximum levels between the ages of 24 and 34 years; beyond the age of 34 years, there was a distinct dip in the mean number of products used. The pattern for use at any time was quite different, with the mean number of products showing a steady increase with increasing age. No consistent trend was evident in Puerto Ricans. Among the subsets of White women from Boston, Black women from Philadelphia and

Puerto Rican women from New York, the patterns were essentially similar.

Socioeconomic Status (Table 18.8)   The mean number of products taken in pregnancy increased with increasing socioeconomic status. This held true both for early use and for use throughout pregnancy. The trends were similar in the single-hospital subsets.

History of Prior Fetal or Neonatal Loss (Table 18.9)   Among White women and Black women, the number of products

Table **18.8**

Mean Number of Products Used in Pregnancy: Socioeconomic Status[1]

Socioeconomic Status (Scale of 0–10)	Lunar Months 1–4			Anytime in Pregnancy			No. of Gravidas		
	W	B	PR	W	B	PR	W	B	PR
<4.0	1.0	1.0	0.5	3.9	3.4	2.6	5,042	12,718	1,860
	(1.0)	(1.0)	(0.3)	(3.7)	(3.5)	(2.4)	(1,176)	(4,068)	(1,434)
4.5–5.9[2]	1.1	1.1	0.5	3.9	3.5	2.8	7,104	8,095	1,203
	(1.2)	(1.1)	(0.4)	(3.9)	(3.6)	(2.4)	(3,193)	(3,197)	(863)
≥6.0	1.7	1.3	0.8	4.6	3.9	3.4	10,665	3,217	378
	(1.5)	(1.3)	(0.5)	(4.1)	(4.0)	(2.7)	(5,838)	(989)	(209)

[1]Data in parentheses refer to White women in Boston, Black women in Philadelphia, and Puerto Rican women at the New York Medical College Metropolitan Hospital.
[2]Includes 855 unknowns

Table **18.9**

Mean number of Products Used in Pregnancy: History of Prior Fetal or Neonatal Loss

	Lunar Months 1–4			Anytime in Pregnancy			No. of Gravidas		
	W	B	PR	W	B	PR	W	B	PR
Prior abortion	1.6	1.4	0.6	4.9	4.4	3.0	4,053	4,406	676
No prior abortion	1.3	1.0	0.5	4.1	3.3	2.7	18,758	19,624	2,765
Prior stillbirth	1.5	1.3	0.5	4.9	4.2	2.9	1,065	1,561	211
No prior stillbirth	1.4	1.0	0.5	4.2	3.5	2.7	21,746	22,469	3,230
Prior neonatal death	1.6	1.3	0.5	4.9	4.0	2.9	805	1,226	143
No prior neonatal death	1.4	1.0	0.5	4.2	3.5	2.7	22,006	22,804	3,298

taken, both early and at any time in pregnancy, was consistently higher when there were histories of prior abortion, stillbirth, or neonatal death.

Duration of Pregnancy (Table 18.10) The mean number of products used in early pregnancy was not related to the duration of gestation. For the entire pregnancy, the mean number of products used was slightly higher in pregnancies lasting 10 or more lunar months. This effect was also evident in the single-hospital subsets.

Toxemia of Pregnancy (Table 18.11) Among women with proteinuria, hypertension, or eclampsia, the mean number of products used was increased for the entire duration of pregnancy. It was also slightly higher during the first four lunar months. The same trend was apparent in the single-hospital subsets, except that

drug use in early pregnancy was not increased among Puerto Rican women.

Vomiting and Hyperemesis Gravidarum (Table 18.12) At all stages of pregnancy, vomiting was related to the number of products taken; the relationship was particularly strong when hyperemesis was recorded, with drug usage in early pregnancy more than doubled. For the entire pregnancy, the mean number of drugs used was also strikingly increased. An analogous pattern was evident in the single-hospital subsets.

Vaginal Bleeding in Pregnancy (Table 18.13) In the table, bleeding is classified by trimester according to its *first* occurrence. First, second, and third trimester bleeding were all associated with higher mean numbers of products used. This was even true for drug use during the first four lunar months when bleeding first

Table **18.10**

Mean Number of Products Used in Pregnancy: Duration of Gestation[1]

Duration of Pregnancy (Lunar Months)	Lunar Months 1–4			Anytime in Pregnancy			No. of Gravidas		
	W	B	PR	W	B	PR	W	B	PR
5	1.8 (1.6)	1.4 (1.1)	0.8 (0.6)	4.0 (3.8)	2.8 (2.5)	1.9 (1.7)	64 (29)	136 (64)	14 (11)
6	1.7 (2.0)	1.2 (1.2)	0.5 (0.3)	4.3 (4.6)	2.8 (2.6)	2.1 (2.1)	114 (52)	218 (95)	13 (10)
7	1.4 (1.2)	1.0 (1.0)	0.6 (0.6)	4.8 (4.9)	3.2 (2.9)	2.2 (2.2)	197 (99)	531 (209)	54 (41)
8	1.5 (1.5)	1.0 (1.1)	0.4 (0.4)	4.3 (4.5)	3.1 (3.1)	2.4 (2.3)	699 (324)	1,616 (612)	195 (144)
9	1.4 (1.3)	1.1 (1.1)	0.6 (0.4)	4.2 (4.0)	3.4 (3.5)	2.7 (2.3)	9,133 (4,175)	11,858 (3,899)	1,612 (1,152)
10	1.3 (1.3)	1.0 (1.2)	0.5 (0.4)	4.2 (4.0)	3.7 (3.8)	2.9 (2.5)	12,160 (5,370)	9,210 (3,193)	1,463 1,073
≥11	1.0 (0.8)	1.0 (1.3)	0.3 (0.3)	4.5 (3.9)	4.1 (4.2)	3.0 (2.7)	444 (158)	461 (164)	90 (75)

[1]Data in parentheses refer to White women in Boston, Black women in Philadelphia, and Puerto Rican women at the New York Medical College Metropolitan Hospital.

Table **18.11**

Mean Number of Products Used in Pregnancy: Toxemia of Pregnancy[1]

	Lunar Months 1–4			Anytime in Pregnancy			No. of Gravidas		
	W	**B**	**PR**	**W**	**B**	**PR**	**W**	**B**	**PR**
Proteinuria and/or hypertension and/or eclampsia	1.5	1.2	0.7	5.5	5.0	4.3	1,015	1,691	128
	(1.4)	(1.5)	(0.3)	(5.3)	(5.9)	(3.6)	(497)	(436)	(55)
No symptoms or edema only	1.4	1.0	0.5	4.1	3.4	2.7	21,796	22,339	3,313
	(1.3)	(1.0)	(0.4)	(3.9)	(3.4)	(2.4)	(9,710)	(7,800)	(2,451)

[1]Data in parentheses refer to White women in Boston, Black women in Philadelphia, and Puerto Rican Women at the New York Medical College Metropolitan Hospital.

Table **18.12**

Mean Number of Products Used in Pregnancy: Vomiting and Hyperemesis Gravidarum[1]

	Lunar Months 1–4			Anytime in Pregnancy			No. of Gravidas		
	W	**B**	**PR**	**W**	**B**	**PR**	**W**	**B**	**PR**
Vomiting during pregnancy	1.4	1.1	0.6	4.5	3.8	3.1	15,541	15,818	1,982
No vomiting	1.0	0.8	0.3	3.5	2.8	2.2	7,270	8,212	1,459
Hyperemesis gravidarum	2.1	2.9	2.4	5.9	6.8	5.3	353	159	28
	(2.0)	(2.8)	(1.6)	(5.8)	(6.7)	(3.4)	(123)	(33)	(5)
No hyperemesis	1.3	1.0	0.5	4.1	3.4	2.7	22,458	23,871	3,413
	(1.2)	(1.1)	(0.4)	(4.0)	(3.6)	(2.4)	(10,084)	(8,203)	(2,501)

[1]Data in parentheses refer to White women in Boston, Black women in Philadelphia, and Puerto Rican women at the New York Medical College Metropolitan Hospital.

occurred in the second or third trimester of pregnancy. An analogous trend was evident in the single-hospital subsets.

Hydramnios (Table 18.14) The mean number of products used during early pregnancy, or at any time during pregnancy, was increased in women with hydramnios. This pattern was also evident in the single-hospital subsets.

Placental Factors (Table 18.15) Among Whites, abruptio placentae was as-sociated with increased drug use, both in early pregnancy and at any time in pregnancy. This relationship was not present in Blacks or Puerto Ricans. Placenta previa gave little evidence of association with increased drug use. Overall, drug use at any time in pregnancy was increased in Whites, but this relationship was not evident among 75 Whites in Boston with placenta previa.

Diabetes Mellitus (Table 18.16) The

Table **18.13**

Mean Number of Products Used in Pregnancy: Vaginal Bleeding in Pregnancy[1]

	Lunar Months 1–4			Anytime in Pregnancy			No. of Gravidas		
	W	**B**	**PR**	**W**	**B**	**PR**	**W**	**B**	**PR**
No bleeding	1.2	0.9	0.5	3.9	3.3	2.6	17,014	17,136	2,938
	(1.2)	(1.0)	(0.4)	(3.8)	(3.3)	(2.3)	(7,994)	(5,602)	(2,197)
First trimester bleeding	2.0	1.6	1.2	4.9	4.2	3.5	1,842	1,653	173
	(1.8)	(1.5)	(0.9)	(4.6)	(4.1)	(2.9)	(783)	(574)	(117)
Second trimester bleeding	1.8	1.4	0.5	5.1	4.2	3.0	1,061	1,396	89
	(1.9)	(1.3)	(0.6)	(5.0)	(4.0)	(2.8)	(424)	(584)	(58)
Third trimester bleeding	1.7	1.2	0.7	5.1	4.1	3.5	2,894	3,845	241
	(1.4)	(1.3)	(0.5)	(4.8)	(4.1)	(2.9)	(1,006)	(1,476)	(134)

[1]Data in parentheses refer to White women in Boston, Black women in Philadelphia, and Puerto Rican women at the New York Medical College Metropolitan Hospital.

Table **18.14**

Mean Number of Products Used in Pregnancy: Hydramnios[1]

	Lunar Months 1–4			Anytime in Pregnancy			No. of Gravidas		
	W	**B**	**PR**	**W**	**B**	**PR**	**W**	**B**	**PR**
Hydramnios	1.7	1.4	1.6	5.9	4.7	4.6	363	315	16
	(1.7)	(1.5)	(0.5)	(5.7)	(4.6)	(2.6)	(223)	(82)	(8)
No hydramnios	1.4	1.1	0.5	4.2	3.5	2.7	22,448	23,715	3,425
	(1.3)	(1.1)	(0.4)	(3.9)	(3.6)	(2.4)	(9,984)	(8,154)	(2,498)

[1]Data in parentheses refer to White women in Boston, Black women in Philadelphia, and Puerto Rican women at the New York Medical College Metropolitan Hospital.

table gives a hierarchical classification of diabetes according to severity. For exposure during the first four lunar months of pregnancy, the mean number of products was highest in gravidas with the most severe diabetes and intermediate in those with treated diabetes lasting less than 5 years. Among gravidas with untreated diabetes of less than 5 years duration, the mean number of products was slightly decreased in White women and slightly increased in Black women. For exposures taking place throughout pregnancy, the mean number of products used was lowest in unaffected women, and there was an increase in the number as the severity of the diabetes increased. For the single-hospital subsets, numbers in each category were rather small. Nevertheless, there was clear evidence that diabetic

271

Table **18.15**

Mean Number of Products Used in Pregnancy: Placental Factors[1]

	Lunar Months 1–4			Anytime in Pregnancy			No. of Gravidas		
	W	B	PR	W	B	PR	W	B	PR
Abruptio placentae	1.9	1.0	0.3	4.9	3.4	2.7	554	450	26
No abruptio placentae	1.3	1.0	0.5	4.2	3.5	2.7	22,257	23,580	3,415
Placenta previa	1.4	0.9	0.3	5.1	3.6	2.3	166	135	17
	(1.3)	(1.1)	(0.4)	(4.0)	(2.8)	(1.8)	(75)	(53)	(11)
No placenta previa	1.4	1.1	0.5	4.2	3.5	2.7	22,645	23,895	3,424
	(1.3)	(0.9)	(0.4)	(4.9)	(3.3)	(1.9)	(10,132)	(8,183)	(2,495)

[1]Data in parentheses refer to White women in Boston, Black women in Philadelphia, and Puerto Rican women at the New York Medical College Metropolitan Hospital.

Table **18.16**

Mean Number of Products Used in Pregnancy: Diabetes Mellitus[1]

	Lunar Months 1–4			Anytime in Pregnancy			No. of Gravidas		
	W	B	PR	W	B	PR	W	B	PR
Treated diabetes ≥ 5 years	3.0	1.9	1.0	9.4	6.1	4.3	65	30	3
	(3.3)	(1.7)	(1.0)	(9.4)	(4.3)	(3.0)	(29)	(3)	(1)
Treated diabetes < 5 years	1.7	1.6	0.8	5.9	6.8	4.3	30	62	4
	(1.5)	(1.9)	(1.0)	(5.8)	(7.8)	(3.5)	(19)	(19)	(2)
Untreated diabetes	1.3	1.3	2.4	4.9	5.1	5.1	67	65	10
	(1.5)	(1.0)	(1.3)	(4.5)	(4.3)	(4.1)	(24)	(23)	(8)
No diabetes	1.4	1.1	0.5	4.2	3.5	2.7	22,649	23,873	3,424
	(1.3)	(1.1)	(0.4)	(4.0)	(3.6)	(2.4)	(10,135)	(8,191)	(2,495)

[1]Data in parentheses refer to White women in Boston, Black women in Philadelphia, and Puerto Rican women at the New York Medical College Metropolitan Hospital.

women used more products than non-diabetics.

Selected Diseases of the Mother (Table 18.17) For some of the diseases listed in the table, numbers among Puerto Ricans were small, with corresponding instability in the mean values. However, trends were consistent among White women and Black women. Drug use in early pregnancy was increased in women with thrombophlebitis, functional cardiovascular disorders, hyperthyroidism, other endocrine disorders, urinary tract infection, convulsive disorder, and bacterial infection. This did not hold true for a recorded diagnosis of anemia or syphilis.

272

Table **18.17**

Mean Number of Products Used in Pregnancy: Selected Diseases of the Mother

	Lunar Months 1–4			Anytime in Pregnancy			No. of Gravidas		
	W	B	PR	W	B	PR	W	B	PR
All gravidas	1.4	1.1	0.5	4.2	3.5	2.7	22,811	24,030	3,441
Thrombophlebitis	2.2	2.0	0.2	7.9	6.0	3.0	88	43	13
Functional cardiovascular disorders	2.1	1.3	0.4	7.1	4.6	3.8	137	172	5
Anemia	1.3	1.0	0.4	4.6	3.6	2.5	2,213	8,299	1,249
Hyperthyroidism	2.0	2.5	5.0	6.0	6.7	6.0	44	42	1
Endocrine disease other than diabetes, hypo-thyroidism, or hyper-thyroidism	1.5	1.4	0.7	4.7	4.2	2.6	547	972	18
Syphilis	1.2	1.1	0.5	4.7	3.8	2.9	71	747	100
Urinary tract infection	1.7	1.3	0.9	7.3	6.3	5.4	271	404	34
Convulsive disorder	2.8	2.4	1.3	6.9	6.5	4.5	160	110	24
Bacterial infection	2.5	1.4	1.0	6.9	5.1	4.9	561	314	24

However, exposure at any time in pregnancy was increased for all of the diagnoses listed in Table 19.17.

Pelvic or Abdominal X-Ray Exposure (Table 18.18) The mean number of products used at any time during pregnancy or during the first four lunar months was increased in gravidas who were X-rayed.

Malformation in the Mother (Table 18.19) Malformed women used more products, both during early pregnancy and at any time.

Malformed Siblings (Table 18.20) The first row in the table gives the mean number of products used by gravidas who were either giving birth for the first time or whose prior offspring were not malformed. When there was a history of prior malformed siblings, drug use in early pregnancy was increased, but it was not materially changed if there was one,

Table **18.18**

Mean Number of Products Used in Pregnancy: Pelvic or Abdominal X-Ray Exposure[1]

	Lunar Months 1–4			Anytime in Pregnancy			No. of Gravidas		
	W	B	PR	W	B	PR	W	B	PR
X-ray	1.7 (1.5)	1.3 (1.7)	0.8 (0.6)	5.0 (4.6)	4.3 (4.8)	3.8 (2.8)	6,416 (2,897)	4,703 (1,144)	281 (97)
No X-ray	1.3 (1.2)	1.0 (1.0)	0.5 (0.4)	4.0 (3.7)	3.3 (3.4)	2.6 (2.4)	16,395 (7,310)	19,327 (7,092)	3,160 (2,409)

[1]Data in parentheses refer to White women in Boston, Black women in Philadelphia, and Puerto Rican women at the New York Medical College Metropolitan Hospital.

Table **18.19**

Mean Number of Products Used in Pregnancy: Malformation in the Mother

	Lunar Months 1–4			Anytime in Pregnancy			No. of Gravidas		
	W	B	PR	W	B	PR	W	B	PR
Mother malformed	1.5	1.3	0.8	4.8	4.1	3.7	741	406	21
Mother not malformed	1.4	1.1	0.5	4.2	3.5	2.7	20,070	23,624	3,420

Table **18.20**

Mean Number of Products Used in Pregnancy: History of Malformations in Prior Siblings[1]

	Lunar Months 1–4			Anytime in Pregnancy			No. of Gravidas		
	W	B	PR	W	B	PR	W	B	PR
Firstborn child or prior siblings normal	1.3	1.0	0.5	4.2	3.5	2.7	20,817	22,449	3,293
	(1.3)	(1.1)	(0.4)	(4.0)	(3.5)	(2.4)	(9,306)	(7,661)	(2,424)
One malformed sibling	1.6	1.3	0.8	4.6	3.9	3.5	1,785	1,397	137
	(1.4)	(1.2)	(0.3)	(4.5)	(3.8)	(2.7)	(816)	(505)	(77)
Two malformed siblings	1.6	1.4	0.6	5.2	4.2	3.6	181	156	10
	(1.7)	(1.3)	(0.2)	(5.3)	(4.2)	(3.0)	(74)	(60)	(5)
Three or more malformed siblings	1.9	0.9	1.0	4.5	3.8	3.0	28	28	1
	(1.5)	(1.4)	(—)	(4.4)	(4.3)	(—)	(11)	(10)	(—)

[1]Data in parentheses refer to White women in Boston, Black women in Philadelphia, and Puerto Rican women at the New York Medical College Metropolitan Hospital.

or more than one, affected sibling. The same trend was apparent for drug exposure throughout pregnancy. An analogous pattern was evident in the single-hospital subsets.

Comments The preceding findings indicate that in general, women with pregnancies at high risk for malformations tended to use more drugs than other women, both during the first trimester as well as throughout pregnancy. These results make it obligatory to control potential confounding if noncausal associations are to be avoided.

In Chapters 3, 19, and 34, the strategy of controlling *late* events in evaluating *early* drug exposure is considered. This strategy can be justified on the grounds that these *late* events may be indicators of antecedent ones that influenced *early* drug use; there would be no need to control *late* events if they were not determinants of *early* drug use. Thus, it is worth emphasizing that some risk factors that are predominantly, or even exclusively, manifestations of *late* pregnancy, were nevertheless related to increased drug use in *early* pregnancy. Certain fac-

274

tors (toxemia, second and third trimester bleeding, and hydramnios) that consistently showed this relationship, are summarized in Table 18.21, which has been excerpted from the preceding tables.

Possible Underascertainment of Drug Exposure

All drug exposure information was collected prior to delivery so that biased recording of drug exposure attributable to knowledge of the outcome was absent. However, since each gravida was questioned about drug use *prior* to registration, and then followed at regular intervals for drug use *after* registration, variable proportions of the information were retrospective and prospective. Thus, a woman who registered in the study at the sixth lunar month initially reported on all of her prior drug ingestion during lunar months one through five, and then at monthly intervals on her drug ingestion (during the preceding month) from the sixth lunar month to term. In the cohort, 27% of the women registered during the first four lunar months of pregnancy, 33% during the fifth and sixth lunar months, and the remainder after the sixth lunar month.

The extent of under-reporting of drug use due to memory loss requires careful assessment. The approach we have taken

has been to compare the rates of exposures to a number of drugs in *early* (LM 1 to 4) and *late* (LM 5+) pregnancy among *early* and *late* registrants to the study. If *early* registrants reported higher rates of exposure to a drug during *early* pregnancy than did the *late* registrants, then the discrepancy might be due to under-reporting of *early* exposure by the *late* registrants. The differences between the two rates might be used to assess roughly the possible magnitude of *early* drug usage not reported by *late* registrants. However, analyses of this sort are not straightforward. It is possible that women requiring medical care for some reason would be more likely to visit an antenatal clinic *early*; it is also possible that they might use drugs more commonly. Depending upon the drug, in evaluation of *early* usage rates in women who registered *early* and in women who registered *late*, it may be difficult, if not impossible, to determine whether differences can be attributed to under-reporting or to medical reasons.

The problems can be illustrated by considering certain drugs. Table 18.22 gives rates of exposure to selected drugs according to when the women were enrolled into the CPP and when they were exposed. Any woman who reported exposure both during *early* and *late* pregnancy is counted twice. The data for exposure during *early* pregnancy were

Table **18.21**

Mean Number of Products Used in Early Pregnancy (LM 1–4) in Relation to Events Occurring Predominantly or Exclusively in Late Pregnancy (LM ⩾ 5)

	Mean No. of Products Used in LM 1–4		
	White	**Black**	**Puerto Rican**
Mean in the entire cohort	1.4	1.1	0.5
Toxemia of pregnancy	1.5	1.2	0.7
Second trimester bleeding	1.8	1.4	0.5
Third trimester bleeding	1.7	1.2	0.7
Hydramnios	1.7	1.4	1.6

Table **18.22**

Percentages of Early and Late Exposure to Selected Drugs According to Time of First Registration Into the Study

	Time of Exposure During Pregnancy	Time of First Registration Into the Study	
		LM 1–4	LM ⩾ 5
Aspirin	LM 1–4	34.9	17.2
	LM ⩾ 5	53.5	41.7
All penicillin preparations	LM 1–4	8.3	6.5
	LM ⩾ 5	8.2	8.3
Killed polio vaccine	LM 1–4	39.9	3.8
	LM ⩾ 5	16.3	28.4
Insulin	LM 1–4	0.4	0.2
	LM ⩾ 5	0.5	0.3
Phenytoin	LM 1–4	3.1	2.2
	LM ⩾ 5	4.8	5.0

obtained relatively close to the time of exposure for women who registered *early*. Memory loss should be minimal in this group. *Early* use in women who registered *late* may be influenced by an imperfect recall of drug use. In contrast, reporting of exposure *late* in pregnancy should have been done with less difference in reliability regardless of whether women registered *early* or *late*.

Aspirin, the most commonly used drug in the cohort, is considered first. Table 18.22 indicates that 34.9% of women who registered *early* used aspirin *early*. By contrast, the corresponding rate of *early* use in women who registered *late* was only 17.2%. The latter rate of 17.2% is no doubt partly a function of memory loss. However, it may also be a function of fewer healthy women tending to register *early* and to use aspirin. In fact, the data lend some support to this possibility; even among *early* registrants, 53.5% used aspirin *late*, whereas only 41.7% of *late* registrants used the drug *late* in pregnancy. Thus, *early* registration was

associated with higher rates of aspirin use throughout pregnancy.

Aspirin is generally used for relatively mild symptoms. Women who register *late* may tend to forget prior use of that drug. Penicillin, on the other hand, is used for infections, which might be less readily forgotten. For this drug, *early* exposure in *early* registrants was 8.3%, which was similar to the 6.5% for *early* exposure in *late* registrants; *late* exposure was also similar in *early* and *late* registrants (8.2% and 8.3%). Thus, as far as can be judged, there was little evidence of memory loss with regard to penicillin exposure.

Interpretation of the data becomes complex when a drug tends to be used in a particular way. Killed poliomyelitis vaccine, for example, tended to be given at, or after registration, but not before. This is clearly reflected in Table 18.22: 39.9% of *early* registrants received the vaccine *early* and 16.3% were given the vaccine *late*, some time after *early* enrollment. Conversely, 28.4% of *late* registrants were vaccinated *late*, while only

3.8% were vaccinated in *early* pregnancy before they entered the study.

Still another pattern emerges when one examines a drug such as insulin: people using this drug are dependent on it for survival, and diabetes is usually present prior to conception. Table 18.22 shows that diabetics tended to register *early*: the rate of insulin use, both *early* and *late,* was higher among *early* registrants than among *late* registrants. However, there was little loss of recall: within the two groups of *early* and *late* registrants, rates of use were similar.

It is a relatively simple matter to evaluate whether there is memory loss in diabetics reporting insulin use; the same does not apply to epileptic women reporting phenytoin use. *Late* use of the drug was higher than *early* use in both *early* and *late* registrants — perhaps because of an adverse influence of pregnancy itself, as it progressed, upon epilepsy. The interaction between pregnancy and epilepsy is so complicated that it is impossible to evaluate the role of memory loss.

From the data presented in Table 18.22, a number of tentative conclusions can be drawn. First, it appears that memory loss was undoubtedly a factor in reporting drug exposure that took place several months earlier. Probably, the less serious the indication, or the more sporadic the use of the drug, the greater the loss of recall. Second, it is possible that discrepancies in *early* drug exposure rates for *early* and *late* registrants may sometimes reflect a tendency for women who were more seriously ill (or who believed that they were) to register *early* and to use more drugs. Third, for certain drugs, such as killed poliomyelitis vaccine, rates of use were largely determined by the time of registration and by what was regarded as good antenatal care. Fourth, *early* use of certain products, such as insulin, taken for relatively serious conditions was probably not appreciably under-reported. Fifth, for some drugs it is

impossible to assess the extent of possible under-reporting. This holds particularly in circumstances where the indication for therapy itself interacts in a complex way with the pregnancy.

The implicit assumption thus far has been that drug usage was, if anything, under-reported rather than over-reported. There is no reason to believe that women would have reported using drugs that they had not taken.

Effects of Under-Reporting of Drug Use on Estimates of Relative Risk of Malformations

Since the possibility of over-reporting of drug use is minimal, the consequences of under-reporting (i.e., false negatives, among the "non-exposed" mother-child pairs) upon the estimation of relative risk must be considered. Most drugs were used by less than a few percent of the gravidas. The rates of most of the malformation classes were on the order of 10 to 20 per 1,000 or less. Consider the case where the "true" relative risk is 2.0, the overall malformation rate is 3 per 1,000, and the observed drug exposure rate is 1.0%. If the "true" drug exposure rate were 2.0% (i.e., if under-reporting were 50%), then the relative risk estimated from the data is about 1% lower than the "true" relative risk of 2.0. This example is presented in Table 18.23. For the same situation, but with a "true" relative risk of 3.0, the estimate from the data is slightly more than 1% lower than the "true" value. As the exposure rate increases, or as the "true" relative risk increases, or as the proportion of under-reported drug exposure increases, so too does the calculated relative risk become increasingly more biased toward 1.0. However, even in the quite extreme case, described in Table 18.24, where the "true" relative risk is 3.0, the "true" drug exposure rate is 30%, the reported drug exposure rate is, say, 15%, and the overall malformation rate is 10 per 1,000, the calculated relative risk is 2.2, which is

277

Table **18.23**

Bias in Estimation of Relative Risk Due to Underascertainment of Drug Exposure. Example 1: Hypothetical Drug with Low Exposure Rate[1]

	No. of Mother-Child Pairs	No. of Malformed Children	Rate/1,000
"True" exposure	1,006	6	5.964
"True" non-exposure	49,276	145	2.943
	"True" relative risk = 2.03		
Recorded exposure	503	3	5.964
Recorded non-exposure	49,779	148	2.973
	Recorded relative risk = 2.01		

[1] "True" relative risk ≃ 2.0
"True" drug exposure rate = 2.0%
Underascertainment = 50%
Hypothetical malformation rate (per 1,000) = 3 (151 malformed children in a cohort of 50,282 mother-child pairs)

Table **18.24**

Bias in Estimation of Relative Risk Due to Underascertainment of Drug Exposure. Example 2: Hypothetical Drug with High Exposure Rate[1]

	No. of Mother-Child Pairs	No. of Malformed Children	Rate/1,000
"True" exposure	15,085	283	18.760
"True" non-exposure	35,197	220	6.251
	"True" relative risk = 3.00		
Recorded exposure	7,542	141	18.695
Recorded non-exposure	42,740	362	8.470
	Recorded relative risk = 2.21		

[1] "True" relative risk ≃ 3.0
"True" drug exposure rate = 30%
Underascertainment = 50%
Hypothetical malformation rate (per 1,000) = 10 (503 malformed children in a cohort of 50,282 mother-child pairs)

appreciably less than the "true" relative risk, but still considerably greater than 1.0. The latter hypothetical case might apply to a drug like aspirin — the most commonly used drug and one for which under-reporting by late entrants may well have been high. In fact, there were no relative risks, for outcomes of reasonable size, that were as high as 2.2 for early aspirin exposure (see Chapter 20). It is thus unlikely that there were actual associations in the cohort of that order of magnitude that escaped detection because of under-reporting. For observed associations of most drugs with malformations, the exposure rates (Appendix 3) were so low that any bias in the estimates of relative risk could have been of the order of no more than a few percent. Such bias is of no practical relevance.

There is no way that a "true" relative risk having a value greater than unity can be *lower* than the recorded one because of random under-reporting of drug use.

Based on the above considerations, it seems reasonable to conclude that while the consequences of under-reporting of drug use would bias the estimates of relative risk toward unity, it is unlikely that associations actually present in the cohort would go completely undetected because of loss of recall of drug exposure in *early* pregnancy by *late* registrants. However, it should be emphasized that all of the discussion so far has ignored the roles of chance, of observer bias, and of possible confounding that was not controlled. In particular, whenever numbers of exposures, or outcomes, were small, teratogenic effects, or even hints of teratogenic effects, could have been missed.

CHAPTER 19

General Approach to the Evaluation of Drugs in Relation to Malformations

In this chapter, the general strategy used to analyze relationships between drugs and malformations is described, together with the format for presenting the results. A detailed consideration of this strategy, together with statistical arguments, has been presented in Chapter 3.

Data Analysis

In principle, it is possible that some teratogens can be rather non-specific, producing malformations in general; some can produce recognizable patterns of deformities; and some may be highly specific. The implication for the present study is that it is necessary to examine malformations in general, malformations classified on the basis of severity, malformations classified in terms of common characteristics, such as anatomical location or other criteria, and, finally, specific malformations.

A similar problem arises when attempts are made to determine whether a particular chemical is teratogenic, or whether a group of chemicals has that effect. For example, compounds that are chemically similar to thalidomide, such as glutethimide, do not appear to harm the fetus.[1,2] Yet a group of chemically dissimilar drugs used for the same indication (such as aminopterin, cyclophosphamide, and other chemotherapeutic agents) all seem to produce birth defects in humans.[3,4] The principle is again clear: it is desirable to evaluate broad groups of drugs (e.g., drugs affecting the autonomic nervous system) and subgroups (e.g., sympathomimetic amines), as well as individual drugs (e.g., pseudoephedrine), in relation to each outcome.

Thus, given the present state of knowledge about teratogens in humans, it seems reasonable to move from the broad to the specific along two axes: drugs and malformations.

All analyses of drugs in this study are based on comparisons of malformation rates between exposed and non-exposed mother-child pairs, with the principal measure of association being the estimate of relative risk. Relative risks must be adjusted for the influence of confounding. The most elaborate standardized estimates of relative risk (SRRs) in the study are derived by multivariate analyses in which the influence of all identified risk factors for the malformations are simultaneously controlled. In circumstances where multivariate analysis is not practical, a less elaborate method (Mantel-Haenszel procedure) is used to adjust the comparisons for confounding.

In the following chapters, drug exposures during the first four lunar months of pregnancy are considered. In each chapter, the procedure is to commence with an examination of an entire drug group (e.g., drugs affecting the autonomic nervous system), together with its subgroups (e.g., sympathomimetic amines), and finally its individual components (e.g., pseudoephedrine) in relation to the entire set of 3,248 malformed children identified in the cohort. In the initial table, three estimates of relative risk are given: the crude estimate, the estimate after adjustment for hospital variability, and the estimate obtained after simultaneous adjustment for the mother's ethnic group and survival of the child. An example is provided by Table 19.1, which presents information on immunizing agents. The two adjustments of the crude relative risk estimate should enable the reader to judge the extent to which hospital variability, ethnic variability, and survival of the child were confounding factors. As can be seen in the sample table, virtually all of the crude relative risks are somewhat altered by the two standardizations. In the text, the *hospital-standardized relative risk* is generally taken to be the most informative of the three, particularly since malformations with appreciable hospital variability are included.

The first table provides only a bird's eye view of the relationship between the entire drug group under consideration and the entire set of 3,248 malformed children. The second table in the sequence presents almost the same information as the first, but slightly narrows the focus by considering the 2,277 children with uniform malformations.

Thereafter, the drug evaluation in each chapter is based on more elaborate control for potential confounding by means of multivariate analysis. The measure of association which is presented is the standardized relative risk (SRR), together with its 95% confidence limits. For this estimate, all potentially confounding factors previously identified are taken into account. The drug group, its subgroups, and individual drugs are examined, in turn, in relation to all malformations to which multiple logistic risk function models were applied. In each instance, the SRR is derived by fitting the model appropriate for the outcome under consideration to the exposed mother-child pairs, and deriving an expected number of malformed children. The expected number is contrasted with the actual number of malformed children observed. The ratio of the observed to the expected number is the SRR. SRRs greater than 1.5 are generally mentioned in the text. Smaller SRRs, although they could also

Children with any Malformation (3,248) in Relation to Exposure to Immunizing Agents During Lunar Months 1–4 Among 50,282 Mother-Child Pairs

	No. of Mother-Child Pairs Exposed	No. of Malformed Children	Crude Relative Risk	Hospital Standardized Relative Risk[1]	Survival and Race Standardized Relative Risk[1]
Immunizing agents	9,222	626	1.06	1.04	1.09
Poliomyelitis vaccine, parenteral	6,774	461	1.06	1.03	1.09
Polio virus vaccine, live oral	1,628	114	1.09	1.11	1.08
Influenza virus vaccine	650	39	0.93	0.91	0.95
Tetanus toxoid	337	24	1.10	1.12	1.20
Smallpox vaccine	172	7	0.63	0.62	0.60
Diphtheria toxoid	75	4	0.83	0.82	0.88
Allergy desensitization vaccine	64	6	1.45	1.32	1.58
Typhoid vaccine	44	1	0.35	0.35	0.38
Polio virus vaccine, n.o.s.	39	1	0.40	0.32	0.47
Measles virus vaccine, live attenuated	37	0	—	—	—
Other virus vaccines[2]	10	0	—	—	—
Specific desensitization vaccine[3]	14	3	3.32	4.25	4.70
Other bacterial vaccines[4]	28	2	1.11	1.06	1.28

[1] Estimated by the Mantel-Haenszel procedure
[2] Measles virus vaccine, inactivated (6); yellow fever vaccine (3); rabies vaccine (1)
[3] House dust extract (10); poison oak extract (3); poison ivy vaccine (2)
[4] Pertussis vaccine (13); typhus vaccine (7); staphylococcus toxoid (2); cholera vaccine (1); tetanus antitoxin (1); paratyphoid vaccine (1); bacterial vaccine (1); bacterial protein, I.V. (1); Rocky Mountain Spotted Fever vaccine (1)

indicate associations, are usually not mentioned.

In each of the chapters, the analyses move along the drug axis from the general to the particular. In successive tables, each exposure group of mother-child pairs is examined in relation to all uniform malformations (2,277 children) and to subsets thereof: major malformations, minor malformations, central nervous malformations, and so on. See Table 19.2 for an example.

Finally, the analyses end with the three non-uniform malformations to which multiple logistic risk function models were applied: inguinal hernia, clubfoot, and pectus excavatum. Here, the information presented is the same as for the uniform malformations, in a slightly con-densed form. See Table 19.3 for an example.

As the number of mother-child pairs exposed to any particular agent becomes smaller, full tabulation of data ceases to serve any useful purpose. Sometimes, data on small numbers are presented for the sake of maintaining uniformity in the tables. However, it can be assumed that when data are not presented, it is because numbers are so sparse as to be uninformative.

Data on all of the drugs in relation to individual malformations are presented in Appendix 4. With few exceptions, evaluation of data at this level is beset by the problem of small numbers. This has dictated the adoption of certain rules in designing the appendix. First, the only

Table **19.2 (Sample)**

Table **19.2 (Sample)**

Multiple Logistic Risk Function Analysis Standardized Relative Risks (SRR) and Their 95% Confidence Intervals (CI_{95}) for Classes of Malformations Showing Uniform Rates by Hospital in Relation to Immunizing Agents Used in Lunar Months 1–4 by 9,222 Pregnant Women

Malformation Classes	No. of Malformed Children		SRR	CI_{95} of SRR
	Observed	Expected		
Any malformation	437	418.7	1.04	0.96–1.13
Major malformations	279	271.4	1.03	0.93–1.14
Minor malformations	158	144.5	1.09	0.96–1.25
Central nervous system	45	49.4	0.91	0.69–1.20
Cardiovascular system	70	72.5	0.96	0.78–1.20
Musculoskeletal (other than polydactyly in Blacks)	101	90.4	1.12	0.94–1.32
Polydactyly in Blacks[1]	47	38.2	1.23	0.96–1.57
Respiratory tract	39	42.7	0.91	0.68–1.23
Gastrointestinal tract	74	62.3	1.19	0.98–1.44
Genitourinary (other than hypospadias)	34	38.3	0.89	0.64–1.23
Hypospadias[2]	29	30.9	0.94	0.66–1.33
Eye and ear	22	23.0	0.96	0.65–1.42
Syndromes (other than Down syndrome)	15	23.8	0.63	0.35–1.04
Down syndrome	12	11.4	1.05	0.54–1.83
Tumors	36	35.8	1.01	0.75–1.36

[1]Drugs used by 2,879 Blacks
[2]Drugs used by 4,649 mothers of male offspring

measures of association to be presented are the relative risks adjusted for hospital variability. Second, data are presented only when numbers are adequate in terms of criteria stipulated in the appendix. Thus, omission of any particular drug or malformation from Appendix 4 indicates that there were insufficient drug exposures and/or malformed children to justify presentation of the data. Third, there are no references to statistical significance in the appendix. In the context of multiple comparisons, the interpretation of "statistical significance" is not clear. In addition, since control for potential confounding is inadequate, with only hospital variability being controlled, it would be improper to present the statistical significance of any particular association.

Each of the chapters evaluating a particular group of drugs ends with a few concluding remarks, and, when appropriate, reference is made to interesting findings in Appendix 4.

Finally, Appendix 1 considers exposures to drugs taken at any time in pregnancy in relation to malformations that may arise during either early or late fetal development. It essentially recapitulates, in condensed form, the procedures described above. In addition, Appendix 5, constructed in exactly the same way as Appendix 4, provides data on relationships between the individual drugs taken at any time during pregnancy and the individual malformations judged to be of this type.

Some Comments on the Methods Used in Drug Evaluation

Simultaneously controlling multiple risk factors in a study of this type has many practical advantages, but one potential drawback, as illustrated by a hypothetical example. Assume that a drug causes hyperemesis gravidarum, which, in turn, causes central nervous malformations. Assume also that the causal mechanism is solely via the path-

Table **19.3 *(Sample)***

Multiple Logistic Risk Function Analysis Standardized Relative Risks (SRR) and Their 95% Confidence Intervals (CI_{95}) for Inguinal Hernia, Clubfoot, and Pectus Excavatum in Relation to Immunizing Agents Used in Lunar Months 1–4

	No. of Users	No. of Malformed Children		SRR	CI_{95} of SRR
		Observed	Expected		
Inguinal hernia					
Immunizing agents	9,222	300	305.8	0.98	0.90–1.07
Poliomyelitis vaccine, parenteral	6,774	227	240.0	0.95	0.85–1.05
Polio virus vaccine, live oral	1,628	49	47.0	1.04	0.80–1.36
Influenza virus vaccine	650	35	29.1	1.20	0.90–1.62
Tetanus toxoid	337	13	11.3	1.16	0.62–1.97
Clubfoot					
Immunizing agents	9,222	90	91.1	0.99	0.85–1.15
Poliomyelitis vaccine, parenteral	6,774	69	72.6	0.95	0.78–1.16
Polio virus vaccine, live oral	1,628	13	11.6	1.12	0.60–1.91
Influenza virus vaccine	650	7	10.3	0.68	0.27–1.39
Tetanus toxoid	337	5	3.2	1.57	0.51–3.65
Pectus excavatum					
Immunizing agents	9,222	57	54.0	1.06	0.88–1.27
Poliomyelitis vaccine, parenteral	6,774	47	46.5	1.01	0.80–1.27
Polio virus vaccine, live oral	1,628	8	4.2	1.92	0.83–3.77
Influenza virus vaccine	650	7	6.6	1.07	0.43–2.20
Tetanus toxoid	337	4	2.0	1.97	0.54–5.20

way of hyperemesis. The effect of controlling hyperemesis in this case would be to conceal the causal association. One can be alerted to this possibility by comparing the crude and adjusted relative risks. In particular, if the SRR is substantially lower than the crude relative risk, the factors bringing about the reduction must be identified, and a judgement made about whether any of them may be part of the causal pathway. Inadvertent *overcontrolling* can thus be avoided. For the overall group of 2,277 children with uniform malformations, there are *four* sets of relative risk estimates presented in each of the drug evaluation chapters which can be compared to check for possible overcontrolling: crude, hospital-standardized, "ethnic group/child survival"–standardized, and the SRR.

It is worth emphasizing that if a given drug causes both hyperemesis and CNS malformations, but by separate pathways, controlling for hyperemesis will not obscure the association with CNS malformations.

Another aspect of the analyses, in which *late* events are controlled in the evaluation of *early* drug exposure, may be confusing. Again, the problem can be illustrated by an example. Assume hydramnios is diagnosed during the seventh lunar month of pregnancy. On the face, there would seem to be little point in controlling hydramnios when examining drug exposure that took place during the first four lunar months, even though it is a risk factor for the malformation in question. However, it is quite possible that hydramnios identified in late pregnancy may reflect antecedent factors that led to a particular drug being used in early pregnancy. Controlling hydramnios may thus have the effect of controlling some unknown antecedent determinant of drug exposure. Failure to control could result in confounding. In fact, Table 18.14 shows that women destined to develop hydramnios used more drugs during early pregnancy.

In this study, a conservative posture has been adopted; as many risk factors as possible, regardless of time of occurrence, have been controlled.

These topics are considered further in Chapter 34.

CHAPTER 20

Analgesic and Antipyretic Drugs

General Evaluation

In this section, the first analysis concerns evaluation of the entire set of 3,248 malformed children in relation to exposure to the entire group of analgesic and antipyretic drugs during the first four lunar months of pregnancy (Table 20.1). The evaluation will then be confined to the 2,277 children whose malformations had uniform hospital distributions (Table 20.2). Three relative risks are given in each table: crude, standardized for hospital variability, and standardized for the mother's ethnic group and survival of the child.

All Malformations in Relation to Analgesic and Antipyretic Drugs (Table 20.1)

There was no evidence of a teratogenic effect for the group of analgesic and antipyretic drugs as a whole or for the two major subgroups, nonaddicting and narcotic analgesics. The hospital-standardized relative risks for these categories equaled or were close to unity. The only hospital-standardized relative risk greater than 1.5 was for opium (1.72), and it was based on a small number of exposed mother-child pairs. The relative risk of 1.27 for codeine, however, was based on a fairly large number of exposed (563).

Table **20.1**

Children (3,248) With Any Malformation in Relation to Exposure to **Analgesic and Antipyretic Drugs** During Lunar Months 1–4 Among 50,282 Mother-Child Pairs

	No. of Mother-Child Pairs Exposed	No. of Malformed Children	Crude Relative Risk	Hospital Standardized Relative Risk[1]	Survival and Race Standardized Relative Risk[1]
Analgesics and antipyretics	15,909	1,064	1.05	1.00	1.04
Non-addicting analgesics	15,463	1,035	1.05	1.00	1.04
Aspirin	14,864	1,006	1.07	1.02	1.06
Phenacetin	5,546	364	1.02	0.98	0.99
Salicylamide	744	47	0.98	0.92	0.95
Acetaminophen	226	17	1.17	1.05	1.19
Analgesic and cold capsules	152	14	1.43	1.33	1.62
Sodium salicylate	54	4	1.15	1.11	1.10
Other non-addicting analgesics and antipyretics[2]	27	1	0.57	0.46	0.54
Narcotic analgesics	1,564	113	1.12	1.06	1.11
Propoxyphene	686	45	1.02	0.94	0.99
Codeine	563	48	1.32	1.27	1.32
Meperidine	268	18	1.04	1.00	0.97
Paregoric	90	8	1.38	1.25	1.30
Morphine	70	5	1.11	1.11	1.10
Ethoheptazine	60	5	1.29	1.26	1.43
Opium	36	4	1.72	1.72	1.51
Other opium alkaloids[3]	46	2	0.67	0.64	0.71
Other narcotic analgesics[4]	13	0	—	—	—

[1]Estimated by the Mantel-Haenszel procedure
[2]Antipyrine (8); acetanilide (7); phenylbutazone (4); dipyrone (3); aminopyrine (2); carbazochrome salicylate (2); dimefadane (1); phenocoll-p-pheneditine (1)
[3]Hydromorphone (12); hydrocodone (12); diacetyl-morphine (11); oxycodone (8); pantopon (3)
[4]Diphenoxylate (7); anileridine (3); methadone (1); alphaprodine (1); levorphanol (1)

Malformations Showing Uniform Rates by Hospital in Relation to Analgesic and Antipyretic Drugs (Table 20.2)

For the drug group as a whole, and for the subgroups of non-addicting and narcotic analgesics, there was no evidence from the hospital-standardized relative risks of a teratogenic effect: all the relative risks were close to unity. The same applied to all the commonly used drugs, and substantial deviations from a relative risk of unity occurred only with a few drugs and were based on limited numbers. Hospital-standardized relative risks greater than 1.5 were seen for analgesic and cold capsules (1.56) and opium (1.84). The hospital-standardized relative

287

Table **20.2**

Children (2,277) With Malformations Showing Uniform Rates by Hospital in Relation to Exposure to **Analgesic and Antipyretic Drugs** During Lunar Months 1–4 Among 50,282 Mother-Child Pairs

	No. of Mother-Child Pairs Exposed	No. of Malformed Children	Crude Relative Risk	Hospital Standardized Relative Risk	Survival and Race Standardized Relative Risk
Analgesics and antipyretics	15,909	720	1.00	0.96	0.99
Non-addicting analgesics	15,463	704	1.01	0.97	1.00
Aspirin	14,864	683	1.02	0.98	1.01
Phenacetin	5,546	250	0.99	0.96	0.97
Salicylamide	744	34	1.01	0.97	0.98
Acetaminophen	226	14	1.37	1.30	1.42
Analgesic and cold capsules	152	11	1.60	1.56	1.90
Sodium salicylate	54	0	—	—	—
Other non-addicting analgesics and antipyretics	27	1	0.82	0.72	0.78
Narcotic analgesics	1,564	75	1.06	1.02	1.03
Propoxyphene	686	31	1.00	0.95	0.97
Codeine	563	32	1.26	1.22	1.22
Meperidine	268	12	0.99	0.96	0.89
Paregoric	90	6	1.47	1.39	1.35
Morphine	70	3	0.95	0.94	0.92
Ethoheptazine	60	3	1.10	1.08	1.25
Opium	36	3	1.84	1.84	1.50
Other opium alkaloids	46	1	0.48	0.47	0.52
Other narcotic analgesics	13	0	—	—	—

risk for 563 mother-child pairs exposed to codeine was 1.22.

Detailed Evaluation of Uniform Malformations

In this section, groups of drugs, followed by individual drugs, are evaluated in relation to various classes or groups of uniform malformations, as well as individual malformations, for which multiple logistic risk function models were developed. In the tables, the observed and expected numbers of malformed children are given for each drug exposure in turn. The measure of association presented is a standardized relative risk (SRR) with its 95% confidence limits. The SRR is the ratio of the observed number to the expected number of malformed children. Since the SRR takes into account potential confounding variables, it represents the best estimate of the relationship between a drug and a malformation. As numbers of exposed mother-child pairs become so small as to be uninformative, data will be omitted.

Any Analgesic or Antipyretic Drug — 15,909 Exposures (Table 20.3)

There was no evidence of association between broad classes of malformations and the drug group as a whole. The same was true of the specific classes of malformations in the table: all SRRs were close to unity.

Non-Addicting Analgesics — 15,463 Exposures (Table 20.4)

There was no evidence, from the SRRs in the table, to suggest that the non-addicting subgroup of drugs is related to any of the listed outcomes.

Aspirin — 14,864 Exposures (Table 20.5) There was no evidence of association of aspirin with any of the malforma-tions listed. The highest SRR was 1.11, for hypospadias.

Phenacetin — 5,546 Exposures (Table 20.6) There was no evidence of association between phenacetin and broad classes of malformations. The highest SRR was 1.18 for malformations of the gastrointestinal tract.

Salicylamide — 744 Exposures (Table 20.7) There was no evidence of association of salicylamide with broad classes of malformations. The highest SRR among these was for minor malformations (1.18). SRRs greater than 1.5 were seen for malformations of the respiratory tract (1.72), genitourinary tract (1.61), and anomalies affecting the eye and ear (1.59).

Narcotic Analgesics — 1,564 Exposures (Table 20.8)

There was no evidence of association between narcotic analgesics and broad

Table **20.3**

Standardized Relative Risks (SRR) and Their 95% Confidence Intervals (CI₉₅) for Classes of Malformations Showing Uniform Rates by Hospital in Relation to Any **Analgesic and Antipyretic Drugs** Used in Lunar Months 1–4 by 15,909 Pregnant Women (Based on Multiple Logistic Risk Function Analysis)

| Malformation Classes | No. of Malformed Children | | SRR | CI₉₅ of SRR |
	Observed	Expected		
Any malformation	720	733.3	0.98	0.92–1.04
Major malformations	436	440.9	0.99	0.92–1.07
Minor malformations	290	296.2	0.98	0.89–1.08
Central nervous	83	82.5	1.01	0.84–1.20
Cardiovascular	125	130.7	0.96	0.82–1.11
Musculoskeletal (other than polydactyly in Blacks)	121	129.2	0.94	0.80–1.09
Polydactyly in Blacks[1]	114	116.1	0.98	0.85–1.14
Respiratory	67	69.4	0.96	0.79–1.18
Gastrointestinal	105	99.2	1.06	0.91–1.24
Genitourinary (other than hypospadias)	62	61.0	1.02	0.83–1.25
Hypospadias[2]	63	57.0	1.11	0.91–1.35
Eye and ear	35	39.5	0.89	0.66–1.19
Syndromes (other than Down syndrome)	37	38.6	0.96	0.73–1.26
Down syndrome	16	19.2	0.83	0.48–1.35
Tumors	53	56.7	0.93	0.74–1.18

[1]Drugs used by 8,323 Blacks
[2]Drugs used by 8,114 mothers of male offspring

Table **20.4**

Standardized Relative Risks (SRR) and Their 95% Confidence Intervals (CI$_{95}$) for Classes of Malformations Showing Uniform Rates by Hospital in Relation to Any **Nonaddicting Analgesic and Antipyretic Drugs** Used in Lunar Months 1–4 by 15,463 Pregnant Women (Based on Multiple Logistic Risk Function Analysis)

Malformation Classes	No. of Malformed Children		SRR	CI$_{95}$ of SRR
	Observed	Expected		
Any malformation	704	711.4	0.99	0.93–1.05
Major malformations	425	426.9	1.00	0.92–1.08
Minor malformations	285	287.7	0.99	0.90–1.09
Central nervous	79	79.7	0.99	0.82–1.19
Cardiovascular	125	126.7	0.99	0.85–1.14
Musculoskeletal (other than polydactyly in Blacks)	118	125.1	0.94	0.81–1.10
Polydactyly in Blacks[1]	114	113.7	1.00	0.86–1.16
Respiratory	66	67.4	0.98	0.80–1.20
Gastrointestinal	101	96.0	1.05	0.90–1.23
Genitourinary (other than hypospadias)	59	59.1	1.00	0.81–1.24
Hypospadias[2]	62	55.2	1.12	0.92–1.37
Eye and ear	35	38.2	0.92	0.68–1.23
Syndromes (other than Down syndrome)	37	37.3	0.99	0.76–1.30
Down syndrome	16	18.6	0.86	0.49–1.40
Tumors	51	55.0	0.93	0.73–1.18

[1]Drugs used by 8,145 Blacks
[2]Drugs used by 7,883 mothers of male offspring

Table **20.5**

Standardized Relative Risks (SRR) and Their 95% Confidence Intervals (CI$_{95}$) for Classes of Malformations Showing Uniform Rates by Hospital in Relation to **Aspirin** Used in Lunar Months 1–4 by 14,864 Pregnant Women (Based on Multiple Logistic Risk Function Analysis)

Malformation Classes	No. of Malformed Children		SRR	CI$_{95}$ of SRR
	Observed	Expected		
Any malformation	683	684.1	1.00	0.94–1.06
Major malformations	413	410.3	1.01	0.93–1.09
Minor malformations	276	276.8	1.00	0.90–1.10
Central nervous	77	76.3	1.01	0.84–1.22
Cardiovascular	122	122.1	1.00	0.86–1.16
Musculoskeletal (other than polydactyly in Blacks)	113	120.1	0.94	0.80–1.11
Polydactyly in Blacks[1]	109	109.8	0.99	0.85–1.16
Respiratory	66	64.8	1.02	0.83–1.25
Gastrointestinal	100	92.1	1.09	0.93–1.27
Genitourinary (other than hypospadias)	58	56.6	1.03	0.83–1.27
Hypospadias[2]	59	52.9	1.11	0.91–1.37
Eye and ear	35	36.7	0.95	0.71–1.27
Syndromes (other than Down syndrome)	36	35.6	1.01	0.77–1.33
Down syndrome	15	17.9	0.84	0.47–1.38
Tumors	51	52.9	0.97	0.76–1.23

[1]Drugs used by 7,877 Blacks
[2]Drugs used by 7,579 mothers of male offspring

Table **20.6**

Standardized Relative Risks (SRR) and Their 95% Confidence Intervals (CI$_{95}$) for Classes of Malformations Showing Uniform Rates by Hospital in Relation to **Phenacetin** Used in Lunar Months 1–4 by 5,546 Pregnant Women (Based on Multiple Logistic Risk Function Analysis)

Malformation Classes	No. of Malformed Children		SRR	CI$_{95}$ of SRR
	Observed	Expected		
Any malformation	250	257.1	0.97	0.86–1.09
Major malformations	155	150.5	1.03	0.89–1.19
Minor malformations	99	107.7	0.92	0.76–1.12
Central nervous	26	28.5	0.91	0.62–1.34
Cardiovascular	35	45.8	0.76	0.53–1.10
Musculoskeletal (other than polydactyly in Blacks)	46	42.8	1.08	0.82–1.40
Polydactyly in Blacks[1]	47	45.3	1.04	0.80–1.35
Respiratory	27	23.6	1.14	0.82–1.59
Gastrointestinal	41	34.8	1.18	0.90–1.54
Genitourinary (other than hypospadias)	18	21.2	0.85	0.50–1.34
Hypospadias[2]	19	19.5	0.97	0.59–1.52
Eye and ear	10	13.6	0.74	0.35–1.35
Syndromes (other than Down syndrome)	13	13.9	0.94	0.50–1.60
Down syndrome	7	6.5	1.07	0.43–2.21
Tumors	13	20.3	0.64	0.34–1.09

[1]Drugs used by 3,253 Blacks
[2]Drugs used by 2,819 mothers of male offspring

Table **20.7**

Standardized Relative Risks (SRR) and Their 95% Confidence Intervals (CI$_{95}$) for Classes of Malformations Showing Uniform Rates by Hospital in Relation to **Salicylamide** Used in Lunar Months 1–4 by 744 Pregnant Women (Based on Multiple Logistic Risk Function Analysis)

Malformation Classes	No. of Malformed Children		SRR	CI$_{95}$ of SRR
	Observed	Expected		
Any malformation	34	34.3	0.99	0.71–1.38
Major malformations	22	21.0	1.05	0.70–1.57
Minor malformations	16	13.5	1.18	0.68–1.91
Central nervous	5	4.2	1.18	0.38–2.74
Cardiovascular	3	5.8	0.51	0.11–1.49
Musculoskeletal (other than polydactyly in Blacks)	6	6.9	0.87	0.32–1.88
Polydactyly in Blacks[1]	6	4.4	1.38	0.51–2.97
Respiratory	6	3.5	1.72	0.63–3.73
Gastrointestinal	4	5.0	0.80	0.22–2.04
Genitourinary (other than hypospadias)	5	3.1	1.61	0.52–3.74
Hypospadias[2]	3	2.9	1.05	0.22–3.03
Eye and ear	3	1.9	1.59	0.33–4.63
Syndromes (other than Down syndrome)	1	2.2	0.46	0.01–2.55
Down syndrome	1	0.7	1.36	0.03–7.55
Tumors	0	2.8	—	0.00–1.30

[1]Drugs used by 301 Blacks
[2]Drugs used by 383 mothers of male offspring

Table **20.8**

Standardized Relative Risks (SRR) and Their 95% Confidence Intervals (CI_{95}) for Classes of Malformations Showing Uniform Rates by Hospital in Relation to **Narcotic Analgesics** Used in Lunar Months 1–4 by 1,564 Pregnant Women (Based on Multiple Logistic Risk Function Analysis)

Malformation Classes	No. of Malformed Children		SRR	CI_{95} of SRR
	Observed	Expected		
Any malformation	75	76.9	0.97	0.78–1.22
Major malformations	47	49.0	0.96	0.72–1.27
Minor malformations	26	29.4	0.88	0.59–1.32
Central nervous	11	9.9	1.11	0.55–1.97
Cardiovascular	10	14.4	0.69	0.33–1.27
Musculoskeletal (other than polydactyly in Blacks)	12	15.8	0.76	0.39–1.32
Polydactyly in Blacks[1]	6	8.6	0.70	0.26–1.51
Respiratory	10	8.7	1.15	0.55–2.10
Gastrointestinal	16	12.7	1.26	0.72–2.03
Genitourinary (other than hypospadias)	9	8.3	1.08	0.50–2.05
Hypospadias[2]	5	5.6	0.90	0.29–2.08
Eye and ear	4	4.2	0.96	0.26–2.46
Syndromes (other than Down syndrome)	2	4.7	0.42	0.05–1.53
Down syndrome	1	1.9	0.52	0.01–2.89
Tumors	7	6.4	1.09	0.44–2.24

[1]Drugs used by 633 Blacks
[2]Drugs used by 798 mothers of male offspring

classes of malformations. The highest SRR was 1.26 for gastrointestinal malformations.

Propoxyphene — 686 Exposures (Table 20.9) There was no evidence of association between propoxyphene and broad classes of malformations. With regard to the specific classes of malformations, the highest SRR was 1.29, for hypospadias.

Codeine — 563 Exposures (Table 20.10) The SRRs in the table give no suggestion of association of codeine with major or minor malformations. The SRR for any malformation was 1.15. SRRs greater than 1.5 were found for respiratory malformations (2.60), genitourinary malformations (2.06), Down syndrome (1.53), and tumors (1.81). With a lower confidence limit of 1.12, the finding for respiratory malformations is statistically significant.

Detailed Evaluation of Non-Uniform Malformations: Inguinal Hernia, Clubfoot, Pectus Excavatum

In this section, the three outcomes are evaluated as in the preceding section dealing with uniform malformations. Instances in which there were fewer than three malformed children exposed to any drug are omitted because they are not informative.

The results of the analysis are given in Table 20.11. For inguinal hernia, the highest SRR was with codeine (1.42). For clubfoot, the drugs with SRRs greater than 1.5 were salicylamide (1.53) and propoxyphene (1.77). There was no evidence of association of this drug group with pectus excavatum.

Table **20.9**

Standardized Relative Risks (SRR) and Their 95% Confidence Intervals (CI$_{95}$) for Classes of Malformations Showing Uniform Rates by Hospital in Relation to **Propoxyphene** Used in Lunar Months 1–4 by 686 Pregnant Women (Based on Multiple Logistic Risk Function Analysis)

| Malformation Classes | No. of Malformed Children | | SRR | CI$_{95}$ of SRR |
	Observed	Expected		
Any malformation	31	34.4	0.90	0.63–1.29
Major malformations	22	21.2	1.04	0.69–1.55
Minor malformations	9	12.8	0.70	0.32–1.33
Central nervous	5	4.4	1.14	0.37–2.66
Cardiovascular	6	6.4	0.94	0.35–2.04
Musculoskeletal (other than polydactyly in Blacks)	3	6.9	0.44	0.09–1.27
Polydactyly in Blacks[1]	3	4.0	0.74	0.15–2.16
Respiratory	4	4.3	0.92	0.25–2.35
Gastrointestinal	6	5.5	1.09	0.40–2.35
Genitourinary (other than hypospadias)	2	3.6	0.55	0.07–1.97
Hypospadias[2]	3	2.3	1.29	0.27–3.74
Eye and ear	2	1.9	1.04	0.13–3.74
Syndromes (other than Down syndrome)	1	2.2	0.46	0.01–2.55
Down syndrome	1	0.9	1.08	0.03–6.02
Tumors	3	3.0	1.00	0.21–2.92

[1]Drugs used by 311 Blacks
[2]Drugs used by 346 mothers of male offspring

Table **20.10**

Standardized Relative Risks (SRR) and Their 95% Confidence Intervals (CI$_{95}$) for Classes of Malformations Showing Uniform Rates by Hospital in Relation to **Codeine** Used in Lunar Months 1–4 by 563 Pregnant Women (Based on Multiple Logistic Risk Function Analysis)

| Malformation Classes | No. of Malformed Children | | SRR | CI$_{95}$ of SRR |
	Observed	Expected		
Any malformation	32	27.8	1.15	0.84–1.57
Major malformations	20	18.5	1.08	0.67–1.66
Minor malformations	12	10.7	1.12	0.58–1.94
Central nervous	5	3.9	1.27	0.41–2.95
Cardiovascular	4	5.4	0.75	0.20–1.90
Musculoskeletal (other than polydactyly in Blacks)	5	5.8	0.86	0.28–1.99
Polydactyly in Blacks[1]	3	2.7	1.11	0.23–3.19
Respiratory	8	3.1	2.60	1.12–5.08
Gastrointestinal	5	4.9	1.02	0.33–2.37
Genitourinary (other than hypospadias)	7	3.4	2.06	0.83–4.22
Hypospadias[2]	1	2.1	0.48	0.01–2.67
Eye and ear	1	1.5	0.68	0.02–3.76
Syndromes (other than Down syndrome)	1	1.9	0.54	0.01–2.98
Down syndrome	1	0.7	1.53	0.04–8.47
Tumors	4	2.2	1.81	0.49–4.61

[1]Drugs used by 202 Blacks
[2]Drugs used by 288 mothers of male offspring

Table **20.11**

Standardized Relative Risks (SRR) and Their 95% Confidence Intervals (CI$_{95}$) for Inguinal Hernia, Clubfoot, and Pectus Excavatum in Relation to **Analgesic and Antipyretic Drugs** Used in Lunar Months 1–4 (Based on Multiple Logistic Risk Function Analysis)

	No. of Users	No. of Malformed Children		SRR	CI$_{95}$ of SRR
		Observed	Expected		
Inguinal hernia					
Analgesics and antipyretics	15,909	241	232.0	1.04	0.94–1.15
Non-addicting analgesics	15,463	231	225.1	1.03	0.92–1.14
Aspirin	14,864	227	216.5	1.05	0.94–1.17
Phenacetin	5,546	72	82.5	0.87	0.69–1.10
Salicylamide	744	7	11.2	0.62	0.25–1.28
Narcotic analgesics	1,564	27	23.9	1.13	0.80–1.60
Propoxyphene	686	7	10.6	0.66	0.26–1.35
Codeine	563	12	8.5	1.42	0.74–2.46
Clubfoot					
Analgesics and antipyretics	15,909	70	65.2	1.07	0.89–1.30
Non-addicting analgesics	15,463	69	63.3	1.09	0.90–1.32
Aspirin	14,864	67	60.5	1.11	0.91–1.34
Phenacetin	5,546	26	22.7	1.14	0.81–1.62
Salicylamide	744	5	3.3	1.53	0.50–3.56
Narcotic analgesics	1,564	10	7.8	1.28	0.62–2.36
Propoxyphene	686	6	3.4	1.77	0.65–3.83
Codeine	563	4	3.0	1.34	0.36–3.40
Pectus excavatum					
Analgesics and antipyretics	15,909	33	38.7	0.85	0.63–1.16
Non-addicting analgesics	15,463	33	37.4	0.88	0.65–1.20
Aspirin	14,864	33	35.8	0.92	0.68–1.25
Phenacetin	5,546	14	13.9	1.01	0.55–1.69
Narcotic analgesics	1,564	3	5.6	0.54	0.11–1.58

Comments

There was little evidence to suggest that analgesics or antipyretics, whether addicting or non-addicting, cause malformations. The data for aspirin, in particular, which accounted for 14,864 exposures, gave no evidence of association with any of the uniform or non-uniform malformation outcomes. Moreover, the confidence limits around the relative risk estimates for aspirin exposure make it unlikely that strong teratogenic effects could have been missed. Similarities between the crude relative risks and all standardized relative risks rule out overcon-

trolling of the analyses as an explanation of the negative findings.

For four other commonly used drugs, phenacetin (5,546 exposures), salicylamide (744), propoxyphene (666), and codeine (563), there was little evidence of association with any of the outcomes — except, perhaps, for a possible association between codeine exposure and respiratory malformations.

With regard to individual malformations (Appendix 4), a large number of associations with aspirin exposure were observed. These associations were derived from multiple comparisons between two groups, one of which (the exposed group) accounted for one-third of the cohort. Many associations would have been expected to occur by chance. Standing alone, the associations cannot be interpreted, and they would have some meaning only if replicated in independent studies.

It should also be remembered that compounds such as aspirin and phenacetin (and caffeine, see Chapter 27) were frequently used by the same women and were often present in the same preparation. Thus, these compounds tended to share associations. For example, there were associations between aspirin and anencephaly (10 malformed-exposed children) and between phenacetin and anencephaly (3 malformed-exposed children); the 3 malformed children accounting for the latter association were also exposed to aspirin.

The data do not accord with the findings in case-control studies[1,2] reporting that a higher proportion of malformed children were exposed to analgesics (mostly aspirin). In addition, Wilson[3] has not found aspirin to be dysmorphogenic in rhesus monkeys.

CHAPTER **21**

Antimicrobial and Antiparasitic Agents

General Evaluation

It should be noted that certain agents in this group are exclusively topical. However, it is possible that topically applied disinfectants and similar substances cause malformations, since many of these substances were taken *per vaginam* and may thus have been absorbed. In Tables 21.1 to 21.5, the entire set of 3,248 malformed children is considered in relation to exposure to the entire group of antimicrobial and antiparasitic drugs during the first four lunar months of pregnancy. In Tables 21.6 to 21.10, the data are confined to the 2,277 children who had malformations which were distributed uniformly across hospitals. Three relative risks are given in each table: crude, standardized for hospital variability, and standardized for the mother's ethnic group and survival of the child. Because of the large number of antimicrobial and antiparasitic drugs, Tables 21.1 and 21.6 present data for the entire group and major subgroups only. Data for specific drugs are found in Tables 21.2 to 21.5 and 21.7 to 21.10, with a separate table for each of the major subgroups.

All Malformations in Relation
to Antimicrobial and
Antiparasitic Agents
(Tables 21.1–21.5)
The hospital-standardized relative risk of all malformations was 1.06 for

Table **21.1**

Children (3,248) With Any Malformation in Relation to Exposure to **Antimicrobial and Antiparasitic Agents** During Lunar Months 1–4 Among 50,282 Mother-Child Pairs

	No. of Mother-Child Pairs Exposed	No. of Malformed Children	Crude Relative Risk	Hospital Standardized Relative Risk[1]	Survival and Race Standardized Relative Risk[1]
Antimicrobials and antiparasitics	8,088	554	1.07	1.06	1.06
Antibiotics	4,444	313	1.10	1.08	1.10
Sulfonamides	1,455	92	0.98	0.97	0.92
Systemic antimicrobials and antiparasitics	981	65	1.03	0.99	0.99
Topical antimicrobials	2,918	203	1.08	1.08	1.07

[1]Estimated by the Mantel-Haenszel procedure

Table **21.2**

Children (3,248) With Any Malformation in Relation to Exposure to **Antibiotics** During Lunar Months 1–4 Among 50,282 Mother-Child Pairs

	No. of Mother-Child Pairs Exposed	No. of Malformed Children	Crude Relative Risk	Hospital Standardized Relative Risk[1]	Survival and Race Standardized Relative Risk[1]
Penicillin derivatives	3,546	244	1.07	1.06	1.07
Tetracycline	341	25	1.14	1.07	1.14
Antibiotic, n.o.s.	202	11	0.84	0.82	0.78
Nystatin	142	14	1.53	1.43	1.61
Streptomycin	135	6	0.69	0.67	0.56
Oxytetracycline	119	15	1.96[3]	1.99[3]	2.02[3]
Chloramphenicol	98	8	1.26	1.17	1.21
Demeclocycline	90	10	1.72	1.54	1.91
Erythromycin	79	8	1.57	1.52	1.50
Gramicidin	61	7	1.78	1.85	1.95
Tyrothricin	31	4	2.00	1.93	1.72
Neomycin	30	2	1.03	0.90	1.04
Novobiocin	21	1	0.74	0.63	0.84
Other antibiotics[2]	79	2	0.39	0.34	0.38

[1]Estimated by the Mantel-Haenszel procedure
[2]Bacitracin (18); dihydrostreptomycin (18); chlortetracycline (14); amphotericin B (9); polymixin (7); oleandomycin (5); troleandomycin (4); griseofulvin (4); cycloserine (3); lincomycin (1); ristocetin (1); cephalothin (1)
[3]X^2_1 = 5.51–6.47; p < 0.025

Table **21.3**

Children (3,248) With Any Malformation in Relation to Exposure to **Sulfonamides** During Lunar Months 1–4 Among 50,282 Mother-Child Pairs

	No. of Mother-Child Pairs Exposed	No. of Malformed Children	Crude Relative Risk	Hospital Standardized Relative Risk[1]	Survival and Race Standardized Relative Risk[1]
Sulfisoxazole	796	56	1.09	1.07	1.04
Sulfa, n.o.s.	318	17	0.83	0.84	0.75
Sulfathiazole	100	5	0.77	0.80	0.67
Sulfadiazine	95	6	0.98	1.00	0.91
Sulfacetamide	93	4	0.67	0.69	0.60
Sulfabenzamide	88	4	0.70	0.73	0.64
Sulfamethoxypyridazine	61	2	0.51	0.49	0.52
Sulfanilamide	55	5	1.41	1.33	1.42
Sulfamerazine	48	3	0.97	0.93	0.81
Sulfamethazine	47	3	0.99	0.94	0.83
Sulfamethoxazole	46	3	1.01	0.98	1.00
Sulfamethizole	37	1	0.42	0.37	0.41
Other sulfonamides[2]	29	1	0.53	0.48	0.48

[1]Estimated by the Mantel-Haenszel procedure

[2]Sulfadimethoxine (16); succinylsulfathiazole (6); sulfaguanidine (2); salicylazosulfapyridine (2); sulfatulamide (1); sulfachlorpyridazine (1); phthalysulfathiazole (1)

antimicrobial and antiparasitic agents as a group (Table 21.1). The relative risks for the four major categories of antimicrobial drugs were all close to unity.

Among the antibiotics (Table 21.2), hospital-standardized relative risks greater than 1.5 were seen for oxytetracycline (1.99), demeclocycline (1.54), erythromycin (1.52), gramicidin (1.85), and tyrothricin (1.93). The finding for oxytetracycline is statistically significant at the 0.025 level.

Among the sulfonamides (Table 21.3), the highest hospital-standardized relative risk was for sulfanilamide (1.33).

Among the systemic antimicrobials and antiparasitics (Table 21.4), hospital-standardized relative risks greater than 1.5 were seen for isoniazid (1.94), aminosalicylic acid (1.92), metronidazole (2.02), and arsenicals (1.62).

Among the topical antimicrobial drugs (Table 21.5), hospital-standardized relative risks greater than 1.5 were seen for thiomersal (2.04), gentian violet (1.57), and phenol (2.06).

Malformations with Uniform Rates by Hospital in Relation to Antimicrobial and Antiparasitic Agents (Tables 21.6–21.10)

As seen in Table 21.1, the hospital-standardized relative risks for each of the categories of antimicrobial and antiparasitic agents were all close to unity.

Hospital-standardized relative risks greater than 1.5 were seen for exposure to the following specific drugs (Tables 21.7–21.10): gramicidin (1.85), tyrothricin (2.09), isoniazid (1.91), aminosalicylic acid (2.20), thiomersal (2.50), thymol (1.67), gentian violet (1.66), and phenol (1.96).

Detailed Evaluation of Uniform Malformations

In this section, groups of drugs, followed by individual drugs, are evaluated in relation to various classes or groups of uniform malformations, as well as individual malformations, for which multiple

Table **21.4**

Children (3,248) With Any Malformation in Relation to Exposure to **Systemic Antimicrobials and Antiparasitics** During Lunar Months 1–4 Among 50,282 Mother-Child Pairs

	No. of Mother-Child Pairs Exposed	No. of Malformed Children	Crude Relative Risk	Hospital Standardized Relative Risk[1]	Survival and Race Standardized Relative Risk[1]
Phenazopyridine	219	13	0.92	0.88	0.90
Diiodohydroxyquin	169	10	0.92	0.88	0.85
Furazolidone	132	9	1.06	1.04	1.02
Quinine	104	2	0.30	0.29	0.28
Isoniazid	85	10	1.82	1.94	1.95
Nitrofurantoin	83	6	1.12	1.07	1.01
Antimony potassium tartrate	75	6	1.24	1.17	1.21
Methenamine	49	4	1.26	1.20	1.19
Aminosalicylic acid	43	5	1.80	1.92	2.12
Metronidazole	31	4	2.00	2.02	2.08
Mandelic acid	30	3	1.55	1.50	1.47
Oxyquinoline	21	0	—	—	—
Hexylresorcinol	20	1	0.77	0.70	0.67
Arsenicals[2]	20	2	1.55	1.62	1.56
Other systemic antimicrobials and antiparasitics[3]	37	0	—	—	—

[1]Estimated by the Mantel-Haenszel procedure
[2]Glycobiarsol (19); acetarsone (2)
[3]Methylene blue (9); pyrvinium pamoate (7); chloroquine (7); piperazine (3); iodochlorhydroxyquin (3); hydroxychloroquine (2); pyrimethamine (2); hexetidine (2); dithiazanine iodide (1); proguanil (1); caprylate sodium (1); nalidixic acid (1); tetrachloroethylene (1)

logistic risk function models were developed. In the tables, the observed and expected numbers of malformed children are given for each drug exposure. The measure of association presented is a standardized relative risk (SRR) with its 95% confidence limits. The SRR is the ratio of the observed number to the expected number of malformed children. Since the SRR takes into account potential confounding variables, it represents the best estimate of the relationship between a drug and a malformation. As numbers of exposed mother-child pairs become so small as to be uninformative, data will be omitted.

All Antimicrobial and Antiparasitic Agents —
8,088 Exposures (Table 21.11)

The SRRs for broad classes of malformations were all close to unity. The highest SRR was 1.35 for defects of the eye and ear.

Antibiotics — 4,444 Exposures (Table 21.12)

As with the total group of antimicrobial and antiparasitic agents, the SRRs for broad classes of malformations did not differ greatly from unity. The highest SRR was 1.31 for syndromes excluding Down syndrome.

Penicillin Derivatives — 3,546 Exposures (Table 21.13) There was no evidence of association of penicillin derivatives with broad classes of malformations. The only SRR greater than 1.5 was seen for syndromes other than Down syndrome (1.73).

Tetracycline — 341 Exposures (Table 21.14) The SRR for minor malformations was 1.65.

Table **21.5**

Children (3,248) With Any Malformation in Relation to Exposure to **Topical Antimicrobial Drugs** During Lunar Months 1–4 Among 50,282 Mother-Child Pairs

	No. of Mother-Child Pairs Exposed	No. of Malformed Children	Crude Relative Risk	Hospital Standardized Relative Risk[1]	Survival and Race Standardized Relative Risk[1]
Antimicrobial agents	2,918	203	1.08	1.08	1.07
Benzethonium	1,131	62	0.85	0.87	0.82
Phenylmercuric acetate	889	47	0.82	0.85	0.80
Cetalkonium	775	62	1.24	1.22	1.25
Cetylpyridinium	326	28	1.33	1.29	1.32
Boric acid	253	19	1.16	1.12	1.13
Nitrofurazone	234	15	0.99	0.99	1.01
Ricinoleic acid	110	7	0.99	0.96	1.03
Aminacrine	59	5	1.31	1.22	1.24
Thiomersal	56	7	1.94	2.04	2.12
Thymol	52	5	1.49	1.42	1.45
Benzalkonium	50	3	0.93	0.87	1.03
Gentian violet	40	4	1.55	1.57	1.82
Chlordantoin	24	0	—	—	—
Phenol	23	3	2.02	2.06	1.89
Other topical antimicrobials[2]	90	6	1.03	1.02	0.95

[1]Estimated by the Mantel-Haenszel procedure
[2]Cresol (16); halazone (14); chlorobutanol (11); propionic acid (7); sodium hypochlorite solution (7); potassium permanganate (6); povidone iodine (6); thonzonium bromide (4); polyethyleneglycoltertdodecylthide (4); dequalinium (3); triclobisonium (3); hydrogen peroxide (2); sodium perborate (2); silver protein (2); chlorhexidine (1); triethanolamine (1); paraformaldehyde (1)

Table **21.6**

Children (2,277) With Malformations Showing Uniform Rates by Hospital in Relation to Exposure to **Antimicrobial and Antiparasitic Agents** During Lunar Months 1–4 Among 50,282 Mother-Child Pairs

	No. of Mother-Child Pairs Exposed	No. of Malformed Children	Crude Relative Risk	Hospital Standardized Relative Risk	Survival and Race Standardized Relative Risk
Antimicrobials and antiparasitics	8,088	360	0.98	0.96	0.97
Antibiotics	4,444	197	0.98	0.96	0.97
Sulfonamides	1,455	64	0.97	0.96	0.90
Systemic antimicrobials and antiparasitics	981	41	0.92	0.90	0.87
Topical antimicrobials	2,918	134	1.01	1.00	1.03

Table **21.7**

Children (2,277) With Malformations Showing Uniform Rates by Hospital in Relation to Exposure to **Antibiotics** During Lunar Months 1–4 Among 50,282 Mother-Child Pairs

	No. of Mother-Child Pairs Exposed	No. of Malformed Children	Crude Relative Risk	Hospital Standardized Relative Risk	Survival and Race Standardized Relative Risk
Penicillin derivatives	3,546	153	0.95	0.94	0.95
Tetracycline	341	16	1.04	1.00	1.02
Antibiotic, n.o.s.	202	7	0.76	0.75	0.67
Nystatin	142	10	1.56	1.48	1.61
Streptomycin	135	5	0.82	0.83	0.64
Oxytetracycline	119	7	1.30	1.28	1.26
Chloramphenicol	98	5	1.13	1.07	1.02
Demeclocycline	90	5	1.23	1.11	1.31
Erythromycin	79	5	1.40	1.37	1.25
Gramicidin	61	5	1.81	1.85	2.03
Tyrothricin	31	3	2.14	2.09	1.68
Neomycin	30	0	—	—	—
Novobiocin	21	1	1.05	0.96	1.30
Other antibiotics	79	0	—	—	—

Table **21.8**

Children (2,277) With Malformations Showing Uniform Rates by Hospital in Relation to Exposure to **Sulfonamides** During Lunar Months 1–4 Among 50,282 Mother-Child Pairs

	No. of Mother-Child Pairs Exposed	No. of Malformed Children	Crude Relative Risk	Hospital Standardized Relative Risk	Survival and Race Standardized Relative Risk
Sulfisoxazole	796	38	1.06	1.04	0.98
Sulfa, n.o.s.	318	15	1.04	1.04	0.94
Sulfathiazole	100	4	0.88	0.90	0.74
Sulfadiazine	95	3	0.70	0.69	0.63
Sulfacetamide	93	3	0.71	0.72	0.63
Sulfabenzamide	88	3	0.75	0.77	0.66
Sulfamethoxypyridazine	61	0	—	—	—
Sulfanilamide	55	3	1.20	1.18	1.22
Sulfamerazine	48	2	0.92	0.91	0.73
Sulfamethazine	47	2	0.94	0.92	0.74
Sulfamethoxazole	46	2	0.96	0.96	0.95
Sulfamethizole	37	1	0.60	0.55	0.60
Other sulfonamides	29	1	0.76	0.72	0.74

Table **21.9**

Children (2,277) With Malformations Showing Uniform Rates by Hospital in Relation to Exposure to **Systemic Antimicrobials and Antiparasitics** During Lunar Months 1–4 Among 50,282 Mother-Child Pairs

	No. of Mother-Child Pairs Exposed	No. of Malformed Children	Crude Relative Risk	Hospital Standardized Relative Risk	Survival and Race Standardized Relative Risk
Phenazopyridine	219	7	0.70	0.69	0.69
Diiodohydroxyquin	169	9	1.18	1.14	1.06
Furazolidone	132	3	0.50	0.48	0.45
Quinine	104	2	0.42	0.42	0.42
Isoniazid	85	7	1.82	1.91	1.98
Nitrofurantoin	83	5	1.33	1.31	1.17
Antimony potassium tartrate	75	3	0.88	0.82	0.76
Methenamine	49	3	1.35	1.32	1.24
Aminosalicylic acid	43	4	2.06	2.20	2.64
Metronidazole	31	2	1.43	1.39	1.31
Mandelic acid	30	2	1.47	1.43	1.31
Oxyquinoline	21	0	—	—	—
Hexylresorcinol	20	1	1.10	1.05	0.90
Arsenicals	20	1	1.10	1.16	1.03
Other antimicrobials and antiparasitics	37	0	—	—	—

Table **21.10**

Children (2,277) With Malformations Showing Uniform Rates by Hospital in Relation to Exposure to **Topical Antimicrobials** During Lunar Months 1–4 Among 50,282 Mother-Child Pairs

	No. of Mother-Child Pairs Exposed	No. of Malformed Children	Crude Relative Risk	Hospital Standardized Relative Risk	Survival and Race Standardized Relative Risk
Benzethonium	1,131	41	0.80	0.80	0.81
Phenylmercuric acetate	889	31	0.77	0.77	0.80
Cetalkonium	775	39	1.11	1.08	1.11
Cetylpyridinium	326	20	1.36	1.33	1.35
Boric acid	253	16	1.40	1.37	1.34
Nitrofurazone	234	7	0.66	0.65	0.67
Ricinoleic acid	110	5	1.00	0.97	1.13
Aminacrine	59	3	1.12	1.09	1.03
Thiomersal	56	6	2.37	2.50	2.69[1]
Thymol	52	4	1.70	1.67	1.62
Benzalkonium	50	1	0.44	0.41	0.50
Gentian violet	40	3	1.66	1.66	2.08
Chlordantoin	24	0	—	—	—
Phenol	23	2	1.92	1.96	1.67
Other topical antimicrobials	90	3	0.74	0.70	0.65

[1] $X^2_1 = 4.36$, $p < 0.05$

Table **21.11**

Standardized Relative Risks (SRR) and Their 95% Confidence Intervals (CI₉₅) for Classes of Malformations Showing Uniform Rates by Hospital in Relation to **Antimicrobial and Antiparasitic Drugs** Used in Lunar Months 1–4 by 8,088 Pregnant Women (Based on Multiple Logistic Risk Function Analysis)

Malformation Classes	No. of Malformed Children		SRR	CI₉₅ of SRR
	Observed	Expected		
Any malformation	360	378.2	0.95	0.87–1.05
Major malformations	205	223.1	0.92	0.81–1.05
Minor malformations	158	155.9	1.01	0.88–1.17
Central nervous	29	42.9	0.68	0.45–1.02
Cardiovascular	69	66.3	1.04	0.84–1.29
Musculoskeletal (other than polydactyly in Blacks)	70	63.0	1.11	0.90–1.36
Polydactyly in Blacks[1]	61	62.0	0.98	0.78–1.24
Respiratory	32	35.7	0.90	0.64–1.25
Gastrointestinal	45	50.5	0.89	0.67–1.18
Genitourinary (other than hypospadias)	22	30.7	0.72	0.45–1.13
Hypospadias[2]	33	29.3	1.13	0.84–1.52
Eye and ear	27	20.0	1.35	1.00–1.83
Syndromes (other than Down syndrome)	21	19.6	1.07	0.73–1.57
Down syndrome	6	10.0	0.60	0.22–1.31
Tumors	26	29.1	0.89	0.61–1.31

[1]Drugs used by 4,467 Blacks
[2]Drugs used by 4,162 mothers of male offspring

Table **21.12**

Standardized Relative Risks (SRR) and Their 95% Confidence Intervals (CI₉₅) for Classes of Malformations Showing Uniform Rates by Hospital in Relation to **Antibiotics** Used in Lunar Months 1–4 by 4,444 Pregnant Women (Based on Multiple Logistic Risk Function Analysis)

Malformation Classes	No. of Malformed Children		SRR	CI₉₅ of SRR
	Observed	Expected		
Any malformation	197	206.8	0.95	0.83–1.09
Major malformations	111	123.9	0.90	0.74–1.08
Minor malformations	85	84.4	1.01	0.82–1.23
Central nervous	19	23.7	0.80	0.48–1.25
Cardiovascular	38	37.0	1.03	0.76–1.39
Musculoskeletal (other than polydactyly in Blacks)	33	35.3	0.93	0.66–1.31
Polydactyly in Blacks[1]	31	32.5	0.95	0.68–1.35
Respiratory	14	20.0	0.70	0.38–1.17
Gastrointestinal	26	27.9	0.93	0.63–1.37
Genitourinary (other than hypospadias)	11	17.1	0.64	0.32–1.15
Hypospadias[2]	21	16.6	1.27	0.88–1.83
Eye and ear	14	10.9	1.28	0.70–2.15
Syndromes (other than Down syndrome)	14	10.7	1.31	0.72–2.20
Down syndrome	4	5.6	0.72	0.20–1.84
Tumors	15	15.6	0.96	0.54–1.58

[1]Drugs used by 2,305 Blacks
[2]Drugs used by 2,259 mothers of male offspring

Table **21.13**

Standardized Relative Risks (SRR) and Their 95% Confidence Intervals (CI$_{95}$) for Classes of Malformations Showing Uniform Rates by Hospital in Relation to **Penicillin Derivatives** Used in Lunar Months 1–4 by 3,546 Pregnant Women (Based on Multiple Logistic Risk Function Analysis)

Malformation Classes	No. of Malformed Children		SRR	CI$_{95}$ of SRR
	Observed	Expected		
Any malformation	153	164.6	0.93	0.79–1.09
Major malformations	88	96.5	0.91	0.74–1.12
Minor malformations	65	68.4	0.95	0.75–1.21
Central nervous	14	18.3	0.76	0.42–1.28
Cardiovascular	29	29.0	1.00	0.70–1.42
Musculoskeletal (other than polydactyly in Blacks)	24	26.6	0.90	0.60–1.36
Polydactyly in Blacks[1]	27	27.8	0.97	0.67–1.40
Respiratory	12	15.2	0.79	0.41–1.38
Gastrointestinal	22	21.6	1.02	0.68–1.52
Genitourinary (other than hypospadias)	10	12.9	0.78	0.37–1.43
Hypospadias[2]	15	13.3	1.13	0.63–1.86
Eye and ear	9	8.5	1.06	0.48–2.00
Syndromes (other than Down syndrome)	14	8.1	1.73	0.95–2.90
Down syndrome	4	4.3	0.93	0.25–2.37
Tumors	11	12.2	0.90	0.45–1.61

[1]Drugs used by 1,985 Blacks
[2]Drugs used by 1,800 mothers of male offspring

Table **21.14**

Standardized Relative Risks (SRR) and Their 95% Confidence Intervals (CI$_{95}$) for Broad Classes of Malformations Showing Uniform Rates by Hospital in Relation to **Tetracycline** Used in Lunar Months 1–4 by 341 Pregnant Women (Based on Multiple Logistic Risk Function Analysis)

	No. of Malformed Children		SRR	CI$_{95}$ of SRR
	Observed	Expected		
Any malformation	16	17.0	0.94	0.54–1.50
Major malformations	6	11.0	0.54	0.20–1.17
Minor malformations	11	6.7	1.65	0.83–2.91

Antibiotics, n.o.s. — 202 Exposures (Table 21.15) There was no evidence of association of antibiotics, n.o.s. with malformations.

Nystatin — 142 Exposures (Table 21.16) The SRR for any malformation was 1.52.

Sulfonamides — 1,455 Exposures (Table 21.17)

The SRRs for broad classes of malformations were all close to unity. SRRs greater than 1.5 were seen for hypospadias (1.51) and syndromes other than Down syndrome (1.64).

Sulfisoxazole — 796 Exposures (Table 21.18) The SRR for minor malformations was 1.35. The only SRR greater than 1.5 was for eye and ear malformations (1.81).

Sulfa, n.o.s. — 318 Exposures (Table 21.19) There was no evidence of a teratogenic effect for these drugs.

Systemic Antimicrobials and Antiparasitics — 981 Exposures (Table 21.20)

The SRRs for broad classes of malformations were all close to unity. The SRR for eye and ear malformations (2.03) was the only one greater than 1.5.

Phenazopyridine — 219 Exposures (Table 21.21) The SRR for minor malformations was 1.24.

Topical Antimicrobials — 2,918 Exposures (Table 21.22)

There was no evidence of association of topical antimicrobials with broad classes of malformations. An SRR of 1.81 was seen for eye and ear malformations.

Table **21.15**

Standardized Relative Risks (SRR) and Their 95% Confidence Intervals (CI$_{95}$) for Broad Classes of Malformations Showing Uniform Rates by Hospital in Relation to **Antibiotics, n.o.s.,** Used in Lunar Months 1–4 by 202 Pregnant Women (Based on Multiple Logistic Risk Function Analysis)

	No. of Malformed Children			
	Observed	Expected	SRR	CI$_{95}$ of SRR
Any malformation	7	9.2	0.76	0.31–1.53
Major malformations	3	6.0	0.50	0.10–1.44
Minor malformations	3	3.6	0.84	0.17–2.43

Table **21.16**

Standardized Relative Risks (SRR) and Their 95% Confidence Intervals (CI$_{95}$) for Broad Classes of Malformations Showing Uniform Rates by Hospital in Relation to **Nystatin** Used in Lunar Months 1–4 by 142 Pregnant Women (Based on Multiple Logistic Risk Function Analysis)

	No. of Malformed Children			
	Observed	Expected	SRR	CI$_{95}$ of SRR
Any malformation	10	6.6	1.52	0.74–2.72
Major malformations	5	4.3	1.15	0.38–2.62
Minor malformations	3	2.2	1.33	0.28–3.82

Table **21.17**

Standardized Relative Risks (SRR) and Their 95% Confidence Intervals (CI_{95}) for Classes of Malformations Showing Uniform Rates by Hospital in Relation to **Sulfonamides** Used in Lunar Months 1–4 by 1,455 Pregnant Women (Based on Multiple Logistic Risk Function Analysis)

Malformation Classes	No. of Malformed Children		SRR	CI_{95} of SRR
	Observed	Expected		
Any malformation	64	71.2	0.90	0.70–1.15
Major malformations	30	43.5	0.69	0.45–1.05
Minor malformations	35	29.2	1.20	0.89–1.61
Central nervous	4	9.0	0.44	0.12–1.13
Cardiovascular	14	12.8	1.09	0.60–1.82
Musculoskeletal (other than polydactyly in Blacks)	11	12.9	0.86	0.43–1.53
Polydactyly in Blacks[1]	7	10.2	0.69	0.28–1.41
Respiratory	8	7.9	1.01	0.44–1.99
Gastrointestinal	8	10.3	0.78	0.34–1.53
Genitourinary (other than hypospadias)	5	6.9	0.72	0.23–1.68
Hypospadias[2]	8	5.3	1.51	0.65–2.97
Eye and ear	5	3.8	1.32	0.43–3.08
Syndromes (other than Down syndrome)	7	4.3	1.64	0.66–3.38
Down syndrome	1	1.9	0.52	0.01–2.91
Tumors	5	6.0	0.83	0.27–1.94

[1]Drugs used by 768 Blacks
[2]Drugs used by 775 mothers of male offspring

Table **21.18**

Standardized Relative Risks (SRR) and Their 95% Confidence Intervals (CI_{95}) for Classes of Malformations Showing Uniform Rates by Hospital in Relation to **Sulfisoxazole** Used in Lunar Months 1–4 by 796 Pregnant Women (Based on Multiple Logistic Risk Function Analysis)

Malformation Classes	No. of Malformed Children		SRR	CI_{95} of SRR
	Observed	Expected		
Any malformation	38	39.9	0.95	0.69–1.31
Major malformations	15	24.6	0.61	0.34–1.00
Minor malformations	23	17.1	1.35	0.95–1.90
Central nervous	4	5.5	0.73	0.20–1.85
Cardiovascular	7	7.0	0.99	0.40–2.04
Musculoskeletal (other than polydactyly in Blacks)	7	7.2	0.98	0.39–2.00
Polydactyly in Blacks[1]	5	6.0	0.83	0.27–1.93
Respiratory	5	5.1	0.98	0.32–2.27
Gastrointestinal	4	6.2	0.65	0.18–1.66
Genitourinary (other than hypospadias)	3	4.2	0.71	0.15–2.08
Hypospadias[2]	4	2.8	1.42	0.39–3.61
Eye and ear	4	2.2	1.81	0.49–4.62
Syndromes (other than Down syndrome)	3	2.7	1.12	0.23–3.27
Down syndrome	0	1.2	—	0.00–2.99
Tumors	3	3.5	0.87	0.18–2.53

[1]Drugs used by 435 Blacks
[2]Drugs used by 422 mothers of male offspring

Table **21.19**

Standardized Relative Risks (SRR) and Their 95% Confidence Intervals (CI_{95}) for Broad Classes of Malformations Showing Uniform Rates by Hospital in Relation to **Sulfa, n.o.s.,** Used in Lunar Months 1–4 by 318 Pregnant Women (Based on Multiple Logistic Risk Function Analysis)

	No. of Malformed Children		SRR	CI_{95} of SRR
	Observed	**Expected**	**SRR**	**CI_{95} of SRR**
Any malformation	15	15.6	0.96	0.54–1.56
Major malformations	8	9.4	0.85	0.37–1.66
Minor malformations	7	6.2	1.13	0.46–2.30

Table **21.20**

Standardized Relative Risks (SRR) and Their 95% Confidence Intervals (CI_{95}) for Classes of Malformations Showing Uniform Rates by Hospital in Relation to **Systemic Antimicrobials and Antiparasitics** Used in Lunar Months 1–4 by 981 Pregnant Women (Based on Multiple Logistic Risk Function Analysis)

Malformation Classes	No. of Malformed Children		SRR	CI_{95} of SRR
	Observed	**Expected**	**SRR**	**CI_{95} of SRR**
Any malformation	41	47.4	0.86	0.63–1.19
Major malformations	23	29.1	0.79	0.50–1.24
Minor malformations	19	18.1	1.05	0.63–1.63
Central nervous	2	5.5	0.36	0.04–1.30
Cardiovascular	4	8.5	0.47	0.13–1.20
Musculoskeletal (other than polydactyly in Blacks)	12	9.2	1.31	0.68–2.28
Polydactyly in Blacks[1]	6	5.8	1.04	0.38–2.25
Respiratory	6	4.8	1.25	0.46–2.72
Gastrointestinal	6	7.0	0.86	0.31–1.86
Genitourinary (other than hypospadias)	5	4.8	1.05	0.34–2.44
Hypospadias[2]	2	3.4	0.59	0.07–2.12
Eye and ear	5	2.5	2.03	0.66–4.72
Syndromes (other than Down syndrome)	0	2.6	—	0.00–1.44
Down syndrome	0	1.3	—	0.00–2.75
Tumors	3	3.9	0.76	0.16–2.22

[1]Drugs used by 438 Blacks
[2]Drugs used by 490 mothers of male offspring

Table **21.21**

Standardized Relative Risks (SRR) and Their 95% Confidence Intervals (CI$_{95}$) for Broad Classes of Malformations Showing Uniform Rates by Hospital in Relation to **Phenazopyridine** Used in Lunar Months 1–4 by 219 Pregnant Women (Based on Multiple Logistic Risk Function Analysis)

| | No. of Malformed Children | | | |
	Observed	Expected	SRR	CI$_{95}$ of SRR
Any malformation	7	10.6	0.66	0.27–1.33
Major malformations	1	6.2	0.16	0.00–0.89
Minor malformations	5	4.0	1.24	0.40–2.85

Table **21.22**

Standardized Relative Risks (SRR) and Their 95% Confidence Intervals (CI$_{95}$) for Classes of Malformations Showing Uniform Rates by Hospital in Relation to **Topical Antimicrobials** Used in Lunar Months 1–4 by 2,918 Pregnant Women (Based on Multiple Logistic Risk Function Analysis)

| | No. of Malformed Children | | | |
Malformation Classes	Observed	Expected	SRR	CI$_{95}$ of SRR
Any malformation	134	135.0	0.99	0.84–1.17
Major malformations	81	76.3	1.06	0.87–1.30
Minor malformations	55	57.7	0.95	0.73–1.24
Central nervous	7	14.8	0.47	0.19–0.98
Cardiovascular	22	23.0	0.96	0.63–1.46
Musculoskeletal (other than polydactyly in Blacks)	30	20.4	1.47[3]	1.10–1.96
Polydactyly in Blacks[1]	28	26.0	1.08	0.76–1.52
Respiratory	10	11.4	0.88	0.42–1.61
Gastrointestinal	19	17.0	1.12	0.68–1.75
Genitourinary (other than hypospadias)	7	10.2	0.68	0.27–1.41
Hypospadias[2]	7	9.9	0.71	0.29–1.46
Eye and ear	13	7.2	1.81	0.97–3.09
Syndromes (other than Down syndrome)	5	6.7	0.75	0.24–1.75
Down syndrome	1	3.5	0.29	0.01–1.60
Tumors	8	10.4	0.77	0.33–1.51

[1]Drugs used by 1,884 Blacks
[2]Drugs used by 1,507 mothers of male offspring
[3]$p < 0.05$

Table **21.23**

Standardized Relative Risks (SRR) and Their 95% Confidence Intervals (CI$_{95}$) for Classes of Malformations Showing Uniform Rates by Hospital in Relation to **Benzethonium** Used in Lunar Months 1–4 by 1,131 Pregnant Women (Based on Multiple Logistic Risk Function Analysis)

Malformation Classes	No. of Malformed Children		SRR	CI$_{95}$ of SRR
	Observed	Expected		
Any malformation	41	51.3	0.80	0.57–1.12
Major malformations	23	26.4	0.87	0.56–1.34
Minor malformations	18	24.2	0.74	0.44–1.17
Central nervous	4	5.5	0.73	0.20–1.86
Cardiovascular	9	8.7	1.04	0.48–1.97
Musculoskeletal (other than polydactyly in Blacks)	6	5.3	1.13	0.42–2.46
Polydactyly in Blacks[1]	10	13.2	0.76	0.36–1.39
Respiratory	5	3.9	1.29	0.42–3.01
Gastrointestinal	5	5.4	0.92	0.30–2.15
Genitourinary (other than hypospadias)	3	3.2	0.95	0.20–2.77
Hypospadias[2]	2	3.5	0.57	0.07–2.04
Eye and ear	2	2.8	0.72	0.09–2.60
Syndromes (other than Down syndrome)	2	2.3	0.87	0.11–3.15
Down syndrome	1	1.3	0.78	0.02–4.35
Tumors	4	3.7	1.08	0.30–2.76

[1]Drugs used by 982 Blacks
[2]Drugs used by 576 mothers of male offspring

The SRR of 1.47 for musculoskeletal malformations was statistically significant at the 0.05 level and had a lower confidence limit of 1.10.

Benzethonium — 1,131 Exposures (Table 21.23) There was no evidence of association of broad classes of malformations with benzethonium. The highest SRR in the table was 1.29, for malformations of the respiratory tract.

Phenylmercuric Acetate — 889 Exposures (Table 21.24) There was no evidence of association of this drug with broad classes of malformations. The only SRR greater than 1.5 was seen for musculoskeletal malformations (1.53).

Cetalkonium — 775 Exposures (Table 21.25) The SRRs for broad classes of malformations were all close to unity. SRRs greater than 1.5 were found for eye and ear malformations (2.20) and syndromes other than Down syndrome (1.69).

Cetylpyridinium — 326 Exposures (Table 21.26) The highest SRR was 1.31, for malformed children.

Boric Acid — 253 Exposures (Table 21.27) The SRR for major malformations was 1.75.

Nitrofurazone — 234 Exposures (Table 21.28) The SRR for minor malformations was 1.25. The negative association of nitrofurazone with major malformations (SRR 0.15) was statistically significant at the 0.05 level, with an upper confidence limit of 0.82.

**Detailed Evaluation of
Non-Uniform Malformations:
Inguinal Hernia, Clubfoot,
Pectus Excavatum**

In this section, the three outcomes are evaluated as in the preceding section dealing with uniform malformations. Instances in which there were fewer than three malformed children exposed to any

Table **21.24**

Standardized Relative Risks (SRR) and Their 95% Confidence Intervals (CI$_{95}$) for Classes of Malformations Showing Uniform Rates by Hospital in Relation to **Phenylmercuric Acetate** Used in Lunar Months 1–4 by 889 Pregnant Women (Based on Multiple Logistic Risk Function Analysis)

Malformation Classes	No. of Malformed Children		SRR	CI$_{95}$ of SRR
	Observed	Expected		
Any malformation	31	39.5	0.79	0.53–1.16
Major malformations	20	26.4	0.87	0.56–1.34
Minor malformations	11	18.8	0.59	0.29–1.04
Central nervous	3	4.2	0.72	0.15–2.09
Cardiovascular	7	6.8	1.03	0.42–2.12
Musculoskeletal (other than polydactyly in Blacks)	6	3.9	1.53	0.56–3.32
Polydactyly in Blacks[1]	5	10.5	0.47	0.15–1.10
Respiratory	4	2.7	1.50	0.41–3.83
Gastrointestinal	5	4.0	1.24	0.40–2.88
Genitourinary (other than hypospadias)	2	2.2	0.92	0.11–3.32
Hypospadias[2]	1	2.7	0.37	0.01–2.06
Eye and ear	2	2.1	0.94	0.11–3.38
Syndromes (other than Down syndrome)	1	1.7	0.59	0.01–3.27
Down syndrome	1	1.0	1.02	0.03–5.65
Tumors	3	2.8	1.08	0.22–3.16

[1]Drugs used by 785 Blacks
[2]Drugs used by 448 mothers of male offspring

Table **21.25**

Standardized Relative Risks (SRR) and Their 95% Confidence Intervals (CI$_{95}$) for Classes of Malformations Showing Uniform Rates by Hospital in Relation to **Cetalkonium** Used in Lunar Months 1–4 by 775 Pregnant Women (Based on Multiple Logistic Risk Function Analysis)

Malformation Classes	No. of Malformed Children		SRR	CI$_{95}$ of SRR
	Observed	Expected		
Any malformation	39	35.5	1.10	0.82–1.47
Major malformations	25	21.3	1.17	0.82–1.68
Minor malformations	16	13.9	1.15	0.66–1.86
Central nervous	2	3.9	0.52	0.06–1.86
Cardiovascular	6	5.9	1.02	0.37–2.20
Musculoskeletal (other than polydactyly in Blacks)	9	6.7	1.34	0.61–2.52
Polydactyly in Blacks[1]	7	5.3	1.33	0.54–2.71
Respiratory	2	3.0	0.67	0.08–2.40
Gastrointestinal	6	4.9	1.24	0.45–2.68
Genitourinary (other than hypospadias)	1	2.9	0.34	0.01–1.90
Hypospadias[2]	3	2.7	1.12	0.23–3.24
Eye and ear	4	1.8	2.20	0.60–5.60
Syndromes (other than Down syndrome)	3	1.8	1.69	0.35–4.93
Down syndrome	0	0.8	—	0.00–4.58
Tumors	0	2.8	—	0.00–1.33

[1]Drugs used by 355 Blacks
[2]Drugs used by 405 mothers of male offspring

Table **21.26**

Standardized Relative Risks (SRR) and Their 95% Confidence Intervals (CI_{95}) for Broad Classes of Malformations Showing Uniform Rates by Hospital in Relation to **Cetylpyridinium** Used in Lunar Months 1–4 by 326 Pregnant Women (Based on Multiple Logistic Risk Function Analysis)

	No. of Malformed Children		SRR	CI_{95} of SRR
	Observed	**Expected**	**SRR**	**CI_{95} of SRR**
Any malformation	20	15.3	1.31	0.81–1.99
Major malformations	10	8.6	1.16	0.56–2.11
Minor malformations	8	6.4	1.25	0.54–2.44

Table **21.27**

Standardized Relative Risks (SRR) and Their 95% Confidence Intervals (CI_{95}) for Broad Classes of Malformations Showing Uniform Rates by Hospital in Relation to **Boric Acid** Used in Lunar Months 1–4 by 253 Pregnant Women (Based on Multiple Logistic Risk Function Analysis)

	No. of Malformed Children		SRR	CI_{95} of SRR
	Observed	**Expected**	**SRR**	**CI_{95} of SRR**
Any malformation	16	12.1	1.32	0.77–2.11
Major malformations	13	7.4	1.75	0.94–2.94
Minor malformations	5	4.6	1.10	0.36–2.53

Table **21.28**

Standardized Relative Risks (SRR) and Their 95% Confidence Intervals (CI_{95}) for Broad Classes of Malformations Showing Uniform Rates by Hospital in Relation to **Nitrofurazone** Used in Lunar Months 1–4 by 234 Pregnant Women (Based on Multiple Logistic Risk Function Analysis)

	No. of Malformed Children		SRR	CI_{95} of SRR
	Observed	**Expected**	**SRR**	**CI_{95} of SRR**
Any malformation	7	11.5	0.61	0.25–1.23
Major malformations	1	6.7	0.15[1]	0.00–0.82
Minor malformations	6	4.8	1.25	0.46–2.67

[1]$p < 0.05$

drug are omitted because they are not informative.

As seen in Table 21.29, the highest SRR for inguinal hernia was 1.33, with cetalkonium. For clubfoot, SRRs greater than 1.5 were observed with topical antimicrobials (1.70) and cetalkonium (2.90). With lower confidence limits exceeding unity, both are statistically significant, as is the SRR of 1.29 with antimicrobials and antiparasitics as a whole. For pectus excavatum, the only SRR greater than 1.5 was with penicillin derivatives (1.81).

Comments

Exposure in early pregnancy to antibiotics, sulfonamides, systemic antimicrobial and antiparasitic agents, and topical antimicrobials gave no overall evidence of associations with malformations in general, uniform malformations, major malformations, or minor malformations. Penicillin derivatives were received by 3,546 women. For the principal outcomes, the narrow confidence limits around the relative risks, which approx-

Table **21.29**

Standardized Relative Risks (SRR) and Their 95% Confidence Intervals (CI_{95}) for Inguinal Hernia, Clubfoot, and Pectus Excavatum in Relation to **Antimicrobial and Antiparasitic Drugs** Used in Lunar Months 1–4 (Based on Multiple Logistic Risk Function Analysis)

	No. of Users	No. of Malformed Children		SRR	CI_{95} of SRR
		Observed	Expected		
Inguinal hernia					
Antimicrobials and antiparasitics	8,088	132	120.4	1.10	0.94–1.27
Antibiotics	4,444	75	66.2	1.13	0.93–1.39
Penicillin derivatives	3,546	55	53.0	1.04	0.81–1.33
Sulfonamides	1,455	24	22.7	1.06	0.72–1.55
Sulfisoxazole	796	16	12.3	1.30	0.74–2.09
Systemic antimicrobials and antiparasitics	981	19	14.5	1.31	0.79–2.04
Topical antimicrobials	2,918	49	43.7	1.12	0.87–1.45
Benzethonium	1,131	16	17.0	0.94	0.54–1.53
Phenylmercuric acetate	889	13	12.7	1.02	0.54–1.74
Cetalkonium	775	15	11.3	1.33	0.75–2.18
Clubfoot					
Antimicrobials and antiparasitics	8,088	43	33.4	1.29	1.01–1.65
Antibiotics	4,444	23	18.8	1.23	0.86–1.75
Penicillin derivatives	3,546	16	14.3	1.12	0.64–1.81
Sulfonamides	1,455	6	6.6	0.90	0.33–1.96
Sulfisoxazole	796	4	4.0	1.00	0.27–2.55
Topical antimicrobials	2,918	19	11.2	1.70	1.03–2.65
Benzethonium	1,131	4	3.4	1.19	0.32–3.03
Cetalkonium	775	9	3.1	2.90	1.33–5.47
Pectus excavatum					
Antimicrobials and antiparasitics	8,088	16	16.1	1.00	0.57–1.62
Antibiotics	4,444	11	9.2	1.20	0.60–2.14
Penicillin derivatives	3,546	11	6.1	1.81	0.90–3.23
Topical antimicrobials	2,918	4	5.1	0.79	0.22–2.03

imated unity, suggest that it is unlikely that penicillin is teratogenic. Tetracycline was used by far fewer women (341) and was associated with minor malformations. With still smaller numbers (119), oxytetracycline was associated with malformations in general at a hospital-standardized relative risk of 1.99. However, the association was much less strong in relation to uniform malformations (relative risk, 1.28). Demeclocycline gave a hint of a similar relationship. The association between nystatin exposure and malformations may exist because this drug was sometimes used as an adjunct to tetracycline therapy. For tetracyclines as a whole, the numbers were too small to justify any conclusions, and further studies are needed, but since it is known that these compounds have an affinity for developing dental and osseous tissues, they should be avoided.[1]

The findings for erythromycin, gramicidin, and tyrothricin were based on small numbers.

Sulfonamides were received by 1,455 women and sulfisoxazole was received by 796; this group of drugs appeared to be devoid of any association with the various malformation outcomes. Strong associations with uniform malformations, major malformations, and minor malformations could be ruled out with reasonable confidence.

Among the systemic antimicrobial agents, there were small numbers of exposures to the antituberculous drugs, isoniazid (85), and aminosalicylic acid (43). In this small series, the risk of malformations was approximately doubled. These findings require independent confirmation. For 104 exposures to quinine, there was no evidence of a teratogenic effect.

With regard to topical agents, 13 out of 253 children exposed to boric acid had major malformations, giving a relative risk of 1.75 with a lower 95% confidence limit of 0.9. This association may merit further investigation. Finally, thiomersal, on the basis of extremely limited numbers (56 exposures) was associated with malformations overall, and with uniform malformations.

CHAPTER 22

Immunizing Agents

General Evaluation

In this section the relationships of immunizing agents to any malformation and to uniform malformations are presented. Crude relative risks and two standardized relative risks obtained by the Mantel-Haenszel procedure are presented. The first standardized risk controls for hospital; the second, for ethnic group of the mother and survival status of the child. In Table 22.1, all 3,248 malformed children are considered in relation to exposure to the entire group of immunizing agents. In Table 22.2, the data are confined to the 2,277 children who had malformations which were uniformly distributed among the hospitals.

All Malformations in Relation
to Immunizing Agents
(Table 22.1)

Among the study pregnancies, 9,222 (183.4 per 1,000) were exposed to immunizing agents during the first four lunar months; 626 (67.9 per 1,000) of the children born from these exposed pregnancies were malformed, giving a hospital-standardized relative risk of 1.04. For those agents to which the pregnancies were most frequently exposed — poliomyelitis vaccine, live oral polio virus vaccine, influenza virus vaccine, and tetanus toxoid — the relative risks for any malformation were quite close to unity. Of the immunizing agents to

Table **22.1**

Children (3,248) With Any Malformation in Relation to Exposure to **Immunizing Agents** During Lunar Months 1–4 Among 50,282 Mother-Child Pairs

	No. of Mother-Child Pairs Exposed	No. of Malformed Children	Crude Relative Risk	Hospital Standardized Relative Risk[1]	Survival and Race Standardized Relative Risk[1]
Immunizing agents	9,222	626	1.06	1.04	1.09
Poliomyelitis vaccine, parenteral	6,774	461	1.06	1.03	1.09
Polio virus vaccine, live oral	1,628	114	1.09	1.11	1.08
Influenza virus vaccine	650	39	0.93	0.91	0.95
Tetanus toxoid	337	24	1.10	1.12	1.20
Smallpox vaccine	172	7	0.63	0.62	0.60
Diphtheria toxoid	75	4	0.83	0.82	0.88
Allergy desensitization vaccine	64	6	1.45	1.32	1.58
Typhoid vaccine	44	1	0.35	0.35	0.38
Polio virus vaccine, n.o.s.	39	1	0.40	0.32	0.47
Measles virus vaccine, live attenuated	37	0	—	—	—
Other virus vaccines[2]	10	0	—	—	—
Specific desensitization vaccine[3]	14	3	3.32	4.25	4.70
Other bacterial vaccines[4]	28	2	1.11	1.06	1.28

[1]Estimated by the Mantel-Haenszel procedure
[2]Measles virus vaccine, inactivated (6); yellow fever vaccine (3); rabies vaccine (1)
[3]House dust extract (10); poison oak extract (3); poison ivy vaccine (2)
[4]Pertussis vaccine (13); typhus vaccine (7); staphylococcus toxoid (2); cholera vaccine (1); tetanus antitoxin (1); paratyphoid vaccine (1); bacterial vaccine (1); bacterial protein, I.V. (1); Rocky Mountain Spotted Fever vaccine (1)

which few women were exposed, the group with the highest hospital-standardized relative risk was the specific desensitization vaccines (4.25), based on three exposed-malformed children.

Malformations Showing Uniform Rates by Hospital in Relation to Immunizing Agents (Table 22.2)

With respect to malformations with uniform rates by hospital, hospital-standardized relative risks for the most commonly used immunizing agents were close to unity. Relative risks for the less commonly used vaccines were all less than unity.

Detailed Evaluation of Uniform Malformations

In this section, groups of drugs, followed by individual drugs, are evaluated in relation to various classes or groups of uniform malformations, as well as individual malformations, for which multiple logistic risk function models were developed. In the tables, the observed and expected numbers of malformed children are given for each drug exposure in turn. The measure of association presented is a standardized relative risk (SRR) with its 95% confidence limits. The SRR is the ratio of the observed number to the expected number of malformed children. Since the SRR takes into account potential

Table **22.2**

Children (2,277) With Malformations Showing Uniform Rates by Hospital in Relation to Exposure to **Immunizing Agents** During Lunar Months 1–4 Among 50,282 Mother-Child Pairs

	No. of Mother-Child Pairs Exposed	No. of Malformed Children	Crude Relative Risk	Hospital Standardized Relative Risk	Survival and Race Standardized Relative Risk
Immunizing agents	9,222	437	1.06	1.02	1.07
Poliomyelitis vaccine, parenteral	6,774	324	1.07	1.02	1.07
Polio virus vaccine, live oral	1,628	77	1.05	1.05	1.05
Influenza virus vaccine	650	27	0.92	0.92	0.91
Tetanus toxoid	337	17	1.11	1.11	1.27
Smallpox vaccine	172	5	0.64	0.62	0.61
Diphtheria toxoid	75	1	0.29	0.29	0.32
Allergy desensitization vaccine	64	2	0.69	0.62	0.66
Typhoid vaccine	44	1	0.50	0.48	0.59
Polio virus vaccine, n.o.s.	39	1	0.57	0.51	0.71
Measles virus vaccine, live attenuated	37	0	—	—	—
Other virus vaccines[2]	10	0	—	—	—
Specific desensitization vaccine[3]	14	0	—	—	—
Other bacterial vaccines[4]	28	1	0.79	0.75	0.95

confounding variables, it represents the best estimate of the relationship between a drug and a malformation. As numbers of exposed mother-child pairs become so small as to be uninformative, data will be omitted.

Any Immunizing Agent —
9,222 Exposures (Table 22.3)

The immunizing agents as a whole were not associated with broad classes of malformations. Of the specific malformation groups, there was no evidence of association with immunizing agents.

Poliomyelitis Vaccine (Parenteral) — 6,774 Exposures (Table 22.4) Poliomyelitis vaccine (parenteral) had no association with broad classes of uniform malformations. The highest SRR was for musculoskeletal malformations other than polydactyly in Blacks (1.16).

Live Oral Polio Virus Vaccine (Table 22.5) Live oral polio virus vaccine had an SRR of 1.24 for minor malformations. There were SRRs greater than 1.5 for gastrointestinal tract malformations (1.67), and Down syndrome (1.60).

Influenza Virus Vaccine — 2,331 Exposures (Table 22.6) Influenza virus vaccine was not positively associated with broad classes of malformations. Based on small numbers, there were SRRs greater than 1.5 for cardiovascular (1.52) and respiratory tract malformations (1.65).

Tetanus Toxoid — 337 Exposures (Table 22.7) The 337 children exposed to tetanus toxoid *in utero* during the first four lunar months had SRRs of 1.36 and 1.60, for major and minor malformations, respectively. Six of the 12 specific malformation groups had relative risks greater than 1.5. These included central nervous (1.67), musculoskeletal other than polydactyly in Blacks (1.90),

Table **22.3**

Standardized Relative Risks (SRR) and their 95% Confidence Intervals (CI$_{95}$) for Classes of Malformations Showing Uniform Rates by Hospital in Relation to **Immunizing Agents** Used in Lunar Months 1–4 by 9,222 Pregnant Women (Based on Multiple Logistic Risk Function Analysis)

Malformation Classes	No. of Malformed Children		SRR	CI$_{95}$ of SRR
	Observed	Expected		
Any malformation	437	418.7	1.04	0.96–1.13
Major malformations	279	271.4	1.03	0.93–1.14
Minor malformations	158	144.5	1.09	0.96–1.25
Central nervous	45	49.4	0.91	0.69–1.20
Cardiovascular	70	72.5	0.96	0.78–1.20
Musculoskeletal (other than polydactyly in Blacks)	101	90.4	1.12	0.94–1.32
Polydactyly in Blacks[1]	47	38.2	1.23	0.96–1.57
Respiratory	39	42.7	0.91	0.68–1.23
Gastrointestinal	74	62.3	1.19	0.98–1.44
Genitourinary (other than hypospadias)	34	38.3	0.89	0.64–1.23
Hypospadias[2]	29	30.9	0.94	0.66–1.33
Eye and ear	22	23.0	0.96	0.65–1.42
Syndromes (other than Down syndrome)	15	23.8	0.63	0.35–1.04
Down syndrome	12	11.4	1.05	0.54–1.83
Tumors	36	35.8	1.01	0.75–1.36

[1]Drugs used by 2,879 Blacks
[2]Drugs used by 4,649 mothers of male offspring

polydactyly in Blacks (2.32), gastrointestinal tract (2.10), eye and ear malformations (2.58), and Down syndrome (2.58).

Detailed Evaluation of Non-Uniform Malformations: Inguinal Hernia, Clubfoot, Pectus Excavatum

In this section, the three outcomes are evaluated as in the preceding section dealing with uniform malformations. Instances in which there were fewer than three malformed children exposed to any drug are omitted because they are not informative.

As shown in Table 22.8, the highest SRRs for inguinal hernia and clubfoot were with polio virus vaccine, live oral (1.13 and 1.24, respectively). For pectus excavatum, the only SRR greater than 1.5 was with polio virus vaccine, live oral (1.88).

Comments

Immunizing agents as a group gave no evidence of being associated with the principal outcomes of the study.

The most commonly used agent was killed poliomyelitis virus vaccine which was generally given by injection as a routine part of antenatal care (6,774 exposures). With regard to the principal outcomes, the findings are reassuring — there was no evidence of association. However, it should be noted (Appendix 4) that there were 24 children with malignant tumors, 7 of whom were exposed in early pregnancy (hospital standardized relative risk, 3.3). The association also held good when exposure during the entire pregnancy was considered (Appendices 1 and 5). The relationship has been more fully documented elsewhere,[1] but it must still be regarded as tentative pending confirmation.

317

Table **22.4**

Standardized Relative Risks (SRR) and Their 95% Confidence Intervals (CI_{95}) for Classes of Malformations Showing Uniform Rates by Hospital in Relation to **Poliomyelitis Vaccine (Parenteral)** Used in Lunar Months 1–4 by 6,774 Pregnant Women (Based on Multiple Logistic Risk Function Analysis)

Malformation Classes	No. of Malformed Children		SRR	CI_{95} of SRR
	Observed	Expected		
Any malformation	324	308.3	1.05	0.95–1.16
Major malformations	214	204.0	1.05	0.93–1.18
Minor malformations	104	99.3	1.05	0.88–1.25
Central nervous	35	36.4	0.96	0.70–1.32
Cardiovascular	51	52.9	0.96	0.74–1.25
Musculoskeletal (other than polydactyly in Blacks)	83	71.3	1.16	0.97–1.40
Polydactyly in Blacks[1]	22	20.3	1.09	0.74–1.60
Respiratory	30	32.6	0.92	0.65–1.30
Gastrointestinal	51	48.3	1.06	0.82–1.36
Genitourinary (other than hypospadias)	27	29.4	0.92	0.64–1.32
Hypospadias[2]	20	21.5	0.93	0.57–1.44
Eye and ear	18	17.0	1.06	0.63–1.67
Syndromes (other than Down syndrome)	11	17.7	0.62	0.31–1.11
Down syndrome	8	8.6	0.94	0.40–1.84
Tumors	28	27.6	1.02	0.72–1.44

[1]Drugs used by 1,601 Blacks
[2]Drugs used by 3,447 mothers of male offspring

"Killed" poliomyelitis vaccine is, in fact, a misnomer. It is known that the vaccine was contaminated with many viruses, including the SV 40 virus, which causes tumors in newborn animals.[2]

In principle, any vaccine containing live viruses should be regarded as a potential teratogen until disproved. Nevertheless, live poliomyelitis vaccine (1,628 exposures) gave little evidence to suggest a teratogenic effect, apart from a hint of association with gastrointestinal malformations and pectus excavatum. In particular, it gave no evidence of association with malignancies.[1] (See also Appendices 1 and 5.)

Among the individual malformations, malrotation of the intestine was associated with exposure to live poliomyelitis vaccine, having a hospital-standardized relative risk of 7.9 (Appendix 4).

For influenza virus vaccine, there were no suggestive associations.

Tetanus toxoid (337 exposures) was associated with over half of the outcomes evaluated in the preceding tables, and the relative risks were modestly increased for major malformations (1.4) and minor malformations (1.6). These findings could readily be due to chance, but they may merit further investigation.

Table **22.5**

Standardized Relative Risks (SRR) and Their 95% Confidence Intervals (Cl$_{95}$) for Classes of Malformations Showing Uniform Rates by Hospital in Relation to **Polio Virus Vaccine (Live Oral)** Used in Lunar Months 1–4 by 1,628 Pregnant Women (Based on Multiple Logistic Risk Function Analysis)

Malformation Classes	No. of Malformed Children		SRR	Cl$_{95}$ of SRR
	Observed	Expected		
Any malformation	77	73.8	1.04	0.84–1.29
Major malformations	40	43.6	0.92	0.67–1.26
Minor malformations	39	31.3	1.24	0.94–1.64
Central nervous	4	8.4	0.48	0.13–1.22
Cardiovascular	12	13.1	0.92	0.47–1.60
Musculoskeletal (other than polydactyly in Blacks)	12	11.9	1.01	0.52–1.76
Polydactyly in Blacks[1]	19	13.6	1.39	0.84–2.17
Respiratory	4	6.8	0.59	0.16–1.51
Gastrointestinal	15	9.0	1.67	0.94–2.75
Genitourinary (other than hypospadias)	6	5.8	1.04	0.38–2.26
Hypospadias[2]	7	6.2	1.12	0.45–2.30
Eye and ear	1	4.0	0.25	0.01–1.40
Syndromes (other than Down syndrome)	3	4.1	0.73	0.15–2.13
Down syndrome	3	1.9	1.60	0.33–4.66
Tumors	7	5.3	1.31	0.53–2.70

[1]Drugs used by 981 Blacks
[2]Drugs used by 785 mothers of male offspring

Table **22.6**

Standardized Relative Risks (SRR) and Their 95% Confidence Intervals (Cl$_{95}$) for Classes of Malformations Showing Uniform Rates by Hospital in Relation to **Influenza Virus Vaccine** Used in Lunar Months 1–4 by 650 Pregnant Women (Based on Multiple Logistic Risk Function Analysis)

Malformation Classes	No. of Malformed Children		SRR	Cl$_{95}$ of SRR
	Observed	Expected		
Any malformation	27	30.2	0.89	0.61–1.32
Major malformations	21	20.7	1.01	0.67–1.53
Minor malformations	11	9.9	1.11	0.56–1.98
Central nervous	4	4.1	0.99	0.27–2.51
Cardiovascular	8	5.3	1.52	0.66–2.98
Musculoskeletal (other than polydactyly in Blacks)	7	6.8	1.03	0.41–2.10
Polydactyly in Blacks[1]	2	1.9	1.08	0.13–3.82
Respiratory	5	3.0	1.65	0.54–3.83
Gastrointestinal	6	4.7	1.29	0.47–2.79
Genitourinary (other than hypospadias)	2	3.1	0.65	0.08–2.34
Hypospadias[2]	1	2.5	0.41	0.01–2.26
Eye and ear	1	1.6	0.61	0.02–3.41
Syndromes (other than Down syndrome)	2	2.0	1.01	0.12–3.62
Down syndrome	1	0.9	1.10	0.03–6.08
Tumors	1	2.6	0.38	0.01–2.12

[1]Drugs used by 143 Blacks
[2]Drugs used by 355 mothers of male offspring

Table **22.7**

Standardized Relative Risks (SRR) and Their 95% Confidence Intervals (CI$_{95}$) for Classes of Malformations Showing Uniform Rates by Hospital in Relation to **Tetanus Toxoid** Used in Lunar Months 1–4 by 337 Pregnant Women (Based on Multiple Logistic Risk Function Analysis)

| Malformation Classes | No. of Malformed Children | | SRR | CI$_{95}$ of SRR |
	Observed	Expected		
Any malformation	17	14.3	1.19	0.70– 1.87
Major malformations	12	8.8	1.36	0.71– 2.35
Minor malformations	9	5.6	1.60	0.74– 2.99
Central nervous	3	1.8	1.67	0.35– 4.84
Cardiovascular	3	2.6	1.16	0.24– 3.35
Musculoskeletal (other than polydactyly in Blacks)	5	2.6	1.90	0.62– 4.40
Polydactyly in Blacks[1]	5	2.2	2.32	0.76– 5.28
Respiratory	2	1.5	1.33	0.16– 4.78
Gastrointestinal	4	1.9	2.10	0.57– 5.32
Genitourinary (other than hypospadias)	0	1.2	—	0.00– 3.01
Hypospadias[2]	1	1.1	0.95	0.02– 5.20
Eye and ear	2	0.8	2.58	0.31– 9.23
Syndromes (other than Down syndrome)	0	0.8	—	0.00– 4.90
Down syndrome	1	0.4	2.58	0.07–14.29
Tumors	0	1.1	—	0.00– 3.23

[1]Drugs used by 145 Blacks
[2]Drugs used by 151 mothers of male offspring

Table **22.8**

Standardized Relative Risks (SRR) and Their 95% Confidence Intervals (CI$_{95}$) for Inguinal Hernia, Clubfoot, and Pectus Excavatum in Relation to **Immunizing Agents** Used in Lunar Months 1–4 (Based on Multiple Logistic Risk Function Analysis)

	No. of Users	No. of Malformed Children		SRR	CI$_{95}$ of SRR
		Observed	Expected		
Inguinal hernia					
Immunizing agents	9,222	124	123.3	1.01	0.86–1.18
Poliomyelitis vaccine, parenteral	6,774	86	88.6	0.97	0.79–1.19
Polio virus vaccine, live oral	1,628	27	23.9	1.13	0.80–1.60
Influenza virus vaccine	650	9	8.8	1.02	0.47–1.93
Clubfoot					
Immunizing agents	9,222	37	37.8	0.98	0.73–1.32
Poliomyelitis vaccine, parenteral	6,774	27	28.8	0.94	0.65–1.36
Polio virus vaccine, live oral	1,628	7	5.7	1.24	0.50–2.55
Pectus excavatum					
Immunizing agents	9,222	31	29.4	1.05	0.77–1.44
Poliomyelitis vaccine, parenteral	6,774	25	24.9	1.00	0.69–1.45
Polio virus vaccine, live oral	1,628	4	2.1	1.88	0.51–4.81

Antinauseants, Antihistamines, and Phenothiazines

General Evaluation

In Table 23.1, all 3,248 malformed children are considered in relation to exposure to the entire group of antinauseants, antihistamines, and phenothiazines during the first four lunar months of pregnancy. In Table 23.2, the data are confined to the 2,277 children who had malformations which were uniformly distributed across the hospitals. Three relative risks are given in each table: crude, standardized for hospital variability, and standardized for the mother's ethnic group and survival of the child.

All Malformations in Relation to Antinauseants, Antihistamines, and Phenothiazines (Table 23.1)

The hospital-standardized relative risk for any malformation associated with this group of drugs was 1.11. The relative risk for all malformations was similar for exposure to antihistamines and antinauseants (1.10). Only the association with brompheniramine (2.34) is statistically significant, at the 0.05 level. This is also the only drug for which the relative risk was greater than 1.5. There was no association with meclizine (relative risk, 1.04), a drug which has been suspected of causing malformations. There was no association between the phenothiazine group and all malformations (relative risk, 1.04),

*Table **23.1***

Children (3,248) With Any Malformation in Relation to Exposure to **Antinauseants, Antihistamines, and Phenothiazines** During Lunar Months 1–4 Among 50,282 Mother-Child Pairs

	No. of Mother-Child Pairs Exposed	No. of Malformed Children	Crude Relative Risk	Hospital Standardized Relative Risk[1]	Survival and Race Standardized Relative Risk[1]
Antinauseants, antihistamines, and phenothiazines	6,194	461	1.18[2]	1.11	1.21[2]
Antihistamines and antinauseants	5,401	404	1.18[2]	1.10	1.21[2]
Doxylamine succinate	1,169	79	1.05	0.96	1.06
Chlorpheniramine	1,070	90	1.31[3]	1.20	1.37[2]
Meclizine	1,014	78	1.20	1.04	1.21
Pheniramine	831	68	1.27[3]	1.24	1.27
Antinauseant, n.o.s.	596	41	1.07	1.07	1.06
Diphenhydramine	595	49	1.28	1.25	1.33
Trimethobenzamide	340	19	0.86	0.79	0.84
Methapyrilene	263	21	1.24	1.20	1.28
Thonzylamine	148	10	1.05	1.02	1.07
Antihistamine, n.o.s.	131	11	1.30	1.27	1.40
Pyrilamine	121	11	1.41	1.22	1.34
Tripelennamine	100	6	0.93	0.81	0.93
Brompheniramine	65	10	2.39[2]	2.34[3]	2.94[2]
Phenyltoloxamine	45	4	1.38	1.13	1.42
Buclizine	44	3	1.06	0.94	1.13
Chlorothen	36	2	0.86	0.77	0.88
Invert sugar	18	0	—	—	—
Other antihistamines[4]	113	5	0.68	0.59	0.74
Phenothiazines	1,309	93	1.10	1.04	1.10
Prochlorperazine	877	66	1.17	1.08	1.18
Chlorpromazine	142	8	0.87	0.82	0.82
Promethazine	114	9	1.22	1.17	1.11
Perphenazine	63	3	0.74	0.73	0.66
Promazine	50	4	1.24	1.25	1.34
Trifluoperazine	42	3	1.11	1.10	1.19
Pipamazine	40	2	0.77	0.77	0.82
Triflupromazine	36	1	0.43	0.44	0.37
Other phenothiazines[5]	71	5	1.09	1.06	1.16

[1]Estimated by the Mantel-Haenszel procedure
[2]$X_1^2 = 7.16 - 11.61$, $p < 0.01$
[3]$X_1^2 = 3.87 - 6.57$, $p < 0.05$
[4]Triprolidine (16); pyrrobutamine (15); cyclizine (15); dexbrompheniramine (14); chlorcyclizine (13); phenindamine (12); thenyldiamine (12); bromodiphenhydramine (10); cyproheptadine (3); carbinoxamine (2); dimethindene (2); diphenylpyraline (1)
[5]Thiethylperazine (19); trimeprazine (14); thioridazine (13); fluphenazine (9); methoxypromazine (5); methdilazine (4); chlorprothixene (3); isothipendyl (2); carphenazine (2); prothipendyl (1)

Table **23.2**

Children (2,277) With Malformations Showing Uniform Rates by Hospital in Relation to Exposure to **Antinauseants, Antihistamines, and Phenothiazines** During Lunar Months 1–4 Among 50,282 Mother-Child Pairs

	No. of Mother-Child Pairs Exposed	No. of Malformed Children	Crude Relative Risk	Hospital Standardized Relative Risk	Survival and Race Standardized Relative Risk
Antinauseants, antihistamines, and phenothiazines	6,194	305	1.10	1.05	1.12
Antihistamines and antinauseants	5,401	261	1.08	1.02	1.10
Doxylamine succinate	1,169	55	1.04	0.97	1.05
Chlorpheniramine	1,070	58	1.20	1.12	1.23
Meclizine	1,014	50	1.09	0.98	1.06
Pheniramine	831	43	1.15	1.10	1.13
Antinauseant, n.o.s.	596	31	1.15	1.15	1.14
Diphenhydramine	595	32	1.19	1.17	1.25
Trimethobenzamide	340	15	0.97	0.93	0.95
Methapyrilene	263	13	1.09	1.06	1.12
Thonzylamine	148	6	0.89	0.86	0.93
Antihistamine, n.o.s.	131	4	0.67	0.63	0.66
Pyrilamine	121	8	1.46	1.33	1.29
Tripelennamine	100	2	0.44	0.40	0.39
Brompheniramine	65	6	2.04	1.98	2.44
Phenyltoloxamine	45	4	1.96	1.80	2.04
Buclizine	44	3	1.51	1.41	1.75
Chlorothen	36	1	0.61	0.57	0.60
Invert sugar	18	0	—	—	—
Other antihistamines, and antinauseants	113	4	0.78	0.71	0.88
Phenothiazines	1,309	66	1.12	1.07	1.09
Prochlorperazine	877	47	1.19	1.13	1.17
Chlorpromazine	142	6	0.93	0.90	0.88
Promethazine	114	7	1.36	1.35	1.20
Perphenazine	63	2	0.70	0.68	0.60
Promazine	50	2	0.88	0.85	0.93
Trifluoperazine	42	3	1.58	1.62	1.85
Pipamazine	40	2	1.10	1.11	1.20
Triflupromazine	36	0	—	—	—
Other phenothiazines	71	5	1.56	1.56	1.73

and only a slight association with certain individual phenothiazines.

Malformations with Uniform
Rates by Hospital in
Relation to Antinauseants,
Antihistamines, and Phenothiazines
(Table 23.2)

There was essentially no association between uniform malformations and the large categories of the drug group. Among individual drugs, hospital-standardized relative risks greater than 1.5 were observed for brompheniramine (1.98), phenyltoloxamine (1.80), trifluoperazine (1.62), and other phenothiazines (1.56).

Detailed Evaluation of Uniform Malformations

In this section, groups of drugs, followed by individual drugs, are evaluated in relation to various classes or groups of uniform malformations, as well as individual malformations, for which multiple logistic risk function models were developed. In the tables, the observed and expected numbers of malformed children are given for each drug exposure in turn. The measure of association presented is a standardized relative risk (SRR) with its 95% confidence limits. The SRR is the ratio of the observed number to the expected number of malformed children. Since the SRR takes into account potential confounding variables, it represents the best estimate of the relationship between a drug and a malformation. As numbers of exposed mother-child pairs become so small as to be uninformative, data will be omitted.

All Antinauseants, Antihistamines,
and Phenothiazines — 6,194
Exposures (Table 23.3)

There was no evidence of association of the drug group as a whole with broad

Table **23.3**

Standardized Relative Risks (SRR) and Their 95% Confidence Intervals (CI_{95}) for Classes of Malformations Showing Uniform Rates by Hospital in Relation to **Antinauseants, Antihistamines, and Phenothiazines** Used in Lunar Months 1–4 by 6,194 Pregnant Women (Based on Multiple Logistic Risk Function Analysis)

Malformation Classes	No. of Malformed Children		SRR	CI_{95} of SRR
	Observed	Expected		
Any malformation	305	281.9	1.08	0.98–1.20
Major malformations	201	182.6	1.10	0.97–1.24
Minor malformations	114	99.4	1.15	0.98–1.36
Central nervous	35	32.0	1.09	0.81–1.48
Cardiovascular	53	48.4	1.10	0.86–1.40
Musculoskeletal (other than polydactyly in Blacks)	61	60.1	1.02	0.81–1.30
Polydactyly in Blacks[1]	37	29.0	1.28	0.97–1.68
Respiratory	30	28.0	1.07	0.77–1.48
Gastrointestinal	51	42.8	1.19	0.93–1.51
Genitourinary (other than hypospadias)	24	26.4	0.91	0.61–1.35
Hypospadias[2]	21	20.3	1.03	0.69–1.56
Eye and ear	19	15.7	1.21	0.72–1.90
Syndromes (other than Down syndrome)	15	15.5	0.97	0.55–1.59
Down syndrome	7	8.0	0.87	0.34–1.82
Tumors	19	24.5	0.78	0.46–1.22

[1]Drugs used by 2,115 Blacks
[2]Drugs used by 3,124 mothers of male offspring

classes of malformations. The highest SRR was for minor malformations (1.15). The highest SRR in the table was 1.28 for polydactyly in Blacks.

Antihistamines and Antinauseants — 5,401 Exposures (Table 23.4)

Since over 80% of the total group of drugs in this chapter is made up of antihistamines and antinauseants, the data in this table are similar to the data in Table 23.3. The only difference to be noted is a somewhat elevated SRR for eye and ear malformations (1.41).

Doxylamine Succinate — 1,169 Exposures (Table 23.5) The SRR for minor malformations was 1.37. There was no association of this drug with major malformations or with the overall group of malformations. The only SRR greater than 1.5 was seen for polydactyly in Blacks (1.68).

Chlorpheniramine — 1,070 Exposures (Table 23.6) The highest SRR among the broad classes of malformations was 1.39 for minor malformations. SRRs greater than 1.5 were found for Black polydactyly (2.05), gastrointestinal malformations (1.67), and eye and ear defects (2.89).

Meclizine — 1,014 Exposures (Table 23.7) None of the SRRs for broad classes of malformations exceeded 1.25. SRRs greater than 1.5 were seen for respiratory malformations (1.64), eye and ear defects (2.79), and Down syndrome (1.56, based on 2 malformed children). The finding for eye and ear malformations is statistically significant, with a lower confidence limit greater than unity.

Pheniramine — 831 Exposures (Table 23.8) None of the SRRs for broad classes of malformations was substantially elevated. SRRs greater than 1.5 were found for respiratory malformations (1.64), malformations of the eye and ear (2.06), and

Table **23.4**

Standardized Relative Risks (SRR) and Their 95% Confidence Intervals (CI$_{95}$) for Classes of Malformations Showing Uniform Rates by Hospital in Relation to **Antihistamines and Antinauseants** Used in Lunar Months 1–4 by 5,401 Pregnant Women (Based on Multiple Logistic Risk Function Analysis)

| Malformation Classes | No. of Malformed Children | | SRR | CI$_{95}$ of SRR |
	Observed	Expected		
Any malformation	261	235.9	1.07	0.96–1.20
Major malformations	172	158.4	1.09	0.95–1.25
Minor malformations	100	86.2	1.16	0.97–1.38
Central nervous	31	27.6	1.12	0.81–1.55
Cardiovascular	40	41.7	0.96	0.71–1.31
Musculoskeletal (other than polydactyly in Blacks)	54	51.9	1.04	0.81–1.34
Polydactyly in Blacks[1]	31	25.1	1.23	0.90–1.68
Respiratory	25	24.0	1.04	0.72–1.51
Gastrointestinal	46	37.3	1.23	0.95–1.59
Genitourinary (other than hypospadias)	19	23.1	0.82	0.49–1.29
Hypospadias[2]	19	17.8	1.07	0.64–1.69
Eye and ear	19	13.4	1.41	0.83–2.23
Syndromes (other than Down syndrome)	13	13.3	0.98	0.53–1.67
Down syndrome	4	6.6	0.60	0.15–1.58
Tumors	13	21.2	0.61	0.31–1.06

[1]Drugs used by 1,840 Blacks
[2]Drugs used by 2,739 mothers of male offspring

Table **23.5**

Standardized Relative Risks (SRR) and Their 95% Confidence Intervals (CI$_{95}$) for Classes of Malformations Showing Uniform Rates by Hospital in Relation to **Doxylamine Succinate** Used in Lunar Months 1–4 by 1,169 Pregnant Women (Based on Multiple Logistic Risk Function Analysis)

Malformation Classes	No. of Malformed Children		SRR	CI$_{95}$ of SRR
	Observed	Expected		
Any malformation	55	51.6	1.07	0.83–1.37
Major malformations	36	33.8	1.06	0.78–1.45
Minor malformations	24	17.5	1.37	0.98–1.93
Central nervous	7	5.7	1.23	0.49–2.52
Cardiovascular	5	8.2	0.61	0.20–1.42
Musculoskeletal (other than polydactyly in Blacks)	13	11.3	1.15	0.61–1.96
Polydactyly in Blacks[1]	8	4.8	1.68	0.73–3.28
Respiratory	7	5.4	1.30	0.52–2.68
Gastrointestinal	12	8.2	1.46	0.76–2.55
Genitourinary (other than hypospadias)	2	5.1	0.39	0.05–1.40
Hypospadias[2]	5	3.5	1.43	0.46–3.31
Eye and ear	2	3.1	0.64	0.08–2.32
Syndromes (other than Down syndrome)	3	2.7	1.10	0.23–3.20
Down syndrome	1	1.3	0.74	0.02–4.14
Tumors	1	4.8	0.21	0.01–1.17

[1]Drugs used by 386 Blacks
[2]Drugs used by 556 mothers of male offspring

syndromes excluding Down syndrome (1.51).

Antinauseants, n.o.s. — 596 Exposures (Table 23.9) The highest SRR among the broad classes of malformations was 1.31 for major malformations. SRRs greater than 1.5 were observed for malformations of the central nervous system (1.82), eye and ear malformations (2.64), and syndromes other than Down syndrome (1.80).

Diphenhydramine — 595 Exposures (Table 23.10) The SRR for major malformations was 1.33. SRRs greater than 1.5 were observed for genitourinary malformations (1.68), hypospadias (1.68), eye and ear defects (1.72), and syndromes excluding Down syndrome (1.67).

Trimethobenzamide — 340 Exposures (Table 23.11) There was no evidence of association between this drug and malformations.

Methapyrilene — 263 Exposures (Table 23.12) There was little evidence of association of methapyrilene with malformations. The highest SRR was for major malformations (1.21).

Phenothiazines — 1,309 Exposures (Table 23.13)

There was little evidence of association between the phenothiazines as a whole and broad classes of malformations. As seen in Table 23.13 only cardiovascular malformations (1.68) and Down syndrome (2.18) had SRRs greater than 1.5.

Prochlorperazine — 877 Exposures (Table 23.14) None of the SRRs for broad classes of malformations exceeded 1.25. SRRs greater than 1.5 were found for cardiovascular (1.85) and genitourinary malformations (1.59) and for Down syndrome (2.38).

Table **23.6**

Standardized Relative Risks (SRR) and Their 95% Confidence Intervals (CI₉₅) for Classes of Malformations Showing Uniform Rates by Hospital in Relation to **Chlorpheniramine** Used in Lunar Months 1–4 by 1,070 Pregnant Women (Based on Multiple Logistic Risk Function Analysis)

| Malformation Classes | No. of Malformed Children | | SRR | CI₉₅ of SRR |
	Observed	Expected		
Any malformation	58	48.3	1.20	0.95–1.51
Major malformations	37	32.1	1.15	0.86–1.55
Minor malformations	22	15.9	1.39	0.97–1.97
Central nervous	8	5.8	1.39	0.60–2.73
Cardiovascular	7	8.1	0.86	0.35–1.76
Musculoskeletal (other than polydactyly in Blacks)	6	10.9	0.55	0.20–1.20
Polydactyly in Blacks[1]	7	3.4	2.05	0.83–4.16
Respiratory	4	4.7	0.84	0.23–2.15
Gastrointestinal	13	7.8	1.67	0.89–2.85
Genitourinary (other than hypospadias)	5	4.7	1.06	0.34–2.47
Hypospadias[2]	4	3.6	1.11	0.30–2.84
Eye and ear	7	2.4	2.89	1.16–5.92
Syndromes (other than Down syndrome)	1	2.8	0.36	0.01–1.98
Down syndrome	0	1.2	—	0.00–2.94
Tumors	3	4.3	0.69	0.14–2.02

[1] Drugs used by 272 Blacks
[2] Drugs used by 549 mothers of male offspring

Table **23.7**

Standardized Relative Risks (SRR) and Their 95% Confidence Intervals (CI₉₅) for Classes of Malformations Showing Uniform Rates by Hospital in Relation to **Meclizine** Used in Lunar Months 1–4 by 1,014 Pregnant Women (Based on Multiple Logistic Risk Function Analysis)

| Malformation Classes | No. of Malformed Children | | SRR | CI₉₅ of SRR |
	Observed	Expected		
Any malformation	50	44.2	1.13	0.88–1.46
Major malformations	36	30.0	1.20	0.90–1.61
Minor malformations	17	13.7	1.24	0.73–1.98
Central nervous	6	4.6	1.30	0.48–2.82
Cardiovascular	8	7.2	1.11	0.48–2.19
Musculoskeletal (other than polydactyly in Blacks)	9	11.1	0.81	0.37–1.54
Polydactyly in Blacks[1]	2	2.4	0.84	0.10–2.98
Respiratory	7	4.3	1.64	0.66–3.37
Gastrointestinal	9	7.2	1.25	0.57–2.36
Genitourinary (other than hypospadias)	4	4.3	0.92	0.25–2.35
Hypospadias[2]	4	2.8	1.42	0.39–3.60
Eye and ear	7	2.5	2.79	1.12–5.73
Syndromes (other than Down syndrome)	3	2.4	1.26	0.26–3.68
Down syndrome	2	1.3	1.56	0.19–5.60
Tumors	2	4.3	0.47	0.06–1.69

[1] Drugs used by 191 Blacks
[2] Drugs used by 479 mothers of male offspring

Table **23.8**

Standardized Relative Risks (SRR) and Their 95% Confidence Intervals (CI$_{95}$) for Classes of Malformations Showing Uniform Rates by Hospital in Relation to **Pheniramine** Used in Lunar Months 1–4 by 831 Pregnant Women (Based on Multiple Logistic Risk Function Analysis)

Malformation Classes	No. of Malformed Children		SRR	CI$_{95}$ of SRR
	Observed	Expected		
Any malformation	43	38.2	1.12	0.85–1.48
Major malformations	28	23.5	1.19	0.85–1.67
Minor malformations	18	14.8	1.22	0.73–1.92
Central nervous	4	4.3	0.94	0.26–2.39
Cardiovascular	7	6.4	1.10	0.44–2.26
Musculoskeletal (other than polydactyly in Blacks)	11	7.5	1.47	0.73–2.61
Polydactyly in Blacks[1]	7	5.4	1.30	0.52–2.65
Respiratory	7	4.3	1.64	0.66–3.37
Gastrointestinal	7	5.5	1.28	0.51–2.62
Genitourinary (other than hypospadias)	2	3.4	0.59	0.07–2.11
Hypospadias[2]	3	2.9	1.05	0.22–3.05
Eye and ear	4	1.9	2.06	0.56–5.26
Syndromes (other than Down syndrome)	3	2.0	1.51	0.31–4.41
Down syndrome	0	0.9	—	0.00–4.29
Tumors	0	3.0	—	0.00–1.22

[1] Drugs used by 361 Blacks
[2] Drugs used by 429 mothers of male offspring

Table **23.9**

Standardized Relative Risks (SRR) and Their 95% Confidence Intervals (CI$_{95}$) for Classes of Malformations Showing Uniform Rates by Hospital in Relation to **Antinauseants, n.o.s.,** Used in Lunar Months 1–4 by 596 Pregnant Women (Based on Multiple Logistic Risk Function Analysis)

Malformation Classes	No. of Malformed Children		SRR	CI$_{95}$ of SRR
	Observed	Expected		
Any malformation	31	27.2	1.14	0.82–1.57
Major malformations	23	17.5	1.31	0.93–1.86
Minor malformations	8	10.8	0.74	0.32–1.45
Central nervous	6	3.3	1.82	0.67–3.94
Cardiovascular	6	4.9	1.22	0.45–2.63
Musculoskeletal (other than polydactyly in Blacks)	3	5.0	0.60	0.12–1.74
Polydactyly in Blacks[1]	2	3.8	0.53	0.06–1.88
Respiratory	3	2.7	1.09	0.23–3.18
Gastrointestinal	6	4.2	1.44	0.53–3.12
Genitourinary (other than hypospadias)	2	2.7	0.73	0.09–2.64
Hypospadias[2]	1	2.3	0.44	0.01–2.46
Eye and ear	4	1.5	2.64	0.72–6.72
Syndromes (other than Down syndrome)	3	1.7	1.80	0.37–5.24
Down syndrome	0	0.8	—	0.00–4.59
Tumors	3	2.1	1.40	0.29–4.07

[1] Drugs used by 278 Blacks
[2] Drugs used by 308 mothers of male offspring

Table **23.10**

Standardized Relative Risks (SRR) and Their 95% Confidence Intervals (CI$_{95}$) for Classes of Malformations Showing Uniform Rates by Hospital in Relation to **Diphenhydramine** Used in Lunar Months 1–4 by 595 Pregnant Women (Based on Multiple Logistic Risk Function Analysis)

| | *No. of Malformed Children* | | | |
Malformation Classes	**Observed**	**Expected**	**SRR**	**CI$_{95}$ of SRR**
Any malformation	32	28.6	1.12	0.77–1.60
Major malformations	25	18.7	1.33	0.88–1.97
Minor malformations	11	9.1	1.21	0.63–2.21
Central nervous	3	3.8	0.80	0.16–2.33
Cardiovascular	8	5.4	1.49	0.64–2.94
Musculoskeletal (other than polydactyly in Blacks)	6	6.0	1.00	0.37–2.18
Polydactyly in Blacks[1]	3	2.8	1.08	0.22–3.15
Respiratory	4	3.3	1.21	0.33–3.09
Gastrointestinal	5	4.6	1.09	0.35–2.54
Genitourinary (other than hypospadias)	5	3.0	1.68	0.54–3.92
Hypospadias[2]	3	1.8	1.68	0.35–4.90
Eye and ear	3	1.7	1.72	0.36–5.04
Syndromes (other than Down syndrome)	3	1.8	1.67	0.34–4.87
Down syndrome	1	0.9	1.15	0.03–6.40
Tumors	0	2.7	—	0.00–1.37

[1] Drugs used by 222 Blacks
[2] Drugs used by 296 mothers of male offspring

Table **23.11**

Standardized Relative Risks (SRR) and Their 95% Confidence Intervals (CI$_{95}$) for Broad Classes of Malformations Showing Uniform Rates by Hospital in Relation to **Trimethobenzamide** Used in Lunar Months 1–4 by 340 Pregnant Women (Based on Multiple Logistic Risk Function Analysis)

| | *No. of Malformed Children* | | | |
	Observed	**Expected**	**SRR**	**CI$_{95}$ of SRR**
Any malformation	15	15.4	0.98	0.55–1.59
Major malformations	9	9.7	0.93	0.43–1.74
Minor malformations	6	5.6	1.07	0.39–2.30

Table **23.12**

Standardized Relative Risks (SRR) and Their 95% Confidence Intervals (CI₉₅) for Broad Classes of Malformations Showing Uniform Rates by Hospital in Relation to **Methapyrilene** Used in Lunar Months 1–4 by 263 Pregnant Women (Based on Multiple Logistic Risk Function Analysis)

| | *No. of Malformed Children* | | | |
	Observed	Expected	SRR	CI₉₅ of SRR
Any malformation	13	12.2	1.07	0.57–1.80
Major malformations	9	7.5	1.21	0.56–2.25
Minor malformations	4	4.6	0.87	0.24–2.21

Table **23.13**

Standardized Relative Risks (SRR) and Their 95% Confidence Intervals (CI₉₅) for Classes of Malformations Showing Uniform Rates by Hospital in Relation to **Phenothiazines** Used in Lunar Months 1–4 by 1,309 Pregnant Women (Based on Multiple Logistic Risk Function Analysis)

| | *No. of Malformed Children* | | | |
Malformation Classes	Observed	Expected	SRR	CI₉₅ of SRR
Any malformation	66	61.4	1.07	0.86–1.35
Major malformations	47	40.6	1.16	0.89–1.50
Minor malformations	23	21.4	1.07	0.73–1.58
Central nervous	7	7.4	0.95	0.38–1.94
Cardiovascular	18	10.7	1.68	1.00–2.65
Musculoskeletal (other than polydactyly in Blacks)	10	13.6	0.74	0.35–1.35
Polydactyly in Blacks[1]	8	5.9	1.33	0.58–2.61
Respiratory	10	6.7	1.50	0.72–2.75
Gastrointestinal	11	9.7	1.14	0.57–2.03
Genitourinary (other than hypospadias)	9	6.1	1.47	0.67–2.78
Hypospadias[2]	3	3.9	0.77	0.16–2.25
Eye and ear	1	4.1	0.25	0.01–1.37
Syndromes (other than Down syndrome)	4	3.6	1.12	0.30–2.85
Down syndrome	5	2.3	2.18	0.71–5.07
Tumors	6	5.6	1.07	0.39–2.32

[1]Drugs used by 435 Blacks
[2]Drugs used by 620 mothers of male offspring

Table **23.14**

Standardized Relative Risks (SRR) and Their 95% Confidence Intervals (CI$_{95}$) for Classes of Malformations Showing Uniform Rates by Hospital in Relation to **Prochlorperazine** Used in Lunar Months 1–4 by 877 Pregnant Women (Based on Multiple Logistic Risk Function Analysis)

Malformation Classes	No. of Malformed Children		SRR	CI$_{95}$ of SRR
	Observed	Expected		
Any malformation	47	41.2	1.14	0.88–1.48
Major malformations	34	27.4	1.24	0.92–1.67
Minor malformations	16	13.5	1.18	0.68–1.91
Central nervous	7	4.9	1.43	0.58–2.94
Cardiovascular	13	7.0	1.85	0.99–3.15
Musculoskeletal (other than polydactyly in Blacks)	6	9.5	0.63	0.23–1.37
Polydactyly in Blacks[1]	4	3.4	1.18	0.32–2.98
Respiratory	7	4.7	1.48	0.60–3.04
Gastrointestinal	7	6.4	1.09	0.44–2.23
Genitourinary (other than hypospadias)	7	4.4	1.59	0.64–3.26
Hypospadias[2]	3	2.4	1.23	0.25–3.57
Eye and ear	1	2.7	0.37	0.01–2.04
Syndromes (other than Down syndrome)	3	2.4	1.24	0.26–3.62
Down syndrome	4	1.7	2.38	0.65–6.07
Tumors	5	3.9	1.28	0.41–2.97

[1]Drugs used by 267 Blacks
[2]Drugs used by 407 mothers of male offspring

Detailed Evaluation of Non-Uniform Malformations: Inguinal Hernia, Clubfoot, Pectus Excavatum

In this section, the three outcomes are evaluated as in the preceding section dealing with uniform malformations. Instances in which there were fewer than three malformed children exposed to any drug are omitted because they are not informative.

As seen in Table 23.15, three drugs had SRRs greater than 1.5 for inguinal hernia: chlorpheniramine (1.53), meclizine (1.59), and diphenhydramine (1.61). The finding for chlorpheniramine is statistically significant, with a lower confidence limit of 1.09. For clubfoot, the following three drugs had SRRs greater than 1.5: doxylamine succinate (1.63), pheniramine (2.86), and diphenhydramine (1.71). The finding for pheniramine is statistically significant

(lower confidence limit, 1.38). For pectus excavatum, only pheniramine (1.65) had an SRR greater than 1.5.

Comments

On the basis of substantial numbers, there was no evidence to suggest that exposure to antihistamines, antinauseants, or to phenothiazines was related to malformations overall, or to large categories of major or minor malformations. In the subgroup of antihistamines and antinauseants (1,169 exposures), there were some suggestions of association (for example, between respiratory malformations and pheniramine; between genitourinary malformations and diphenhydramine; or between inguinal hernia and both meclizine and diphenhydramine). However, there was little in the way of consistently discernible patterns.

Table **23.15**

Standardized Relative Risks (SRR) and Their 95% Confidence Intervals (CI$_{95}$) for Inguinal Hernia, Clubfoot, and Pectus Excavatum in Relation to **Antinauseants, Antihistamines, and Phenothiazines** Used in Lunar Months 1–4 (Based on Multiple Logistic Risk Function Analysis)

	No. of Users	No. of Malformed Children		SRR	CI$_{95}$ of SRR
		Observed	Expected		
Inguinal hernia					
Antinauseants, antihistamines, and phenothiazines	6194	101	82.8	1.22	1.00–1.44
Antihistamines and antinauseants	5401	90	72.0	1.25	1.04–1.49
Doxylamine succinate	1169	12	15.3	0.78	0.41–1.36
Chlorpheniramine	1070	22	14.4	1.53	1.09–2.14
Meclizine	1014	18	11.3	1.59	0.95–2.50
Pheniramine	831	15	11.9	1.26	0.71–2.07
Antinauseants, n.o.s.	596	9	8.5	1.06	0.48–1.99
Diphenhydramine	595	13	8.1	1.61	0.86–2.75
Phenothiazines	1309	23	17.0	1.35	0.96–1.92
Prochlorperazine	877	16	11.0	1.45	0.83–2.34
Clubfoot					
Antinauseants, antihistamines, and phenothiazines	6194	35	28.1	1.25	0.94–1.66
Antihistamines and antinauseants	5401	33	24.4	1.35	0.97–1.79
Doxylamine succinate	1169	9	5.5	1.63	0.75–3.09
Meclizine	1014	5	5.1	0.97	0.32–2.27
Pheniramine	831	10	3.5	2.86	1.38–5.24
Diphenhydramine	595	5	2.9	1.71	0.56–3.98
Phenothiazines	1309	5	6.2	0.80	0.26–1.87
Prochlorperazine	877	3	4.5	0.67	0.14–1.96
Pectus excavatum					
Antinauseants, antihistamines, and phenothiazines	6194	25	23.7	1.05	0.73–1.51
Antihistamines and antinauseants	5401	22	21.4	1.03	0.70–1.54
Doxylamine succinate	1169	4	5.5	0.73	0.20–1.87
Chlorpheniramine	1070	5	5.2	0.97	0.31–2.25
Meclizine	1014	6	6.9	0.86	0.32–1.87
Pheniramine	831	4	2.4	1.65	0.45–4.21
Diphenhydramine	595	3	2.0	1.47	0.30–4.30
Phenothiazines	1309	5	4.9	1.01	0.33–2.35
Prochlorperazine	877	3	3.8	0.78	0.16–2.27

Experimental data favor the hypothesis that cyclizine and meclizine may produce a variety of defects, particularly cleft anomalies.[1] However, contradictory findings have been reported in humans.[2,3] Most recently, McBride[4] was unable to identify an increase in clefts in exposed children when nausea and vomiting were controlled. The data in this study gave no evidence of association with cleft anomalies.

Exposure to phenothiazines as a group, and to prochlorperazine (877 exposures), which was the most commonly used phenothiazine, was associated with cardiovascular deformities, and Appendix 4 shows that the latter drug was associated, in particular, with ventricular septal defects. In one study, no evidence of association was found;[5] and, as in this study, other antinauseants gave no evidence of being teratogenic.

CHAPTER 24

Sedatives, Tranquilizers and Anti-depressant Drugs

General Evaluation

In this first section, data are presented for two classes of malformations — all 3,248 malformed children and the 2,277 children with uniform malformation rates by hospital. The relative risks for these malformations are presented for the total group of drugs, for three subgroups (barbiturates, tranquilizers and non-barbiturate sedatives, and antidepressants), and for individual drugs comprising each of these subgroups. Crude relative risks are presented as well as two Mantel-Haenszel-standardized summary relative risks; the first standardization is with respect to hospital; the second, with respect to the survival of the child and the ethnic group of the mother.

All Malformations in Relation to Sedatives, Tranquilizers, and Antidepressant Drugs (Table 24.1)

The hospital-standardized relative risk for any malformation associated with this group of drugs was 1.17. This result is statistically significant at the 0.05 level. Hospital-standardized relative risks greater than 1.5 were found for the following specific drugs or groups of drugs: butabarbital (1.80), chloral hydrate (1.68), glutethimide (1.63), hydroxyzine (1.57), and monoamine oxidase inhibitors (2.26). The last finding is based on only three malformed children.

335

Table **24.1**

Children (3,248) With Any Malformation in Relation to Exposure to **Sedatives, Tranquilizers, and Antidepressants** During Lunar Months 1–4 Among 50,282 Mother-Child Pairs

	No. of Mother-Child Pairs Exposed	No. of Malformed Children	Crude Relative Risk	Hospital Standardized Relative Risk[1]	Survival and Race Standardized Relative Risk[1]
Sedatives, tranquilizers, and antidepressants	3,122	244	1.23[2]	1.17[3]	1.22[2]
Barbiturates	2,413	177	1.14	1.08	1.12
Phenobarbital	1,415	99	1.09	1.06	1.03
Secobarbital	378	30	1.23	1.20	1.16
Amobarbital	298	24	1.25	0.99	1.30
Pentobarbital	250	15	0.93	0.88	0.90
Thiopental	152	9	0.92	0.89	0.94
Butalbital	112	8	1.11	0.99	1.07
Butabarbital	109	14	1.99[3]	1.80	2.25[2]
Methohexital	41	2	0.76	0.70	0.71
Thiamylal	21	1	0.74	0.71	0.69
Other barbiturates[4]	16	0	—	—	—
Tranquilizers and non-barbiturate sedatives	946	80	1.32[3]	1.24	1.36[3]
Meprobamate	356	27	1.18	1.09	1.22
Chlordiazepoxide	257	20	1.21	1.11	1.24
Sedative/tranquilizer, n.o.s.	165	12	1.13	1.14	1.15
Chloral hydrate	71	8	1.75	1.68	1.86
Glutethimide	67	8	1.85	1.63	2.29[3]
Hydroxyzine	50	5	1.55	1.57	1.44
Other tranquilizers/non-barbiturate sedatives[5]	68	6	1.37	1.25	1.33
Antidepressants	59	5	1.31	1.24	1.29
Amitriptyline	21	0	—	—	—
Monoamine oxidase inhibitors[6]	21	3	2.21	2.26	2.62
Other tricyclic antidepressants[7]	20	2	1.55	1.50	1.43

[1]Estimated by the Mantel-Haenszel procedure
[2]$X^2_1 = 7.12 - 9.89$, $p < 0.01$
[3]$X^2_1 = 3.99 - 6.36$, $p < 0.05$
[4]Mephobarbital (8); barbital (5); barbiturate, n.o.s. (2); vinbarbital (1)
[5]Benactyzine (15); ethchlorvynol (12); diazepam (10); methyprylon (8); phenaglycodol (5); chlormezanone (5); carbromal (4); ethinamate (3); chloral betaine (1); mephenoxalone (1); hydroxyphenamate (1); emylcamate (1); paraldehyde (1); oxazepam (1); tybamate (1); ectylurea (1); thalidomide (1);
[6]Tranylcypromine (13); phenelzine (3); etryptamine (2); isocarboxazid (1); nialamide (1); cyprolidol (1);
[7]Imipramine (19); nortriptylene (1)

Malformations with Uniform Rates by Hospital in Relation to Sedatives, Tranquilizers, and Antidepressant Drugs (Table 24.2)

A somewhat similar pattern emerges for the 2,277 children with uniform mal-formations. The hospital-standardized relative risk for the whole group of seda-tives, tranquilizers, and antidepressants was 1.15. Hospital-standardized relative risks greater than 1.5 were seen for chloral hydrate (2.19), other tranquilizers and non-barbiturate sedatives (1.55), and

336

Table **24.2**

Children (2,277) With Malformations Showing Uniform Rates by Hospital in Relation to Exposure to **Sedatives, Tranquilizers, and Antidepressants** During Lunar Months 1–4 Among 50,282 Mother-Child Pairs

	No. of Mother-Child Pairs Exposed	No. of Malformed Children	Crude Relative Risk	Hospital Standardized Relative Risk	Survival and Race Standardized Relative Risk
Sedatives, tranquilizers, and antidepressants	3,122	167	1.20[1]	1.15	1.16
Barbiturates	2,413	122	1.12	1.08	1.08
Phenobarbital	1,415	74	1.16	1.14	1.08
Secobarbital	378	23	1.35	1.32	1.22
Amobarbital	298	16	1.19	1.02	1.20
Pentobarbital	250	6	0.53	0.50	0.50
Thiopental	152	9	1.31	1.30	1.38
Butalbital	112	4	0.79	0.72	0.74
Butabarbital	109	7	1.42	1.29	1.55
Methohexital	41	2	1.08	1.04	1.05
Thiamylal	21	0	—	—	—
Other barbiturates	16	0	—	—	—
Tranquilizers and nonbarbiturate sedatives	946	53	1.24	1.19	1.26
Meprobamate	356	20	1.24	1.18	1.29
Chlordiazepoxide	257	11	0.94	0.88	0.94
Sedative/tranquilizer, n.o.s.	165	11	1.47	1.48	1.54
Chloral hydrate	71	7	2.18	2.19	2.27
Glutethimide	67	2	0.66	0.57	0.79
Hydroxyzine	50	1	0.44	0.43	0.38
Other tranquilizers/non-barbiturate sedatives	68	5	1.63	1.55	1.55
Antidepressants	59	4	1.50	1.47	1.43
Amitriptyline	21	0	—	—	—
Monoamine oxidase inhibitors	21	3	3.16	3.41	4.00
Other tricyclic antidepressants	20	1	1.10	1.06	0.88

[1]$X_1^2 = 4.99$, $p < 0.05$

monoamine oxidase inhibitors (3.41 — again, based on three malformed children).

Detailed Evaluation of Uniform Malformations

In this section, groups of drugs, followed by individual drugs, are evaluated in relation to various classes or groups of uniform malformations, as well as individual malformations, for which multiple logistic risk function models were developed. In the tables, the observed and expected numbers of malformed children are given for each drug exposure in turn. The measure of association presented is a standardized relative risk (SRR) with its 95% confidence limits. The SRR is the ratio of the observed number to the expected number of malformed children. Since the SRR takes into account potential confounding variables, it represents the best estimate of the relationship between a drug and a malformation. As numbers of exposed mother-child pairs become so small as to be uninformative, data will be omitted.

Sedatives, Tranquilizers, and Antidepressants — 3,122 Exposures (Table 24.3)

There was no evidence of association of the drug group as a whole with broad classes of malformations. The highest SRR among the malformations was 1.35 (Down syndrome).

Barbiturates — 2,413 Exposures (Table 24.4)

Since almost 80% of the exposures to the group of drugs discussed in this chapter are to barbiturates, the data in these tables are similar to the data in Table 24.3. There were no SRRs greater than 1.5. The

relative risk of 1.40 for cardiovascular system malformations is statistically significant, with a lower confidence limit of 1.05.

Phenobarbital — 1,415 Exposures (Table 24.5) The SRRs of the largest outcome classes — any malformation, major malformations, and minor malformations — were all close to unity. Of the remaining SRRs, only that of Down syndrome (1.62) was greater than 1.5.

Secobarbital — 378 Exposures (Table 24.6) No association was evident between this drug and any of the broad classes of malformations. The SRR for cardiovascular malformations was 1.90.

Amobarbital — 298 Exposures (Table 24.7) The SRRs of major and minor malformations were 1.40 and 1.69, respectively. For any malformation, the SRR was much less (1.16). Among the specific classes of malformations, SRRs greater than 1.5 were seen for cardiovascular

Table **24.3**

Standardized Relative Risks (SRR) and Their 95% Confidence Intervals (CI$_{95}$) for Classes of Malformations Showing Uniform Rates by Hospital in Relation to **Sedatives, Tranquilizers, and Antidepressants** Used in Lunar Months 1–4 by 3,122 Pregnant Women (Based on Multiple Logistic Risk Function Analysis)

Malformation Classes	No. of Malformed Children		SRR	CI$_{95}$ of SRR
	Observed	Expected		
Any malformation	167	158.6	1.05	0.91–1.21
Major malformations	111	104.5	1.06	0.89–1.26
Minor malformations	61	55.9	1.09	0.86–1.38
Central nervous	19	20.8	0.91	0.55–1.43
Cardiovascular	39	29.7	1.31	1.00–1.71
Musculoskeletal (other than polydactyly in Blacks)	31	32.3	0.96	0.67–1.36
Polydactyly in Blacks[1]	22	16.4	1.34	0.95–1.91
Respiratory	13	15.2	0.85	0.46–1.46
Gastrointestinal	24	24.2	0.99	0.67–1.47
Genitourinary (other than hypospadias)	16	14.4	1.11	0.64–1.81
Hypospadias[2]	12	11.1	1.08	0.56–1.89
Eye and ear	4	9.1	0.44	0.12–1.13
Syndromes (other than Down syndrome)	6	9.8	0.61	0.22–1.33
Down syndrome	7	5.2	1.35	0.54–2.79
Tumors	10	13.8	0.72	0.35–1.33

[1]Drugs used by 1,185 Blacks
[2]Drugs used by 1,610 mothers of male offspring

338

Table **24.4**

Standardized Relative Risks (SRR) and Their 95% Confidence Intervals (CI$_{95}$) for Classes of Malformations Showing Uniform Rates by Hospital in Relation to **Barbiturates** Used in Lunar Months 1–4 by 2,413 Pregnant Women (Based on Multiple Logistic Risk Function Analysis)

Malformation Classes	No. of Malformed Children		SRR	CI$_{95}$ of SRR
	Observed	Expected		
Any malformation	122	123.5	0.99	0.83–1.17
Major malformations	84	80.9	1.04	0.85–1.27
Minor malformations	41	43.9	0.93	0.68–1.27
Central nervous	14	16.1	0.87	0.48–1.46
Cardiovascular	32	22.9	1.40	1.05–1.86
Musculoskeletal (other than polydactyly in Blacks)	22	24.4	0.90	0.58–1.39
Polydactyly in Blacks[1]	17	13.9	1.22	0.71–1.95
Respiratory	9	11.9	0.76	0.35–1.44
Gastrointestinal	18	18.3	0.98	0.58–1.55
Genitourinary (other than hypospadias)	12	11.2	1.07	0.55–1.87
Hypospadias[2]	6	8.1	0.74	0.27–1.60
Eye and ear	2	7.2	0.28	0.03–1.01
Syndromes (other than Down syndrome)	5	7.5	0.66	0.21–1.54
Down syndrome	5	3.7	1.36	0.44–3.16
Tumors	7	11.0	0.64	0.26–1.31

[1]Drugs used by 1,023 Blacks
[2]Drugs used by 1,224 mothers of male offspring

Table **24.5**

Standardized Relative Risks (SRR) and Their 95% Confidence Intervals (CI$_{95}$) for Classes of Malformations Showing Uniform Rates by Hospital in Relation to **Phenobarbital** Used in Lunar Months 1–4 by 1,415 Pregnant Women (Based on Multiple Logistic Risk Function Analysis)

Malformation Classes	No. of Malformed Children		SRR	CI$_{95}$ of SRR
	Observed	Expected		
Any malformation	74	75.2	0.98	0.79–1.23
Major malformations	47	48.5	0.97	0.73–1.28
Minor malformations	25	27.6	0.91	0.60–1.36
Central nervous	10	10.1	0.99	0.48–1.82
Cardiovascular	18	14.0	1.29	0.77–2.03
Musculoskeletal (other than polydactyly in Blacks)	12	12.9	0.93	0.48–1.62
Polydactyly in Blacks[1]	13	10.3	1.27	0.68–2.15
Respiratory	5	6.9	0.73	0.24–1.70
Gastrointestinal	9	10.8	0.83	0.38–1.58
Genitourinary (other than hypospadias)	7	6.5	1.08	0.44–2.23
Hypospadias[2]	1	4.5	0.22	0.01–1.24
Eye and ear	2	4.4	0.45	0.05–1.63
Syndromes (other than Down syndrome)	1	4.4	0.23	0.01–1.27
Down syndrome	4	2.5	1.62	0.44–4.13
Tumors	7	6.7	1.04	0.42–2.14

[1]Drugs used by 751 Blacks
[2]Drugs used by 717 mothers of male offspring

Table **24.6**

Standardized Relative Risks (SRR) and Their 95% Confidence Intervals (Cl₉₅) for Classes of Malformations Showing Uniform Rates by Hospital in Relation to **Secobarbital** Used in Lunar Months 1–4 by 378 Pregnant Women (Based on Multiple Logistic Risk Function Analysis)

Malformation Classes	No. of Malformed Children		SRR	CI_{95} of SRR
	Observed	Expected		
Any malformation	23	22.0	1.05	0.71–1.54
Major malformations	18	15.8	1.14	0.68–1.77
Minor malformations	6	7.5	0.79	0.29–1.71
Central nervous	3	3.6	0.85	0.17–2.45
Cardiovascular	9	4.8	1.90	0.87–3.56
Musculoskeletal (other than polydactyly in Blacks)	5	5.0	1.00	0.33–2.32
Polydactyly in Blacks[1]	2	1.5	1.34	0.16–4.73
Respiratory	1	3.0	0.33	0.01–1.84
Gastrointestinal	5	3.7	1.34	0.43–3.10
Genitourinary (other than hypospadias)	2	2.7	0.73	0.09–2.63
Hypospadias[2]	1	1.5	0.67	0.02–3.70
Eye and ear	0	1.5	—	0.00–2.51
Syndromes (other than Down syndrome)	1	1.8	0.56	0.01–3.10
Down syndrome	0	0.7	—	0.00–5.37
Tumors	0	1.8	—	0.00–2.01

[1]Drugs used by 121 Blacks
[2]Drugs used by 196 mothers of male offspring

Table **24.7**

Standardized Relative Risks (SRR) and Their 95% Confidence Intervals (Cl₉₅) for Classes of Malformations Showing Uniform Rates by Hospital in Relation to **Amobarbital** Used in Lunar Months 1–4 by 298 Pregnant Women (Based on Multiple Logistic Risk Function Analysis)

Malformation Classes	No. of Malformed Children		SRR	CI_{95} of SRR
	Observed	Expected		
Any malformation	16	13.8	1.16	0.67–1.85
Major malformations	14	10.0	1.40	0.77–2.31
Minor malformations	7	4.1	1.69	0.68–3.44
Central nervous	1	1.6	0.63	0.02– 3.49
Cardiovascular	7	2.7	2.55	1.03– 5.19
Musculoskeletal (other than polydactyly in Blacks)	3	3.9	0.78	0.16– 2.24
Polydactyly in Blacks[1]	2	0.4	5.04	0.62–16.55
Respiratory	1	1.4	0.71	0.02– 3.91
Gastrointestinal	3	2.5	1.21	0.25– 3.51
Genitourinary (other than hypospadias)	3	1.3	2.35	0.49– 6.81
Hypospadias[2]	1	1.1	0.96	0.02– 5.24
Eye and ear	0	0.8	—	0.00– 4.73
Syndromes (other than Down syndrome)	1	0.8	1.18	0.03– 6.52
Down syndrome	1	0.3	3.08	0.08–17.02
Tumors	0	1.4	—	0.00– 2.69

[1]Drugs used by 29 Blacks
[2]Drugs used by 149 mothers of male offspring

malformations (2.55), polydactyly in Blacks (5.04), genitourinary malformations excluding hypospadias (2.35), and Down syndrome (3.08). The SRR for cardiovascular malformations is statistically significant, with a lower confidence limit greater than unity. The SRRs for Black polydactyly, genitourinary malformations other than hypospadias, and Down syndrome are all based on three or fewer malformed children.

Pentobarbital — 250 Exposures (Table 24.8) All SRRs in the table were below unity.

Tranquilizers and Nonbarbiturate
Sedatives — 946 Exposures
(Table 24.9)

The SRR for minor malformations was 1.34. The only SRR greater than 1.5 was for hypospadias (1.86).

Meprobamate — 356 Exposures (Table 24.10) The SRR of minor malformations was 1.78. The component of the minor malformation class which appears to contribute most to the elevated SRR is hypospadias, where the SRR was 3.37 with 95% confidence limits of 1.10–7.72, thus attaining statistical significance. The only other SRR greater than 1.5 was for Black polydactyly (2.27 — based on two malformed children).

Chlordiazepoxide — 257 Exposures (Table 24.11) For the outcomes in the table, all SRRs were close to or below unity.

**Detailed Evaluation of
Non-Uniform Malformations:
Inguinal Hernia, Clubfoot,
Pectus Excavatum**

In this section, the three outcomes are evaluated as in the preceding section dealing with uniform malformations. Instances in which there were fewer than three malformed children exposed to any drug are omitted because they are not informative.

As shown in Table 24.12, the following drugs had relative risks greater than 1.5 for inguinal hernia: amobarbital (2.20), tranquilizers and non-barbiturate sedatives (1.67), meprobamate (1.61), glutethimide (4.37), and hydroxyzine (3.86).* The findings for amobarbital, tranquilizers and non-barbiturate sedatives, and glutethimide are statistically significant, with lower confidence limits exceeding unity, as is the SRR of 1.31 for the drug group as a whole. For clubfoot, only amobarbital (2.15) had an SRR greater than 1.5. For pectus excavatum, the relative risks were well below unity. The SRR of 0.41 with the whole group of sedatives, tranquilizers, and antidepressants was statistically significant, with an upper confidence limit below unity.

---

*The results of the multiple logistic risk function analysis of uniform malformations for glutethimide and hydroxyzine were not presented in the previous section because there were not sufficient numbers of exposed-malformed children to be informative.

Table **24.8**

Standardized Relative Risks (SRR) and Their 95% Confidence Intervals (CI$_{95}$) for Broad Classes of Malformations Showing Uniform Rates by Hospital in Relation to **Pentobarbital** Used in Lunar Months 1–4 by 250 Pregnant Women (Based on Multiple Logistic Risk Function Analysis)

	No. of Malformed Children			
	Observed	Expected	SRR	CI$_{95}$ of SRR
Any malformation	6	12.7	0.47	0.17–1.01
Major malformations	3	8.5	0.35	0.07–1.03
Minor malformations	3	4.6	0.66	0.14–1.90

Table **24.9**

Standardized Relative Risks (SRR) and Their 95% Confidence Intervals (CI95) for Classes of Malformations Showing Uniform Rates by Hospital in Relation to **Tranquilizers and Nonbarbiturate Sedatives** Used in Lunar Months 1–4 by 946 Pregnant Women (Based on Multiple Logistic Risk Function Analysis)

Malformation Classes	No. of Malformed Children		SRR	CI95 of SRR
	Observed	Expected		
Any malformation	53	47.0	1.13	0.88–1.44
Major malformations	33	31.9	1.04	0.75–1.44
Minor malformations	21	15.7	1.34	0.93–1.93
Central nervous	5	6.2	0.81	0.26–1.89
Cardiovascular	12	9.2	1.31	0.68–2.27
Musculoskeletal (other than polydactyly in Blacks)	10	10.7	0.94	0.45–1.71
Polydactyly in Blacks[1]	5	3.3	1.50	0.49–3.45
Respiratory	3	4.4	0.68	0.14–1.99
Gastrointestinal	7	7.6	0.92	0.37–1.89
Genitourinary (other than hypospadias)	3	4.3	0.70	0.15–2.05
Hypospadias[2]	7	3.8	1.86	0.75–3.81
Eye and ear	2	2.5	0.79	0.10–2.83
Syndromes (other than Down syndrome)	1	3.1	0.32	0.01–1.80
Down syndrome	2	1.9	1.06	0.13–3.82
Tumors	3	4.0	0.74	0.15–2.16

[1]Drugs used by 230 Blacks
[2]Drugs used by 509 mothers of male offspring

Table **24.10**

Standardized Relative Risks (SRR) and Their 95% Confidence Intervals (CI95) for Classes of Malformations Showing Uniform Rates by Hospital in Relation to **Meprobamate** Used in Lunar Months 1–4 by 356 Pregnant Women (Based on Multiple Logistic Risk Function Analysis)

Malformation Classes	No. of Malformed Children		SRR	CI95 of SRR
	Observed	Expected		
Any malformation	20	17.4	1.15	0.71–1.75
Major malformations	9	12.1	0.74	0.34–1.39
Minor malformations	10	5.6	1.78	0.86–3.23
Central nervous	0	2.3	—	0.00–1.58
Cardiovascular	4	3.4	1.17	0.32–2.96
Musculoskeletal (other than polydactyly in Blacks)	3	4.2	0.72	0.15–2.09
Polydactyly in Blacks[1]	2	0.9	2.27	0.28–7.92
Respiratory	0	1.6	—	0.00–2.31
Gastrointestinal	3	2.7	1.12	0.23–3.25
Genitourinary (other than hypospadias)	0	1.5	—	0.00–2.46
Hypospadias[2]	5	1.5	3.37	1.10–7.72
Eye and ear	1	0.9	1.02	0.03–5.64
Syndromes (other than Down syndrome)	0	1.1	—	0.00–3.39
Down syndrome	1	0.8	1.25	0.03–6.94
Tumors	1	1.5	0.66	0.02–3.64

[1]Drugs used by 77 Blacks
[2]Drugs used by 186 mothers of male offspring

Table **24.11**

Standardized Relative Risks (SRR) and Their 95% Confidence Intervals (CI$_{95}$) for Broad Classes of Malformations Showing Uniform Rates by Hospital in Relation to **Chlordiazepoxide** Used in Lunar Months 1–4 by 257 Pregnant Women (Based on Multiple Logistic Risk Function Analysis)

| | No. of Malformed Children | | | |
	Observed	Expected	SRR	CI$_{95}$ of SRR
Any malformation	11	13.3	0.83	0.42–1.46
Major malformations	6	8.9	0.67	0.25–1.44
Minor malformations	5	4.3	1.16	0.38–2.68

Table **24.12**

Standardized Relative Risks (SRR) and Their 95% Confidence Intervals (CI$_{95}$) for Inguinal Hernia, Clubfoot, and Pectus Excavatum in Relation to **Sedatives, Tranquilizers, and Antidepressants** Used in Lunar Months 1–4 (Based on Multiple Logistic Risk Function Analysis)

| | No. of Users | No. of Malformed Children | | SRR | CI$_{95}$ of SRR |
		Observed	Expected		
Inguinal hernia					
Sedatives, tranquilizers, antidepressants	3122	61	46.4	1.31	1.06–1.63
Barbiturates	2413	43	36.2	1.19	0.91–1.55
Phenobarbital	1415	22	21.6	1.02	0.68–1.54
Secobarbital	378	8	6.6	1.22	0.53–2.38
Amobarbital	298	9	4.1	2.20	1.01–4.11
Tranquilizers and non-barbiturate sedatives	946	23	13.7	1.67	1.22–2.29
Meprobamate	356	8	5.0	1.61	0.70–3.13
Glutethimide	67	5	1.2	4.37	1.44–9.68
Hydroxyzine	50	3	0.8	3.86	0.81–10.63
Clubfoot					
Sedatives, tranquilizers, antidepressants	3122	18	14.8	1.22	0.72–1.92
Barbiturates	2413	12	11.5	1.04	0.54–1.81
Phenobarbital	1415	6	6.3	0.95	0.35–2.06
Amobarbital	298	4	1.9	2.15	0.59–5.44
Tranquilizers and non-barbiturate sedatives	946	5	4.4	1.14	0.37–2.65
Pectus excavatum					
Sedatives, tranquilizers, antidepressants	3122	5	12.2	0.41	•0.13–0.95
Barbiturates	2413	4	9.0	0.44	0.12–1.13

Comments

There was little evidence of an overall teratogenic effect attributable to the combined group of sedatives, tranquilizers, and antidepressants. However, there was some suggestion of association between barbiturates (2,413 exposures) and cardiovascular malformations. This was not evident for all of the barbiturate drugs. In addition, the SRR was only modestly elevated (1.29) for exposure to phenobarbital, which was the most commonly used barbiturate (1,415 exposures). Secobarbital and amobarbital were more strongly associated, in terms of relative risk, with cardiovascular malformations. With regard to individual malformations, phenobarbital exposure was associated with ventricular septal defect and coarctation of the aorta (Appendix 4). Amobarbital exposure was related to inguinal hernia and clubfoot. The findings for the barbiturate group of drugs require independent confirmation.

Among the tranquilizers and non-barbiturate sedatives, meprobamate (356 exposures) was associated with hypospadias, but the finding was based on small numbers. No other suggestive associations were found for meprobamate or chlordiazepoxide. These two drugs have been more fully analyzed elsewhere.[1] The present findings conflict with those reported in another study.[2]

For limited data on glutethimide (67 exposures), there were no prominent associations. Lack of evidence of an overt teratogenic effect of this drug is of interest because of its chemical resemblance to thalidomide. Experimentally, the drug does not appear to be teratogenic.[3,4]

Numbers were too limited to justify any comment on the antidepressant drugs (other than phenothiazines, which were classified together with antihistamines and antinauseants). The literature on whether tricyclic antidepressants are teratogenic in humans is conflicting.[5]

CHAPTER **25**

Drugs
Affecting the
Autonomic
Nervous
System

General Evaluation

In Table 25.1, the entire set of 3,248
malformed children is considered in relation to exposure to the entire group of
drugs affecting the autonomic nervous
system during the first four lunar months
of pregnancy. In Table 25.2, the data are
confined to the 2,277 children who had
malformations which were distributed
uniformly among hospitals. Three relative risks are given in each table: crude,
standardized for hospital variability, and
standardized for the mother's ethnic
group and survival of the child.

All Malformations in Relation
to All Drugs Affecting
the Autonomic Nervous System
(Table 25.1)

Overall, the hospital-standardized relative risk for any malformation in relation
to all drugs affecting the autonomic nervous system was 1.12. There is a statistically significant association ($p < 0.05$) for
sympathomimetic drugs, with a relative
risk of 1.19. Among these drugs, hospital-standardized relative risks greater
than 1.5 were observed for epinephrine (1.71 — statistically significant
at the 0.05 level), and levonordefrin
(1.53). The hospital-standardized relative
risk of 1.40 for phenylpropanolamine is
statistically significant at the 0.01 level.
There is essentially no association with
parasympatholytic drugs. There was not

345

Table **25.1**

Children (3,248) With Any Malformation in Relation to Exposure to **Drugs Affecting the Autonomic Nervous System** During Lunar Months 1–4 Among 50,282 Mother-Child Pairs

	No. of Mother-Child Pairs Exposed	No. of Malformed Children	Crude Relative Risk	Hospital Standardized Relative Risk[1]	Survival and Race Standardized Relative Risk[1]
Drugs affecting the autonomic nervous system	4,657	354	1.20[2]	1.12	1.22[2]
Sympathomimetic drugs	3,082	249	1.27[2]	1.19[3]	1.30[2]
Phenylephrine	1,249	102	1.27[3]	1.23	1.31[3]
Phenylpropanolamine	726	71	1.53[2]	1.40[4]	1.57[2]
Ephedrine	373	26	1.08	1.07	1.05
Dextroamphetamine	367	29	1.23	0.96	1.29
Amphetamines	215	17	1.23	1.13	1.21
Epinephrine	189	22	1.81[4]	1.71[3]	1.99[4]
Methamphetamine	89	5	0.87	0.81	0.82
Phenmetrazine	58	4	1.07	0.99	1.10
Isoxsuprine	54	3	0.86	0.74	0.77
Diethylpropion	40	3	1.16	0.93	1.27
Pseudoephedrine	39	1	0.40	0.35	0.36
Isoproterenol	31	2	1.00	0.94	1.02
Levonordefrin	26	3	1.79	1.53	1.76
Naphazoline	20	1	0.77	0.61	0.89
Other sympathomimetics[5]	96	7	1.13	0.96	1.08
Parasympatholytic drugs	2,323	168	1.13	1.04	1.14
Dicyclomine	1,024	68	1.03	0.93	1.05
Belladonna	554	46	1.29	1.23	1.35
Atropine	401	25	0.96	0.92	0.96
Hyoscyamine	322	19	0.91	0.86	0.88
Scopolamine	309	21	1.05	1.00	1.03
Isopropamide iodide	180	15	1.29	1.09	1.18
Scopolamine aminoxide hydrobromide	79	5	0.98	0.96	0.92
Hyoscyamus	41	1	0.38	0.36	0.40
Propantheline bromide	33	2	0.94	0.82	0.98
Homatropine	26	1	0.60	0.51	0.60
Other parasympatholytics[6]	60	3	0.77	0.66	0.75
Parasympathomimetic drugs	30	2	1.03	0.89	0.93
Neostigmine bromide	22	1	0.70	0.56	0.79
Other parasympathomimetics[7]	8	1	1.94	2.07	1.24

[1]Estimated by the Mantel-Haenszel procedure
[2]$x^2_1 = 10.87 - 13.97$, $p < 0.001$
[3]$X^2_1 = 4.96 - 6.25$, $p < 0.05$
[4]$X^2_1 = 6.67 - 8.13$, $p < 0.01$
[5]Levarterenol (18); cyclopentamine (17); methylphenidate (11); xylometazoline (8); isometheptene (8); benzphetamine (6); methoxamine (5); propylhexadrine (5); tetrahydrozoline (3); methoxyphenamine (3); pipradol (3); etafedrine (2); hydroxyamphetamine hydrobromide (2); oxymetazoline (2); metaraminol (2); ethylnorepinephrine (1); phendimetrazine (1)
[6]Piperidolate (16); trihexyphenidyl (9); tridihexethyl (6); benztropine mesylate (4); adiphenine (4); glycopyrrolate (4); clidinium bromide (4); anisotropine methylbromide (2); methscopolamine bromide (2); methantheline bromide (2); methylatropine (2); poldine methylsulfate (1); cyclopentolate (1); oxyphencyclimine (1); mepenzolate bromide (1); ambutonium bromide (1);
[7]Edrophonium bromide (4); bethanechol (3); pyridostigmine bromide (1); ambenonium (1)

Table **25.2**

Children (2,277) With Malformations Showing Uniform Rates by Hospital in Relation to Exposure to **Drugs Affecting the Autonomic Nervous System** During Lunar Months 1–4 Among 50,282 Mother-Child Pairs

	No. of Mother-Child Pairs Exposed	No. of Malformed Children	Crude Relative Risk	Hospital Standardized Relative Risk	Survival and Race Standardized Relative Risk
Drugs affecting the autonomic nervous system	4,657	233	1.12	1.06	1.13
Sympathomimetic drugs	3,082	159	1.15	1.09	1.15
Phenylephrine	1,249	66	1.17	1.13	1.20
Phenylpropanolamine	726	45	1.38[1]	1.29	1.37
Ephedrine	373	17	1.01	0.98	0.95
Dextroamphetamine	367	18	1.08	0.92	1.11
Amphetamines	215	10	1.03	0.96	0.95
Epinephrine	189	14	1.64	1.57	1.75
Methamphetamine	89	4	0.99	0.94	0.92
Phenmetrazine	58	3	1.14	1.09	1.16
Isoxsuprine	54	2	0.82	0.77	0.72
Diethylpropion	40	3	1.66	1.47	1.95
Pseudoephedrine	39	1	0.57	0.51	0.55
Isoproterenol	31	1	0.71	0.68	0.66
Levonordefrin	26	2	1.70	1.49	1.58
Naphazoline	20	0	—	—	—
Other sympathomimetics	96	4	0.92	0.81	0.83
Parasympatholytic drugs	2,323	114	1.09	1.03	1.09
Dicyclomine	1,024	48	1.04	0.96	1.05
Belladonna	554	34	1.36	1.32	1.45
Atropine	401	17	0.94	0.91	0.94
Hyoscyamine	322	14	0.96	0.93	0.94
Scopolamine	309	14	1.00	0.97	0.98
Isopropamide iodide	180	9	1.10	0.98	0.90
Scopolamine aminoxide hydrobromide	79	2	0.56	0.53	0.43
Hyoscyamus	41	1	0.54	0.53	0.63
Propantheline bromide	33	1	0.67	0.60	0.70
Homatropine	26	1	0.85	0.78	0.86
Other parasympatholytics	60	2	0.74	0.68	0.71
Parasympathomimetic drugs	30	2	1.47	1.40	1.35
Neostigmine bromide	22	1	1.00	0.91	1.23
Other para-sympathomimetics	8	1	2.76	3.04	1.56

[1]$X^2_1 = 4.37$, p $<$ 0.05

sufficient exposure to parasympathomimetic drugs to permit an assessment of their teratogenic potential.

Malformations Showing Uniform Rates by Hospital in Relation to Drugs Affecting the Autonomic Nervous System (Table 25.2)

As seen in the table, the association of these drugs with malformations showing uniform rates by hospitals is considerably less. The only relative risk greater than 1.5 was for epinephrine (1.57). Relative risks for levonordefrin (1.49), and phenylpropanolamine (1.29) were again elevated, along with diethylpropion (1.47).

Detailed Evaluation of Uniform Malformations

In this section, groups of drugs, followed by individual drugs, are evaluated in relation to various classes or groups of uniform malformations, as well as individual malformations, for which multiple logistic risk function models were developed. In the tables, the observed and expected numbers of malformed children are given for each drug exposure in turn. The measure of association presented is a standardized relative risk (SRR) with its 95% confidence limits. The SRR is the ratio of the observed number to the expected number of malformed children. Since the SRR takes into account potential confounding variables, it represents the best estimate of the relationship between a drug and a malformation. As numbers of exposed mother-child pairs become so small as to be uninformative, data will be omitted.

All Drugs Affecting the Autonomic Nervous System — 4,657 Exposures (Table 25.3)

The SRR for minor malformations was 1.30. A lower confidence limit of 1.11 in-

Table *25.3*

Standardized Relative Risks (SRR) and Their 95% Confidence Intervals (CI$_{95}$) for Classes of Malformations Showing Uniform Rates by Hospital in Relation to **Drugs Affecting the Autonomic Nervous System** Used in Lunar Months 1–4 by 4,657 Pregnant Women (Based on Multiple Logistic Risk Function Analysis)

Malformation Classes	No. of Malformed Children		SRR	CI$_{95}$ of SRR
	Observed	Expected		
Any malformation	233	214.0	1.09	0.97–1.22
Major malformations	140	136.7	1.02	0.88–1.20
Minor malformations	100	76.7	1.30	1.11–1.54
Central nervous	25	24.2	1.03	0.71–1.50
Cardiovascular	36	37.8	0.95	0.69–1.31
Musculoskeletal (other than polydactyly in Blacks)	45	45.3	0.99	0.75–1.32
Polydactyly in Blacks[1]	34	23.7	1.43	1.09–1.88
Respiratory	23	20.9	1.10	0.76–1.59
Gastrointestinal	35	31.5	1.11	0.82–1.50
Genitourinary (other than hypospadias)	14	19.4	0.72	0.39–1.21
Hypospadias[2]	18	15.3	1.17	0.70–1.85
Eye and ear	15	11.6	1.30	0.73–2.13
Syndromes (other than Down syndrome)	10	11.5	0.87	0.42–1.59
Down syndrome	4	5.8	0.69	0.19–1.76
Tumors	13	18.1	0.72	0.38–1.22

[1]Drugs used by 1,712 Blacks
[2]Drugs used by 2,346 mothers of male offspring

dicates that this finding is statistically significant. Of the specific classes of malformations, none had SRRs greater than 1.5. A lower confidence limit greater than unity indicates that the SRR for Black polydactyly (1.43) is statistically significant.

Sympathomimetic Drugs —
3,082 Exposures (Table 25.4)

Among all sympathomimetic drugs, the highest relative risk in the broad classes of malformations was seen for minor malformations (1.35). A lower confidence limit exceeding unity indicates that this finding is statistically significant. An SRR greater than 1.5 was found for eye and ear malformations (1.77).

Phenylephrine — 1,249 Exposures (Table 25.5) The association of malformations with phenylephrine, the most common of the sympathomimetic drugs, was somewhat similar to that of the overall group. Thus, the relative risk for minor malfor-

mations (1.23) was higher than for major (1.12). Among the specific classes of malformations, the only SRR greater than 1.5 was for eye and ear defects (2.74). This relative risk is statistically significant, as indicated by a confidence interval which does not include unity.

Phenylpropanolamine — 726 Exposures (Table 25.6) For phenylpropanolamine, the relative risk was also higher for minor malformations (1.67) than for major (1.16). Both the finding for minor malformations and that for any malformation (1.35) had lower confidence limits exceeding unity. Among the specific classes of malformations, relative risks greater than 1.5 were seen for hypospadias (1.63) and eye and ear malformations (4.04). The latter SRR, with a lower confidence limit of 1.63 is statistically significant.

Ephedrine — 373 Exposures (Table 25.7) Overall, there was no evidence of association between ephedrine and malformations.

Table **25.4**

Standardized Relative Risks (SRR) and Their 95% Confidence Intervals (CI$_{95}$) for Classes of Malformations Showing Uniform Rates by Hospital in Relation to **Sympathomimetic Drugs** Used in Lunar Months 1–4 by 3,082 Pregnant Women (Based on Multiple Logistic Risk Function Analysis)

Malformation Classes	No. of Malformed Children		SRR	CI$_{95}$ of SRR
	Observed	Expected		
Any malformation	159	141.9	1.12	0.97–1.29
Major malformations	93	90.2	1.03	0.85–1.25
Minor malformations	69	51.1	1.35	1.11–1.64
Central nervous	18	16.1	1.12	0.66–1.77
Cardiovascular	23	25.1	0.92	0.60–1.39
Musculoskeletal (other than polydactyly in Blacks)	31	29.7	1.04	0.74–1.46
Polydactyly in Blacks[1]	22	15.9	1.38	0.98–1.96
Respiratory	16	13.4	1.20	0.68–1.94
Gastrointestinal	23	20.7	1.11	0.76–1.62
Genitourinary (other than hypospadias)	9	12.6	0.71	0.33–1.35
Hypospadias[2]	12	10.6	1.14	0.59–1.98
Eye and ear	13	7.4	1.77	0.94–3.01
Syndromes (other than Down syndrome)	8	7.7	1.04	0.45–2.05
Down syndrome	2	3.6	0.56	0.07–2.03
Tumors	11	11.7	0.94	0.47–1.67

[1]Drugs used by 1,114 Blacks
[2]Drugs used by 1,591 mothers of male offspring

Table **25.5**

Standardized Relative Risks (SRR) and Their 95% Confidence Intervals (Cl$_{95}$) for Classes of Malformations Showing Uniform Rates by Hospital in Relation to **Phenylephrine** Used in Lunar Months 1–4 by 1,249 Pregnant Women (Based on Multiple Logistic Risk Function Analysis)

| Malformation Classes | No. of Malformed Children | | SRR | Cl$_{95}$ of SRR |
	Observed	Expected		
Any malformation	66	57.2	1.15	0.93–1.44
Major malformations	39	34.8	1.12	0.84–1.50
Minor malformations	27	22.0	1.23	0.88–1.72
Central nervous	4	6.2	0.65	0.18–1.66
Cardiovascular	9	9.7	0.93	0.43–1.76
Musculoskeletal (other than polydactyly in Blacks)	14	10.8	1.30	0.71–2.17
Polydactyly in Blacks[1]	11	8.4	1.31	0.66–2.33
Respiratory	2	4.9	0.41	0.05–1.47
Gastrointestinal	10	7.7	1.30	0.63–2.39
Genitourinary (other than hypospadias)	2	4.7	0.43	0.05–1.54
Hypospadias[2]	4	4.3	0.92	0.25–2.35
Eye and ear	8	2.9	2.74	1.18–5.38
Syndromes (other than Down syndrome)	3	2.9	1.02	0.21–2.99
Down syndrome	1	1.5	0.65	0.02–3.64
Tumors	2	4.6	0.44	0.05–1.58

[1]Drugs used by 578 Blacks
[2]Drugs used by 657 mothers of male offspring

Dextroamphetamine — 367 Exposures (Table 25.8) The relative risk of 1.46 for minor malformations in children exposed to dextroamphetamine is similar to that for all drugs in this class.

Parasympatholytic Drugs —
2,323 Exposures (Table 25.9)

As with the sympathomimetic drugs, there was no association with major malformations (SRR, 1.02), and a statistically significant association with minor malformations (SRR, 1.31 — lower confidence limit of 1.03). There were no SRRs greater than 1.5 among the various classes of malformations.

Dicyclomine — 1,024 Exposures (Table 25.10) A statistically significant SRR of 1.46 was found for minor malformations (lower confidence limit of 1.02). Black polydactyly (1.89) had an SRR greater than 1.5.

Belladonna — 554 Exposures (Table 25.11) Belladonna was found to be associated with malformations as a whole

(SRR, 1.37) and with minor malformations (1.84). Both of these relative risks are statistically significant, with lower confidence limits exceeding unity. SRRs greater than 1.5 were seen for respiratory tract (1.88), hypospadias (1.70), and eye and ear defects (4.64). The latter finding is statistically significant, with a lower confidence limit of 1.70.

Atropine — 401 Exposures (Table 25.12), Hyoscyamine — 322 Exposures (Table 25.13), Scopolamine — 309 Exposures (Table 25.14) There was no evidence for an association between malformations and atropine, hyoscyamine, or scopolamine.

**Detailed Evaluation of
Non-Uniform Malformations:
Inguinal Hernia, Clubfoot,
Pectus Excavatum**

In this section, the three outcomes are evaluated as in the preceding section dealing with uniform malformations. In-

Table **25.6**

Standardized Relative Risks (SRR) and Their 95% Confidence Intervals (CI$_{95}$) for Classes of Malformations Showing Uniform Rates by Hospital in Relation to **Phenylpropanolamine** Used in Lunar Months 1–4 by 726 Pregnant Women (Based on Multiple Logistic Risk Function Analysis)

| | No. of Malformed Children | | | |
Malformation Classes	Observed	Expected	SRR	CI$_{95}$ of SRR
Any malformation	45	33.4	1.35	1.05–1.72
Major malformations	26	22.3	1.16	0.82–1.65
Minor malformations	19	11.3	1.67	1.01–2.59
Central nervous	6	4.2	1.42	0.52–3.08
Cardiovascular	5	5.8	0.86	0.28–1.99
Musculoskeletal (other than polydactyly in Blacks)	9	7.3	1.24	0.57–2.33
Polydactyly in Blacks[1]	3	2.8	1.05	0.22–3.04
Respiratory	4	3.6	1.11	0.30–2.82
Gastrointestinal	6	5.4	1.10	0.41–2.39
Genitourinary (other than hypospadias)	2	3.5	0.57	0.07–2.04
Hypospadias[2]	4	2.5	1.63	0.44–4.13
Eye and ear	7	1.7	4.04	1.63–8.29
Syndromes (other than Down syndrome)	1	2.1	0.48	0.01–2.66
Down syndrome	1	0.9	1.11	0.03–6.17
Tumors	4	2.9	1.38	0.38–3.52

[1]Drugs used by 213 Blacks
[2]Drugs used by 360 mothers of male offspring

Table **25.7**

Standardized Relative Risks (SRR) and Their 95% Confidence Intervals (CI$_{95}$) for Broad Classes of Malformations Showing Uniform Rates by Hospital in Relation to **Ephedrine** Used in Lunar Months 1–4 by 373 Pregnant Women (Based on Multiple Logistic Risk Function Analysis)

| | No. of Malformed Children | | | |
	Observed	Expected	SRR	CI$_{95}$ of SRR
Any malformation	17	17.0	1.00	0.59–1.58
Major malformations	8	10.7	0.75	0.32–1.46
Minor malformations	8	6.8	1.18	0.51–2.30

stances in which there were fewer than three malformed children exposed to any drug are omitted because they are not informative.

The results of the analysis are given in Table 25.15. For inguinal hernia, only phenylpropanolamine (1.51) had an SRR greater than 1.5. However, the SRRs with the drug group as a whole (1.26) and with sympathomimetic drugs (1.34) were statistically significant, as indicated by lower confidence limits exceeding unity. For clubfoot, the following drugs (or groups) had SRRs greater than 1.5, all with lower confidence limits exceeding unity: the drug group as a whole (1.61),

Table **25.8**

Standardized Relative Risks (SRR) and Their 95% Confidence Intervals (CI$_{95}$) for Broad Classes of Malformations Showing Uniform Rates by Hospital in Relation to **Dextroamphetamine** Used in Lunar Months 1–4 by 367 Pregnant Women (Based on Multiple Logistic Risk Function Analysis)

| | No. of Malformed Children | | | |
	Observed	Expected	SRR	CI$_{95}$ of SRR
Any malformation	18	16.7	1.08	0.65–1.68
Major malformations	15	11.6	1.29	0.73–2.10
Minor malformations	7	4.8	1.46	0.59–2.98

Table **25.9**

Standardized Relative Risks (SRR) and Their 95% Confidence Intervals (CI$_{95}$) for Classes of Malformations Showing Uniform Rates by Hospital in Relation to **Parasympatholytic Drugs** Used in Lunar Months 1–4 by 2,323 Pregnant Women (Based on Multiple Logistic Risk Function Analysis)

| | No. of Malformed Children | | | |
Malformation Classes	Observed	Expected	SRR	CI$_{95}$ of SRR
Any malformation	114	106.9	1.07	0.90–1.27
Major malformations	71	69.6	1.02	0.82–1.28
Minor malformations	49	37.5	1.31	1.03–1.66
Central nervous	15	12.5	1.20	0.67–1.97
Cardiovascular	17	18.7	0.91	0.53–1.46
Musculoskeletal (other than polydactyly in Blacks)	20	23.3	0.86	0.52–1.32
Polydactyly in Blacks[1]	15	10.9	1.38	0.78–2.26
Respiratory	13	11.4	1.14	0.61–1.94
Gastrointestinal	16	16.4	0.97	0.56–1.58
Genitourinary (other than hypospadias)	7	10.5	0.67	0.27–1.37
Hypospadias[2]	9	7.1	1.27	0.58–2.40
Eye and ear	8	6.0	1.33	0.57–2.61
Syndromes (other than Down syndrome)	4	6.0	0.67	0.18–1.70
Down syndrome	3	3.1	0.98	0.20–2.85
Tumors	5	9.4	0.53	0.17–1.24

[1]Drugs used by 826 Blacks
[2]Drugs used by 1,117 mothers of male offspring

Table **25.10**

Standardized Relative Risks (SRR) and Their 95% Confidence Intervals (CI$_{95}$) for Classes of Malformations Showing Uniform Rates by Hospital in Relation to **Dicyclomine** Used in Lunar Months 1–4 by 1,024 Pregnant Women (Based on Multiple Logistic Risk Function Analysis)

Malformation Classes	No. of Malformed Children		SRR	CI$_{95}$ of SRR
	Observed	Expected		
Any malformation	48	44.9	1.07	0.82–1.40
Major malformations	32	30.2	1.06	0.76–1.47
Minor malformations	21	14.4	1.46	1.02–2.07
Central nervous	7	5.0	1.39	0.56–2.86
Cardiovascular	6	7.2	0.84	0.31–1.81
Musculoskeletal (other than polydactyly in Blacks)	12	10.5	1.14	0.59–1.99
Polydactyly in Blacks[1]	6	3.2	1.89	0.70–4.06
Respiratory	7	4.8	1.45	0.58–2.97
Gastrointestinal	9	7.4	1.21	0.56–2.29
Genitourinary (other than hypospadias)	2	4.7	0.43	0.05–1.54
Hypospadias[2]	4	2.9	1.38	0.38–3.50
Eye and ear	1	2.7	0.37	0.01–2.04
Syndromes (other than Down syndrome)	3	2.5	1.22	0.25–3.56
Down syndrome	1	1.2	0.84	0.02–4.65
Tumors	1	4.2	0.24	0.01–1.31

[1]Drugs used by 277 Blacks
[2]Drugs used by 473 mothers of male offspring

Table **25.11**

Standardized Relative Risks (SRR) and Their 95% Confidence Intervals (CI$_{95}$) for Classes of Malformations Showing Uniform Rates by Hospital in Relation to **Belladonna** Used in Lunar Months 1–4 by 554 Pregnant Women (Based on Multiple Logistic Risk Function Analysis)

Malformation Classes	No. of Malformed Children		SRR	CI$_{95}$ of SRR
	Observed	Expected		
Any malformation	34	24.8	1.37	1.03– 1.82
Major malformations	18	15.3	1.18	0.70– 1.84
Minor malformations	16	8.7	1.84	1.06– 2.86
Central nervous	4	2.7	1.46	0.40– 3.71
Cardiovascular	5	4.0	1.23	0.40– 2.86
Musculoskeletal (other than polydactyly in Blacks)	2	4.8	0.42	0.05– 1.49
Polydactyly in Blacks[1]	4	3.0	1.31	0.36– 3.31
Respiratory	4	2.1	1.88	0.51– 4.78
Gastrointestinal	4	3.4	1.19	0.32– 3.02
Genitourinary (other than hypospadias)	2	2.0	1.01	0.12– 3.62
Hypospadias[2]	3	1.8	1.70	0.35– 4.93
Eye and ear	6	1.3	4.64	1.70–10.03
Syndromes (other than Down syndrome)	0	1.2	—	0.00– 2.99
Down syndrome	1	0.8	1.32	0.03– 7.32
Tumors	3	2.10	1.43	0.30– 4.16

[1]Drugs used by 229 Blacks
[2]Drugs used by 273 mothers of male offspring

Table **25.12**

Standardized Relative Risks (SRR) and Their 95% Confidence Intervals (CI_{95}) for Broad Classes of Malformations Showing Uniform Rates by Hospital in Relation to **Atropine** Used in Lunar Months 1–4 by 401 Pregnant Women (Based on Multiple Logistic Risk Function Analysis)

| | No. of Malformed Children | | | |
	Observed	Expected	SRR	CI_{95} of SRR
Any malformation	17	19.4	0.88	0.51–1.39
Major malformations	11	12.1	0.91	0.46–1.61
Minor malformations	6	7.5	0.80	0.29–1.72

Table **25.13**

Standardized Relative Risks (SRR) and Their 95% Confidence Intervals (CI_{95}) for Broad Classes of Malformations Showing Uniform Rates by Hospital in Relation to **Hyoscyamine** Used in Lunar Months 1–4 by 322 Pregnant Women (Based on Multiple Logistic Risk Function Analysis)

| | No. of Malformed Children | | | |
	Observed	Expected	SRR	CI_{95} of SRR
Any malformation	14	15.8	0.88	0.49–1.46
Major malformations	8	9.6	0.83	0.36–1.62
Minor malformations	6	6.0	1.00	0.37–2.15

Table **25.14**

Standardized Relative Risks (SRR) and Their 95% Confidence Intervals (CI_{95}) for Broad Classes of Malformations Showing Uniform Rates by Hospital in Relation to **Scopolamine** Used in Lunar Months 1–4 by 309 Pregnant Women (Based on Multiple Logistic Risk Function Analysis)

| | No. of Malformed Children | | | |
	Observed	Expected	SRR	CI_{95} of SRR
Any malformation	1	1.3	0.75	0.02–4.15
Major malformations	2	1.7	1.17	0.14–4.18
Minor malformations	3	2.9	1.02	0.21–2.96

Table **25.15**

Standardized Relative Risks (SRR) and Their 95% Confidence Intervals (CI₉₅) for Inguinal Hernia, Clubfoot, and Pectus Excavatum in Relation to **Drugs Affecting the Autonomic Nervous System** Used in Lunar Months 1–4 (Based on Multiple Logistic Risk Function Analysis)

	No. of Users	No. of Malformed Children		SRR	CI₉₅ of SRR
		Observed	Expected		
Inguinal hernia					
Drugs affecting the autonomic nervous system	4657	82	65.0	1.26	1.05–1.52
Sympathomimetic drugs	3082	59	44.0	1.34	1.08–1.66
Phenylephrine	1249	22	18.1	1.21	0.83–1.77
Phenylpropanolamine	726	15	9.9	1.51	0.85–2.47
Parasympatholytic drugs	2323	38	31.3	1.21	0.91–1.61
Dicyclomine	1024	9	12.7	0.71	0.32–1.34
Belladonna	554	10	7.6	1.32	0.64–2.41
Clubfoot					
Drugs affecting the autonomic nervous system	4657	34	21.1	1.61	1.25–2.08
Sympathomimetic drugs	3082	27	14.3	1.89	1.45–2.48
Phenylephrine	1249	14	5.3	2.65	1.45–4.43
Parasympatholytic drugs	2323	11	10.7	1.03	0.52–1.84
Dicyclomine	1024	7	4.9	1.43	0.57–2.93
Pectus excavatum					
Drugs affecting the autonomic nervous system	4657	15	18.1	0.83	0.46–1.36
Sympathomimetic drugs	3082	11	12.6	0.87	0.44–1.56
Phenylephrine	1249	3	3.3	0.92	0.19–2.68
Phenylpropanolamine	726	7	3.6	1.92	0.77–3.94
Parasympatholytic drugs	2323	8	9.5	0.84	0.36–1.65
Dicyclomine	1024	5	5.2	0.96	0.31–2.24

sympathomimetic drugs (1.89), and phenylephrine (2.65). For pectus excavatum, as for inguinal hernia, only phenylpropanolamine (1.92) had an SRR greater than 1.5.

Comments

The patterns that emerged were quite striking: minor malformations were associated with exposure to the sympathomimetic amines, phenylephrine, phenylpropanolamine, ephedrine, and dextroamphetamine. With the exception of ephedrine, exposure to these drugs was also related to deformities of the eye or ear. In addition, sympathomimetic drug exposure was associated with the non-uniform malformations, inguinal hernia and clubfoot.

The findings with sympathomimetic drugs were based on large numbers (3,082 exposures). These drugs were commonly ingredients in nosedrops and inhalants and in a variety of commercially available preparations taken orally to alleviate symptoms of upper respiratory infection. Quite often, more than one compound was present in the same preparation.

Exposure to parasympatholytic drugs

was also associated with minor malformations. These agents were also commonly components of proprietary "cold" tablets and were frequently taken together with preparations containing sympathomimetic amines. Again, the findings were based on large numbers (2,323 exposures).

The occurrence in pregnancy of viral infections of the upper respiratory tract was not recorded in this study. Either infections, or some agent or agents used to treat them, could have caused malformations. Further suspicion that viral infections of the respiratory tract may be causal can be adduced from absence of association between cough medicines and malformations. Presumably, infections not accompanied by severe cough were predominantly viral. An extensive and conflicting literature on the topic of influenza as a possible cause of malformations has most recently been summarized by Shepard.[1]

Data on parasympathomimetic drugs were too sparse to justify comment.

CHAPTER **26**

Anesthetics, Anti-convulsants, Muscle Relaxants, and Stimulants

General Evaluation

In Table 26.1, all 3,248 malformed children are considered in relation to exposure to the entire group of anesthetics, anticonvulsants, muscle relaxants, and stimulants during the first four lunar months of pregnancy. In Table 26.2, the data are confined to the 2,277 children who had malformations which were uniformly distributed among the hospitals. Three relative risks are given in each table: crude, standardized for hospital variability, and standardized for the mother's ethnic group and survival of the child.

All Malformations in Relation to Anesthetics, Anticonvulsants, Muscle Relaxants, and Stimulants (Table 26.1)

The hospital-standardized relative risk of any malformation was 0.97 for this group of drugs. Relative risks greater than 1.5 were seen for the following groups and specific drugs: mepivacaine (1.98), benzocaine (1.53), other local anesthetics (1.95), other general anesthetics (1.78 — based on 2 malformed children), non-barbiturate anticonvulsants (1.95), phenytoin (1.71), other non-barbiturate anticonvulsants (2.53), central nervous system stimulants (1.57), and

357

Table **26.1**

Children (3,248) With Any Malformation in Relation to Exposure to **Anesthetics, Anticonvulsants, Muscle Relaxants, and Other Stimulants** During Lunar Months 1–4 Among 50,282 Mother-Child Pairs

	No. of Mother-Child Pairs Exposed	No. of Malformed Children	Crude Relative Risk	Hospital Standardized Relative Risk[1]	Survival and Race Standardized Relative Risk[1]
Anesthetics, anticonvulsants, muscle relaxants, and other stimulants	2,657	175	1.02	0.97	1.02
Local anesthetics	2,165	137	0.98	0.93	0.98
Procaine	1,340	78	0.90	0.87	0.90
Local anesthetic, n.o.s.	386	23	0.92	0.89	0.90
Lidocaine	293	16	0.84	0.76	0.85
Mepivacaine	82	12	2.27[2]	1.98	2.66[2]
Benzocaine	47	5	1.65	1.53	1.48
Propoxycaine	41	5	1.89	1.49	1.76
Tetracaine	23	1	0.67	0.63	0.67
Other local anesthetics[4]	30	4	2.07	1.95	2.53
General anesthetics and oxygen	218	9	0.64	0.60	0.66
General anesthetic, n.o.s.	98	3	0.47	0.45	0.47
Nitrous oxide	76	4	0.81	0.75	0.86
Oxygen	52	2	0.60	0.55	0.60
Halothane	25	2	1.24	1.18	1.33
Other general anesthetics[5]	39	2	0.79	1.78	0.87
Non-barbiturate anticonvulsants	151	18	1.85[3]	1.95[3]	1.83[3]
Phenytoin	132	14	1.64	1.71	1.56
Other non-barbiturate anticonvulsants[6]	34	5	2.28	2.53	2.29
Central nervous system stimulants	60	6	1.55	1.57	1.42
Lobelia	38	4	1.63	1.70	1.50
Other central nervous system stimulants[7]	22	2	1.41	1.36	1.27
Muscle relaxants	83	4	0.75	0.68	0.78
Succinylcholine	26	0	—	—	—
Methocarbamol	22	1	0.70	0.67	0.74
Other centrally acting muscle relaxants[8]	29	3	1.60	1.49	1.77
Other neuromuscular blockers[9]	13	0	—	—	—
Smooth muscle stimulants	57	5	1.36	1.31	1.43
Ergotamine	25	2	1.24	1.18	1.43
Other ergot derivatives[10]	32	3	1.45	1.44	1.43
Other smooth muscle stimulants (sparteine)	1	0	—	—	—

lobelia (1.70). The finding for non-barbiturate anticonvulsants is statistically significant at the 0.05 level.

Malformations with Uniform
Rates by Hospital in
Relation to Anesthetics,
Anticonvulsants, Muscle Relaxants,
and Stimulants (Table 26.2)

A somewhat similar pattern emerged for the uniform malformations. The hospital-standardized relative risk for the entire group of drugs was 0.88. Hospital-standardized relative risks greater than 1.5 were found for mepivacaine (1.96), benzocaine (1.82), propoxycaine (1.89), halothane (1.80), non-barbiturate anticonvulsants (1.64), other non-barbiturate anticonvulsants (2.81), other central nervous system stimulants (2.05), and ergotamine (1.74). The findings for halothane, other central nervous system stimulants, and ergotamine were each based on only two malformed children.

**Detailed Evaluation of
Uniform Malformations**

In this section, groups of drugs, followed by individual drugs, are evaluated in relation to various classes or groups of uniform malformations, as well as individual malformations, for which multiple logistic risk function models were developed. In the tables, the observed and expected numbers of malformed children are given for each drug exposure in turn. The measure of association presented is a standardized relative risk (SRR) with its

95% confidence limits. The SRR is the ratio of the observed number to the expected number of malformed children. Since the SRR takes into account potential confounding variables, it represents the best estimate of the relationship between a drug and a malformation. As numbers of exposed mother-child pairs become so small as to be uninformative, data will be omitted.

Anesthetics, Anticonvulsants,
Muscle Relaxants, and Stimulants —
2,657 Exposures (Table 26.3)

There was no evidence of an association of this group of drugs with broad classes of malformations. The highest SRR among the malformations was 1.34 for eye and ear defects.

Local Anesthetics —
2,165 Exposures (Table 26.4)

Over 80% of the total exposures to the entire drug group are to the subgroup of local anesthetics. Not surprisingly, the data for the subgroup show essentially the same features as for the entire group.

Procaine — 1,340 Exposures (Table 26.5) For this preparation, as for the subgroup to which it belongs, there was no evidence of association with broad classes of malformations. Only the outcome eye and ear malformations (1.79), had an SRR greater than 1.5.

Local Anesthetic, n.o.s. —386 Exposures (Table 26.6) There is no evidence of an overall teratogenic effect of this drug category. Three SRRs of over 1.5 may be noted: for respiratory malformations

← ────────────────────────────────

[1] Estimated by the Mantel-Haenszel procedure
[2] $X^2_1 = 7.78 - 8.76$, $p < 0.01$
[3] $X^2_1 = 5.09 - 6.60$, $p < 0.05$
[4] Dibucaine (9); metabutoxycaine (9); butethamine (3); oxethazaine (3); piperocaine (3); pyrrocaine (1); salicyl alcohol (1); cocaine (1)
[5] Cyclopropane (17); ether (8); ethyl chloride (4); vinyl ether (3); acetamidoeugenol (3); methoxyflurane (2); chloroform (2); trichloroethylene (2)
[6] Primidone (15); mephenytoin (8); magnesium sulfate (6); methsuximide (4); ethotoin (2); trimethadione (2); ethosuximide (1); phenacemide (1)
[7] Ammonia spirit (14); gelsemium (8)
[8] Carisoprodol (14); mephenesin (6); orphenadrine (3); chlorzoxazone (2); metaxalone (2); procyclidine (2)
[9] Gallamine triethiodide (10); curare (3)
[10] Ergonovine (18); methylergonovine maleate (5); ergot (5); dihydroergotamine (3); methysergide (1)

Table **26.2**

Children (2,277) With Malformations Showing Uniform Rates by Hospital in Relation to Exposure to **Anesthetics, Anticonvulsants, Muscle Relaxants, and Stimulants** During Lunar Months 1–4 Among 50,282 Mother-Child Pairs

	No. of Mother-Child Pairs Exposed	No. of Malformed Children	Crude Relative Risk	Hospital Standardized Relative Risk	Survival and Race Standardized Relative Risk
Anesthetics, anticonvulsants, muscle relaxants, and stimulants	2,657	111	0.92	0.88	0.90
Local anesthetics	2,165	87	0.88	0.84	0.87
Procaine	1,340	49	0.80	0.77	0.78
Local anesthetic, n.o.s.	386	15	0.86	0.83	0.84
Lidocaine	293	8	0.60	0.54	0.59
Mepivacaine	82	8	2.16	1.96	2.46[1]
Benzocaine	47	4	1.88	1.82	1.60
Propoxycaine	41	4	2.16	1.89	1.82
Tetracaine	23	1	0.96	0.92	0.96
Other local anesthetics	30	2	1.47	1.39	1.84
General anesthetics and oxygen	218	7	0.71	0.69	0.76
General anesthetic, n.o.s.	98	3	0.68	0.66	0.68
Nitrous oxide	76	3	0.87	0.83	0.96
Oxygen	52	0	—	—	—
Halothane	25	2	1.77	1.80	2.01
Other general anesthetics	39	1	0.57	0.54	0.67
Non-barbiturate anticonvulsants	151	11	1.61	1.64	1.48
Phenytoin	132	8	1.34	1.35	1.15
Other non-barbiturate anticonvulsants	34	4	2.60	2.81	2.46
Central nervous system stimulants	60	4	1.47	1.47	1.29
Lobelia	38	2	1.16	1.14	1.01
Other central nervous system stimulants	22	2	2.01	2.05	1.87
Muscle relaxants	83	2	0.53	0.50	0.56
Succinylcholine	26	0	—	—	—
Methocarbamol	22	0	—	—	—
Other centrally acting muscle relaxants	29	2	1.52	1.47	1.72
Other neuromuscular blockers	13	0	—	—	—
Smooth muscle stimulants	57	3	1.16	1.12	1.21
Ergotamine	25	2	1.77	1.74	2.22
Other ergot derivatives	32	1	0.69	0.66	0.63
Other smooth muscle stimulants	1	0	—	—	—

[1] $X^2_1 = 4.53$, $p < 0.05$

Table **26.3**

Standardized Relative Risks (SRR) and Their 95% Confidence Intervals (CI$_{95}$) for Classes of Malformations Showing Uniform Rates by Hospital in Relation to **Anesthetics, Anticonvulsants, Muscle Relaxants, and Stimulants** Used in Lunar Months 1–4 by 2,657 Pregnant Women (Based on Multiple Logistic Risk Function Analysis)

| | No. of Malformed Children | | | |
Malformation Classes	Observed	Expected	SRR	CI$_{95}$ of SRR
Any malformation	111	128.6	0.86	0.71–1.05
Major malformations	73	84.2	0.87	0.68–1.10
Minor malformations	37	45.2	0.82	0.58–1.16
Central nervous	11	16.4	0.67	0.33–1.20
Cardiovascular	20	22.5	0.89	0.54–1.37
Musculoskeletal (other than polydactyly in Blacks)	18	23.2	0.78	0.46–1.22
Polydactyly in Blacks[1]	13	12.5	1.04	0.55–1.77
Respiratory	16	12.3	1.30	0.74–2.10
Gastrointestinal	12	19.7	0.61	0.32–1.06
Genitourinary (other than hypospadias)	9	11.0	0.82	0.38–1.55
Hypospadias[2]	9	10.1	0.89	0.41–1.69
Eye and ear	9	6.7	1.34	0.61–2.53
Syndromes (other than Down syndrome)	4	7.4	0.54	0.15–1.38
Down syndrome	0	3.1	—	0.00–1.18
Tumors	9	10.5	0.86	0.39–1.63

[1]Drugs used by 890 Blacks
[2]Drugs used by 1,391 mothers of male offspring

(2.66), genitourinary malformations other than hypospadias (2.12, based on three malformed children), and hypospadias (1.64, based on two malformed children).

Lidocaine — 293 Exposures (Table 26.7) There was no evidence of an association of this drug with broad classes of malformations. SRRs greater than 1.5 were found for the following malformations: respiratory tract (2.02, based on three malformed children), and tumors (1.89, based on two malformed children).

General Anesthetics and Oxygen — 218 Exposures (Table 26.8)

There was no evidence of any association between this group or any of its components and any class of malformations or individual defect.

Nonbarbiturate Anticonvulsants — 151 Exposures (Table 26.9)

In view of the condition for which these drugs are principally used, the rela-

tive risks calculated by the multiple logistic risk function approach are appreciably lower than the crude relative risks or those derived by the simpler standardization technique. The SRR for any malformations was thus 0.94.

Detailed Evaluation of Non-Uniform Malformations: Inguinal Hernia, Clubfoot, Pectus Excavatum

In this section, the three outcomes are evaluated as in the preceding section dealing with uniform malformations. Instances in which there were fewer than three malformed children exposed to any drug are omitted because they are not informative.

As indicated in Table 26.10, the only SRR greater than 1.5 for inguinal hernia was with lidocaine (1.78). The SRRs for clubfoot were all below unity, while the highest SRR for pectus excavatum was with procaine (1.20).

Table **26.4**

Standardized Relative Risks (SRR) and Their 95% Confidence Intervals (CI$_{95}$) for Classes of Malformations Showing Uniform Rates by Hospital in Relation to **Local Anesthetics** Used in Lunar Months 1–4 by 2,165 Pregnant Women (Based on Multiple Logistic Risk Function Analysis)

| | No. of Malformed Children | | | |
Malformation Classes	Observed	Expected	SRR	CI$_{95}$ of SRR
Any malformation	87	101.0	0.86	0.69–1.07
Major malformations	55	65.0	0.85	0.64–1.12
Minor malformations	32	36.0	0.89	0.62–1.27
Central nervous	6	12.2	0.49	0.18–1.07
Cardiovascular	17	18.0	0.94	0.55–1.51
Musculoskeletal (other than polydactyly in Blacks)	13	21.2	0.61	0.33–1.05
Polydactyly in Blacks[1]	10	9.4	1.06	0.51–1.94
Respiratory	13	9.5	1.37	0.73–2.34
Gastrointestinal	11	15.1	0.73	0.36–1.30
Genitourinary (other than hypospadias)	8	9.1	0.88	0.38–1.73
Hypospadias[2]	8	8.1	0.99	0.43–1.94
Eye and ear	7	5.4	1.29	0.52–2.66
Syndromes (other than Down syndrome)	4	6.0	0.66	0.18–1.70
Down syndrome	0	2.4	—	0.00–1.54
Tumors	8	7.8	1.03	0.44–2.02

[1]Drugs used by 666 Blacks
[2]Drugs used by 1,123 mothers of male offspring

Table **26.5**

Standardized Relative Risks (SRR) and Their 95% Confidence Intervals (CI$_{95}$) for Classes of Malformations Showing Uniform Rates by Hospital in Relation to **Procaine** Used in Lunar Months 1–4 by 1,340 Pregnant Women (Based on Multiple Logistic Risk Function Analysis)

| | No. of Malformed Children | | | |
Malformation Classes	Observed	Expected	SRR	CI$_{95}$ of SRR
Any malformation	49	62.0	0.79	0.58–1.07
Major malformations	32	41.1	0.78	0.53–1.14
Minor malformations	16	19.9	0.80	0.46–1.30
Central nervous	3	7.5	0.40	0.08–1.16
Cardiovascular	9	11.0	0.81	0.37–1.54
Musculoskeletal (other than polydactyly in Blacks)	8	14.0	0.57	0.25–1.12
Polydactyly in Blacks[1]	4	3.2	1.24	0.34–3.15
Respiratory	5	5.8	0.86	0.28–2.00
Gastrointestinal	6	9.4	0.64	0.23–1.38
Genitourinary (other than hypospadias)	3	5.5	0.55	0.11–1.59
Hypospadias[2]	5	5.3	0.95	0.31–2.21
Eye and ear	6	3.3	1.79	0.66–3.88
Syndromes (other than Down syndrome)	4	3.5	1.16	0.32–2.95
Down syndrome	0	1.5	—	0.00–2.49
Tumors	4	4.9	0.82	0.22–2.10

[1]Drugs used by 268 Blacks
[2]Drugs used by 705 mothers of male offspring

Table **26.6**

Standardized Relative Risks (SRR) and Their 95% Confidence Intervals (CI$_{95}$) for Classes of Malformations Showing Uniform Rates by Hospital in Relation to **Local Anesthetics, n.o.s.,** Used in Lunar Months 1–4 by 386 Pregnant Women (Based on Multiple Logistic Risk Function Analysis)

Malformation Classes	No. of Malformed Children		SRR	CI$_{95}$ of SRR
	Observed	Expected		
Any malformation	15	17.8	0.84	0.47–1.37
Major malformations	7	10.2	0.68	0.28–1.40
Minor malformations	10	8.2	1.23	0.59–2.23
Central nervous	1	1.9	0.52	0.01–2.88
Cardiovascular	2	3.1	0.64	0.08–2.31
Musculoskeletal (other than polydactyly in Blacks)	1	2.5	0.40	0.01–2.20
Polydactyly in Blacks[1]	4	4.3	0.93	0.25–2.35
Respiratory	4	1.5	2.66	0.73–6.76
Gastrointestinal	3	2.2	1.40	0.29–4.05
Genitourinary (other than hypospadias)	3	1.4	2.12	0.44–6.15
Hypospadias[2]	2	1.2	1.64	0.20–5.84
Eye and ear	0	0.9	—	0.00–3.93
Syndromes (other than Down syndrome)	0	0.9	—	0.00–4.22
Down syndrome	0	0.4	—	0.00–8.62
Tumors	0	1.3	—	0.00–2.83

[1]Drugs used by 273 Blacks
[2]Drugs used by 186 mothers of male offspring

Table **26.7**

Standardized Relative Risks (SRR) and Their 95% Confidence Intervals (CI$_{95}$) for Classes of Malformations Showing Uniform Rates by Hospital in Relation to **Lidocaine** Used in Lunar Months 1–4 by 293 Pregnant Women (Based on Multiple Logistic Risk Function Analysis)

Malformation Classes	No. of Malformed Children		SRR	CI$_{95}$ of SRR
	Observed	Expected		
Any malformation	8	14.3	0.56	0.24– 1.08
Major malformations	4	9.0	0.44	0.12– 1.12
Minor malformations	3	5.3	0.56	0.12– 1.62
Central nervous	1	1.9	0.52	0.01– 2.86
Cardiovascular	0	2.4	—	0.00– 1.50
Musculoskeletal (other than polydactyly in Blacks)	1	2.9	0.34	0.01– 1.89
Polydactyly in Blacks[1]	1	1.4	0.74	0.02– 4.03
Respiratory	3	1.5	2.02	0.42– 5.85
Gastrointestinal	0	2.4	—	0.00– 1.52
Genitourinary (other than hypospadias)	2	1.5	1.30	0.16– 4.64
Hypospadias[2]	0	1.2	—	0.00– 3.08
Eye and ear	0	0.8	—	0.00– 4.84
Syndromes (other than Down syndrome)	0	1.3	—	0.00– 2.90
Down syndrome	0	0.3	—	0.00–11.71
Tumors	2	1.1	1.89	0.23– 6.75

[1]Drugs used by 88 Blacks
[2]Drugs used by 161 mothers of male offspring

Table **26.8**

Standardized Relative Risks (SRR) and Their 95% Confidence Intervals (CI$_{95}$) for Broad Classes of Malformations Showing Uniform Rates by Hospital in Relation to **General Anesthetics and Oxygen** Used in Lunar Months 1–4 by 218 Pregnant Women (Based on Multiple Logistic Risk Function Analysis)

| | No. of Malformed Children | | | |
	Observed	Expected	SRR	CI$_{95}$ of SRR
Any malformation	7	10.0	0.71	0.29–1.43
Major malformations	4	6.1	0.66	0.18–1.66
Minor malformations	3	3.8	0.78	0.16–2.26

Table **26.9**

Standardized Relative Risks (SRR) and Their 95% Confidence Intervals (CI$_{95}$) for Broad Classes of Malformations Showing Uniform Rates by Hospital in Relation to **Nonbarbiturate Anticonvulsants** Used in Lunar Months 1–4 by 151 Pregnant Women (Based on Multiple Logistic Risk Function Analysis)

| | No. of Malformed Children | | | |
	Observed	Expected	SRR	CI$_{95}$ of SRR
Any malformation	11	11.7	0.94	0.48–1.63
Major malformations	9	9.6	0.94	0.44–1.73
Minor malformations	1	2.8	0.36	0.01–1.99

Comments

There was no evidence to suggest that exposure early in pregnancy to local anesthetics was related to an increased risk of any particular malformation. Procaine was received by 1,340 women; the confidence limits around the relative risks for the larger outcomes were reasonably narrow and the data suggest that this agent is unlikely to have a powerful teratogenic effect.

Data for exposure to general anesthesia were relatively sparse, but, again, there was no hint of teratogenicity.

The non-barbiturate anticonvulsants — principally phenytoin, 132 exposures — are of interest. The initial comparisons which did not standardize for the influence of epilepsy in the mother suggested an approximate twofold increase in the risk. Once the influence of all identified risk factors for malformations, including maternal epilepsy, was controlled, the relative risk estimates for uniform malformations, major malformations, and minor malformations were reduced to approximately unity or less. Elsewhere, we have published more detailed data suggesting that the determinant of malformations may be parental epilepsy (in either the mother or the father), rather

Table **26.10**

Standardized Relative Risks (SRR) and Their 95% Confidence Intervals (CI_{95}) for Inguinal Hernia, Clubfoot, and Pectus Excavatum in Relation to **Anesthetics, Anticonvulsants, Muscle Relaxants, and Stimulants** Used in Lunar Months 1–4 (Based on Multiple Logistic Risk Function Analysis)

	No. of Users	No. of Malformed Children		SRR	CI_{95} of SRR
		Observed	Expected		
Inguinal hernia					
Anticonvulsants, anesthetics, muscle relaxants, and stimulants	2657	48	37.9	1.27	0.99–1.62
Local anesthetics	2165	36	30.3	1.19	0.88–1.59
Procaine	1340	23	18.2	1.26	0.88–1.81
Local anesthetics, n.o.s.	386	5	5.6	0.89	0.29–2.06
Lidocaine	293	8	4.5	1.78	0.77–3.46
Clubfoot					
Anesthetics, anticonvulsants, muscle relaxants, and stimulants	2657	9	11.4	0.79	0.36–1.50
Local anesthetics	2165	7	9.2	0.76	0.30–1.56
Procaine	1340	3	5.4	0.56	0.12–1.63
Pectus excavatum					
Anesthetics, anticonvulsants, muscle relaxants, and stimulants	2657	9	8.9	1.01	0.46–1.91
Local anesthetics	2165	8	7.0	1.15	0.50–2.26
Procaine	1340	5	4.2	1.20	0.39–2.78

than its treatment.[1] The findings with regard to phenytoin do not accord with experimental work[2,3] or with a number of epidemiological studies in humans.[4] Some of the latter studies, however, compared children born to treated epileptics with children born to non-epileptic controls.

Data for central nervous stimulants, muscle relaxants, and smooth muscle stimulants were scanty, but no evidence of teratogenic effects was apparent.

CHAPTER 27

Caffeine and Other Xanthine Derivatives

General Evaluation

In Table 27.1, all 3,248 malformed children are considered in relation to exposure to the entire group of caffeine and other xanthine derivatives during the first four lunar months of pregnancy. In Table 27.2, the data are confined to the 2,277 children who had malformations which were uniformly distributed among the hospitals. Three relative risks are given in each table: crude, standardized for hospital variability, and standardized for the mother's ethnic group and survival of the child.

All Malformations in Relation
to Caffeine and Other
Xanthine Derivatives (Table 27.1)
The hospital-standardized relative risk for any malformation associated with this group of drugs as a whole was 0.98. The largest relative risk was for theophylline, with 117 exposures (1.38).

Malformations with Uniform
Rates by Hospital in Relation
to Caffeine and Other
Xanthine Derivatives (Table 27.2)
The relative risks presented in this table were all close to unity.

Detailed Evaluation of Uniform Malformations

In this section, groups of drugs, followed by individual drugs, are evaluated

Table **27.1**

Children (3,248) With Any Malformation in Relation to Exposure to **Caffeine and Other Xanthine Derivatives** During Lunar Months 1–4 Among 50,282 Mother-Child Pairs

	No. of Mother-Child Pairs Exposed	No. of Malformed Children	Crude Relative Risk	Hospital Standardized Relative Risk[1]	Survival and Race Standardized Relative Risk[1]
Caffeine and other xanthine derivatives	5,773	380	1.02	0.98	0.99
Caffeine	5,378	350	1.01	0.97	0.98
Chlorotheophylline (dimenhydrinate)	319	24	1.17	1.14	1.24
Theophylline	117	10	1.32	1.38	1.29
Aminophylline	76	6	1.22	1.20	1.20
Other xanthine derivatives[2]	4	0	—	—	—

[1] Estimated by the Mantel-Haenszel procedure
[2] Theobromine (3); ambuphylline (1)

Table **27.2**

Children (2,277) With Malformations Showing Uniform Rates by Hospital in Relation to Exposure to **Caffeine and Other Xanthine Derivatives** During Lunar Months 1–4 Among 50,282 Mother-Child Pairs

	No. of Mother-Child Pairs Exposed	No. of Malformed Children	Crude Relative Risk	Hospital Standardized Relative Risk	Survival and Race Standardized Relative Risk
Caffeine and other xanthine derivatives	5,773	254	0.97	0.93	0.95
Caffeine	5,378	239	0.98	0.95	0.96
Chlorotheophylline (dimenhydrinate)	319	13	0.90	0.86	0.94
Theophylline	117	5	0.94	0.96	0.84
Aminophylline	76	4	1.16	1.13	1.11
Other xanthine derivatives	4	0	—	—	—

in relation to various classes or groups of uniform malformations, as well as individual malformations, for which multiple logistic risk function models were developed. In the tables, the observed and expected numbers of malformed children are given for each drug exposure in turn. The measure of association presented is a standardized relative risk (SRR) with its 95% confidence limits. The SRR is the ratio of the observed number to the expected number of malformed children. Since the SRR takes into account potential confounding variables, it represents the best estimate of the relationship between a drug and a malformation. As numbers of exposed mother-child pairs becomes so small as to be uninformative, data will be omitted.

Caffeine and Other Xanthine Derivatives — 5,773 Exposures (Table 27.3)

There was no evidence of association of the drug group as a whole with broad classes or with specific classes of malformations. The highest SRR among the malformations was 1.16 for Down syndrome.

Caffeine — 5,378 Exposures (Table 27.4) This preparation comprises 93% of the entire drug group. There was no evidence of association with either broad classes or with specific classes of malformations.

Chlorotheophylline — 319 Exposures (Table 27.5) The relative risks for broad classes of malformations were all close to or below unity. Among specific classes of malformations, SRRs greater than 1.5

were found for cardiovascular malformations (2.01) and Down syndrome (2.05, based on 1 malformed child).

Detailed Evaluation of Non-Uniform Malformations: Inguinal Hernia, Clubfoot, Pectus Excavatum

In this section, the three outcomes are evaluated as in the preceding section dealing with uniform malformations. Instances in which there were fewer than three malformed children exposed to any drug are omitted because they are not informative.

Table 27.6 indicates that the only SRR greater than 1.5 for inguinal hernia was with chlorotheophylline (2.00). This also held true for clubfoot, where the corresponding SRR was 1.99. There was no evidence of association of caffeine and other xanthine derivatives with pectus excavatum.

Table **27.3**

Standardized Relative Risks (SRR) and Their 95% Confidence Intervals (CI$_{95}$) for Classes of Malformations Showing Uniform Rates by Hospital in Relation to **Caffeine and Other Xanthine Derivatives** Used in Lunar Months 1–4 by 5,773 Pregnant Women (Based on Multiple Logistic Risk Function Analysis)

Malformation Classes	No. of Malformed Children		SRR	CI$_{95}$ of SRR
	Observed	Expected		
Any malformation	254	266.8	0.95	0.85–1.07
Major malformations	158	156.7	1.01	0.87–1.17
Minor malformations	101	111.0	0.91	0.75–1.10
Central nervous	27	29.8	0.91	0.62–1.32
Cardiovascular	41	47.3	0.87	0.63–1.18
Musculoskeletal (other than polydactyly in Blacks)	42	45.0	0.93	0.69–1.26
Polydactyly in Blacks[1]	48	46.0	1.04	0.81–1.35
Respiratory	27	24.5	1.10	0.79–1.54
Gastrointestinal	41	36.3	1.13	0.86–1.48
Genitourinary (other than hypospadias)	18	22.2	0.81	0.48–1.28
Hypospadias[2]	20	20.2	0.99	0.61–1.53
Eye and ear	10	14.3	0.70	0.34–1.28
Syndromes (other than Down syndrome)	14	14.4	0.97	0.53–1.63
Down syndrome	8	6.9	1.16	0.50–2.28
Tumors	15	21.2	0.71	0.40–1.16

[1]Drugs used by 3,307 Blacks
[2]Drugs used by 2,937 mothers of male offspring

Table **27.4**

Standardized Relative Risks (SRR) and Their 95% Confidence Intervals (CI$_{95}$) for Classes of Malformations Showing Uniform Rates by Hospital in Relation to **Caffeine** Used in Lunar Months 1–4 by 5,378 Pregnant Women (Based on Multiple Logistic Risk Function Analysis)

Malformation Classes	No. of Malformed Children		SRR	CI$_{95}$ of SRR
	Observed	Expected		
Any malformation	239	248.5	0.96	0.85–1.09
Major malformations	148	145.0	1.02	0.88–1.19
Minor malformations	95	104.2	0.91	0.75–1.11
Central nervous	26	27.4	0.95	0.65–1.38
Cardiovascular	34	43.9	0.77	0.54–1.12
Musculoskeletal (other than polydactyly in Blacks)	40	41.3	0.97	0.72–1.31
Polydactyly in Blacks[1]	45	43.8	1.03	0.78–1.34
Respiratory	26	22.8	1.14	0.81–1.60
Gastrointestinal	39	33.6	1.16	0.88–1.53
Genitourinary (other than hypospadias)	17	20.3	0.84	0.49–1.34
Hypospadias[2]	20	19.0	1.05	0.64–1.62
Eye and ear	10	13.1	0.76	0.37–1.40
Syndromes (other than Down syndrome)	13	13.4	0.97	0.52–1.66
Down syndrome	7	6.3	1.11	0.45–2.29
Tumors	13	19.6	0.66	0.35–1.13

[1]Drugs used by 3,158 Blacks
[2]Drugs used by 2,741 mothers of male offspring

Table **27.5**

Standardized Relative Risks (SRR) and Their 95% Confidence Intervals (CI$_{95}$) for Classes of Malformations Showing Uniform Rates by Hospital in Relation to **Chlorotheophylline (Dimenhydrinate)** Used in Lunar Months 1–4 by 319 Pregnant Women (Based on Multiple Logistic Risk Function Analysis)

Malformation Classes	No. of Malformed Children		SRR	CI$_{95}$ of SRR
	Observed	Expected		
Any malformation	13	14.3	0.91	0.49– 1.53
Major malformations	11	9.3	1.19	0.60– 2.10
Minor malformations	4	5.1	0.78	0.21– 1.98
Central nervous	2	1.8	1.08	0.13– 3.87
Cardiovascular	5	2.5	2.01	0.65– 4.65
Musculoskeletal (other than polydactyly in Blacks)	2	3.2	0.63	0.08– 2.25
Polydactyly in Blacks[1]	1	1.2	0.80	0.02– 4.35
Respiratory	2	1.4	1.41	0.17– 5.04
Gastrointestinal	3	2.5	1.22	0.25– 3.54
Genitourinary (other than hypospadias)	2	1.5	1.33	0.16– 4.76
Hypospadias[2]	1	0.9	1.05	0.03– 5.78
Eye and ear	0	1.0	—	0.00– 3.84
Syndromes (other than Down syndrome)	1	0.8	1.29	0.03– 7.12
Down syndrome	1	0.5	2.05	0.05–11.35
Tumors	0	1.4	—	0.00– 2.66

[1]Drugs used by 101 Blacks
[2]Drugs used by 161 mothers of male offspring

Table **27.6**

Standardized Relative Risks (SRR) and Their 95% Confidence Intervals (CI$_{95}$) for Inguinal Hernia, Clubfoot, and Pectus Excavatum in Relation to **Caffeine and Other Xanthine Derivatives** Used in Lunar Months 1–4 (Based on Multiple Logistic Risk Function Analysis)

| | No. of Users | No. of Malformed Children | | SRR | CI$_{95}$ of SRR |
		Observed	Expected		
Inguinal hernia					
Caffeine and other xanthine derivatives	5773	78	85.2	0.92	0.74–1.14
Caffeine	5378	68	80.1	0.85	0.67–1.08
Chlorotheophylline	319	8	4.0	2.00	0.87–3.90
Clubfoot					
Caffeine and other xanthine derivatives	5773	31	23.7	1.31	0.97–1.75
Caffeine	5378	26	21.9	1.19	0.85–1.67
Chlorotheophylline	319	3	1.5	1.99	0.41–5.78
Pectus excavatum					
Caffeine and other xanthine derivatives	5773	14	14.3	0.98	0.54–1.64
Caffeine	5378	14	13.1	1.07	0.58–1.79

Comments

Caffeine and other xanthine derivatives gave no evidence of a teratogenic effect. For the large number of exposures to caffeine (5,773), in particular, it was possible to confidently rule out an association with most malformation outcomes of reasonable size. Caffeine was usually taken as an ingredient in medications also containing aspirin and phenacetin. In Appendix 4, it can be seen that the association of this drug and craniosynostosis was also present for aspirin and phenacetin. This was due to overlapping of the three drugs. The absence of evidence linking caffeine to malformations should be interpreted with caution since it can be assumed that most of the women drank coffee.

Based on small numbers, chlorotheophylline (319 exposures) was associated with cardiovascular defects and with inguinal hernia. This drug gave no evidence of being related to other outcomes.

Data for aminophylline were sparse (76 exposures), but there was no evidence of association with malformations in general.

CHAPTER 28

Diuretics and Drugs Taken for Cardiovascular Disorders

General Evaluation

In this section, data are presented for two malformation groups — all 3,248 malformed children and the 2,277 children with uniform malformation rates by hospital. Crude relative risks and two Mantel-Haenszel summary relative risks for these malformations are presented for the total group of diuretics and drugs taken for cardiovascular disorders; for the subgroups diuretics, antihypertensive agents, vasodilators, and digitalis glycosides; and for the individual drugs making up the subgroups. One Mantel-Haenszel estimate standardizes for hospital, the other for survival of the child together with ethnic group of the mother.

All Malformations in Relation
to Diuretics and Drugs
Taken for Cardiovascular
Disorders (Table 28.1)

The hospital-standardized relative risk for any malformation for diuretics and drugs taken for cardiovascular disorders was 1.32. The relative risks for chlorthalidone (2.19), mercury diuretics (3.62), other thiazide diuretics (2.07), vasodilators (2.53), vasodilators other than ethyl nitrite (5.08), and digitalis glycosides (1.54), exceeded 1.5. The association with vasodilators other than ethyl nitrite was significant at the 0.02 level.

371

Table **28.1**

Children (3,248) With Any Malformation in Relation to Exposure to **Diuretics and Drugs Taken for Cardiovascular Disorders** During Lunar Months 1–4 Among 50,282 Mother-Child Pairs

	No. of Mother-Child Pairs Exposed	No. of Malformed Children	Crude Relative Risk	Hospital Standardized Relative Risk[1]	Survival and Race Standardized Relative Risk[1]
Diuretics and drugs taken for cardiovascular disorders	392	35	1.39	1.32	1.33
Diuretics	280	23	1.27	1.18	1.23
Hydrochlorothiazide	107	9	1.30	1.20	1.16
Chlorothiazide	63	5	1.23	1.16	1.28
Diuretic, n.o.s.	38	1	0.41	0.39	0.40
Chlorthalidone	20	3	2.32	2.19	2.42
Mercury diuretics[4]	14	3	3.32	3.62	4.25
Carbonic anhydrase inhibitors[5]	13	0	—	—	—
Other thiazide diuretics[6]	35	5	2.21	2.07	2.32
Other miscellaneous diuretics[7]	13	0	—	—	—
Antihypertensive agents	53	5	1.46	1.41	1.45
Reserpine and other rauwolfia alkaloids	48	4	1.29	1.24	1.23
Other antihypertensive agents[8]	13	1	1.19	1.13	1.34
Vasodilators	39	6	2.38	2.53	2.45
Ethyl nitrite	24	2	1.29	1.25	1.00
Other vasodilators[9]	15	4	4.13[2]	5.08[3]	6.03[3]
Digitalis glycosides	52	5	1.49	1.54	1.42

[1]Estimated by the Mantel-Haenszel procedure
[2]$p < 0.05$
[3]$X_1^2 = 6.56–8.69$, $p < 0.02$
[4]Mercaptomerin (7); meralluride (5); mersalyl (2)
[5]Acetazolamide (12); ethoxyzolamide (1)
[6]Bendroflumethiazide (13); polythiazide (10); benzthiazide (5); methyclothiazide (3); trichloromethiazide (2); cyclothiazide (1); hydroflumethiazide (1); flumethiazide (1)
[7]Quinethazone (8); triamterene (5)
[8]Hydralazine (8); guanethidine (2); methyldopa (1); protoveratrine A & B (1); mecamylamine (1); phentolamine (1);
[9]Nitroglycerin and amyl nitrite (7); pentaerythritol tetranitrate (3); papaverine (2); tolazoline (2); nicotinyl alcohol (1)

Malformations with Uniform Rates by Hospital in Relation to Diuretics and Drugs Taken for Cardiovascular Disorders (Table 28.2)

The hospital-standardized relative risk for the drug group as a whole was 1.37. The highest relative risk for an individual drug was 3.10 for vasodilators other than ethyl nitrite, based on 2 exposed-malformed children. Other hospital-standardized relative risks greater than 1.5 were seen for chlorthalidone (2.17), mercury diuretics (1.56), other thiazide diuretics (1.76), antihypertensive agents (2.06), reserpine and other rauwolfia alkaloids (1.79), other antihypertensive agents (1.67), vasodilators (2.30), and ethyl nitrite (1.82). Most of the findings

Table **28.2**

Children (2,277) With Malformations Showing Uniform Rates by Hospital in Relation to Exposure to **Diuretics and Drugs Taken for Cardiovascular Disorders** During Lunar Months 1–4 Among 50,282 Mother-Child Pairs

	No. of Mother-Child Pairs Exposed	No. of Malformed Children	Crude Relative Risk	Hospital Standardized Relative Risk	Survival and Race Standardized Relative Risk
Diuretics and drugs taken for cardiovascular disorders	392	25	1.41	1.37	1.30
Diuretics	280	15	1.18	1.13	1.09
Hydrochlorothiazide	107	7	1.45	1.37	1.21
Chlorothiazide	63	2	0.70	0.67	0.72
Diuretic, n.o.s.	38	1	0.58	0.57	0.57
Chlorthalidone	20	2	2.21	2.17	2.06
Mercury diuretics	14	1	1.58	1.56	1.58
Carbonic anhydrase inhibitors	13	0	—	—	—
Other thiazide diuretics	36	3	1.84	1.76	1.77
Other miscellaneous diuretics	13	0	—	—	—
Antihypertensive agents	53	5	2.09	2.06	2.14
Reserpine and other rauwolfia alkaloids	48	4	1.84	1.79	1.82
Other antihypertensive agents	13	1	1.70	1.67	2.12
Vasodilators	39	4	2.27	2.30	2.20
Ethyl nitrite	24	2	1.84	1.82	1.42
Other vasodilators	15	2	2.95	3.10	3.94
Digitalis glycosides	52	2	0.85	0.84	0.73

were based on three or fewer exposed-malformed children.

Detailed Evaluation of Uniform Malformations

In this section, groups of drugs, followed by individual drugs, are evaluated in relation to various classes or groups of uniform malformations, as well as individual malformations, for which multiple logistic risk function models were developed. In the tables, the observed and expected numbers of malformed children are given for each drug exposure in turn. The measure of association presented is a standardized relative risk (SRR) with its 95% confidence limits. The SRR is the ratio of the observed number to the expected number of malformed children. Since the SRR takes into account potential confounding variables, it represents the best estimate of the relationship between a drug and a malformation. As numbers of exposed mother-child pairs become so small as to be uninformative, data will be omitted.

Diuretics and Drugs Taken for Cardiovascular Disorders — 392 Exposures (Table 28.3)

There was no evidence of association between the drug group as a whole and broad classes of malformations. SRRs exceeding 1.5 were found for musculoskeletal malformations other than

Table **28.3**

Standardized Relative Risks (SRR) and Their 95% Confidence Intervals (CI$_{95}$) for Classes of Malformations Showing Uniform Rates by Hospital in Relation to **Diuretics and Drugs Taken for Cardiovascular Disorders** Used in Lunar Months 1–4 by 392 Pregnant Women (Based on Multiple Logistic Risk Function Analysis)

| Malformation Classes | No. of Malformed Children | | SRR | CI$_{95}$ of SRR |
	Observed	Expected		
Any malformation	25	24.0	1.04	0.72–1.50
Major malformations	19	17.9	1.06	0.64–1.63
Minor malformations	10	8.8	1.14	0.55–2.07
Central nervous	4	3.7	1.08	0.30–2.74
Cardiovascular	5	5.7	0.88	0.29–2.05
Musculoskeletal (other than polydactyly in Blacks)	8	5.3	1.51	0.65–2.95
Polydactyly in Blacks[1]	3	2.2	1.34	0.28–3.84
Respiratory	5	3.4	1.48	0.48–3.44
Gastrointestinal	6	4.3	1.40	0.51–3.01
Genitourinary (other than hypospadias)	7	3.4	2.03	0.82–4.14
Hypospadias[2]	0	1.4	—	0.00–2.59
Eye and ear	0	1.3	—	0.00–2.79
Syndromes (other than Down syndrome)	2	1.9	1.07	0.13–3.84
Down syndrome	0	1.0	—	0.00–3.58
Tumors	3	2.1	1.43	0.30–4.15

[1]Drugs used by 155 Blacks
[2]Drugs used by 203 mothers of male offspring

polydactyly in Blacks (1.51), and genitourinary system malformations other than hypospadias (2.03).

Diuretics — 280 Exposures
(Table 28.4)

Diuretics accounted for about 70% of the exposures to the group of drugs described in this chapter. There was no evidence of association with broad classes of malformations. SRRs greater than 1.5 were seen for respiratory tract (1.98), genitourinary malformations other than hypospadias (1.99), and syndromes other than Down syndrome (1.77, based on two malformed children).

Antihypertensive Agents —
53 Exposures (Table 28.5)

The SRR for any malformation was 1.31.

Detailed Evaluation of Non-Uniform Malformations: Inguinal Hernia, Clubfoot, Pectus Excavatum

In this section, the three outcomes are evaluated as in the preceding section dealing with uniform malformations. Instances in which there were fewer than three malformed children exposed to any drug are omitted because they are not informative.

As seen in Table 28.6, the highest SRR for inguinal hernia was with diuretics (1.33). For clubfoot, the SRRs with the drug group as a whole (2.15) and diuretics (2.75) both exceeded 1.5. Numbers were too small to identify any association with pectus excavatum.

Comments

In this study, diuretics and digitalis glycosides were taken in early pregnancy

Table **28.4**

Standardized Relative Risks (SRR) and Their 95% Confidence Intervals (CI$_{95}$) for Classes of Malformations Showing Uniform Rates by Hospital in Relation to **Diuretics** Used in Lunar Months 1–4 by 280 Pregnant Women (Based on Multiple Logistic Risk Function Analysis)

Malformation Classes	No. of Malformed Children		SRR	CI$_{95}$ of SRR
	Observed	Expected		
Any malformation	15	16.5	0.91	0.15–1.47
Major malformations	12	12.6	0.96	0.50–1.64
Minor malformations	6	5.5	1.09	0.40–2.35
Central nervous	4	3.7	1.08	0.30–2.74
Cardiovascular	3	3.8	0.79	0.16–2.28
Musculoskeletal (other than polydactyly in Blacks)	5	3.9	1.28	0.42–2.96
Polydactyly in Blacks[1]	2	1.4	1.48	0.18–5.22
Respiratory	4	2.0	1.98	0.54–5.02
Gastrointestinal	3	2.6	1.16	0.24–3.37
Genitourinary (other than hypospadias)	4	2.0	1.99	0.54–5.04
Hypospadias[2]	0	0.9	—	0.00–4.09
Eye and ear	0	0.9	—	0.00–4.01
Syndromes (other than Down syndrome)	2	1.1	1.77	0.21–6.32
Down syndrome	0	0.7	—	0.00–5.57
Tumors	1	1.5	0.67	0.02–3.69

[1]Drugs used by 103 Blacks
[2]Drugs used by 146 mothers of male offspring

Table **28.5**

Standardized Relative Risks (SRR) and Their 95% Confidence Intervals (CI$_{95}$) for Broad Classes of Malformations Showing Uniform Rates by Hospital in Relation to **Antihypertensive Agents** Used in Lunar Months 1–4 by 53 Pregnant Women (Based on Multiple Logistic Risk Function Analysis)

	No. of Malformed Children		SRR	CI$_{95}$ of SRR
	Observed	Expected		
Any malformation	5	3.8	1.31	0.43–2.86
Major malformations	3	2.7	1.11	0.23–3.07
Minor malformations	2	1.8	1.09	0.13–3.73

Table **28.6**

Standardized Relative Risks (SRR) and Their 95% Confidence Intervals (CI$_{95}$) for Inguinal Hernia Clubfoot, and Pectus Excavatum in Relation to **Diuretics and Drugs Taken for Cardiovascular Disorders** Used in Lunar Months 1–4 (Based on Multiple Logistic Risk Function Analysis)

| | No. of Users | No. of Malformed Children | | SRR | CI$_{95}$ of SRR |
		Observed	Expected		
Inguinal hernia					
Diuretics and drugs taken for					
cardiovascular disorders	392	8	6.9	1.16	0.50–2.26
Diuretics	280	6	4.5	1.33	0.49–2.87
Clubfoot					
Diuretics and drugs taken for					
cardiovascular disorders	392	5	2.3	2.15	0.70–4.99
Diuretics	280	4	1.5	2.75	0.75–6.96
Pectus excavatum	—	—	—	—	—

predominantly for cardiovascular disorders (diuretic use increased greatly, due to edema, as pregnancy progressed).

Early exposure to diuretics (280 mother-child pairs) gave no evidence of association with any outcomes except respiratory malformations, and numbers were small.

Based on only 48 exposures and 4 malformed children, the relative risk for uniform malformations among children exposed to rauwolfia alkaloids was 1.8. Taken in conjunction with other findings (Appendices 1 and 4), the hypothesis that rauwolfia compounds may be teratogenic deserves further exploration. In animal experiments, reserpine is an established teratogen.[1,2]

With very scanty numbers indeed, vasodilators (39 exposures) were associated with malformations in general and with uniform malformations.

CHAPTER 29

Cough Medicines

General Evaluation

In this section, the first analysis is concerned with the evaluation of all 3,248 malformed children in relation to exposure to all cough medicines during the first four lunar months of pregnancy (Table 29.1). In Table 29.2, only the 2,277 children who had a malformation distributed uniformly among the hospitals are considered. In each of the tables, the exposed and nonexposed children are compared using the crude relative risk, the hospital-standardized relative risks, and the relative risk standardized for ethnic group of the mother and survival status of the child.

All Malformations in Relation
to Cough Medicines (Table 29.1)
The hospital-standardized relative risk for all malformations in relation to all cough medicines was 1.10. The hospital-standardized relative risks for two drugs were greater than 1.5: potassium iodide (1.98) and caramiphen (1.78).

Malformations with Uniform
Rates by Hospital in
Relation to Cough Medicines
(Table 29.2)
The hospital-standardized relative risk for the uniform malformations in relation to all cough medicines was 1.00. Again, the relative risks were greater than 1.5 for potassium iodide (1.56) and caramiphen (1.58).

Table **29.1**

Children (3,248) With Any Malformation in Relation to Exposure to **Cough Medicines** During Lunar Months 1–4 Among 50,282 Mother-Child Pairs

	No. of Mother-Child Pairs Exposed	No. of Malformed Children	Crude Relative Risk	Hospital Standardized Relative Risk[1]	Survival and Race Standardized Relative Risk[1]
Cough medicines	948	71	1.16	1.10	1.14
Expectorants	864	65	1.17	1.12	1.14
Chloroform, p.o.	421	35	1.29	1.25	1.30
Ammonium chloride	365	26	1.10	1.05	1.07
Glyceryl guaiacolate	197	14	1.10	1.03	1.08
Elixir terpin hydrate	146	13	1.38	1.29	1.47
Ipecac	68	5	1.14	1.10	1.02
Potassium iodide	56	7	1.94	1.98	1.72
Other expectorants[2]	30	1	0.52	0.51	0.48
Antitussives	344	29	1.31	1.24	1.28
Dextromethorphan hydrobromide	300	24	1.24	1.18	1.20
Caramiphen	38	5	2.04	1.78	2.34
Other antitussives[3]	8	0	—	—	—
Unspecified cough medicines	55	4	1.13	1.08	1.14

[1]Estimated by the Mantel-Haenszel procedure
[2]Pine tar (14); desmethylemetine (7); scilla (7); euphorbia pilulifera (6); cocillana (2); apomorphine (1)
[3]Benzonatate (2); levopropoxyphene (2); homarylamine (1); chlophedianol (1); pipazethate (1); dimethoxyanate (1)

Detailed Evaluation of Uniform Malformations

In this section, groups of drugs, followed by individual drugs, are evaluated in relation to various classes or groups of uniform malformations, as well as individual malformations, for which multiple logistic risk function models were developed. In the tables, the observed and expected numbers of malformed children are given for each drug exposure in turn. The measure of association presented is a standardized relative risk (SRR) with its 95% confidence limits. The SRR is the ratio of the observed number to the expected number of malformed children. Since the SRR takes into account potential confounding variables, it represents the best estimate of the relationship between a drug and a malformation. As numbers of exposed mother-child pairs become so small as to be uninformative, data will be omitted.

Cough Medicines — 948 Exposures (Table 29.3)

None of the broad classes of malformations was associated with cough medicines. Among the specific classes, the only relative risk greater than 1.5 was 2.00 for eye and ear malformations.

Expectorants — 864 Exposures (Table 29.4)

As shown in the table, none of the major groups of malformations had a relative risk substantially different from 1.0. Among the specific classes, only eye and ear malformations (2.21) had an SRR greater than 1.5.

378

Table **29.2**

Children (2,277) With Malformations Showing Uniform Rates by Hospital in Relation to Exposure to **Cough Medicines** During Lunar Months 1–4 Among 50,282 Mother-Child Pairs

	No. of Mother-Child Pairs Exposed	No. of Malformed Children	Crude Relative Risk	Hospital Standardized Relative Risk	Survival and Race Standardized Relative Risk
Cough medicines	948	45	1.05	1.00	1.00
Expectorants	864	40	1.02	0.98	0.98
Chloroform, p.o.	421	18	0.94	0.90	0.93
Ammonium chloride	365	15	0.91	0.86	0.85
Glyceryl guaiacolate	197	6	0.67	0.63	0.60
Elixir terpin hydrate	146	10	1.51	1.47	1.65
Ipecac	68	2	0.65	0.62	0.55
Potassium iodide	56	4	1.58	1.56	1.26
Other expectorants	30	0	—	—	—
Antitussives	344	20	1.29	1.24	1.25
Dextromethorphan hydrobromide	300	17	1.25	1.21	1.20
Caramiphen	38	3	1.74	1.58	1.88
Other antitussives	8	0	—	—	—
Unspecified cough medicines	55	3	1.20	1.16	1.26

Table **29.3**

Standardized Relative Risks (SRR) and Their 95% Confidence Intervals (CI_{95}) for Classes of Malformations Showing Uniform Rates by Hospital in Relation to **Cough Medicines** Used in Lunar Months 1–4 by 948 Pregnant Women (Based on Multiple Logistic Risk Function Analysis)

	No. of Malformed Children			
Malformation Classes	**Observed**	**Expected**	**SRR**	**CI_{95} of SRR**
Any malformation	45	45.3	0.99	0.75–1.32
Major malformations	29	28.0	1.03	0.73–1.48
Minor malformations	15	18.2	0.82	0.46–1.35
Central nervous	6	5.7	1.06	0.39–2.29
Cardiovascular	8	7.9	1.01	0.44–1.98
Musculoskeletal (other than polydactyly in Blacks)	7	8.5	0.83	0.33–1.70
Polydactyly in Blacks[1]	5	6.5	0.76	0.25–1.77
Respiratory	2	4.9	0.41	0.05–1.47
Gastrointestinal	8	6.6	1.21	0.52–2.38
Genitourinary (other than hypospadias)	4	4.3	0.93	0.25–2.37
Hypospadias[2]	3	3.4	0.88	0.18–2.56
Eye and ear	5	2.5	2.00	0.65–4.65
Syndromes (other than Down syndrome)	1	3.0	0.33	0.01–1.86
Down syndrome	1	1.3	0.76	0.02–4.25
Tumors	5	3.9	1.29	0.42–3.00

[1]Drugs used by 948 Blacks
[2]Drugs used by 481 mothers of male offspring

Table **29.4**

Standardized Relative Risks (SRR) and Their 95% Confidence Intervals (CI$_{95}$) for Classes of Malformations Showing Uniform Rates by Hospital in Relation to **Expectorants** Used in Lunar Months 1–4 by 864 Pregnant Women (Based on Multiple Logistic Risk Function Analysis)

| | No. of Malformed Children | | | |
Malformation Classes	Observed	Expected	SRR	CI$_{95}$ of SRR
Any malformation	40	41.5	0.96	0.71–1.31
Major malformations	25	25.6	0.98	0.66–1.44
Minor malformations	14	16.7	0.84	0.46–1.40
Central nervous	4	5.3	0.76	0.21–1.94
Cardiovascular	7	7.3	0.96	0.39–1.97
Musculoskeletal (other than polydactyly in Blacks)	7	7.6	0.92	0.37–1.88
Polydactyly in Blacks[1]	5	6.1	0.81	0.26–1.88
Respiratory	1	4.5	0.22	0.01–1.24
Gastrointestinal	6	6.0	1.00	0.37–2.17
Genitourinary (other than hypospadias)	3	3.9	0.76	0.16–2.22
Hypospadias[2]	3	3.1	0.97	0.20–2.81
Eye and ear	5	2.3	2.21	0.72–5.14
Syndromes (other than Down syndrome)	1	2.8	0.36	0.01–1.99
Down syndrome	1	1.2	0.81	0.02–4.52
Tumors	4	3.5	1.13	0.31–2.87

[1]Drugs used by 436 Blacks
[2]Drugs used by 442 mothers of male offspring

Table **29.5**

Standardized Relative Risks (SRR) and Their 95% Confidence Intervals (CI$_{95}$) for Broad Classes of Malformations Showing Uniform Rates by Hospital in Relation to **Chloroform, p.o.** Used in Lunar Months 1–4 by 421 Pregnant Women (Based on Multiple Logistic Risk Function Analysis)

| | No. of Malformed Children | | | |
	Observed	Expected	SRR	CI$_{95}$ of SRR
Any malformation	18	19.7	0.91	0.55–1.43
Major malformations	12	11.8	1.02	0.53–1.76
Minor malformations	6	7.8	0.75	0.28–1.62

Chloroform, p.o. — 421 Exposures (Table 29.5) None of the major groups of malformations was associated with exposure to chloroform, p.o.

Ammonium Chloride — 365 Exposures (Table 29.6) None of the major groups of malformations was associated with exposure to ammonium chloride.

Antitussives — 344 Exposures (Table 29.7)

As seen in the table, the SRR for any malformation was slightly elevated (1.25). The SRR for major malformations was 1.27. Although many of the SRRs for the specific classes of malformations are greater than 1.5, most are based on three

Table **29.6**

Standardized Relative Risks (SRR) and Their 95% Confidence Intervals (CI$_{95}$) for Broad Classes of Malformations Showing Uniform Rates by Hospital in Relation to **Ammonium Chloride** Used in Lunar Months 1–4 by 365 Pregnant Women (Based on Multiple Logistic Risk Function Analysis)

| | No. of Malformed Children | | | |
	Observed	Expected	SRR	CI$_{95}$ of SRR
Any malformation	15	18.0	0.83	0.47–1.36
Major malformations	9	11.2	0.80	0.37–1.50
Minor malformations	5	7.0	0.71	0.25–1.65

Table **29.7**

Standardized Relative Risks (SRR) and Their 95% Confidence Intervals (CI$_{95}$) for Classes of Malformations Showing Uniform Rates by Hospital in Relation to **Antitussives** Used in Lunar Months 1–4 by 344 Pregnant Women (Based on Multiple Logistic Risk Function Analysis)

| | No. of Malformed Children | | | |
Malformation Classes	Observed	Expected	SRR	CI$_{95}$ of SRR
Any malformation	20	16.0	1.25	0.77– 1.89
Major malformations	12	9.4	1.27	0.66– 2.19
Minor malformations	8	6.8	1.18	0.51– 2.30
Central nervous	3	1.8	1.67	0.35– 4.85
Cardiovascular	1	0.4	2.21	0.06–11.79
Musculoskeletal (other than polydactyly in Blacks)	4	2.7	1.51	0.41– 3.82
Polydactyly in Blacks[1]	2	2.7	0.74	0.09– 2.63
Respiratory	1	1.7	0.58	0.01– 3.18
Gastrointestinal	5	2.3	2.14	0.69– 4.94
Genitourinary (other than hypospadias)	2	1.5	1.36	0.17– 4.89
Hypospadias[2]	2	1.3	1.55	0.19– 5.53
Eye and ear	2	0.9	2.31	0.28– 8.28
Syndromes (other than Down syndrome)	0	0.9	—	0.00– 4.09
Down syndrome	0	0.4	—	0.00–10.24
Tumors	3	1.3	2.25	0.47– 6.53

[1]Drugs used by 198 Blacks
[2]Drugs used by 184 mothers of male offspring

or fewer children. They included central nervous system (1.67), cardiovascular system (2.21), musculoskeletal malformations (4 malformed children, SRR 1.51), gastrointestinal malformations (5 malformed children, SRR 2.14), hypospadias (1.55), eye and ear malformations (2.31), and tumors (2.25).

Dextromethorphan hydrobromide — 300 Exposures (Table 29.8) The SRR for minor malformations was 1.30.

Detailed Evaluation of Non-Uniform Malformations: Inguinal Hernia, Clubfoot, Pectus Excavatum

In this section, the three outcomes are evaluated as in the preceding section dealing with uniform malformations. Instances in which there were fewer than three malformed children exposed to any drug are omitted because they are not informative.

Table **29.8**

Standardized Relative Risks (SRR) and Their 95% Confidence Intervals (CI$_{95}$) for Broad Classes of Malformations Showing Uniform Rates by Hospital in Relation to **Dextromethorphan Hydrobromide** Used in Lunar Months 1–4 by 300 Pregnant Women (Based on Multiple Logistic Risk Function Analysis)

| | No. of Malformed Children | | | |
	Observed	**Expected**	**SRR**	**CI$_{95}$ of SRR**
Any malformation	17	14.2	1.19	0.70–1.88
Major malformations	9	8.2	1.10	0.50–2.05
Minor malformations	8	6.2	1.30	0.56–2.52

Table **29.9**

Standardized Relative Risks (SRR) and Their 95% Confidence Intervals (CI$_{95}$) for Inguinal Hernia, Clubfoot, and Pectus Excavatum in Relation to **Cough Medicines** Used in Lunar Months 1–4 (Based on Multiple Logistic Risk Function Analysis)

| | **No. of Users** | No. of Malformed Children | | **SRR** | **CI$_{95}$ of SRR** |
		Observed	**Expected**		
Inguinal hernia					
Cough medicines	948	20	14.5	1.38	0.85–2.12
Expectorants	864	20	13.3	1.51	0.92–2.31
Clubfoot					
Cough medicines	948	6	4.5	1.33	0.49–2.89
Expectorants	864	4	4.0	0.99	0.27–2.53
Pectus excavatum	—	—	—	—	—

For inguinal hernia, the SRR with expectorants (1.51) was greater than 1.5, compared with a relative risk of 1.38 with the overall group of cough medicines (Table 29.9). For clubfoot, the highest SRR was 1.33, with the drug group as a whole. There were not sufficient numbers for any association to be identified with pectus excavatum.

Comments

There was little evidence to suggest that cough medicines were teratogenic. Relative risks for expectorants (864 exposures) and antitussives (344 exposures) were close to unity. The lack of a relationship between cough medicines and malformations, as against the association identified for "cold preparations" (Chapter 25) is of interest. Based on the drug exposure frequencies (Chapter 25), upper respiratory infections without severe cough were common. Such infections were, presumably, more of viral origin, and their potential teratogenicity needs to be studied further.

CHAPTER 30

Drugs Taken for Gastro- intestinal Disturbances

General Evaluation

In this first section, data are presented for two classes of malformations — all 3,248 malformed children and the 2,277 children with uniform malformation rates by hospital. The relative risks for these malformations are presented for the total group of drugs and for individual drugs comprising the group. Crude relative risks are presented as well as two Mantel-Haenszel-standardized summary relative risks: The first standardization is with respect to hospital; the second, with respect to the survival of the child and ethnic group of the mother.

All Malformations (Table 30.1)

The hospital-standardized relative risk of any malformation was 0.94 for this group of drugs. Only taka-diastase, with 33 exposures (1.95), and casanthranol, with 21 exposures (1.90), had relative risks greater than 1.5.

Malformations with Uniform Rates by Hospital (Table 30.2)

The results for this outcome are very similar to those in the previous section. The relative risks were close to unity for the entire group and for its largest component, phenolphthalein. The only relative risk greater than 1.5 was for casanthranol (1.90).

Table **30.1**

Children (3,248) With Any Malformation in Relation to Exposure to **Drugs Used for Gastrointestinal Disturbances** During Lunar Months 1–4 Among 50,282 Mother-Child Pairs

	No. of Mother-Child Pairs Exposed	No. of Malformed Children	Crude Relative Risk	Hospital Standardized Relative Risk[1]	Survival and Race Standardized Relative Risk[1]
Drugs taken for gastro-intestinal disturbances	440	28	0.99	0.94	1.01
Phenolphthalein	236	17	1.12	1.09	1.20
Cascara	53	4	1.17	1.15	1.09
Black draught	39	1	0.40	0.42	0.37
Taka-Diastase	33	4	1.88	1.95	2.25
Dioctyl sodium sulfosuccinate	30	3	1.55	1.33	1.32
Casanthranol	21	3	2.21	1.90	2.16
Other peroral enzymes[2]	21	0	—	—	—
Miscellaneous gastro-intestinal drugs[3]	50	1	0.31	0.27	0.33

[1] Estimated by the Mantel-Haenszel procedure
[2] Papain (14); bromelain (3); pancreatin (3); proteolytic enzymes (1)
[3] Podophyllum (14); bismuth subgallate (13); bile salts (11); dehydrocholic acid (6); potassium bitartrate (4); bismuth subcarbonate (1); dihydroxyaluminum aminoacetate (1); rhubarb (1); milk of bismuth (1)

Table **30.2**

Children (2,277) With Malformations Showing Uniform Rates by Hospital in Relation to Exposure to **Drugs Used for Gastrointestinal Disturbances** During Lunar Months 1–4 Among 50,282 Mother-Child Pairs

	No. of Mother-Child Pairs Exposed	No. of Malformed Children	Crude Relative Risk	Hospital Standardized Relative Risk	Survival and Race Standardized Relative Risk
Drugs taken for gastrointestinal disturbances	440	20	1.00	0.98	1.07
Phenolphthalein	236	13	1.22	1.21	1.40
Cascara	53	3	1.25	1.25	1.15
Black draught	39	1	0.57	0.58	0.56
Taka-Diastase	33	2	1.34	1.36	1.65
Dioctyl sodium sulfosuccinate	30	2	1.47	1.34	1.11
Casanthranol	21	2	2.10	1.90	1.85
Other peroral enzymes	21	0	—	—	—
Miscellaneous gastrointestinal drugs	50	1	0.44	0.41	0.52

Detailed Evaluation of Uniform Malformations

In this section, groups of drugs, followed by individual drugs, are evaluated in relation to various classes or groups of uniform malformations, as well as individual malformations, for which multiple logistic risk function models were developed. In the tables, the observed and expected numbers of malformed children are given for each drug exposure in turn. The measure of association presented is a standardized relative risk (SRR) with its 95% confidence limits. The SRR is the ratio of the observed number to the expected number of malformed children. Since the SRR takes into account potential confounding variables, it represents the best estimate of the relationship between a drug and a malformation. As numbers of exposed mother-child pairs become so small as to be uninformative, data will be omitted. In this case, only the entire group of drugs taken for gastrointestinal disturbances and phenolphthalein will be examined.

Drugs Taken for Gastrointestinal Disturbances — 440 Exposures (Table 30.3)

The SRRs for broad classes of uniform malformations do not indicate any association with drugs taken for gastrointestinal disturbances. Central nervous system malformations (1.91), genitourinary malformations other than hypospadias (2.11), and eye and ear defects (2.95) were found to have SRRs greater than 1.5.

Phenolphthalein — 236 Exposures (Table 30.4) There is no suggestion of any substantial association between this drug and any of the outcomes in the table.

Table **30.3**

Standardized Relative Risks (SRR) and Their 95% Confidence Intervals (CI$_{95}$) for Classes of Malformations Showing Uniform Rates by Hospital in Relation to **Drugs Taken for Gastrointestinal Disturbances** Used in Lunar Months 1–4 by 440 Pregnant Women (Based on Multiple Logistic Risk Function Analysis)

Malformation Classes	No. of Malformed Children		SRR	CI$_{95}$ of SRR
	Observed	Expected		
Any malformation	20	20.3	0.99	0.61–1.51
Major malformations	13	12.0	1.08	0.58–1.83
Minor malformations	7	8.5	0.82	0.33–1.68
Central nervous	4	2.1	1.91	0.52–4.86
Cardiovascular	0	3.5	—	0.00–1.05
Musculoskeletal (other than polydactyly in Blacks)	3	3.2	0.92	0.19–2.71
Polydactyly in Blacks[1]	3	4.0	0.76	0.16–2.19
Respiratory	1	1.6	0.61	0.02–3.39
Gastrointestinal	2	2.4	0.82	0.10–2.93
Genitourinary (other than hypospadias)	3	1.4	2.11	0.44–6.14
Hypospadias[2]	0	1.5	—	0.00–2.45
Eye and ear	3	1.0	2.95	0.61–8.56
Syndromes (other than Down syndrome)	1	1.1	0.93	0.02–5.15
Down syndrome	0	0.6	—	0.00–6.22
Tumors	2	1.7	1.21	0.15–4.33

[1]Drugs used by 261 Blacks
[2]Drugs used by 232 mothers of male offspring

**Detailed Evaluation of
Non-Uniform Malformations:
Inguinal Hernia, Clubfoot,
Pectus Excavatum**

In this section, the three outcomes are evaluated as in the preceding section dealing with uniform malformations. Instances in which there were fewer than three malformed children exposed to any drug are omitted because they are not informative.

Table 30.5 shows that there was no association between the drug group as a whole and inguinal hernia. For clubfoot,

the corresponding SRR was 1.61. There were insufficient numbers to identify any association with pectus excavatum.

Comments

There was no evidence to suggest that exposure to drugs taken for gastrointestinal disturbances (440 mother-child pairs) increases the risk of malformations. However, numbers were small and associations between specific drugs and various malformations could not be ruled out.

Table **30.4**

Standardized Relative Risks (SRR) and Their 95% Confidence Intervals (CI_{95}) for Broad Classes of Malformations Showing Uniform Rates by Hospital in Relation to **Phenolphthalein** Used in Lunar Months 1–4 by 236 Pregnant Women (Based on Multiple Logistic Risk Function Analysis)

	No. of Malformed Children		SRR	CI_{95} of SRR
	Observed	**Expected**	**SRR**	**CI_{95} of SRR**
Any malformation	13	10.8	1.21	0.65–2.02
Major malformations	7	6.2	1.14	0.46–2.30
Minor malformations	6	4.6	1.31	0.48–2.80

Table **30.5**

Standardized Relative Risks (SRR) and Their 95% Confidence Intervals (CI_{95}) for Inguinal Hernia, Clubfoot, and Pectus Excavatum in Relation to **Drugs Taken for Gastrointestinal Disturbances** in Lunar Months 1–4 (Based on Multiple Logistic Risk Function Analysis)

	No. of Users	No. of Malformed Children		SRR	CI_{95} of SRR
	No. of Users	**Observed**	**Expected**	**SRR**	**CI_{95} of SRR**
Inguinal hernia					
Drugs taken for gastrointestinal disturbances	440	6	6.5	0.92	0.34–1.99
Clubfoot					
Drugs taken for gastrointestinal disturbances	440	3	1.9	1.61	0.33–4.61
Pectus excavatum	—	—	—	—	—

CHAPTER **31**

Hormones, Hormone Antagonists, and Contraceptives

General Evaluation

Initially, the entire set of 3,248 malformed children is considered in relation to exposure to the entire group of hormones, hormone antagonists, oral contraceptives, and local contraceptives during the first four lunar months of pregnancy (Table 31.1). Oral contraceptives have been split into their components as well as evaluated as combination products. In Table 31.2, the data are confined to the 2,277 children who had malformations which were distributed uniformly among hospitals. Three relative risks are given in each table: crude, standardized for hospital variability, and standardized for the mother's ethnic group and survival of the child.

All Malformations in
Relation to All Hormones,
Hormone Antagonists, and
Contraceptives (Table 31.1)

The hospital-standardized relative risk of any malformation for exposure to all hormones, hormone antagonists, and contraceptives was 1.25; this association is statistically significant at the 5% level. For the major components of this mixed category of drugs, the hospital-standardized relative risks were as follows: progestational agents, 1.27; estrogenic agents, 1.06; thyroid hormones, 1.26; corticosteroids and corticotropins, 0.67; antidiabetic drugs, 3.10;

388

Table *31.1*

Children (3,248) With Any Malformation in Relation to Exposure to **Hormones, Hormone Antagonists, and Contraceptives** During Lunar Months 1–4 Among 50,282 Mother-Child Pairs

	No. of Mother-Child Pairs Exposed	No. of Malformed Children	Crude Relative Risk	Hospital Standardized Relative Risk[1]	Survival and Race Standardized Relative Risk[1]
Hormones, hormone antagonists, and contraceptives	2,327	193	1.30[2]	1.25[3]	1.24[3]
Progestational agents	866	75	1.35[2]	1.27	1.31[3]
Progesterone	253	20	1.23	1.13	1.18
Hydroxyprogesterone	162	9	0.86	0.85	0.75
Norethynodrel	154	11	1.11	1.05	1.10
Norethindrone	132	14	1.64	1.53	1.80
Medroxyprogesterone	130	18	2.15[2]	1.91[3]	2.12[2]
Progestational agents, n.o.s.	96	5	0.81	0.83	0.78
Ethisterone	29	2	1.07	0.92	1.12
Other progestational agents[6]	10	1	1.55	1.23	1.35
Estrogenic agents	614	44	1.11	1.06	1.07
Mestranol	179	13	1.12	1.06	1.11
Diethylstilbestrol	164	13	1.23	1.18	1.04
Estrogen, n.o.s.	110	5	0.70	0.71	0.68
Ethinyl estradiol	89	9	1.57	1.38	1.78
Estradiol	48	2	0.64	0.62	0.55
Dienestrol	36	2	0.86	0.77	0.86
Other estrogenic agents[7]	13	1	1.19	1.07	1.42
Thyroid hormones	560	48	1.33	1.26	1.29
Thyroxin and thyroid	537	45	1.30	1.23	1.26
Liothyronine	34	4	1.82	1.55	1.87
Corticosteroids and corticotropins	145	7	0.75	0.67	0.73
Prednisone	43	2	0.72	0.66	0.62
Cortisone	34	1	0.46	0.42	0.46
Hydrocortisone	21	3	2.21	2.18	2.79
Other corticosteroids and corticotropins[8]	56	2	0.55	0.47	0.51
Antidiabetic drugs	139	24	2.69[4]	3.10[4]	1.99[5]
Insulin	121	22	2.83[4]	3.28[4]	2.09[5]
Oral hypoglycemic agents[9]	21	2	1.47	1.60	1.10
Miscellaneous hormones	131	7	0.83	0.78	0.79
Hormone, n.o.s.	105	5	0.74	0.71	0.67
Infrequently used hormones[10]	26	2	1.19	1.05	1.39
Thyroid suppressants[11]	25	4	2.48	2.64	2.05

Table *31.1* (continued)

	No. of Mother- Child Pairs Exposed	No. of Malformed Children	Crude Relative Risk	Hospital Standardized Relative Risk[1]	Survival and Race Standardized Relative Risk[1]
Oral contraceptives	278	18	1.00	0.97	0.99
Mestranol and norethynodrel	154	11	1.11	1.05	1.10
Oral contra- ceptives, n.o.s.	96	5	0.81	0.83	0.78
Mestranol and norethindrone	25	1	0.62	0.55	0.67
Other oral contraceptives[12]	5	1	3.10	3.04	3.11
Local contraceptives	462	31	1.04	1.02	1.00
Nonoxynol 9	342	23	1.04	1.01	0.98
P-Diisobutylphenoxy- Polyethoxy E	84	4	0.74	0.71	0.76
Local contraceptive, n.o.s. and other[13]	37	4	1.67	1.83	1.67

[1] Estimated by the Mantel-Haenszel procedure
[2] $X_1^2 = 6.70–10.58$, $p < 0.01$
[3] $X_1^2 = 4.67–5.56$, $p < 0.05$
[4] $X_1^2 = 25.18–26.49$, $p < 0.001$
[5] $X_1^2 = 8.75–9.19$, $p < 0.01$
[6] Dydrogesterone (9); ethynodiol (1)
[7] Estrogens, conjugated (11); estrone (3)
[8] Methylprednisolone (16); prednisolone (15); triamcinolone (8); dexamethasone (8); corticotropin (6); paramethasone (2); desoxycorticosterone (2); aldosterone (1); betamethasone (1)
[9] Tolbutamide (13); chlorpropamide (5); acetohexamide (2); phenformin (1)
[10] Oxytocin (6); lututrin (5); methandrostenolone (4); testosterone (3); gonadotropin chorionic (2); clomiphene (2); vasopressin (1); fluoxymesterone (1); male hormone, n.o.s. (1); methyltestosterone (1)
[11] Propylthiouracil (16); methimazole (9); methylthiouracil (1); iodothiouracil (1)
[12] Ethinyl estradiol and medroxyprogesterone (5); mestranol and ethynodiol (1)
[13] Local contraceptives, n.o.s. (35); p-triisopropylphenoxypolyethylor (1); chlorindanol (1)

miscellaneous hormones, 0.78; thyroid suppressants, 2.64; oral contraceptives, 0.97; and local contraceptives, 1.02. Only the association with antidiabetic drugs is statistically significant (at the 0.001 level).

Relative risks above 1.5, based on two or more exposed-malformed children, were seen for the following drugs: norethindrone (1.53), medroxyprogesterone (1.91, statistically significant at the 5% level), liothyronine (1.55), hydrocortisone (2.18), insulin (3.18, statistically significant at the 0.001 level), oral hypoglycemic agents (1.60), and local contraceptives, n.o.s. (1.83).

Malformations Showing Uniform Rates by Hospital in Relation to Hormones, Hormone Antagonists, and Contraceptives (Table 31.2)

The hospital-standardized relative risks of the uniform malformations did not differ greatly from those of all malformations. The risk relative to all drugs in this category was 1.28.

Relative risks above 1.5, based on two or more exposed-malformed children, were seen for norethindrone (1.79), diethylstilbestrol (1.56), ethinyl estradiol (1.89), hydrocortisone (2.09), insulin

Table **31.2**

Children (2,277) With Malformations Showing Uniform Rates by Hospital in Relation to Exposure to **Hormones, Hormone Antagonists, and Contraceptives** During Lunar Months 1–4 Among 50,282 Mother-Child Pairs

	No. of Mother-Child Pairs Exposed	No. of Malformed Children	Crude Relative Risk	Hospital Standardized Relative Risk	Survival and Race Standardized Relative Risk
Hormones, hormone antagonists, and contraceptives	2,327	137	1.32	1.28	1.28
Progestational agents	866	47	1.20	1.15	1.11
Progesterone	253	9	0.78	0.72	0.70
Hydroxyprogesterone	162	6	0.82	0.79	0.64
Norethynodrel	154	7	1.00	0.96	0.96
Norethindrone	132	11	1.84	1.79	2.05
Medroxyprogesterone	130	8	1.36	1.21	1.18
Progestational agents, n.o.s.	96	5	1.15	1.21	1.15
Ethisterone	29	2	1.52	1.44	1.74
Other progestational agents	10	1	2.21	1.99	2.08
Estrogenic agents	614	35	1.26	1.22	1.19
Mestranol	179	8	0.99	0.94	0.94
Diethylstilbestrol	164	12	1.62	1.56	1.27
Estrogen, n.o.s.	110	5	1.00	1.04	1.02
Ethinyl estradiol	89	8	1.99	1.89	2.35
Estradiol	48	1	0.46	0.43	0.32
Dienestrol	36	1	0.61	0.58	0.64
Other estrogenic agents	13	1	1.70	1.63	2.18
Thyroid hormones	560	35	1.39	1.33	1.27
Thyroxin and thyroid	537	34	1.40	1.35	1.29
Liothyronine	34	1	0.65	0.55	0.52
Corticosteroids and corticotropins	145	6	0.91	0.85	0.88
Prednisone	43	1	0.51	0.48	0.39
Cortisone	34	1	0.65	0.62	0.65
Hydrocortisone	21	2	2.10	2.09	2.74
Other corticosteroids and corticotropins	56	2	0.79	0.72	0.73
Antidiabetic drugs	139	18	2.87	3.17	1.77
Insulin	121	17	3.12	3.48	1.92
Oral hypoglycemic agents	21	1	1.05	1.05	0.61
Miscellaneous hormones	131	4	0.67	0.64	0.63
Hormone, n.o.s.	105	4	0.84	0.82	0.75
Infrequently used hormones	26	0	—	—	—
Thyroid suppressants	25	4	3.54	3.83	2.65
Oral contraceptives	278	13	1.03	1.02	1.00
Mestranol and norethynodrel	154	7	1.00	0.96	0.96

Table *31.2* (continued)

	No. of Mother- Child Pairs Exposed	No. of Malformed Children	Crude Relative Risk	Hospital Standardized Relative Risk	Survival and Race Standardized Relative Risk
Oral contraceptives, n.o.s.	96	5	1.15	1.21	1.15
Mestranol and norethindrone	25	0	—	—	—
Other oral contraceptives	5	1	4.42	4.75	4.71
Local contraceptives	462	23	1.10	1.09	1.08
Nonoxynol 9	342	17	1.10	1.08	1.05
P-Diisobutylphenoxy- Polyethoxy E	84	3	0.79	0.76	0.89
Local contraceptives, n.o.s.	37	3	1.79	1.88	1.85

(3.48), and local contraceptives, n.o.s. (1.88).

Detailed Evaluation of Uniform Malformations

In this section, groups of drugs, followed by individual drugs, are evaluated in relation to various classes or groups of uniform malformations, as well as individual malformations, for which multiple logistic risk function models were developed. In the tables, the observed and expected numbers of malformed children are given for each drug exposure in turn. The measure of association presented is a standardized relative risk (SRR) with its 95% confidence limits. The SRR is the ratio of the observed number to the expected number of malformed children. Since the SRR takes into account potential confounding variables, it represents the best estimate of the relationship between a drug and a malformation. As numbers of exposed mother-child pairs become so small as to be uninformative, data will be omitted.

All Hormones, Hormone Antagonists, and Contraceptives — 2,327 Exposures (Table 31.3)

The overall relative risk of any malformation was 1.05. The highest SRRs were for Down syndrome (1.39) and cardiovascular malformations (1.21).

Progestational Agents — 866 Exposures (Table 31.4)

The overall association of uniform malformations with progestational agents was minimal. However, the SRRs of two malformation classes were greater than 1.5: cardiovascular (1.80) and hypospadias (1.70).

The SRR of 1.80 for cardiovascular malformations is statistically significant as indicated by its lower confidence limit.

Progesterone — 253 Exposures (Table 31.5) No positive association of uniform malformations was seen with progesterone.

Estrogenic Agents — 614 Exposures (Table 31.6)

A somewhat similar pattern to that of progestational agents was seen with estrogenic agents. The association with broad classes of malformations was minimal. Relative risks greater than 1.5 were seen for cardiovascular malformations (1.89), hypospadias (1.60), eye and ear malformations (1.71), and Down syndrome (1.61).

Diethylstilbestrol — 164 Exposures (Table 31.7) The association of malformations with diethylstilbestrol was minimal.

Table **31.3**

Standardized Relative Risks (SRR) and Their 95% Confidence Intervals (CI$_{95}$) for Classes of Malformations Showing Uniform Rates by Hospital in Relation to **Hormones, Hormone Antagonists, and Contraceptives** Used in Lunar Months 1–4 by 2,327 Pregnant Women (Based on Multiple Logistic Risk Function Analysis)

Malformation Classes	No. of Malformed Children		SRR	CI$_{95}$ of SRR
	Observed	Expected		
Any malformation	137	130.4	1.05	0.90–1.23
Major malformations	97	92.8	1.04	0.87–1.26
Minor malformations	44	46.6	0.94	0.70–1.27
Central nervous	10	18.3	0.55	0.26–1.00
Cardiovascular	32	26.4	1.21	0.89–1.64
Musculoskeletal (other than polydactyly in Blacks)	28	27.9	1.00	0.70–1.44
Polydactyly in Blacks[1]	13	12.0	1.08	0.58–1.84
Respiratory	10	15.8	0.63	0.30–1.16
Gastrointestinal	19	21.1	0.90	0.54–1.40
Genitourinary (other than hypospadias)	11	16.6	0.66	0.33–1.18
Hypospadias[2]	9	9.1	0.99	0.45–1.87
Eye and ear	7	6.3	1.11	0.45–2.28
Syndromes (other than Down syndrome)	7	8.9	0.78	0.32–1.61
Down syndrome	6	4.3	1.39	0.51–3.02
Tumors	6	9.8	0.61	0.22–1.32

[1]Drugs used by 874 Blacks
[2]Drugs used by 1,194 mothers of male offspring

Thyroid Hormones — 560
Exposures (Table 31.8)

The SRR for major malformations in association with all thyroid hormones was 1.19. SRRs greater than 1.5 were seen for cardiovascular malformations (1.61), polydactyly in Blacks (2.42), and Down syndrome (2.36).

Thyroxin and Thyroid — 537 Exposures (Table 31.9) Since over 95% of the exposure to all thyroid hormones was to thyroxin or thyroid, the pattern in the table is similar to that in the preceding table.

Antidiabetic Drugs —
139 Exposures (Table 31.10)
No association was observed between the uniform malformations and antidiabetic drugs.

Oral Contraceptives —
278 Exposures (Table 31.11)
There was no association of the broad classes of uniform malformations with oral contraceptives. SRRs greater than 1.5 were seen for cardiovascular malformations (2.41) and hypospadias (2.66).

Local Contraceptives —
462 Exposures (Table 31.12)
The association of broad classes of malformations with local contraceptives was minimal. The only SRR greater than 1.5 was for polydactyly in Blacks (1.76).

Nonoxynol 9 — 342 Exposures (Table 31.13) The, SRR for minor malformations was 1.29.

Table **31.4**

Standardized Relative Risks (SRR) and Their 95% Confidence Intervals (CI$_{95}$) for Classes of Malformations Showing Uniform Rates by Hospital in Relation to **Progestational Agents** Used in Lunar Months 1–4 by 866 Pregnant Women (Based on Multiple Logistic Risk Function Analysis)

| | No. of Malformed Children | | | |
| | Observed | Expected | | |
Malformation Classes	**Observed**	**Expected**	**SRR**	**CI$_{95}$ of SRR**
Any malformation	47	45.4	1.04	0.79–1.36
Major malformations	35	30.9	1.13	0.84–1.53
Minor malformations	17	16.8	1.01	0.59–1.61
Central nervous	3	6.1	0.49	0.10–1.44
Cardiovascular	16	8.9	1.80	1.04–2.91
Musculoskeletal (other than polydactyly in Blacks)	10	10.1	0.99	0.48–1.82
Polydactyly in Blacks[1]	1	3.4	0.29	0.01–1.62
Respiratory	2	5.2	0.39	0.05–1.39
Gastrointestinal	7	8.0	0.87	0.35–1.79
Genitourinary (other than hypospadias)	3	5.3	0.57	0.12–1.65
Hypospadias[2]	6	3.5	1.70	0.67–3.67
Eye and ear	3	2.4	1.24	0.26–3.62
Syndromes (other than Down syndrome)	7	8.9	0.78	0.32–1.61
Down syndrome	2	1.5	1.33	0.16–4.78
Tumors	1	3.6	0.28	0.01–1.53

[1] Drugs used by 274 Blacks
[2] Drugs used by 441 mothers of male offspring

Table **31.5**

Standardized Relative Risks (SRR) and Their 95% Confidence Intervals (CI$_{95}$) for Broad Classes of Malformations Showing Uniform Rates by Hospital in Relation to **Progesterone** Used in Lunar Months 1–4 by 253 Pregnant Women (Based on Multiple Logistic Risk Function Analysis)

	No. of Malformed Children			
	Observed	**Expected**	**SRR**	**CI$_{95}$ of SRR**
Any malformation	9	12.3	0.73	0.34–1.37
Major malformations	7	8.0	0.88	0.35–1.78
Minor malformations	4	4.4	0.92	0.25–2.32

Table **31.6**

Standardized Relative Risks (SRR) and Their 95% Confidence Intervals (CI$_{95}$) for Classes of Malformations Showing Uniform Rates by Hospital in Relation to **Estrogenic Agents** Used in Lunar Months 1–4 by 614 Pregnant Women (Based on Multiple Logistic Risk Function Analysis)

Malformation Classes	No. of Malformed Children		SRR	CI$_{95}$ of SRR
	Observed	Expected		
Any malformation	35	32.3	1.08	0.80–1.43
Major malformations	27	22.5	1.20	0.86–1.68
Minor malformations	8	11.5	0.69	0.30–1.36
Central nervous	2	4.3	0.47	0.06–1.67
Cardiovascular	12	6.3	1.89	0.98–3.28
Musculoskeletal (other than polydactyly in Blacks)	8	7.3	1.10	0.48–2.16
Polydactyly in Blacks[1]	0	2.3	—	0.00–1.60
Respiratory	1	3.6	0.28	0.01–1.54
Gastrointestinal	4	5.5	0.73	0.20–1.85
Genitourinary (other than hypospadias)	1	3.8	0.26	0.01–1.47
Hypospadias[2]	4	2.5	1.60	0.44–4.04
Eye and ear	3	1.7	1.71	0.35–4.97
Syndromes (other than Down syndrome)	2	2.1	0.96	0.12–3.46
Down syndrome	2	1.2	1.61	0.20–5.80
Tumors	2	2.6	0.78	0.09–2.80

[1]Drugs used by 192 Blacks
[2]Drugs used by 299 mothers of male offspring

Table **31.7**

Standardized Relative Risks (SRR) and Their 95% Confidence Intervals (CI$_{95}$) for Broad Classes of Malformations Showing Uniform Rates by Hospital in Relation to **Diethylstilbestrol** Used in Lunar Months 1–4 by 164 Pregnant Women (Based on Multiple Logistic Risk Function Analysis)

	No. of Malformed Children		SRR	CI$_{95}$ of SRR
	Observed	Expected		
Any malformation	12	1.04	1.16	0.61–1.96
Major malformations	9	8.0	1.12	0.52–2.07
Minor malformations	2	3.6	0.56	0.07–1.97

Detailed Evaluation of Non-Uniform Malformations: Inguinal Hernia, Clubfoot, Pectus Excavatum

In this section, the three outcomes are evaluated as in the preceding section dealing with uniform malformations. Instances in which there were fewer than three malformed children exposed to any drug are omitted because they are not informative.

As seen in Table 31.14, the only SRR greater than 1.5 for inguinal hernia was with progestational agents (1.52). This

395

Table **31.8**

Standardized Relative Risks (SRR) and Their 95% Confidence Intervals (CI$_{95}$) for Classes of Malformations Showing Uniform Rates by Hospital in Relation to **Thyroid Hormones** Used in Lunar Months 1–4 by 560 Pregnant Women (Based on Multiple Logistic Risk Function Analysis)

Malformation Classes	No. of Malformed Children		SRR	CI$_{95}$ of SRR
	Observed	Expected		
Any malformation	35	30.2	1.16	0.86–1.56
Major malformations	27	22.7	1.19	0.85–1.66
Minor malformations	8	9.7	0.83	0.36–1.62
Central nervous	2	4.2	0.47	0.06–1.69
Cardiovascular	9	5.6	1.61	0.74–3.03
Musculoskeletal (other than polydactyly in Blacks)	7	7.2	0.97	0.39–1.99
Polydactyly in Blacks[1]	3	1.2	2.42	0.50–6.86
Respiratory	3	3.5	0.86	0.18–2.50
Gastrointestinal	7	5.3	1.31	0.53–2.69
Genitourinary (other than hypospadias)	1	3.2	0.32	0.01–1.75
Hypospadias[2]	1	2.2	0.46	0.01–2.52
Eye and ear	2	1.4	1.42	0.17–5.10
Syndromes (other than Down syndrome)	2	2.6	0.77	0.09–2.76
Down syndrome	3	1.3	2.36	0.49–6.85
Tumors	1	2.6	0.39	0.01–2.15

[1]Drugs used by 93 Blacks
[2]Drugs used by 298 mothers of male offspring

association is statistically significant, with a lower confidence limit of 1.10. For clubfoot, local contraceptives (1.62) had an SRR greater than 1.5. Pectus excavatum did not appear to be positively associated with the drugs in this group.

Comments

In this study, exposure to progestational agents (866 mother-child pairs), estrogenic agents (614), and oral contraceptives (278) was associated with cardiovascular malformations, with the relative risk being almost doubled. For the largest exposure group of progestational agents, the association was statistically significant. While the association was not significant in the case of estrogen exposures, numbers were smaller and the SRR was of the same magnitude. With still smaller numbers, the SRR was also increased for oral contraceptive exposure — most of which was, presumably, inadvertent. Because of the methods of classification used in the study, the ingredients of oral contraceptives were also classified as progestational or estrogenic agents. In addition, some women received estrogens, together with progestogens, for poor obstetrical histories and other indications. When the classification was made mutually exclusive, the findings were not materially changed.[1]

Female hormones were mainly used when there were poor obstetrical histories; it is possible that the associations found in this study reflect this fact. However, this explanation is unlikely since history of prior abortion or stillbirth was taken into account. Moreover, poor obstetrical histories would not explain the association with oral contraceptives. The findings suggesting an association between female hormones and cardiovascular malformations are consistent

Table **31.9**

Standardized Relative Risks (SRR) and Their 95% Confidence Intervals (CI_{95}) for Classes of Malformations Showing Uniform Rates by Hospital in Relation to **Thyroxin and Thyroid** Used in Lunar Months 1–4 by 537 Pregnant Women (Based on Multiple Logistic Risk Function Analysis)

Malformation Classes	No. of Malformed Children		SRR	CI_{95} of SRR
	Observed	Expected		
Any malformation	34	28.7	1.19	0.88–1.60
Major malformations	27	21.4	1.26	0.91–1.75
Minor malformations	7	8.8	0.80	0.32–1.63
Central nervous	2	3.8	0.53	0.06–1.90
Cardiovascular	9	5.2	1.72	0.79–3.23
Musculoskeletal (other than polydactyly in Blacks)	7	6.8	1.03	0.42–2.11
Polydactyly in Blacks[1]	3	1.2	2.47	0.51–7.01
Respiratory	3	3.3	0.92	0.19–2.67
Gastrointestinal	6	4.6	1.29	0.47–2.79
Genitourinary (other than hypospadias)	1	2.8	0.35	0.01–1.95
Hypospadias[2]	1	2.1	0.48	0.01–2.63
Eye and ear	2	1.3	1.50	0.18–5.39
Syndromes (other than Down syndrome)	2	2.3	0.87	0.11–3.14
Down syndrome	3	1.3	2.36	0.49–6.85
Tumors	1	2.4	0.41	0.01–2.26

[1] Drugs used by 91 Blacks
[2] Drugs used by 288 mothers of male offspring

Table **31.10**

Standardized Relative Risks (SRR) and Their 95% Confidence Intervals (CI_{95}) for Broad Classes of Malformations Showing Uniform Rates by Hospital in Relation to **Antidiabetic Drugs** Used in Lunar Months 1–4 by 139 Pregnant Women (Based on Multiple Logistic Risk Function Analysis)

	No. of Malformed Children		SRR	CI_{95} of SRR
	Observed	Expected		
Any malformation	18	18.8	0.96	0.58–1.46
Major malformations	18	18.4	0.98	0.59–1.49
Minor malformations	3	5.2	0.58	0.12–1.65

with limited data published elsewhere.[2-5] Further studies are needed, but there appear to be legitimate grounds for suspecting that this association may be causal.

The data also suggest that exposure to progestational agents may increase the risk of inguinal hernia. No evidence of association between female hormone exposure and limb reduction defects was found.[6]

The findings with respect to insulin (121 exposures) illustrate one instance of

Table *31.11*

Standardized Relative Risks (SRR) and Their 95% Confidence Intervals (CI$_{95}$) for Classes of Malformations Showing Uniform Rates by Hospital in Relation to **Oral Contraceptives** Used in Lunar Months 1–4 by 278 Pregnant Women (Based on Multiple Logistic Risk Function Analysis)

Malformation Classes	No. of Malformed Children		SRR	CI$_{95}$ of SRR
	Observed	Expected		
Any malformation	13	13.5	0.96	0.52– 1.62
Major malformations	10	8.5	1.17	0.57– 2.12
Minor malformations	5	4.8	1.04	0.34– 2.41
Central nervous	1	1.5	0.67	0.02– 3.69
Cardiovascular	6	2.5	2.41	0.89– 5.18
Musculoskeletal (other than polydactyly in Blacks)	2	2.8	0.71	0.09– 2.55
Polydactyly in Blacks[1]	0	1.2	—	0.00– 2.99
Respiratory	1	1.2	0.80	0.02– 4.40
Gastrointestinal	2	2.2	0.91	0.11– 3.27
Genitourinary (other than hypospadias)	1	1.2	0.87	0.02– 4.82
Hypospadias[2]	3	1.1	2.66	0.55– 7.61
Eye and ear	1	0.7	1.41	0.04– 7.81
Syndromes (other than Down syndrome)	0	0.6	—	0.00– 5.86
Down syndrome	0	0.3	—	0.00–13.92
Tumors	0	1.0	—	0.00– 3.70

[1]Drugs used by 91 Blacks
[2]Drugs used by 134 mothers of male offspring

complete overlap between a disease and its treatment. Initially, strong associations were identified for exposure to insulin in relation to either malformations in general or uniform malformations. However, the associations were eliminated in the final analyses — mainly because of diabetes. Since insulin-dependent diabetics must use the drug in order to survive, it is impossible to evaluate the separate effects of diabetes and its treatment in this study. On the basis of experiments in animals, Tuchmann-Duplessis believes that diabetes itself is more likely to be the causal factor.[7] However, the matter is controversial, and it is possible that repeated bouts of hypoglycemia may adversely affect the fetus.[8] There were no individual malformations associated with the insulin use, suggesting that the teratogenic effect, regardless of whether it should be attrib-

uted to the disease or the treatment, is rather non-specific.

Based on very limited numbers (4 malformed children out of 25 exposed), the data for exposure to thyroid suppressant drugs were consistent with one report suggesting that this group of drugs is teratogenic.[9]

Exposure to thyroxin or thyroid hormone (537 mother-child pairs) was associated with cardiac malformations. Again, this was based on small numbers.

Corticosteroids and corticotropins gave no evidence of association with malformations. Numbers, however, were limited. Primates are resistant to *in utero* exposure to cortisone, although there is evidence that it produces clefts and other anomalies in other species.[7]

Finally, miscellaneous hormones and local contraceptives gave no evidence of association with malformations.

Table **31.12**

Standardized Relative Risks (SRR) and Their 95% Confidence Intervals (CI$_{95}$) for Classes of Malformations Showing Uniform Rates by Hospital in Relation to **Local Contraceptives** Used in Lunar Months 1–4 by 462 Pregnant Women (Based on Multiple Logistic Risk Function Analysis)

| | No. of Malformed Children | | | |
Malformation Classes	Observed	Expected	SRR	CI$_{95}$ of SRR
Any malformation	23	21.5	1.07	0.72–1.58
Major malformations	10	11.4	0.88	0.42–1.60
Minor malformations	13	10.2	1.28	0.68–2.16
Central nervous	1	2.2	0.44	0.01–2.46
Cardiovascular	3	3.6	0.84	0.17–2.45
Musculoskeletal (other than polydactyly in Blacks)	3	2.9	1.05	0.22–3.05
Polydactyly in Blacks[1]	9	5.1	1.76	0.81–3.30
Respiratory	3	2.0	1.50	0.31–4.35
Gastrointestinal	1	2.6	0.38	0.01–2.12
Genitourinary (other than hypospadias)	2	1.6	1.24	0.15–4.47
Hypospadias[2]	1	1.6	0.61	0.02–3.39
Eye and ear	0	1.1	—	0.00–3.30
Syndromes (other than Down syndrome)	1	0.9	1.05	0.03–5.81
Down syndrome	1	0.6	1.79	0.05–9.91
Tumors	1	1.6	0.61	0.02–3.38

[1]Drugs used by 351 Blacks
[2]Drugs used by 240 mothers of male offspring

Table **31.13**

Standardized Relative Risks (SRR) and Their 95% Confidence Intervals (CI$_{95}$) for Broad Classes of Malformations Showing Uniform Rates by Hospital in Relation to **Nonoxynol 9** Used in Lunar Months 1–4 by 342 Pregnant Women (Based on Multiple Logistic Risk Function Analysis)

| | No. of Malformed Children | | | |
	Observed	Expected	SRR	CI$_{95}$ of SRR
Any malformation	17	16.4	1.04	0.61–1.64
Major malformations	7	8.9	0.79	0.32–1.60
Minor malformations	10	7.7	1.29	0.63–2.35

Nora and Nora have suggested that oral contraceptive exposure may be related to the "Vacterl" group of anomalies (vertebral, anal, cardiac, tracheal, esophageal, renal, and limb).[4] Apart from cardiac malformations, there was no evidence that oral contraceptives, in particular, or female hormones, in general, were related to the remaining components of the "Vacterl" group.

Table *31.14*

Standardized Relative Risks (SRR) and Their 95% Confidence Intervals (CI$_{95}$) for Inguinal Hernia, Clubfoot, and Pectus Excavatum in Relation to **Hormones, Hormone Antagonists, and Contraceptives** Used in Lunar Months 1–4 (Based on Multiple Logistic Risk Function Analysis)

	No. of Users	No. of Malformed Children		SRR	CI$_{95}$ of SRR
		Observed	Expected		
Inguinal hernia					
Hormones, hormone antago-nists, and contraceptives	2,327	48	39.7	1.21	0.94–1.55
Progestational agents	866	23	15.1	1.52	1.10–2.11
Estrogenic agents	614	8	10.2	0.79	0.34–1.54
Thyroid hormones	560	11	8.3	1.32	0.66–2.34
Thyroxin and thyroid	537	10	8.0	1.25	0.60–2.29
Local contraceptives	462	6	7.3	0.82	0.30–1.77
Clubfoot					
Hormones, hormone antago-nists, and contraceptives	2,327	9	11.6	0.78	0.36–1.47
Progestational agents	866	3	4.8	0.62	0.13–1.81
Local contraceptives	462	3	1.8	1.62	0.34–4.72
Pectus excavatum					
Hormones, hormone antago-nists, and contraceptives	2,327	4	7.8	0.51	0.14–1.31
Progestational agents	866	3	4.1	0.74	0.15–2.15

CHAPTER 32

Inorganic Compounds and Certain Vitamins

General Evaluation

In Table 32.1, all 3,248 malformed children are considered in relation to exposure to the entire group of inorganic compounds and certain vitamins during the first four lunar months of pregnancy. In Table 32.2, the data are confined to the 2,277 children who had malformations which were distributed uniformly among hospitals. Three relative risks are given in each table: crude, standardized for hospital variability, and standardized for the mother's ethnic group and survival of the child.

All Malformations in Relation
to Inorganic Compounds and
Certain Vitamins (Table 32.1)

The hospital-standardized relative risk for all malformations in relation to inorganic compounds and certain vitamins was 1.07. The only elevated hospital-standardized relative risk was for inorganic fluorides (1.39).

Malformations with Uniform
Rates by Hospital in
Relation to Inorganic
Compounds and Certain Vitamins
(Table 32.2)

The hospital-standardized relative risk for the uniform malformations in relation to inorganic compounds and certain vitamins was 1.10. The relative risk for these malformations in relation to fluorides was 1.65.

Table **32.1**

Children (3,248) With Any Malformation in Relation to Exposure to **Inorganic Compounds and Certain Vitamins** During Lunar Months 1–4 Among 50,282 Mother-Child Pairs

	No. of Mother-Child Pairs Exposed	No. of Malformed Children	Crude Relative Risk	Hospital Standardized Relative Risk[1]	Survival and Race Standardized Relative Risk[1]
Inorganic compounds and certain vitamins	2,542	184	1.13	1.07	1.10
Bromides, fluorides, and iodides	1,526	121	1.24[2]	1.17	1.20
Fluorides	122	11	1.40	1.39	1.39
Iodides	489	38	1.21	1.11	1.10
Bromides	986	77	1.21	1.16	1.22
Calcium (parenteral), iron, and vitamins	1,091	65	0.92	0.87	0.91
Calcium compounds (salts)	1,007	61	0.94	0.88	0.93
Iron, i.m.	66	3	0.70	0.68	0.66
Vitamins B_{12} and K[3]	28	1	0.55	0.50	0.45

[1]Estimated by the Mantel-Haenszel procedure
[2]$X^2_1 = 5.38$, $p < 0.05$
[3]Phytonadione (14); cyanocobalamin (11); liver extract, i.m. (6)

Table **32.2**

Children (2,277) With Malformations Showing Uniform Rates by Hospital in Relation to Exposure to **Inorganic Compounds and Certain Vitamins** During Lunar Months 1–4 Among 50,282 Mother-Child Pairs

	No. of Mother-Child Pairs Exposed	No. of Malformed Children	Crude Relative Risk	Hospital Standardized Relative Risk	Survival and Race Standardized Relative Risk
Inorganic compounds and some vitamins	2,542	130	1.14	1.10	1.11
Bromides, fluorides, and iodides	1,526	86	1.25[1]	1.21	1.19
Fluorides	122	9	1.63	1.65	1.62
Iodides	489	27	1.22	1.16	1.04
Bromides	986	54	1.21	1.18	1.22
Calcium (parenteral), iron, and vitamins	1,091	45	0.91	0.88	0.93
Iron, i.m.	66	2	0.67	0.66	0.63
Vitamins B_{12} and K	28	1	0.79	0.75	0.70
Calcium compounds	1,007	42	0.92	0.89	0.95

[1]$X^2_1 = 4.20$, $p < 0.05$

402

Detailed Evaluation of Uniform Malformations

In this section, groups of drugs, followed by individual drugs, are evaluated in relation to various classes or groups of uniform malformations, as well as individual malformations, for which multiple logistic risk function models were developed. In the tables, the observed and expected numbers of malformed children are given for each drug exposure in turn. The measure of association presented is a standardized relative risk (SRR) with its 95% confidence limits. The SRR is the ratio of the observed number to the expected number of malformed children. Since the SRR takes into account potential confounding variables, it represents the best estimate of the relationship between a drug and a malformation. As numbers of exposed mother-child pairs become so small as to be uninformative, data will be omitted.

Inorganic Compounds and Certain Vitamins — 2,542 Exposures (Table 32.3)

The relative risk for major malformations was 1.16. Relative risks greater than 1.5 were observed for central nervous system malformations (1.63) and eye and ear malformations (1.64). The lower confidence limit of 1.20 for central nervous system malformations indicates that this finding is statistically significant.

Bromides, Fluorides, and Iodides — 1,526 Exposures (Table 32.4)

The relative risk for major malformations was 1.28. The only SRR greater than 1.5 was for musculoskeletal malformations (1.56). Both of these findings are statistically significant, as indicated by the lower confidence limits of 1.04 (major malformations), and 1.13 (musculoskeletal malformations).

Iodides — 489 Exposures (Table 32.5)

Table **32.3**

Standardized Relative Risks (SRR) and Their 95% Confidence Intervals (CI_{95}) for Classes of Malformations Showing Uniform Rates by Hospital in Relation to **Inorganic Compounds and Certain Vitamins** Used in Lunar Months 1–4 by 2,542 Pregnant Women (Based on Multiple Logistic Risk Function Analysis)

Malformation Classes	No. of Malformed Children		SRR	CI_{95} of SRR
	Observed	Expected		
Any malformation	130	122.8	1.06	0.90–1.24
Major malformations	88	75.8	1.16	0.96–1.40
Minor malformations	52	50.0	1.04	0.80–1.35
Central nervous	24	14.7	1.63	1.20–2.21
Cardiovascular	19	22.5	0.84	0.51–1.32
Musculoskeletal (other than polydactyly in Blacks)	25	21.7	1.15	0.80–1.65
Polydactyly in Blacks[1]	24	19.3	1.24	0.88–1.76
Respiratory	11	12.1	0.90	0.45–1.61
Gastrointestinal	16	17.8	0.90	0.52–1.46
Genitourinary (other than hypospadias)	14	11.7	1.20	0.66–2.01
Hypospadias[2]	10	8.7	1.15	0.55–2.11
Eye and ear	11	6.7	1.64	0.82–2.92
Syndromes (other than Down syndrome)	4	7.2	0.56	0.15–1.42
Down syndrome	1	3.8	0.26	0.01–1.47
Tumors	9	10.1	0.89	0.41–1.70

[1] Drugs used by 1,349 Blacks
[2] Drugs used by 1,268 mothers of male offspring

Table 32.4

Standardized Relative Risks (SRR) and Their 95% Confidence Intervals (CI$_{95}$) for Classes of Malformations Showing Uniform Rates by Hospital in Relation to **Bromides, Fluorides, and Iodides** Used in Lunar Months 1–4 by 1,526 Pregnant Women (Based on Multiple Logistic Risk Function Analysis)

Malformation Classes	No. of Malformed Children		SRR	CI$_{95}$ of SRR
	Observed	Expected		
Any malformation	86	76.5	1.12	0.93–1.36
Major malformations	64	49.8	1.28	1.04–1.58
Minor malformations	28	29.4	0.95	0.66–1.38
Central nervous	14	9.8	1.42	0.78–2.38
Cardiovascular	11	14.3	0.77	0.38–1.37
Musculoskeletal (other than polydactyly in Blacks)	23	14.8	1.56	1.13–2.16
Polydactyly in Blacks[1]	11	9.2	1.19	0.60–2.11
Respiratory	6	8.4	1.07	0.49–2.03
Gastrointestinal	12	12.1	0.99	0.51–1.72
Genitourinary (other than hypospadias)	10	8.2	1.22	0.59–2.23
Hypospadias[2]	4	5.3	0.75	0.20–1.91
Eye and ear	6	4.2	1.41	0.52–3.06
Syndromes (other than Down syndrome)	2	5.0	0.40	0.05–1.44
Down syndrome	1	2.5	0.41	0.01–2.27
Tumors	6	6.5	0.93	0.34–2.01

[1]Drugs used by 648 Blacks
[2]Drugs used by 775 mothers of male offspring

The relative risk for major malformations was 1.47. The lower confidence limit of 1.08 indicates that this SRR is statistically significant. Relative risks greater than 1.5 were 1.63 for central nervous system malformations and 3.55 for eye and ear malformations. The latter finding is statistically significant at the 0.05 level, and has a lower confidence limit of 1.15.

Bromides — 986 Exposures (Table 32.6) The SRRs for broad classes of malformations were close to unity. The SRR for musculoskeletal malformations was 1.64 and for gastrointestinal malformations 1.41.

Calcium, Parenteral Iron,
and Vitamins — 1,091
Exposures (Table 32.7)
The SRRs for broad classes of malfor-

mations were all close to unity. SRRs greater than 1.5 were seen for malformations of the central nervous system (1.91), hypospadias (1.68), and eye and ear defects (1.89).

Calcium Compounds — 1,007 Exposures (Table 32.8) Since calcium compounds comprised over 90% of the subgroup (calcium, parenteral iron, and vitamins), it is not surprising to note that a similar pattern emerged. The SRRs for broad classes of malformations all approached unity. Again, relative risks greater than 1.5 were seen for malformations of the central nervous system (2.11), for hypospadias (1.57), and for eye and ear malformations (1.62). The lower confidence limit of 1.02 for central nervous system malformations indicates that the finding is statistically significant.

Table **32.5**

Standardized Relative Risks (SRR) and Their 95% Confidence Intervals (CI_{95}) for Classes of Malformations Showing Uniform Rates by Hospital in Relation to **Iodides** Used in Lunar Months 1–4 by 489 Pregnant Women (Based on Multiple Logistic Risk Function Analysis)

| Malformation Classes | No. of Malformed Children | | SRR | CI_{95} of SRR |
	Observed	Expected		
Any malformation	27	25.3	1.07	0.75–1.52
Major malformations	26	17.7	1.47	1.08–2.00
Minor malformations	4	9.1	0.44	0.12–1.11
Central nervous	6	3.7	1.63	0.60–3.51
Cardiovascular	3	4.7	0.64	0.13–1.86
Musculoskeletal (other than polydactyly in Blacks)	8	5.6	1.44	0.62–2.81
Polydactyly in Blacks[1]	1	1.4	0.69	0.02–3.79
Respiratory	3	3.1	0.97	0.20–2.83
Gastrointestinal	3	4.5	0.66	0.14–1.92
Genitourinary (other than hypospadias)	1	3.3	0.30	0.01–1.66
Hypospadias[2]	1	1.9	0.54	0.01–2.98
Eye and ear	5	1.4	3.55[3]	1.15–8.22
Syndromes (other than Down syndrome)	1	1.9	0.53	0.01–2.96
Down syndrome	1	1.0	0.97	0.02–5.38
Tumors	1	2.3	0.44	0.01–2.43

[1]Drugs used by 118 Blacks
[2]Drugs used by 246 mothers of male offspring
[3]$p < 0.05$

Table **32.6**

Standardized Relative Risks (SRR) and Their 95% Confidence Intervals (CI_{95}) for Classes of Malformations Showing Uniform Rates by Hospital in Relation to **Bromides** Used in Lunar Months 1–4 by 986 Pregnant Women (Based on Multiple Logistic Risk Function Analysis)

| Malformation Classes | No. of Malformed Children | | SRR | CI_{95} of SRR |
	Observed	Expected		
Any malformation	54	47.9	1.13	0.88–1.44
Major malformations	34	29.8	1.14	0.85–1.55
Minor malformations	22	19.1	1.15	0.78–1.69
Central nervous	7	5.9	1.18	0.47–2.42
Cardiovascular	8	8.9	0.90	0.39–1.76
Musculoskeletal (other than polydactyly in Blacks)	14	8.6	1.64	0.90–2.74
Polydactyly in Blacks[1]	8	7.2	1.11	0.48–2.17
Respiratory	5	5.0	1.00	0.32–2.33
Gastrointestinal	10	7.1	1.41	0.68–2.59
Genitourinary (other than hypospadias)	5	4.8	1.03	0.34–2.40
Hypospadias[2]	3	3.4	0.89	0.18–2.59
Eye and ear	1	2.6	0.38	0.01–2.10
Syndromes (other than Down syndrome)	1	2.9	0.34	0.01–1.91
Down syndrome	1	1.4	0.72	0.02–3.97
Tumors	4	4.0	1.01	0.27–2.57

[1]Drugs used by 506 Blacks
[2]Drugs used by 498 mothers of male offspring

Table **32.7**

Standardized Relative Risks (SRR) and Their 95% Confidence Intervals (CI$_{95}$) for Classes of Malformations Showing Uniform Rates by Hospital in Relation to **Calcium, Parenteral Iron, and Vitamins** Used in Lunar Months 1–4 by 1,091 Pregnant Women (Based on Multiple Logistic Risk Function Analysis)

Malformation Classes	No. of Malformed Children		SRR	CI$_{95}$ of SRR
	Observed	Expected		
Any malformation	45	49.5	0.91	0.67–1.23
Major malformations	25	27.8	0.90	0.60–1.35
Minor malformations	24	22.0	1.09	0.75–1.59
Central nervous	10	5.2	1.91	0.92–3.51
Cardiovascular	8	8.8	0.91	0.39–1.78
Musculoskeletal (other than polydactyly in Blacks)	3	7.5	0.40	0.08–1.17
Polydactyly in Blacks[1]	13	10.9	1.20	0.64–2.03
Respiratory	2	4.0	0.50	0.06–1.79
Gastrointestinal	4	6.1	0.66	0.18–1.69
Genitourinary (other than hypospadias)	4	3.7	1.09	0.30–2.79
Hypospadias[2]	6	3.6	1.68	0.62–3.62
Eye and ear	5	2.7	1.89	0.61–4.35
Syndromes (other than Down syndrome)	2	2.3	0.85	0.10–3.07
Down syndrome	0	1.4	—	0.00–2.58
Tumors	3	3.8	0.78	0.16–2.28

[1]Drugs used by 748 Blacks
[2]Drugs used by 535 mothers of male offspring

Table **32.8**

Standardized Relative Risks (SRR) and Their 95% Confidence Intervals (CI$_{95}$) for Classes of Malformations Showing Uniform Rates by Hospital in Relation to **Calcium Compounds** Used in Lunar Months 1–4 by 1,007 Pregnant Women (Based on Multiple Logistic Risk Function Analysis)

Malformation Classes	No. of Malformed Children		SRR	CI$_{95}$ of SRR
	Observed	Expected		
Any malformation	42	45.6	0.97	0.68–1.25
Major malformations	22	25.3	0.87	0.56–1.35
Minor malformations	23	20.4	1.13	0.77–1.65
Central nervous	10	4.7	2.11	1.02–3.87
Cardiovascular	7	8.2	0.86	0.34–1.76
Musculoskeletal (other than polydactyly in Blacks)	3	6.8	0.44	0.09–1.28
Polydactyly in Blacks[1]	13	10.3	1.26	0.67–2.13
Respiratory	2	3.7	0.54	0.07–1.94
Gastrointestinal	4	5.6	0.72	0.20–1.84
Genitourinary (other than hypospadias)	3	3.3	0.90	0.19–2.62
Hypospadias[2]	5	3.2	1.57	0.51–3.63
Eye and ear	4	2.5	1.62	0.44–4.12
Syndromes (other than Down syndrome)	2	2.2	0.92	0.11–3.32
Down syndrome	0	1.2	—	0.00–3.11
Tumors	3	3.6	0.84	0.17–2.45

[1]Drugs used by 703 Blacks
[2]Drugs used by 489 mothers of male offspring

Table **32.9**

Standardized Relative Risks (SRR) and Their 95% Confidence Intervals (CI$_{95}$) for Inguinal Hernia, Clubfoot, and Pectus Excavatum in Relation to **Inorganic Compounds and Certain Vitamins** Used in Lunar Months 1–4 (Based on Multiple Logistic Risk Function Analysis)

	No. of Users	No. of Malformed Children		SRR	CI$_{95}$ of SRR
		Observed	Expected		
Inguinal hernia					
Inorganic compounds and certain vitamins	2542	43	37.9	1.13	0.86–1.49
Bromides, fluorides, and iodides	1526	24	22.9	1.05	0.71–1.54
Iodides	489	7	7.3	0.95	0.38–1.95
Bromides	986	16	14.7	1.09	0.62–1.75
Calcium, parenteral iron, and vitamins	1091	19	16.2	1.18	0.71–2.35
Calcium compounds	1007	19	14.7	1.29	0.78–2.00
Clubfoot					
Inorganic compounds and certain vitamins	2542	12	11.4	1.05	0.55–1.84
Bromides, fluorides, and iodides	1526	9	7.3	1.23	0.56–2.32
Bromides	986	7	4.3	1.62	0.65–3.32
Calcium, parenteral iron, and vitamins	1091	4	4.4	0.92	0.25–2.35
Calcium compounds	1007	3	4.0	0.75	0.15–2.18
Pectus excavatum					
Inorganic compounds and certain vitamins	2542	5	6.5	0.77	0.25–1.78
Bromides, fluorides, and iodides	1526	5	4.9	1.02	0.33–2.37
Iodides	489	3	2.4	1.27	0.26–3.69

Detailed Evaluation of Non-Uniform Malformations: Inguinal Hernia, Clubfoot, Pectus Excavatum

In this section, the three outcomes are evaluated as in the preceding section dealing with uniform malformations. Instances in which there were fewer than three malformed children exposed to any drug are omitted because they are not informative.

As seen in Table 32.9, the highest SRR for inguinal hernia was with calcium compounds (1.29). For clubfoot, the SRR with bromides (1.62) was greater than 1.5. For pectus excavatum, the highest SRR was with iodides (1.27).

Comments

In this study, an attempt was made to evaluate preparations containing

407

halogens (other than chlorine) and calcium. These preparations overlap drugs also considered elsewhere in this book. The strongest association was between iodine-containing drugs (489 exposures) and malformations affecting the eye or ear. There were only five children with such malformations, but four of them (Appendix 4) had the same malformation, cataract. The data are clearly insufficient to justify anything more than a suspicion of possible teratogenicity which requires confirmation. Iodides and bromides (986 exposures) were also associated with central nervous deformities.

Fluorides (122 exposures) gave minimal, if any, evidence of association with malformations, but numbers were small.

Strong associations between calcium-containing compounds (1,007 exposures) and uniform, major or minor malformations could be ruled out with confidence. However, there was an association between this group of drugs and central nervous malformations. The relationship was not confined to any specific deformity. The association requires independent confirmation.

CHAPTER 33

Diagnostic Aids, Technical Aids, and Rare Drugs

General Evaluation

In Table 33.1, all 3,248 malformed children are considered in relation to exposure to the entire group of diagnostic aids, technical aids, and rare drugs during the first four lunar months of pregnancy. In Table 33.2, the data are confined to the 2,277 children who had malformations which were uniformly distributed among the hospitals. Three relative risks are given in each table: crude, standardized for hospital variability, and standardized for the mother's ethnic group and survival of the child.

All Malformations in Relation to Diagnostic Aids, Technical Aids, and Rare Drugs (Table 33.1)

Because there is no logical association of these three groups of drugs, no overall grouping is provided. The hospital-standardized relative risks for each group are diagnostic aids, 1.45; technical aids, 1.15; and rare drugs and drugs with unknown ingredients, 0.92.

Among the diagnostic aids, the hospital-standardized relative risk for all malformations is 1.58 for radiopaque media and 2.37 for intravenous dilution test agents. These relative risks are based on small numbers of malformed children.

Among the technical aids, the only relative risks greater than 1.5 are 2.08 for

Table **33.1**

Children (3,248) With Any Malformation in Relation to Exposure to **Diagnostic Aids, Technical Aids, and Rare Drugs** During Lunar Months 1–4 Among 50,282 Mother-Child Pairs

	No. of Mother-Child Pairs Exposed	No. of Malformed Children	Crude Relative Risk	Hospital Standardized Relative Risk[1]	Survival and Race Standardized Relative Risk[1]
Diagnostic aids	108	10	1.43	1.45	1.17
Radiopaque media[3]	69	7	1.57	1.58	1.34
Intravenous dilution test					
agents[4]	22	3	2.11	2.37	1.46
Radioactive material[5]	21	1	0.74	0.72	0.66
Technical aids	431	33	1.19	1.15	1.15
Local irritants and					
keratolytics	386	30	1.21	1.18	1.17
Camphor[6]	168	10	0.92	0.88	0.85
Sodium tetradecyl sulfate	95	12	1.96[2]	2.08[2]	2.15[2]
Allantoin	51	4	1.21	1.12	1.19
Pulsatilla nigra	38	2	0.81	0.83	0.71
Other local irritants					
and keratolytics[7]	36	2	0.86	0.80	0.86
Enzymes[8]	19	0	—	—	—
Agents for wound protection					
(aluminum powder)	27	3	1.72	1.68	1.63
Rare drugs and drugs with					
unknown ingredients	300	19	0.98	0.92	0.88
Miscellaneous infrequently					
used drugs[9]	50	3	0.93	0.88	0.70
Drugs with unknown					
ingredients	250	5	0.89	0.81	0.85

[1]Estimated by the Mantel-Haenszel procedure
[2]$X^2 = 4.63$–5.02, $p < 0.05$
[3]IV—Pyelography, n.o.s. (42); bunamiodyl (10); diatrizoate sodium (9); iopanoic acid (8); diatrizoate meglumine (3); iodohippurate (1); iophendylate (1)
[4]Phenolsulfonphthalein (12); sulfobromophthalein (9); sodium thiosulfate (1)
[5]Sodium iodine I131 (19); albumin, iodinated I131 serum (2)
[6]Camphor (167); paregoric (90); camphor monobromated (1)
[7]Methyl salicylate (19); resorcinol (8); ferric chloride (5); eugenol (3); capsicum (1)
[8]Trypsin and chymotrypsin, crystalline (14); streptokinase and streptodornase (5); hyaluronidase (1)
[9]Anticoagulants (10); chelating agents (8); asthma medications, n.o.s. (7); infrequently used IV (7); antiarrythmic drugs (7); Uricosuric agents (4); narcotic antagonists (4); intravenous nutrients (3); antineoplastic agents (2); hallucinogenic drugs (2)

sodium tetradecyl sulfate and 1.68 for aluminum powder.

There were too few exposures to rare drugs to permit reliable assessment of their teratogenic potential. It is of interest that one of the two children who were exposed to antineoplastic agents had multiple malformations, and this child died *in utero*.

Malformations with Uniform Rates by Hospital in Relation to Diagnostic Aids, Technical Aids, and Rare Drugs (Table 33.2)

The relative risks in this table, while based on small numbers of malformed children, are similar to those in Table 33.1. Hospital-standardized relative risks

Table **33.2**

Children (2,277) With Malformations Showing Uniform Rates by Hospital in Relation to Exposure to **Diagnostic Aids, Technical Aids, and Rare Drugs** During Lunar Months 1–4 Among 50,282 Mother-Child Pairs

	No. of Mother-Child Pairs Exposed	No. of Malformed Children	Crude Relative Risk	Hospital Standardized Relative Risk	Survival and Race Standardized Relative Risk
Diagnostic aids	108	7	1.43	1.44	1.05
Radiopaque media	69	5	1.60	1.61	1.25
Intravenous dilution test agents	22	2	2.01	2.09	1.14
Radioactive material	21	1	1.05	1.04	0.94
Technical aids	431	24	1.23	1.20	1.18
Local irritants and keratolytics	386	22	1.26	1.23	1.20
Sodium tetradecyl sulfate	95	10	2.33[1]	2.36[1]	2.50[1]
Allantoin	51	2	0.87	0.83	0.82
Pulsatilla nigra	38	0	—	—	—
Camphor	168	8	1.05	1.02	0.96
Other local irritants and keratolytics	36	2	1.23	1.19	1.36
Enzymes	19	0	—	—	—
Agents for wound protection (aluminum powder)	27	2	1.64	1.63	1.48
Rare drugs and drugs with unknown ingredients	300	14	1.03	0.99	0.90
Miscellaneous infrequently used drugs	50	2	0.88	0.86	0.58
Drugs with unknown ingredients	250	12	1.06	1.02	0.98

[1] $X^2_1 = 5.50\text{–}6.59, p < 0.05$

greater than 1.5, based on at least two malformed children, are present for radiopaque media (1.61), intravenous dilution test agents (2.09), sodium tetradecyl sulfate (2.36), and aluminum powder (1.63).

Detailed Evaluation of Uniform Malformations

In this section, groups of drugs, followed by individual drugs, are evaluated in relation to various classes or groups of uniform malformations, as well as individual malformations, for which multiple logistic risk function models were developed. In the tables, the observed and expected numbers of malformed children are given for each drug exposure in turn. The measure of association presented is a standardized relative risk (SRR) with its 95% confidence limits. The SRR is the ratio of the observed number to the expected number of malformed children. Since the SRR takes into account potential confounding variables, it represents the best estimate of the relationship between a drug and a malformation. As numbers of exposed mother-child pairs become so small as to be uninformative, data will be omitted.

411

Diagnostic Aids —
108 Exposures (Table 33.3)

In contrast to the data in Tables 33.1 and 33.2, the SRR for any malformation in relation to diagnostic aids is only 1.04. SRRs greater than 1.5 were present for malformations of the gastrointestinal tract (2.29), and for syndromes other than Down syndrome (4.02).

Technical Aids —
431 Exposures (Table 33.4)

The SRR was greater than 1.5 for minor malformations (1.56). Specific classes of malformations with SRRs greater than 1.5 were cardiovascular (2.10), musculoskeletal (1.63), genitourinary (2.40), hypospadias (2.64), eye and ear malformations (2.52), and tumors (1.74).

Local Irritants and Keratolytics — 386 Exposures (Table 33.5) There was little evidence of association with broad classes of malformations. SRRs greater than 1.5 were seen for cardiovascular malformations (2.32), musculoskeletal malformations (1.78), respiratory malformations (1.50), gastrointestinal malformations (1.60), genitourinary malformations (2.01), hypospadias (2.87), eye and ear malformations (1.85), and tumors (1.91).

Rare Drugs and Drugs
with Unknown Ingredients
— 300 Exposures (Table 33.6)

The SRRs for broad classes of malformations were all close to unity. The only SRR greater than 1.5 was for eye and ear malformations (4.02).

Drugs with Unknown Ingredients — 250 Exposures (Table 33.7) For 250 exposures to drugs with unknown ingredients, there was no evidence of association with broad classes of malformations.

Table **33.3**

Standardized Relative Risks (SRR) and Their 95% Confidence Intervals (CI95) for Classes of Malformations Showing Uniform Rates by Hospital in Relation to **Diagnostic Aids** Used in Lunar Months 1–4 by 108 Pregnant Women (Based on Multiple Logistic Risk Function Analysis)

	No. of Malformed Children			
Malformation Classes	**Observed**	**Expected**	**SRR**	**CI95 of SRR**
Any malformation	7	6.7	1.04	0.42– 2.07
Major malformations	6	4.6	1.29	0.48– 2.72
Minor malformations	2	3.0	0.67	0.08– 2.35
Central nervous	1	1.1	0.93	0.02– 5.09
Cardiovascular	2	1.3	1.50	0.18– 5.30
Musculoskeletal (other than polydactyly in Blacks)	0	1.4	—	0.00– 2.64
Polydactyly in Blacks[1]	0	0.7	—	0.00– 5.12
Respiratory	1	1.1	0.88	0.02– 4.79
Gastrointestinal	3	1.3	2.29	0.48– 6.52
Genitourinary (other than hypospadias)	2	1.3	1.50	0.18– 5.30
Hypospadias[2]	1	0.4	2.22	0.06–11.85
Eye and ear	0	0.4	—	0.00– 9.06
Syndromes (other than Down syndrome)	2	0.5	4.02	0.49–14.15
Down syndrome	0	0.3	—	0.00–10.62
Tumors	1	0.7	1.45	0.04– 7.88

[1]Drugs used by 50 Blacks
[2]Drugs used by 54 mothers of male offspring

Table **33.4**

Standardized Relative Risks (SRR) and Their 95% Confidence Intervals (CI$_{95}$) for Classes of Malformations Showing Uniform Rates by Hospital in Relation to **Technical Aids** Used in Lunar Months 1–4 by 431 Pregnant Women (Based on Multiple Logistic Risk Function Analysis)

Malformation Classes	No. of Malformed Children		SRR	CI$_{95}$ of SRR
	Observed	Expected		
Any malformation	24	20.1	1.19	0.83– 1.71
Major malformations	14	12.6	1.11	0.61– 1.84
Minor malformations	12	7.7	1.56	0.81– 2.70
Central nervous	1	2.3	0.43	0.01– 2.40
Cardiovascular	7	3.3	2.10	0.84– 4.28
Musculoskeletal (other than polydactyly in Blacks)	6	3.7	1.63	0.60– 3.51
Polydactyly in Blacks[1]	1	2.6	0.39	0.01– 2.14
Respiratory	3	2.2	1.34	0.28– 3.89
Gastrointestinal	4	2.7	1.45	0.40– 3.70
Genitourinary (other than hypospadias)	4	1.6	2.40	0.66– 6.11
Hypospadias[2]	4	1.5	2.64	0.72– 6.67
Eye and ear	3	1.2	2.52	0.52– 7.31
Syndromes (other than Down syndrome)	0	1.2	—	0.00– 3.05
Down syndrome	1	0.5	1.85	0.05–10.23
Tumors	3	1.7	1.74	0.36– 5.04

[1]Drugs used by 185 Blacks
[2]Drugs used by 227 mothers of male offspring

Table **33.5**

Standardized Relative Risks (SRR) and Their 95% Confidence Intervals (CI$_{95}$) for Classes of Malformations Showing Uniform Rates by Hospital in Relation to **Local Irritants and Keratolytics** Used in Lunar Months 1–4 by 386 Pregnant Women (Based on Multiple Logistic Risk Function Analysis)

Malformation Classes	No. of Malformed Children		SRR	CI$_{95}$ of SRR
	Observed	Expected		
Any malformation	22	18.1	1.22	0.84– 1.77
Major malformations	13	11.4	1.14	0.61– 1.93
Minor malformations	0	0.6	—	0.00– 5.91
Central nervous	1	2.1	0.48	0.01– 2.68
Cardiovascular	7	3.0	2.32	0.94– 4.74
Musculoskeletal (other than polydactyly in Blacks)	6	3.4	1.78	0.66– 3.84
Polydactyly in Blacks[1]	0	2.1	—	0.00– 1.71
Respiratory	3	2.0	1.50	0.31– 4.33
Gastrointestinal	4	2.5	1.60	0.44– 4.05
Genitourinary (other than hypospadias)	3	1.5	2.01	0.42– 5.83
Hypospadias[2]	4	1.4	2.87	0.79– 7.25
Eye and ear	2	1.1	1.85	0.22– 6.62
Syndromes (other than Down syndrome)	0	1.1	—	0.00– 3.31
Down syndrome	1	0.5	1.99	0.05–11.02
Tumors	3	1.6	1.91	0.39– 5.54

[1]Drugs used by 158 Blacks
[2]Drugs used by 208 mothers of male offspring

Table **33.6**

Standardized Relative Risks (SRR) and Their 95% Confidence Intervals (CI$_{95}$) for Classes of Malformations Showing Uniform Rates by Hospital in Relation to **Rare Drugs and Drugs with Unknown Ingredients** Used in Lunar Months 1–4 by 300 Pregnant Women (Based on Multiple Logistic Risk Function Analysis)

Malformation Classes	No. of Malformed Children		SRR	CI$_{95}$ of SRR
	Observed	Expected		
Any malformation	14	14.5	0.96	0.53– 1.59
Major malformations	8	8.6	0.93	0.40– 1.71
Minor malformations	6	6.2	0.97	0.36– 2.09
Central nervous	2	1.6	1.25	0.15– 4.46
Cardiovascular	3	2.5	1.22	0.25– 3.52
Musculoskeletal (other than polydactyly in Blacks)	1	2.5	0.40	0.01– 2.22
Polydactyly in Blacks[1]	1	2.4	0.42	0.01– 2.28
Respiratory	1	1.5	0.68	0.02– 3.74
Gastrointestinal	0	2.0	—	0.00– 1.84
Genitourinary (other than hypospadias)	1	1.2	0.82	0.02– 4.56
Hypospadias[2]	1	1.2	0.82	0.02– 4.51
Eye and ear	3	0.7	4.02	0.83–11.65
Syndromes (other than Down syndrome)	0	0.8	—	0.00– 4.53
Down syndrome	0	0.5	—	0.00– 8.01
Tumors	1	1.9	0.92	0.02– 5.07

[1]Drugs used by 157 Blacks
[2]Drugs used by 156 mothers of male offspring

Table **33.7**

Standardized Relative Risks (SRR) and Their 95% Confidence Intervals (CI$_{95}$) for Broad Classes of Malformations Showing Uniform Rates by Hospital in Relation to **Drugs With Unknown Ingredients** Used in Lunar Months 1–4 by 250 Pregnant Women (Based on Multiple Logistic Risk Function Analysis)

	No. of Malformed Children		SRR	CI$_{95}$ of SRR
	Observed	Expected		
Any malformation	12	11.9	1.01	0.53–1.73
Major malformations	6	6.9	0.86	0.32–1.85
Minor malformations	6	5.2	1.14	0.42–2.46

Detailed Evaluation of Non-Uniform Malformations: Inguinal Hernia, Clubfoot, Pectus Excavatum

In this section, the three outcomes are evaluated as in the preceding section dealing with uniform malformations. Instances in which there were fewer than three malformed children exposed to any particular drug are omitted because they are not informative.

Table 33.8 indicates that numbers were

414

Table **33.8**

Standardized Relative Risks (SRR) and Their 95% Confidence Intervals (CI$_{95}$) for Inguinal Hernia, Clubfoot, and Pectus Excavatum in Relation to **Diagnostic Aids, Technical Aids, and Rare Drugs** Used in Lunar Months 1–4 (Based on Multiple Logistic Risk Function Analysis)

	No. of Users	No. of Malformed Children		SRR	CI$_{95}$ of SRR
		Observed	Expected		
Inguinal hernia					
Diagnostic Aids	108	3	1.9	1.56	0.32–4.42
Technical Aids	431	7	6.7	1.04	0.42–2.13
Rare Drugs and Drugs with Unknown Ingredients	300	4	4.6	0.87	0.24–2.20
Clubfoot	—	—	—	—	—
Pectus Excavatum	—	—	—	—	—

too small to identify any associations with clubfoot or pectus excavatum. For inguinal hernia, the only SRR greater than 1.5 was with diagnostic aids (1.56).

Comments

There was no evidence to suggest that diagnostic aids cause malformations. Included in this miscellaneous group were 21 exposures to radioactive material. Numbers were obviously too small to confidently rule out a teratogenic effect. However, there is ample evidence to suggest that radioactive compounds should be avoided. This applies particularly to I^{131} which can cause hypothyroidism in the newborn.[1]

Exposure to sodium tetradecyl sulfate (75 mother-child pairs) was related to malformations in general. This drug was given by injection into varicose veins as a sclerosing agent. Although the findings must be confirmed, the use in pregnancy of an intravenously injected agent whose action depends on a toxic effect, is clearly contraindicated, even in the absence of firm evidence that it is teratogenic.

CHAPTER **34**

Considerations Concerning the Evaluation and Control of Risk Factors Other Than Drugs

Evaluation of Possible Overcontrolling

This study is unique in that an attempt has been made to control simultaneously a variety of potentially confounding factors while carrying out multiple comparisons. Models based on multiple logistic risk function analysis were the chief analytical tools used for this purpose. The principle was to control *all* factors found to be related to the outcome under consideration. The reasoning was that all identifiable, potentially confounding factors would be controlled without designing the many thousands of separate analyses that would otherwise have been needed to evaluate each drug in relation to each outcome.

It is worth stressing that only a small fraction of birth defects are explicable on the basis of current knowledge. Given the lack of insight that exists, it seemed conservative to control all of those variables that could be identified as predicting any given outcome so that some control for unsuspected or unrecorded confounding factors could thereby be achieved. For this reason, events occurring in late pregnancy (e.g., toxemia) or factors identified only at birth (e.g., low birthweight) were controlled. However, this strategy requires an evaluation of whether some analyses may have been inadvertently overcontrolled.

The issue can be illustrated with a few examples, the first being single umbilical artery. Is it more legitimate to regard this factor as a malformation in its own right or as an indicator of antecedent events in pregnancy that may have influenced drug use? To give another example — hydramnios is an event that is diagnosed only in the third trimester. Is hydramnios a link in the chain of causation leading to any particular malformation or an indicator of prior events that caused deformities on the one hand and hydramnios on the other? In neither example is there a clear-cut answer.

To the extent that single umbilical artery or hydramnios were components in a causal chain, controlling these variables would have tended to obscure a causal association. Conversely, to the extent that they may have been independently related to some prior event on which there were no recorded data, controlling them was desirable.

In this study, the strategy was to control variables of this type at the risk of overcontrolling the analyses. However, the possibility of overcontrolling could be checked in three ways. The first method was to compare crude and standardized relative risks (SRRs). If any SRR was substantially lower than the crude relative risk, the factors bringing about the reduction could be identified.

The second method was to estimate the SRRs for various drugs in relation to a large number of outcomes when factors such as single umbilical artery, pre-eclampsia, prematurity, etc. were controlled and when they were not. No SRRs were found to be materially altered.

The third and most definitive way was to treat drugs identified as being associated with malformations as independent risk factors and then to include them as additional risk factors in the appropriate multivariate models described in the first half of this book. It was then possible to determine whether the relative risk estimates derived by including the drugs in the models differed appreciably from the SRRs. Three outcomes were selected for this purpose: central nervous, musculoskeletal, and cardiovascular malformations. The drugs most strongly related to these outcomes were evaluated. In Table 34.1, the computed SRRs (also presented in the appropriate drug chapters) are compared with the relative risk estimates obtained in the multiple logistic risk function models. For example, in Chapter 32, the SRR of CNS malformations among 1,007 exposures to calcium-containing compounds was estimated to be 2.11 (Table 32.8). When calcium exposure was included as a risk factor in the multiple logistic risk function analysis of CNS malformations, the relative risk estimate was almost unchanged at 2.20 when all the factors identified in Chapter 8 (Table 8.28) were present in the same model. These factors included hydramnios, single umbilical artery, low birthweight, pre-eclampsia, and low placental weight. Had the association between calcium and CNS malformations been overcontrolled, the effect, in the model, would have been to alter substantially the relative risk of calcium exposure. In fact, the relative risk was hardly changed at all.

Table 34.1 also shows that the two types of relative risk estimates agreed well for exposure to female hormones, thyroid hormones, and phenothiazines in relation to cardiovascular deformities, and for pheniramine exposure in relation to musculoskeletal anomalies.

In summary, no instances of possible overcontrolling in this study were detected.

Table **34.1**

Comparisons of Standardized Relative Risks (SRR) and Estimated Relative Risks Obtained by Multiple Logistic Risk Function Analysis

	SRR	Relative Risk Estimated by Multiple Logistic Risk Function Analysis
Central nervous system		
Calcium compounds	2.11	2.20
Cardiovascular system		
Phenothiazines	1.68	1.51
Barbiturates	1.40	1.21
Progestational agents	1.80	1.45
Estrogenic agents	1.89	1.23
Thyroxin and thyroid	1.72	1.65
Oral contraceptives	2.41	2.03
Musculoskeletal system		
Pheniramine	1.47	1.35

The General Epidemiology of Risk Factors Other Than Drugs

In this study it was not possible to evaluate drugs as potential teratogens without first investigating the epidemiology of malformations in a more general sense. This was necessary to ensure that potential confounding had been controlled as adequately as was feasible. Thus the first half of this book has dealt with general epidemiological data.

The multiple logistic risk function analyses presented in Chapters 8 through 17 represent estimates of the extent to which the presented risk factors predicted the outcomes under consideration when all other factors in the tables were simultaneously controlled. For example, in Table 8.28, the adjusted relative risk of central nervous malformations, given hydramnios, was 8.5, and the ratio of the risk function coefficient to its standard error was so high (2.14/0.21) that the association was unlikely to be due to chance. All other factors in the table were taken into account in estimating the strength of the association between hydramnios and CNS deformities (and inclusion of drugs as risk factors in the model was without material effect). Moreover, in Table 8.20, it can be seen that the crude relative risk, given hydramnios, was 9.0 (i.e., virtually identical to the multivariate estimate of 8.5). The univariate findings with regard to hydramnios can therefore be accepted as reasonably reliable since potentially confounding factors had virtually no effect on the association.

In other circumstances, when the strength of any particular univariate association was appreciably changed in multivariate analysis, the univariate findings cannot be accepted at face value and must be interpreted with caution. For example, factors such as low placental weight, low birthweight, or short duration of pregnancy were closely correlated for obvious reasons. The univariate and multivariate estimates of association sometimes differed appreciably. It was beyond the scope of this study to explore fully interactions among factors of this type. The task involved in assessing such interactions would have called for a large study in its own right.

Some further limitations to the interpretability of what might be termed the general epidemiological aspects of this study must also be stressed. It was impossible to pursue questions that could have been addressed if drugs had not been the principal focus of this study. For example, multivariate models could have been devised to evaluate, say, diabetes mellitus as a predictor of hydramnios or pre-eclampsia. Or, although numbers were modest, more detailed data on predictors of outcomes such as cranio-spinal fusion defects, cleft anomalies, etc. might have been of general epidemiological interest.

The focus on drugs also required that certain puzzling findings had to remain partly or completely unexplored. For example, as shown in Chapters 5, 6, 8, 9, 11 and 13, the relative risks, given very low birthweight or short gestation, were elevated in both the White and the Black ethnic groups for uniform, major, central nervous, cardiovascular, respiratory, and genitourinary malformations. However, these relative risks tended to be much higher among Whites. On further exploration, the results appeared to be due to more complete ascertainment of malformations in prematurely born White children who survived. Analyses designed to explore all such anomalous features in the data were impractical when they did not bear directly on the question of whether drugs cause birth defects.

Of course, it is obvious that the basic data files, as organized in this study, can be readily explored for the above purposes. However, even the data presented in this volume are informative, and many of the findings concerning maternal characteristics, prior obstetrical history, characteristics of the pregnancy, complications of pregnancy, maternal illnesses, environmental factors, and genetic factors, can be readily interpreted as they stand.

Certain factors were of particular interest, sometimes because they were positively related to malformations, sometimes not. For example, the data suggested that nausea and vomiting of pregnancy was not usually an important risk factor for most malformations — and certainly, in the sense that the majority of the gravidas were affected, vomiting was "normal." Conversely, other factors such as diabetes mellitus or toxemia were impressive predictors, with the risk of malformations appearing monotonically related to their severity. There were also some surprises. Thus, bleeding in early pregnancy did not, on the whole, appear to be a strong risk factor; by contrast, factors such as hemorrhagic shock, coagulation defect, or the vena cava syndrome gave hints of association that might merit further research.

One overwhelming conclusion emerges: The large series of successive analyses has suggested that congenital deformities can seldom be attributed predominantly to a single factor. Occasionally some overwhelming factor (e.g., rubella, thalidomide) can be identified, but it appears to be much more the rule that birth defects have a multifactorial etiology.

419

CHAPTER 35

Summary of
the Study

Drugs as Potential Teratogens

No commonly used drugs were identified whose potency as teratogens could be regarded as even remotely comparable to thalidomide. In that sense the findings of this study are reassuring. However, it is immediately necessary to emphasize that less easily identifiable drug teratogens may have escaped detection.

Even in a cohort as massive as this one, it was usually the rule that numbers were inadequate for analyzing a specific drug in relation to a specific deformity. Sampling variation alone could have obscured even quite strong associations. Because of the problem of small numbers, because teratogenicity may be the property of a group of compounds, and because a teratogenic effect need not necessarily be specific, groups and subgroups of drugs, as well as individual drugs, were considered in relation to categories and subcategories of malformations, as well as individual malformations. Even in these circumstances, however, small numbers were frequently a problem.

There is an important difference, sometimes not appreciated, between *failure to find evidence of association* (i.e., a relative risk of unity with *wide* confidence limits) and *evidence suggesting that there is no association* (i.e., a relative risk of unity with *narrow* confidence limits). In the latter circumstance, there is reason to believe that a drug may be safe; in the former, the matter of safety is left unresolved. If the goal is to set narrow confidence limits around a relative risk of unity, large numbers are required. The study was large enough to enable evaluation of safety for some of the more commonly used drugs, or drug groups, in relation to large coalesced outcomes. Thus, it was encouraging to find that agents such as non-addicting analgesics, sulfonamides, vaccines, antinauseants, and sedatives, when evaluated against large outcomes, appeared to be reasonably safe. However, such evaluations must not be allowed to induce a false sense of security since sampling variation could readily have obscured specific relationships. Moreover, while malformations in general may not have been associated with some particular exposure, specific malformations sometimes were.

Certain drugs were not used by a sufficient number of women to assess safety, even in relation to the larger malformation categories. Nevertheless, the impression was one of relative safety — the marked secular increase in drug use between the years 1958 and 1965 was not accompanied by a secular change in the malformation rate. If any common and relatively powerful drug teratogen had been introduced over those years, a corresponding increase in the malformation rate might have been expected.

With regard to the positive associations identified in this study, none of them can be considered as more than hypotheses requiring independent confirmation. They have been described or documented in the appropriate chapters and appendices, and no association will be singled out for further mention here.

The Need for Surveillance

The fetus is most susceptible to the teratogenic effects of drugs (or other agents) prior to the 45th day after conception. Pregnancy cannot be confidently diagnosed before the 28th day and is frequently diagnosed later. Thus, women may be taking drugs when neither they nor their medical attendants are aware that they are pregnant. This consideration, together with the secular pattern of increasing drug use found over successive years of recruitment to this study, leads to the depressing thought that if a powerful teratogen had been made available for some common indication, it would probably have been used. There is no reason to believe that the situation is any different today.

From a public health point of view there will always be a need for surveillance of birth defects as they relate to drugs as well as other environmental factors. Moreover, the relationship between vaginal adenocarcinoma and female hormone exposure in pregnancy indicates that many outcomes other than those conventionally considered as birth defects need to be monitored.[1,2]

The experience acquired in analyzing the Collaborative Perinatal data has been helpful in developing methods to deal with the complex problems involved in evaluating drugs as potential teratogens. It is unlikely that a study of this scale will soon be repeated. However, it should now be possible to design less ambitious and more focused follow-up studies, or case-control studies that can provide the surveillance needed to protect pregnant women and their offspring.

Evaluation of Drugs in Relation to Malformations Which May Originate During Early or Late Embryogenesis

Classical malformations, such as cleft anomalies, can arise only at very specific, and early, susceptible periods during embryogenesis. Most malformations are considered to be of this type. If a drug is causing any such malformation, exposure must take place during the early development of the fetus. In this study, the indicator of early exposure was taken to be drug use during the first four lunar months of pregnancy. Consequently, the major part of the analysis in this book has been concentrated on early drug exposure.

However, it is clear that certain malformations may arise not only during early embryogenesis, but also at later points in development. For some malformations, the exact time of origin may not be at all clear. It is important to judge which malformations are of this type since they may be associated with drug exposure taking place after the conventional susceptible period of embryogenesis. In this study, we have considered that the malformations listed in Table A1.1 may arise at any time during pregnancy. All of the malformations listed in the table are components of the uniform set of malformations and are here designated as the set of "anytime" malformations. They affected 911 children.

In the following two sections, anytime malformations are evaluated in the same way as the other malformation outcomes. We also judged that the non-uniform malformations — inguinal hernia, clubfoot, pectus excavatum, and urethral obstruction — may sometimes arise after the first trimester. Both sets of malformations are considered together in relation to drug exposure throughout pregnancy, in a later section of this appendix. It must be emphasized that drugs are in general more likely to have teratogenic effects when the embryo is undergoing its most radical metamorphoses, and that there is an arbitrary element in deciding whether certain malformations can be designated as belonging to the "anytime" category. Consequently, we consider the analyses in this appendix to be more tentative than those of drug exposure that took place during early pregnancy.

Risk Factors Other Than Drugs for Anytime Malformations

Administrative Data
Number of Antenatal Visits (Table A1.2) The relative risks for 1 to 4 visits and 15 or more visits were 1.3 and 1.5, respectively.

Characteristics of the Mother
Ethnic Group (Table A1.3) In White children, the relative risk of anytime malformations was 1.5.

Maternal Age (Table A1.4) For children of Black and Puerto Rican mothers over the age of 40 years, the relative risks were 2.9 and 3.8, respectively. However, for children of White mothers over 40 the

corresponding relative risk was 0.2. The results for Whites and Puerto Ricans were based on 2 malformed children.

Religion (Table A1.5) In children of Black Catholic women, the relative risk of anytime malformations was 1.4.

Characteristics and Survival of the Offspring
Birthweight (Table A1.6) In babies weighing less than 2 kg, and 2 to 2.4 kg, the relative risks for anytime malformations were 3.3 and 2.1, respectively.

Sex of Child (Table A1.7) The rates of anytime malformations were similar in male and female children.

Survival of the Child (Table A1.8) All mortality categories were associated with increased rates of anytime malformations; the relative risks ranged from 4.8 to 11.1.

Reproductive History of the Mother
Prior Premature Births (Table A1.9) For children whose mothers had had three or more prior premature births, the relative risk was 1.2.

Prior Stillbirth and Neonatal Death (Table A1.10) The relative risks for prior stillbirth and prior neonatal death were 1.2 and 1.5, respectively.

Characteristics and Complications of the Pregnancy
Duration of Pregnancy (Table A1.11) The relative risks for short pregnancies (less than 9 lunar months) and long pregnancies (over 10 lunar months) were 2.1 and 1.5, respectively.

Placental Weight (Table A1.12) Children had an increased rate of anytime malformations when the placenta weighed less than 300 gm, giving a relative risk of 2.4.

Single Umbilical Artery (Table A1.13) For children with single umbilical artery, the relative risk was 5.9.

Signs of Toxemia (Table A1.14) Rates of anytime malformations were elevated in children whose mothers had

423

*Table **A1.1***

Malformations Which May Have Their Origin
Anytime During Pregnancy (911 Children)

	No. of Children
Central nervous system	
Hydrocephaly	75
Microcephaly	77
Hypoplasia/atrophy of brain	10
Macrocephaly	18
Anomalies of pituitary gland	7
Atrophy/hypoplasia of optic nerve	7
Cardiovascular system	
Ductus arteriosus persistens	45
Musculoskeletal system	
Hypoplasia of limb or part thereof	51
Congenital dislocation of hip	92
Miscellaneous foot abnormalities	
(e.g., Rocker bottom feet)	10
Other musculoskeletal anomalies	
(e.g., hemihypertrophy)	10
Respiratory tract	
Malformations of the thoracic wall	
(e.g., pigeon breast, asymmetry)	18
Hiatal hernia	8
Anomalies of teeth	19
Other respiratory anomalies	
(e.g., macroglossia, single nostril)	19
Gastrointestinal tract	
Hirschsprung's disease	13
Pyloric stenosis	95
Umbilical hernia	51
Ventral, epigastric, and femoral hernia	5
Genitourinary system	
Stenotic ureter	26
Hypoplasia of penis	4
Abnormal testis	15
Abnormal ovary	8
Hydronephrosis	23
Hydroureter	21
Ambiguous genitalia	5
Hydrocele	10
Malformation of female genitalia	36
Eye and ear	
Coloboma	13
Cataract	44
Glaucoma/buphthalmos	10
Corneal opacity	8

*Table **A1.1** (continued)*

	No. of Children
Syndromes	
Hypoplasia/atrophy of adrenals	26
Other adrenal anomalies	
(e.g., necrosis, abnormal shape, malposition)	16
Adrenogenital syndrome	4
Tumors	
Benign tumors	140
Malignant tumors	24

*Table **A1.2***

Distribution of Children with Anytime Malformations by Number of Antenatal Visits

No. of Antenatal Visits	No. of Children	Children with Anytime Malformations		Relative Risk
		No.	Rate/1,000	
1–4	8,624	191	22.1	1.3
5–14	37,958	630	16.6	1.0*
≥15	3,700	90	24.3	1.5

*Reference category

*Table **A1.3***

Distribution of Children with Anytime Malformations by Ethnic Group

	No. of Children	Children with Anytime Malformations		Relative Risk
		No.	Rate/1,000	
White	22,811	507	22.2	1.5
Black	24,030	352	14.6	1.0*
Puerto Rican	3,441	52	15.1	1.0

*Reference category

Table **A1.4**

Race-Specific Distribution of Children with Anytime Malformations by Mother's Age at Registration

| | Mother's Age | No. of Children | Children with Anytime Malformations | | Relative Risk |
			No.	Rate/1,000	
White	<20	4,074	77	18.9	0.8
	20–39	18,351	428	23.3	1.0*
	≥40	386	2	5.2	0.2
Black	<20	6,978	94	13.5	0.9
	20–39	16,700	243	14.6	1.0*
	≥40	352	15	42.6	2.9
Puerto Rican	<20	852	10	11.7	0.7
	20–39	2,555	40	15.7	1.0*
	≥40	34	2	58.8	3.8

*Reference category

Table **A1.5**

Race-Specific Distribution of Children with Anytime Malformations by Mother's Religion

| | | No. of Children | Children with Anytime Malformations | | Relative Risk |
			No.	Rate/1,000	
White	Protestant	9,031	195	21.6	1.0*
	Catholic	11,943	272	22.8	1.0
	Other	1,837	40	21.8	1.0
Black	Protestant	20,620	291	14.1	1.0*
	Catholic	2,833	56	19.8	1.4
	Other	577	5	8.7	0.6
Puerto Rican	Protestant	279	7	25.1	1.0*
	Catholic	3,136	45	14.3	0.6
	Other	26	0	0	—

*Reference category

426

Table **A1.6**

Distribution of Children with Anytime Malformations by Child's Birthweight

| Birthweight (grams) | No. of Children | Children with Anytime Malformations | | Relative Risk |
		No.	Rate/1,000	
<2,000	1,976	102	51.6	3.3
2,000–2,499	3,704	121	32.7	2.1
≥2,500	44,602	688	15.4	1.0*

*Reference category

Table **A1.7**

Distribution of Children with Anytime Malformations by Sex of Child

| | No. of Children | Children with Anytime Malformations | | Relative Risk |
		No.	Rate/1,000	
Male	25,542	467	18.3	1.0*
Female	24,740	444	17.9	1.0

*Reference category

Table **A1.8**

Distribution of Children with Anytime Malformations by Survival of the Child

| Survival of Child | No. of Children | Children with Anytime Malformations | | Relative Risk |
		No.	Rate/1,000	
Stillbirth	798	55	68.9	4.8
Neonatal death	806	71	88.1	6.2
Infant death	384	61	158.9	11.1
Childhood death	239	38	159.0	11.1
Survived	48,055	686	14.3	1.0*

*Reference category

427

Table **A1.9**

Distribution of Children with Anytime Malformations by History of Prior Premature Births

| No. of Prior Premature Births | No. of Children | Children with Any Malformations | | Relative Risk |
		No.	Rate/1,000	
None	26,707[1]	476	17.8	1.0*
1	5,443	97	17.8	1.0
2	1,677	30	17.9	1.0
≥3	901	19	21.1	1.2
No prior liveborn	15,554	289	18.6	1.0

*Reference category
[1]Includes 952 unknowns

Table **A1.10**

Distribution of Children with Anytime Malformations by History of Prior Stillbirth and Neonatal Death

| | No. of Children | Children with Anytime Malformations | | Relative Risk |
		No.	Rate/1,000	
Prior stillbirth	2,837	61	21.5	1.2
No prior stillbirth	32,280	571	17.7	1.0*
No prior pregnancies 20 weeks or over	15,165	279	18.4	1.0
Prior neonatal death	2,174	55	25.3	1.5
No prior neonatal death	32,554	567	17.4	1.0*
No prior liveborn	15,554	289	18.6	1.1

*Reference category

Table **A1.11**

Distribution of Children with Anytime Malformations by Duration of Pregnancy

| Length of Gestation (lunar months) | No. of Children | Children with Anytime Malformations | | Relative Risk |
		No.	Rate/1,000	
≤8	3,851	135	35.1	2.1
9–10	45,436	751	16.5	1.0*
≥11	995	25	25.1	1.5

*Reference category

*Table **A1.12***

Distribution of Children with Anytime Malformations by Placental Weight

| Placental Weight (grams) | No. of Children | Children with Anytime Malformations | | Relative Risk |
		No.	Rate/1,000	
≤299	2,483	98	39.5	2.4
300–399	13,115	248	18.9	1.1
≥400	28,270	470	16.6	1.0*
Unknown	6,414	95	14.8	0.9

*Reference category

*Table **A1.13***

Distribution of Children with Anytime Malformations by Number of Umbilical Arteries

| No. of Umbilical Arteries | No. of Children | Children with Anytime Malformations | | Relative Risk |
		No.	Rate/1,000	
One	341	36	105.6	5.9
Two	44,851	798	17.8	1.0*
Unknown	5,090	77	15.1	0.9

*Reference category

*Table **A1.14***

Distribution of Children with Anytime Malformations by Signs of Toxemia[1]

| | No. of Children | Children with Anytime Malformations | | Relative Risk |
		No.	Rate/1,000	
Eclampsia	22	0	—	—
Chronic hypertension	669	18	26.9	1.5
Acute hypertension (BP ≥ 160/110 after LM 6)	930	31	33.3	1.9
Proteinuria with or without edema	1,213	31	25.6	1.4
Generalized edema only	11,425	189	16.5	0.9
None	36,023	642	17.8	1.0*

*Reference category
[1]This classification is hierarchical and based on severity—for example, a pregnancy complicated by chronic hypertension is classified as such, even though proteinuria and edema may also be present.

Distribution of Children with Anytime Malformations by Placental Factors

	No. of Children	Children with Anytime Malformations		Relative Risk*
		No.	Rate/1,000	
Marginal sinus rupture	639	19	29.7	1.7
Abruptio placentae	1,030	35	34.0	1.9
Placental infarct ≥ 3 cm	1,501	39	26.0	1.4

*For each condition, the reference category is those without the condition.

proteinuria or hypertension, with relative risks ranging between 1.4 and 1.9.

Placental Factors (Table A1.15) Rates of anytime malformations were elevated in children whose mothers had marginal sinus rupture, abruptio placentae, and large placental infarct, giving relative risks of 1.7, 1.9, and 1.4, respectively.

Complications and Diseases of Pregnancy (Table A1.16) Hyperemesis gravidarum and anemia were both negatively related to anytime malformations (relative risk, 0.7). Hydramnios (relative risk, 4.0), hemorrhagic shock (2.9), vena cava syndrome (2.7), diabetes (2.2), hyper-

thyroidism (2.6), syphilis (mostly inactive) (1.1), urinary tract infection (1.3), convulsive disorder (2.3), and septic shock (12.3) were all positively associated with anytime malformations.

Environmental Factors

Pelvic or Abdominal X-Ray Exposure During Pregnancy (Table A1.17) For children whose mothers were exposed to X-rays, the relative risk was 1.3.

Genetic Factors

Prior Malformed Siblings (Table A1.18) Given a history of malformed sib-

Distribution of Children with Anytime Malformations by Various Diseases and Complications of Pregnancy

	No. of Children	Children with Anytime Malformations		Relative Risk*
		No.	Rate/1,000	
Hyperemesis gravidarum	540	7	13.0	0.7
Hydramnios	694	48	69.1	4.0
Hemorrhagic shock	99	5	50.5	2.9
Vena cava syndrome	144	7	48.6	2.7
Anemia	11,761	157	13.3	0.7
Diabetes mellitus	333	13	39.0	2.2
Hyperthyroidism	87	4	46.0	2.6
Syphilis	918	18	19.6	1.1
Urinary tract infection (fever ≥ 100.4°F)	709	17	24.0	1.3
Convulsive disorder	294	12	40.8	2.3
Septic shock	9	2	222.2	12.3

*For each condition, the reference category is those without the condition.

430

Distribution of Children with Anytime Malformations by Pelvic and/or Abdominal X-Ray
Exposure During Pregnancy

Pelvic and/or Abdominal X-Ray Exposure	No. of Children	Children with Anytime Malformations		Relative Risk
		No.	Rate/1,000	
Present	11,400	258	22.6	1.3
Absent	38,882	653	16.8	1.0*

*Reference category

lings, the relative risks for anytime malformations ranged from 1.5 to 1.7, depending on the malformation in the sibling.

Erythroblastosis Fetalis (Table A1.19) All incompatibilities resulting in clinical erythroblastosis fetalis were positively related to anytime malformations, with relative risks ranging from 1.8 to 7.9.

Multivariate Analysis

Based on the preceding comparisons, 33 factors were selected for multivariate analysis and scaled as dichotomous variables. The following variables were eliminated after linear discriminant function analysis because of low coefficients: prior stillbirths, prior neonatal deaths, prior premature children, marginal sinus rupture, abruptio placentae, syphilis, urinary tract infection, and prior sibling with a head/spine malformation. The results of the multiple logistic risk function analysis for the remaining 24 factors are presented in Table A1.20.

Variables with a relative risk greater than 3 were septic shock (5.7), single umbilical artery (4.8), and hydramnios (3.2). The association with septic shock was not statistically significant. Variables with relative risks between 2 and 3 were maternal age at least 40 years among non-Whites (2.4), vena cava syndrome (2.4), low birthweight (2.3), convulsive disorder (2.2), and hyperthyroidism (2.0). Only the association with hyperthyroidism was not statistically

Table **A1.18**

Distribution of Children with Any Malformation by History of Selected Malformations in Prior Siblings

Malformation in Prior Sibling(s)	No. of Children	Children with Any Malformations		Relative Risk
		No.	Rate/1,000	
Finger/toe	453	12	26.5	1.5
Head/spine	466	13	27.9	1.6
Miscellaneous other defects[1]	1,301	38	29.2	1.7
No defects	30,613	526	17.2	1.0*
No prior liveborn	15,166	279	18.4	1.1

*Reference category
[1]Not including cardiac malformations, clubfoot, or cleft palate

Table **A1.19**

Distribution of Children with Anytime Malformations by Erythroblastosis Fetalis

Type of Erythroblastosis	No. of Children	Children with Anytime Malformations		Relative Risk
		No.	Rate/1,000	
Rh	266	10	37.6	2.1
ABO	155	5	32.3	1.8
Other	7	1	142.9	7.9
None/Unknown	49,585	891	18.0	1.0*

*Reference category

Table **A1.20**

Factors Related to the Risk of Malformations Which Can Originate at Anytime During Pregnancy, Based Upon Multiple Logistic Risk Function Analysis

	Estimated Risk Function Coefficient	Standard Error of Coefficient	Estimated Standardized Relative Risk
Septic shock during pregnancy	1.75	0.89	5.7
Single umbilical artery	1.57	0.19	4.8
Hydramnios	1.18	0.16	3.2
Maternal age $\geq$ 40 among non-Whites	0.89	0.26	2.4
Vena cava syndrome	0.88	0.39	2.4
Birthweight $\leq$ 2,500 gm	0.85	0.09	2.3
Convulsive disorder	0.77	0.30	2.2
Hyperthyroidism	0.69	0.52	2.0
Diabetes mellitus	0.51	0.32	1.7
Length of gestation $\geq$ 11 lunar months	0.45	0.21	1.6
White ethnic group	0.45	0.08	1.6
Prior sibling with miscellaneous malformations[1]	0.40	0.15	1.5
Erythroblastosis fetalis	0.38	0.26	1.5
Catholic religion among Blacks	0.34	0.15	1.4
Hypertension/eclampsia	0.33	0.15	1.4
Sibling with finger/toe abnormalities	0.33	0.30	1.4
Hemorrhagic shock during pregnancy	0.29	0.49	1.3
Placental weight < 300 gm	0.27	0.13	1.3
At least 15 antenatal visits	0.24	0.12	1.3
Placental infarcts $\geq$ 3 cm	0.23	0.17	1.3
Less than 5 antenatal visits	0.18	0.09	1.2
Pelvic/abdominal X-ray exposure during pregnancy	0.15	0.08	1.2
Anemia	−0.25	0.09	0.8
Hyperemesis gravidarum	−0.47	0.38	0.6

[1]Not including malformations of the fingers/toes, head/spine, heart, clubfoot, and cleft lip/palate.

significant. Of the remaining variables, the following had a statistically significant association with anytime malformations: duration of pregnancy at least 11 lunar months (1.6), White ethnic group (1.6), sibling with one or more miscellaneous malformations (1.5), Catholic religion among Blacks (1.4), chronic hypertension (1.4), placental weight less than 300 gm (1.3), fewer than 5 antenatal visits (1.2), and maternal anemia (0.8).

As seen in Table A1.21, stratification of the 911 children with anytime malformations according to risk score showed good agreement between the observed and expected numbers of malformations. The ratio of the numbers in the highest to the lowest decile was over 6, indicating that the model was satisfactory in discriminating between degrees of risk.

Evaluation of Drugs

In this section, multiple logistic risk function analysis will be used to evaluate the drug exposure experience of the cohort, throughout pregnancy, in relation to the set of anytime malformations. To reduce the data to a manageable amount, no information will be provided on any drug when there were fewer than three exposed and malformed children. In addition, Appendix 5 gives data, standardized for hospital variability, on the relationships between individual drugs taken at any time during pregnancy and individual anytime malformations. Once again it must be emphasized that any of the associations listed here, or in Appendix 5, even when nominally "significant" and even when powerful in

Table **A1.21**

Distribution of Observed and Expected Numbers of Children with Anytime Malformations Which Can Originate at Any Stage in Pregnancy by Multiple Logistic Risk Function Scores

Risk Score Percentile[1]	Observed Number of Children with Anytime Malformations	Expected Number of Children with Anytime Malformations
99–100	88	93.3
97–98	49	49.7
95–96	50	40.3
93–94	34	35.4
91–92	23	31.2
Subtotal (91–100)	244	249.9
81–90	122	122.7
71–80	86	96.5
61–70	88	85.8
51–60	80	78.5
41–50	90	74.6
31–40	61	60.8
21–30	54	51.8
11–20	48	49.8
1–10	38	40.6
Total	911	911.0

[1]Each decile contains 5,025 pregnancies, except the lowest which contains 5,057 pregnancies.

terms of relative risk, may reflect nothing more than random variation. It is intended that these associations should be interpreted either as hypotheses for further research or as data to be checked against other independently collected material. On their own, they do not justify causal inferences. A further point must be stressed: proper evaluation of the data presented in these appendices requires that the associations be examined in conjunction with the data dealing with first trimester exposure presented in the preceding chapters and Appendix 4.

Analgesic and Antipyretic Drugs (Table A1.22) It is noteworthy that aspirin, which was received by over 60% of the gravidas, gave no evidence of association with the set of anytime malformations (SRR 0.98). SRRs greater than 1.5 were noted for ethoheptazine (1.57), opium (1.87), hydromorphone (2.04), and hydrocodone (2.45). The SRR of 1.17 for narcotic analgesics had a lower confidence limit of 1.02, thus attaining statistical significance.

Antimicrobial and Antiparasitic Drugs (Table A1.23) SRRs for the drug group as a whole (0.95) and for its subgroups — antibiotics (0.92), sulfonamides (0.92), miscellaneous drugs (0.94), and topical agents (1.09) — were all close to unity. SRRs in excess of 1.5 were noted for tyrothricin (1.50) and gramicidin (2.14) among the antibiotics; for sulfathiazole (1.60); for methenamine (2.25), mandelic acid (1.77), diiodohydroxyquin (1.68), and methylene blue (3.43), among the miscellaneous agents; and for cetylpyridinium (1.53), boric acid (1.69), thymol (2.08), and thiomersal (3.13) among the topical agents. The lower

Table **A1.22**

Standardized Relative Risks (SRR) and their 95% Confidence Intervals (CI$_{95}$) for Anytime Malformations Showing Uniform Rates by Hospital in Relation to **Analgesic and Antipyretic Drugs** Used Anytime During Pregnancy (Based on Multiple Logistic Risk Function Analysis)

	No. of Users	No. of Malformed Children		SRR	CI$_{95}$ of SRR
		Observed	Expected		
Analgesics and antipyretics	33,841	605	615.95	0.98	0.94–1.03
Nonaddicting analgesics and antipyretics	32,856	576	594.86	0.97	0.92–1.02
Aspirin	32,164	570	582.35	0.98	0.93–1.03
Phenacetin	13,031	228	233.83	0.98	0.87–1.09
Salicylamide	1,623	38	31.92	1.19	0.89–1.59
Acetaminophen	781	18	14.24	1.26	0.75–1.98
Analgesic and cold capsules, n.o.s.	644	14	11.99	1.17	0.64–1.94
Narcotic analgesics	6,745	161	138.08	1.17	1.02–1.33
Propoxyphene	2,914	73	60.11	1.21	0.99–1.49
Codeine	2,522	57	50.81	1.12	0.88–1.43
Meperidine	1,100	30	25.54	1.17	0.85–1.63
Paregoric	562	10	10.10	0.99	0.48–1.81
Morphine	448	15	12.34	1.22	0.69–1.98
Ethoheptazine	300	10	6.37	1.57	0.76–2.84
Opium	181	7	3.75	1.87	0.76–3.76
Hydromorphone	61	3	1.47	2.04	0.43–5.68
Hydrocodone	60	4	1.63	2.45	0.68–5.94

Table **A1.23**

Standardized Relative Risks (SRR) and Their 95% Confidence Intervals (CI$_{95}$) for Anytime Malformations Showing Uniform Rates by Hospital in Relation to **Antimicrobial and Antiparasitic Agents** Used Anytime During Pregnancy (Based on Multiple Logistic Risk Function Analysis)

	No. of Users	No. of Malformed Children		SRR	CI$_{95}$ of SRR
		Observed	Expected		
Antimicrobial and antiparasitic agents	17,538	302	317.72	0.95	0.87–1.04
Antibiotics	9,560	163	176.95	0.92	0.80–1.06
Tetracycline	1,336	21	26.94	0.78	0.48–1.26
Antibiotic, n.o.s.	390	7	7.90	0.89	0.36–1.81
Streptomycin	355	7	7.03	1.00	0.40–2.03
Chloramphenicol	348	8	6.73	1.19	0.52–2.31
Oxytetracycline	328	4	6.20	0.65	0.18–1.64
Demeclocycline	280	3	7.39	0.41	0.08–1.17
Nystatin	230	4	4.89	0.82	0.22–2.07
Erythromycin	230	6	4.79	1.25	0.46–2.68
Tyrothricin	130	4	2.67	1.50	0.41–3.74
Gramicidin	96	4	1.87	2.14	0.59–5.30
Penicillin derivatives	7,171	119	128.87	0.92	0.78–1.10
Sulfonamides	5,689	93	100.82	0.92	0.76–1.13
Sulfisoxazole	4,287	74	74.14	1.00	0.80–1.24
Sulfa, n.o.s.	653	8	13.34	0.60	0.26–1.17
Sulfamethoxypyridazine	358	3	6.51	0.46	0.10–1.34
Sulfadiazine	293	3	5.16	0.58	0.12–1.68
Sulfamethoxazole	210	4	3.79	1.05	0.29–2.66
Sulfathiazole	124	4	2.50	1.60	0.44–4.00
Systemic antimicrobials and antiparasitic agents	3,185	54	57.19	0.94	0.72–1.23
Phenazopyridine	1,109	15	17.85	0.84	0.47–1.38
Nitrofurantoin	590	14	10.74	1.30	0.72–2.17
Antimony potassium tartrate	394	9	8.18	1.10	0.51–2.07
Methenamine	299	12	5.34	2.25	1.17–3.87
Mandelic acid	224	7	3.96	1.77	0.71–3.58
Diiodohydroxyquin	172	6	3.57	1.68	0.62–3.58
Isoniazid	146	4	2.84	1.41	0.39–3.52
Methylene blue	46	3	0.88	3.43	0.72–9.39
Topical antimicrobial agents	4,792	94	85.86	1.09	0.91–1.32
Cetalkonium	2,195	45	40.91	1.10	0.84–1.45
Benzethonium	1,134	14	17.04	0.82	0.45–1.37
Phenylmercuric acetate	930	12	13.59	0.88	0.46–1.53
Cetylpyridinium	490	14	9.14	1.53	0.84–2.55
Boric acid	463	15	8.86	1.69	0.95–2.76
Thymol	117	4	1.92	2.08	0.57–5.18
Thiomersal	60	4	1.28	3.13	0.87–7.60

confidence limit for methenamine (1.17) indicates that the association reaches nominal statistical significance.

Immunizing Agents (Table A1.24) The highest relative risk (1.20) was noted for tetanus toxoid.

Antinauseants, Antihistamines, and Phenothiazines (Table A1.25) Among antihistamines and antinauseants (overall SRR, 1.09), SRRs greater than 1.5 were noted for thonzylamine (1.65), pyrilamine (1.58), phenyltoloxamine (2.32), and buclizine (2.45). Overall, phenothiazines gave no evidence of being related to anytime malformations (SRR, 0.98), and an SRR greater than 1.5 was observed for only one of them (trimeprazine; 1.62).

Sedatives, Tranquilizers, and Antidepressants (Table A1.26) The SRR for all barbiturates was 0.92, and none of the individual barbiturate drugs gave any evidence of association. Among the tranquilizers and non-barbiturate sedatives, only chlormezanone (7.47) had a relative risk greater than 1.5. This finding is statistically significant, with a lower confidence limit exceeding unity. For 152 exposures to antidepressants, there were only 2 children with anytime malformations.

Drugs Affecting the Autonomic Nervous System (Table A1.27) SRRs greater than 1.5 were seen for other sympathomimetic drugs (1.51) and homatropine (1.55).

Anesthetics, Anticonvulsants, Muscle Relaxants, and Smooth Muscle Stimulants (Table A1.28) Among local anesthetics, SRRs in excess of 1.5 were found for mepivacaine (1.55) and the category of other local anesthetics (4.03). The latter finding had a lower confidence limit of 1.12. General anesthetics (SRR, 0.68), non-barbiturate anticonvulsants (SRR, 1.02), central nervous system stimulants (SRR, 1.25), muscle relaxants (SRR, 0.77), and smooth muscle stimulants (SRR, 1.12), gave no evidence of association.

Caffeine and Other Xanthine Derivatives (Table A1.29) All SRRs were close to unity.

Diuretics and Drugs Taken for Cardiovascular Disorders (Table A1.30) Among the diuretics, SSRs greater than 1.5 were noted for polythiazide (1.53) and mercaptomerin (1.65). It should be noted that based on substantial numbers (1,310 exposures), the SRR for chlorthalidone was 1.41 with a lower confidence limit of 1.06. Among the antihypertensives, the SRR for hydralazine was 2.09; and among the

Table **A1.24**

Standardized Relative Risks (SRR) and Their 95% Confidence Intervals (CI$_{95}$) for Anytime Malformations Showing Uniform Rates by Hospital in Relation to **Immunizing Agents** Used Anytime During Pregnancy (Based on Multiple Logistic Risk Function Analysis)

	No. of Users	No. of Malformed Children		SRR	CI$_{95}$ of SRR
		Observed	Expected		
Immunizing agents	22,707	446	424.61	1.05	0.98–1.12
Poliomyelitis vaccine—parenteral	18,219	374	345.89	1.08	1.00–1.17
Polio virus vaccine, live oral	3,059	44	54.06	0.81	0.59–1.12
Influenza virus vaccine	2,283	47	42.60	1.10	0.84–1.44
Tetanus toxoid	853	19	15.79	1.20	0.73–1.87
Smallpox vaccine	281	3	5.02	0.60	0.12–1.73

Table **A1.25**

Standardized Relative Risks (SRR) and Their 95% Confidence Intervals (CI$_{95}$) for Anytime Malformations Showing Uniform Rates by Hospital in Relation to **Antinauseants, Antihistamines, and Phenothiazines** Used Anytime During Pregnancy (Based on Multiple Logistic Risk Function Analysis)

	No. of Users	No. of Malformed Children		SRR	CI$_{95}$ of SRR
		Observed	Expected		
Antinauseants, antihistamines, and phenothiazines	14,641	298	279.13	1.07	0.97–1.17
Antihistamines and antinauseants	12,678	263	241.61	1.09	0.98–1.20
Chlorpheniramine	3,931	82	77.54	1.06	0.86–1.30
Diphenhydramine	2,948	64	58.47	1.09	0.87–1.37
Pheniramine	2,442	51	45.44	1.12	0.87–1.45
Doxylamine succinate	1,700	34	32.67	1.04	0.75–1.44
Meclizine	1,463	28	29.04	0.96	0.66–1.40
Antinauseant, n.o.s.	774	19	14.20	1.34	0.81–2.08
Trimethobenzamide	700	13	13.25	0.98	0.52–1.67
Methapyrilene	525	12	10.24	1.17	0.61–2.03
Tripelennamine	490	8	9.17	0.87	0.38–1.70
Thonzylamine	444	13	7.89	1.65	0.88–2.79
Brompheniramine	412	6	6.94	0.87	0.32–1.87
Pyrilamine	392	12	7.59	1.58	0.82–2.73
Antihistamine, n.o.s.	326	4	6.71	0.60	0.16–1.51
Phenyltoloxamine	142	7	3.01	2.32	0.94–4.66
Buclizine	62	3	1.22	2.45	0.51–6.83
Phenothiazines	3,675	71	72.79	0.98	0.78–1.22
Prochlorperazine	2,023	40	39.71	1.01	0.74–1.36
Promethazine	746	12	14.08	0.85	0.44–1.48
Promazine	347	10	9.63	1.04	0.50–1.89
Chlorpromazine	284	6	5.40	1.11	0.41–2.39
Perphenazine	166	4	3.60	1.11	0.30–2.79
Trimeprazine	140	5	3.09	1.62	0.53–3.69

Table **A1.26**

Standardized Relative Risks (SRR) and Their 95% Confidence Intervals (CI$_{95}$) for Anytime Malformations Showing Uniform Rates by Hospital in Relation to **Sedatives, Tranquilizers, and Antidepressant Drugs** Used Anytime During Pregnancy (Based on Multiple Logistic Risk Function Analysis)

	No. of Users	No. of Malformed Children		SRR	CI$_{95}$ of SRR
		Observed	Expected		
Sedatives, tranquilizers, and antidepressants	14,278	273	294.41	0.93	0.84–1.03
Barbiturates	12,639	241	262.26	0.92	0.82–1.03
Phenobarbital	8,037	164	168.08	0.98	0.85–1.12
Secobarbital	4,248	93	95.77	0.97	0.80–1.18
Pentobarbital	1,523	38	34.94	1.09	0.81–1.47
Amobarbital	867	16	18.54	0.86	0.50–1.39
Butabarbital	305	7	6.28	1.12	0.45–2.27
Tranquilizers and nonbarbiturate sedatives	3,231	62	70.67	0.88	0.68–1.13
Meprobamate	1,204	16	25.63	0.62	0.36–1.01
Chlordiazepoxide	740	13	17.18	0.76	0.40–1.29
Glutethimide	640	8	13.36	0.60	0.26–1.17
Chloral hydrate	358	9	9.19	0.98	0.45–1.84
Sedative-tranquilizer, n.o.s.	256	7	5.45	1.28	0.52–2.61
Hydroxyzine	187	6	4.43	1.35	0.50–2.89
Chlormezanone	26	3	0.40	7.47	1.58–19.42

vasodilators (overall SRR, 2.32), there was a significant association for ethyl nitrite (SRR, 3.15; lower confidence limit, 1.28). Digitalis gave no evidence of association.

Cough Medicines (Table A1.31) None of the expectorants or unidentified cough medicines was associated with anytime malformations. For antitussives, the SRR, overall, was 1.59, and the result was statistically significant. The major contributions to this elevated SRR were from caramiphen (SRR, 1.65) and dextromethorphan hydrobromide (SRR, 1.39).

Drugs Taken for Gastrointestinal Disturbances (Table A1.32) SRRs greater than 1.5 were observed for cascara sagrada (2.03) and taka-diastase (1.87).

Hormones, Hormone Antagonists, and Contraceptives (Table A1.33) SRRs greater than 1.5 were noted for norethindrone (1.95), progestational agents, n.o.s. (1.54), hydrocortisone (1.70), tolbutamide (1.68), thyroid suppressants (1.55), and oral contraceptives, n.o.s. (1.54).

Inorganic Compounds and Certain Vitamins (Table A1.34) The highest SRR (1.25) was seen for iodides.

Standardized Relative Risks (SRR) and Their 95% Confidence Intervals (CI_{95}) for Anytime Malformations Showing Uniform Rates by Hospital in Relation to **Drugs Affecting the Autonomic Nervous System** Used Anytime During Pregnancy (Based on Multiple Logistic Risk Function Analysis)

	No. of Users	No. of Malformed Children		SRR	CI_{95} of SRR
		Observed	Expected		
Drugs affecting the autonomic nervous system	12,502	238	235.90	1.01	0.90–1.13
Sympathomimetic drugs	9,719	187	183.50	1.02	0.90–1.16
Phenylephrine	4,194	86	77.55	1.11	0.91–1.35
Phenylpropanolamine	2,489	52	49.43	1.05	0.81–1.36
Dextroamphetamine	1,069	23	22.04	1.04	0.70–1.55
Ephedrine	873	14	16.01	0.87	0.48–1.46
Isoxsuprine	858	12	15.58	0.77	0.40–1.34
Amphetamines	509	12	10.57	1.13	0.59–1.96
Epinephrine	508	11	9.85	1.12	0.56–1.98
Methamphetamine	320	6	5.23	1.15	0.42–2.47
Phenmetrazine	257	5	5.09	0.98	0.32–2.26
Diethylpropion	225	4	4.27	0.94	0.26–2.36
Pseudoephedrine	194	3	3.22	0.93	0.19–2.68
Other sympathomimetic drugs	120	4	2.65	1.51	0.42–3.77
Parasympatholytic drugs	5,623	112	109.88	1.02	0.86–1.21
Dicyclomine	1,593	28	31.03	0.90	0.61–1.33
Belladonna	1,355	29	25.97	1.12	0.79–1.57
Atropine	1,198	22	24.52	0.90	0.58–1.39
Isopropamide iodide	1,071	23	22.36	1.03	0.69–1.53
Homatropine	86	3	1.94	1.55	0.32–4.38
Scopolamine aminoxide hydrobromide	172	3	3.22	0.93	0.19–2.67
Scopolamine	881	24	17.32	1.39	0.99–1.94
Hyoscyamine	1,067	22	19.38	1.14	0.77–1.68

Diagnostic Aids, Technical Aids, and Rare Drugs (Table A1.35) The SRR for diagnostic aids was 1.95, with a lower confidence limit of 1.15. Within this group, SRRs greater than 1.5 were seen for radiopaque media (2.35; lower confidence limit, 1.09) and radioactive material (1.99). Among the technical aids, the SRR for resorcinol was 1.64.

Comments

As already mentioned, the data concerning drug exposure at any time during

Table **A1.28**

Standardized Relative Risks (SRR) and Their 95% Confidence Intervals (CI$_{95}$) for Anytime Malformations, Showing Uniform Rates by Hospital in Relation to **Anesthetics, Anticonvulsants, Muscle Relaxants, and Stimulants** Used Anytime During Pregnancy (Based on Multiple Logistic Risk Function Analysis)

	No. of Users	No. of Malformed Children		SRR	CI$_{95}$ of SRR
		Observed	Expected		
Anesthetics, anticonvulsants, muscle relaxants, and stimulants	6,990	142	144.45	0.98	0.84–1.15
Local anesthetics	5,703	113	114.71	0.99	0.83–1.17
Local anesthetic, n.o.s.	998	11	17.05	0.65	0.32–1.15
Lidocaine	947	20	20.15	0.99	0.61–1.52
Benzocaine	238	5	4.59	1.09	0.35–2.51
Mepivacaine	224	7	4.51	1.55	0.63–3.15
Propoxycaine	90	3	2.05	1.46	0.30–4.14
Procaine	3,395	71	70.46	1.01	0.80–1.26
Other local anesthetics	49	4	0.99	4.03	1.12–9.66
General anesthetics and oxygen	492	7	10.34	0.68	0.27–1.38
General anesthetic, n.o.s.	169	4	3.46	1.16	0.32–2.91
Nonbarbiturate anticonvulsants	425	14	13.72	1.02	0.56–1.69
Diphenylhydantoin	273	9	9.97	0.90	0.42–1.69
Magnesium sulfate	141	3	3.35	0.89	0.19–2.56
Central nervous system stimulants	228	5	3.98	1.25	0.41–2.89
Muscle relaxants	266	4	5.19	0.77	0.21–1.95
Smooth muscle stimulants	196	5	4.45	1.12	0.37–2.58
Sparteine	96	3	2.30	1.31	0.27–3.70

Table **A1.29**

Standardized Relative Risks (SRR) and Their 95% Confidence Intervals (CI$_{95}$) for Anytime Malformations Showing Uniform Rates by Hospital in Relation to **Caffeine and Other Xanthine Derivatives** Used Anytime During Pregnancy (Based on Multiple Logistic Risk Function Analysis)

	No. of Users	No. of Malformed Children		SRR	CI$_{95}$ of SRR
		Observed	Expected		
Caffeine and other xanthine derivatives	13,509	239	242.99	0.98	0.88–1.10
Caffeine	12,696	225	228.24	0.99	0.88–1.11
Theophylline	394	8	6.80	1.18	0.51–2.29
Aminophylline	259	4	5.20	0.77	0.21–1.95
Chlorotheophylline (dimenhydrinate)	697	12	13.32	0.90	0.47–1.56

Table **A1.30**

Standardized Relative Risks (SRR) and Their 95% Confidence Intervals (CI$_{95}$) for Anytime Malformations Showing Uniform Rates by Hospital in Relation to **Diuretics and Drugs Taken for Cardiovascular Disorders** Used Anytime During Pregnancy (Based on Multiple Logistic Risk Function Analysis)

	No. of Users	No. of Malformed Children		SRR	CI$_{95}$ of SRR
		Observed	Expected		
Diuretics and drugs taken for cardiovascular disorders	15,887	297	290.22	1.02	0.93–1.12
Diuretics	15,671	281	283.64	0.99	0.90–1.09
Hydrochlorothiazide	7,575	144	148.07	0.97	0.83–1.13
Chlorothiazide	5,283	88	88.02	1.00	0.82–1.22
Chlorthalidone	1,310	33	23.41	1.41	1.06–1.88
Bendroflumethiazide	1,156	20	21.15	0.95	0.58–1.45
Acetazolamide	1,024	18	18.06	1.00	0.59–1.57
Methyclothiazide	942	21	16.33	1.29	0.88–1.87
Diuretic, n.o.s.	735	8	13.99	0.57	0.25–1.12
Polythiazide	505	16	10.48	1.53	0.88–2.45
Trichlormethiazide	405	5	7.47	0.67	0.22–1.55
Meralluride	390	13	12.00	1.08	0.58–1.83
Quinethazone	316	8	6.99	1.15	0.50–2.23
Triamterene	271	5	5.39	0.93	0.30–2.14
Mercaptomerin	121	6	3.64	1.65	0.61–3.49
Antihypertensive agents	525	19	16.79	1.13	0.69–1.75
Hydralazine	136	8	3.83	2.09	0.91–4.00
Reserpine and other rauwolfia alkaloids	475	15	15.49	0.97	0.55–1.58
Vasodilators	129	7	3.02	2.32	0.94–4.63
Ethyl nitrite	98	7	2.22	3.15	1.28–6.24
Digitalis glycosides	129	3	3.48	0.86	0.18–2.46

pregnancy in relation to malformations that may arise at any time are presented in a tentative spirit. We feel particularly tentative about combining the "anytime" malformations for evaluation as a single outcome group. We wish to reiterate that the legitimacy of this approach is open to question; evaluation of potential late-acting teratogens in human populations is largely unexplored.

The preceding tables and Appendix 5 contain a large number of associations that may be of interest either in terms of providing clues for further research or, perhaps, in terms of comparisons with data obtained elsewhere. Here, we allude to only the most prominent associations.

Table A1.36 summarizes all associations having SRRs of 2.0 or greater for the combined set of anytime malformations. Seven of the associations were based on critical cells of only three or four exposed and malformed children. On the basis of only three exposed and malformed children, the SRR for chlormezanone exposure was 7.47; although the finding reaches formal "statistical significance," its meaning is questionable. Even with

Table **A1.31**

Standardized Relative Risks (SRR) and Their 95% Confidence Intervals (Cl$_{95}$) for Anytime Malformations Showing Uniform Rates by Hospital in Relation to **Cough Medicines** Used Anytime During Pregnancy (Based on Multiple Logistic Risk Function Analysis)

	No. of Users	No. of Malformed Children		SRR	Cl$_{95}$ of SRR
		Observed	Expected		
Cough medicines	7,941	161	149.22	1.08	0.94–1.24
Expectorants	6,277	131	119.80	1.09	0.94–1.28
Ammonium chloride	3,401	75	68.95	1.09	0.88–1.34
Chloroform, p.o.	2,181	46	41.32	1.11	0.85–1.46
Elixir terpin hydrate	1,762	29	30.60	0.95	0.66–1.37
Glyceryl guaiacolate	1,336	26	25.26	1.03	0.71–1.50
Ipecac	379	3	6.27	0.48	0.10–1.39
Potassium iodide	221	7	5.43	1.29	0.52–2.61
Antitussives	867	26	16.40	1.59	1.17–2.15
Dextromethorphan hydrobromide	580	15	10.75	1.39	0.78–2.28
Caramiphen	236	8	4.85	1.65	0.72–3.20
Cough medicine, n.o.s.	1,789	33	31.04	1.06	0.77–1.47

Table **A1.32**

Standardized Relative Risks (SRR) and Their 95% Confidence Intervals (Cl$_{95}$) for Anytime Malformations Showing Uniform Rates by Hospital in Relation to **Drugs Taken for Gastrointestinal Disturbances** Used Anytime During Pregnancy (Based on Multiple Logistic Risk Function Analysis)

	No. of Users	No. of Malformed Children		SRR	Cl$_{95}$ of SRR
		Observed	Expected		
Drugs taken for gastrointestinal disturbances	1,500	31	26.22	1.18	0.86–1.63
Phenolphthalein	806	12	13.28	0.90	0.47–1.57
Cascara	188	7	3.45	2.03	0.82–4.10
Bismuth subgallate	144	4	2.98	1.34	0.37–3.36
Dioctyl sodium sulfosuccinate	116	3	2.23	1.35	0.28–3.84
Casanthranol	109	3	2.04	1.47	0.30–4.18
Taka-diastase	97	3	1.61	1.87	0.39–5.29

Table **A1.33**

Standardized Relative Risks (SRR) and Their 95% Confidence Intervals (CI_{95}) for Anytime Malformations Showing Uniform Rates by Hospital in Relation to **Hormones, Hormone Antagonists and Contraceptives** Used Anytime During Pregnancy (Based on Multiple Logistic Risk Function Analysis)

	No. of Users	No. of Malformed Children		SRR	CI_{95} of SRR
		Observed	Expected		
Hormones, hormone antagonists and contraceptives	3,506	90	88.05	1.02	0.84–1.24
Progestational agents	1,399	41	37.63	1.09	0.82–1.45
Progesterone	527	7	14.63	0.48	0.19–0.98
Hydroxyprogesterone	495	17	16.17	1.05	0.62–1.67
Medroxyprogesterone	217	9	6.89	1.31	0.60–2.43
Norethynodrel	180	3	4.44	0.68	0.14–1.94
Norethindrone	148	6	3.08	1.95	0.72–4.14
Progestational agent, n.o.s.	99	3	1.94	1.54	0.32–4.38
Estrogenic agents	761	18	19.52	0.92	0.55–1.45
Diethylstilbestrol	233	7	7.15	0.98	0.40–1.99
Mestranol	206	4	5.02	0.80	0.22–2.01
Estrogen, n.o.s.	118	3	2.34	1.28	0.27–3.66
Ethinyl estradiol	98	3	2.17	1.38	0.29–3.93
Thyroid hormones	825	18	20.97	0.86	0.51–1.35
Thyroxin and thyroid	780	18	20.11	0.90	0.53–1.41
Corticosteroids and corticotropins	275	5	5.90	0.85	0.28–1.95
Hydrocortisone	74	3	1.76	1.70	0.35–4.79
Antidiabetic drugs	234	12	12.44	0.96	0.50–1.65
Insulin	198	11	11.37	0.97	0.49–1.69
Tolbutamide	42	3	1.78	1.68	0.35–4.58
Miscellaneous hormones	433	13	10.75	1.21	0.65–2.05
Oxytocin	255	9	6.16	1.46	0.67–2.73
Hormone, n.o.s.	119	3	2.58	1.16	0.24–3.32
Thyroid suppressants	38	3	1.93	1.55	0.33–4.19
Oral contraceptives	309	7	7.09	0.99	0.40–2.01
Mestranol and norethynodrel	180	3	4.44	0.68	0.14–1.94
Oral contraceptives, n.o.s.	99	3	1.94	1.54	0.32–4.38
Local contraceptives	466	4	7.74	0.52	0.14–1.31
Nonoxynol 9	346	4	6.03	0.66	0.18–1.68

443

Table **A1.34**

Standardized Relative Risks (SRR) and Their 95% Confidence Intervals (CI$_{95}$) for Anytime Malformations Showing Uniform Rates by Hospital in Relation to **Inorganic Compounds and Certain Vitamins** Used Anytime During Pregnancy (Based on Multiple Logistic Risk Function Analysis)

	No. of Users	No. of Malformed Children		SRR	CI$_{95}$ of SRR
		Observed	Expected		
Inorganic compounds and certain vitamins	10,116	188	180.94	1.04	0.92–1.18
Bromides, fluorides, and iodides	5,312	114	103.24	1.10	0.94–1.30
Fluorides	1,422	23	26.86	0.86	0.55–1.32
Iodides	1,635	44	35.18	1.25	0.96–1.62
Bromides	2,610	57	48.62	1.17	0.93–1.48
Calcium, parenteral iron, and vitamins	5,598	88	91.42	0.96	0.79–1.18
Iron, i.m.	1,864	31	29.10	1.07	0.76–1.49
Calcium compounds	3,739	59	60.26	0.98	0.76–1.26

Table **A1.35**

Standardized Relative Risks (SRR) and Their 95% Confidence Intervals (CI$_{95}$) for Anytime Malformations Showing Uniform Rates by Hospital in Relation to **Diagnostic Aids, Technical Aids, and Rare Drugs** Used Anytime During Pregnancy (Based on Multiple Logistic Risk Function Analysis)

	No. of Users	No. of Malformed Children		SRR	CI$_{95}$ of SRR
		Observed	Expected		
Diagnostic aids	313	17	8.72	1.95	1.15–3.07
Radiopaque media	150	9	3.83	2.35	1.09–4.34
Intravenous dilution test agent	127	5	3.93	1.27	0.42–2.89
Radioactive material	50	3	1.51	1.99	0.42–5.47
Technical aids	1,736	35	33.86	1.03	0.75–1.43
Local irritants and keratolytics	1,661	32	32.46	0.99	0.70–1.39
Sodium tetradecyl sulfate	606	13	13.62	0.95	0.51–1.62
Resorcinol	118	4	2.44	1.64	0.45–4.08
Camphor	763	13	13.65	0.95	0.51–1.62
Rare drugs	777	13	15.02	0.87	0.46–1.47
Miscellaneous infrequently used drugs	148	4	3.68	1.09	0.30–2.72
Drugs with unknown ingredients	632	9	11.41	0.79	0.36–1.49

Summary of Associations Between Drugs and Anytime Malformations[1]

Category	Drug	No. of Exposed and Malformed Children	SRR
Narcotic analgesics	Hydromorphone	3	2.04
	Hydrocodone	4	2.45
Antibiotics	Gramicidin	4	2.14
Systemic antimicrobials	Methenamine	7	2.25
	Methylene blue	3	3.43
Topical antimicrobial agents	Thiomersal	4	3.13
Antihistamines and antinauseants	Phenyltoloxamine	7	2.32
	Buclizine	3	2.45
Tranquilizers and non-barbiturate sedatives	Chlormezanone	3	7.47
Antihypertensive agents	Hydralazine	8	2.09
Vasodilators	Ethyl nitrite	7	3.15
Drugs taken for gastrointestinal disorders	Cascara	7	2.03
Radiopaque media		9	2.35

[1]Only relative risks of 2.0 or greater are included. With the exception of radiopaque media, only individual drugs are tabulated.

regard to the remaining findings, it is impossible to interpret the associations without independent confirmation.

As for individual malformations, specific attention will be drawn to only two (Appendix 5). The first is between killed poliomyelitis vaccination and malignant tumors, particularly neural tumors and leukemia. This finding has been more fully reported, and we have suggested that the association may be attributable to SV 40 virus contamination of batches of killed polio vaccine.[1] The SV 40 virus is known to be carcinogenic when given by injection to experimental animals.[2] Batch contamination could explain time clustering in the affected children who were exposed (data on clustering are not given here).[1] Failure to observe an association between live attenuated polio virus vaccine exposure and malignancy may be due to the latter vaccine being administered orally rather than parenterally, because it, too, was contaminated with the SV 40 virus.[3] The findings require independent confirmation.

The second association is between exposure to rauwolfia alkaloids and microcephaly. The hospital-standardized relative risk for this outcome was 8.0 (Appendix 5). While this finding is quite striking, it should again be stressed that it has been made within the context of multiple comparisons and needs to be independently confirmed. However, there are experimental data implicating rauwolfia alkaloids as teratogens.[4,5]

Complete Listing of Malformations Found in the Offspring of 50,282 Women

The following is a complete listing, by anatomic class, of the malformations analyzed in this book. In addition to individual malformations, some combinations are listed. Each malformation and combination has been assigned a code number. The combinations and their constituents are given as coalition codes. The six non-uniform malformations (described in Chapter 17) are listed last.

Malformations of the Central Nervous System (CNS)

Code			No. of Children
1	Anencephaly	Major	26
2	Encephalocele	Major	5
3	Meningomylocele	Major	36
4	Spina bifida without CNS involvement	Minor	7
5	Spina bifida with meningomylocele	Major	9
6	Absent corpus callosum	Major	4
7	Hydrocephaly	Major	75
8	Microcephaly	Major	77
9	Hypoplasia/atrophy brain—secondary	Major	10
10	Miscellaneous brain abnormalities[1]	Major	8
11	Malformed medulla	Major	3
12	Craniosynostosis	Major	26
13	Macrocephaly	Major	18
14	Absence olfactory nerve/arhinencephaly	Major	6
15	Cerebral hypoplasia—primary	Major	11
16	Porencephaly/hydrancephaly	Major	4
17	Anomalies pituitary[2]	Major	7
18	Rachischisis/cranioschisis	Major	8
19	Miscellaneous sinus tract abnormalities[3]	Minor	10
20	Arnold Chiari/Dandy Walker	Major	8
21	Atrophy/hypoplasia optic nerve	Major	7
22	Craniospinal fusion defects without anencephaly	Major	53
23	Any cranial nerve malformation	Major	10
24	Any brain malformation	Major	241
25	Any spinal malformation	Major	58
26	Craniospinal fusion defects with anencephaly	Major	69
	Total number of children with CNS malformations		266
	Total number of CNS malformations		365

Coalition codes: 22 = 2, 3, 4, 5, 18
23 = 14, 21 (partially)
24 = 1, 2, 6, 7, 8, 9, 10, 11,
12, 13, 14, 15, 16, 17, 20, 21
25 = 3, 4, 5, 18, 19
26 = 1, 2, 3, 4, 5, 18

[1]Brain malformation, n.o.s. (5); hypertrophy of brain (3)
[2]Hypoplasia pituitary (3); agenesis pituitary (2); hypertrophy pituitary (1); hypoplasia capsule pituitary (1)
[3]Pilonidal sinus (4); pilonidal dimple (2); other midline sinus (1); pre-sacral dimple (1); lumbar-sacral dimple/sinus (1); suboccipital sinus tract (1)

Malformations of the Cardiovascular System (CVS)

Classification of cardiovascular malformations presents some rather unique problems. Cardiovascular malformations can exist alone, in a variety of well-known combinations (e.g., Tetralogy of Fallot), or in combinations that are not well recognized. In addition, there are now believed to be embryological entities that cover a variety of specific pathological diagnoses. Three such entities have been used in this classification:

Code 60: Conus Arteriosus Syndrome
  Tetralogy of Fallot
  Eisenmenger
  Transposition of great arteries
  Truncus arteriosus
  Double outlet ventricle
Code 61: Endocardial Cushion Defect (ECD)
  Atrial septal defect, primum
  (partial ECD)

447

Atrioventricular canal (complete ECD)

Cleft mitral valve (partial ECD)

Code 79: Hypoplastic Left Heart Syndrome

Aortic and mitral valve atresia

Hypoplastic left heart

The above three entities can be considered as embryological syndromes. Well-recognized clinical syndromes (e.g., Tetralogy) have also been assigned code numbers. Finally, when appropriate, individual malformations are identified as being either isolated or existing in combination with other cardiovascular malformations. For example, the code for any atrial septal defect-secundum is 31. When the same defect is not associated with any other cardiovascular anomaly, the code is 32. When the defect is one of multiple cardiovascular anomalies, the code is 33.

Malformations of the Cardiovascular System (CVS)

Code			No. of Children
1	Any atrial septal defect (secundum or primum)	Major	52
2	Any ventricular septal defect (open or closing)	Major	171
3	Atrioventricular canal	Major	18
4	Aortic valve malformation (stenosis or atresia)	Major	28
5	Pulmonic valve malformation	Major	75
6	Mitral valve malformation	Major	17
7	Tricuspid valve malformation	Major	10
8	Any malposition of great vessels (union)	Major	29
9	Transposition of great arteries	Major	17
10	Anomalous venous drainage	Major	7
11	Abnormalities of coronary arteries, isolated	Major	3
12	Ductus arteriosus persistens	Major	45
13	Any coarctation of aorta—pre-ductal or post-ductal	Major	36
14	Truncus arteriosus	Major	6
15	Vascular ring	Major	9
16	Coarctation of aorta—pre-ductal	Major	26
17	Coarctation of aorta—post-ductal	Major	10
18	Abnormalities of coronary arteries	Major	6
19	Endocardial fibroelastosis	Major	12
20	Endomyocardial fibrosis	Major	2
21	Single atrium	Major	3
22	Single ventricle	Major	6
23	Tetralogy of Fallot	Major	15
24	Aortic and mitral valve atresia	Major	13
25	Ventricular septal defect and pulmonic stenosis (VSD open or closing and PS or PPS)[1]	Major	10
26	Abnormalities of coronary arteries, multiple	Major	3
27	Truncus arteriosus, isolated	Major	2
28	Truncus arteriosus, multiple	Major	4
29	Single ventricle, isolated	Major	1
30	Single ventricle, multiple	Major	5
31	Atrial septal defect—secundum	Major	38
32	Atrial septal defect—secundum, isolated	Major	28
33	Atrial septal defect—secundum, multiple	Major	10
34	Atrial septal defect—primum	Major	15
35	Atrial septal defect—primum, isolated	Major	9
36	Atrial septal defect—primum, multiple	Major	6
37	Any atrial septal defect—secundum or primum, isolated	Major	37
38	Any atrial septal defect—secundum or primum, multiple	Major	15
39	Ventricular septal defect (open)	Major	129
40	Ventricular septal defect (open), isolated	Major	76
41	Ventricular septal defect (open), multiple	Major	61

Code			No. of Children
42	Ventricular septal defect—spontaneously closing	Major	34
43	Any ventricular septal defect (open or closing), isolated	Major	109
44	Any ventricular septal defect (open or closing), multiple	Major	62
45	Atrioventricular canal, isolated	Major	12
46	Atrioventricular canal, multiple	Major	6
47	Aortic stenosis	Major	16
48	Aortic stenosis, isolated	Major	11
49	Aortic stenosis, multiple	Major	5
50	Vascular ring, isolated	Major	3
51	Vascular ring, multiple	Major	6
52	Hypoplasia left ventricle	Major	11
53	Left vena cava	Minor	7
54	Wolff-Parkinson-White syndrome	Minor	3
55	Anomalous right subclavian artery	Minor	5
56	Hypoplasia left atrium	Major	9
57	Hypoplasia cordis	Minor	19
58	Endocardial disease (union)	Major	14
59	Aortic insufficiency	Major	2
60	Conus arteriosus syndrome	Major	44
61	Endocardial cushion defect	Major	34
62	Aortic valve malformation (stenosis or atresia), isolated	Major	13
63	Aortic valve malformation (stenosis or atresia), multiple	Major	5
64	Pulmonic valvular or unspecified stenosis	Major	56
65	Pulmonic valvular or unspecified stenosis, isolated	Major	29
66	Pulmonic valvular or unspecified stenosis, multiple	Major	27
67	Peripheral pulmonic stenosis	Major	8
68	Peripheral pulmonic stenosis, isolated	Major	5
69	Peripheral pulmonic stenosis, multiple	Major	3
70	Pulmonary atresia	Major	11
71	Pulmonary atresia, isolated	Major	1
72	Pulmonary atresia, multiple	Major	10
73	Tricuspid valve malformation, isolated	Major	2
74	Pulmonic valve malformation, isolated	Major	35
75	Pulmonic valve malformation, multiple	Major	40
76	Mitral insufficiency	Major	3
77	Tricuspid valve malformation, multiple	Major	8
78	Rare single malformation[2]	Minor	6
79	Hypoplastic left heart syndrome	Major	24
80	Transposition of great arteries, isolated	Major	1
81	Transposition of great arteries, multiple	Major	16
82	Double outlet of right ventricle	Major	5
83	Double outlet of right ventricle, isolated	Major	2
84	Double outlet of right ventricle, multiple	Major	3
85	Hypoplasia pulmonary artery	Minor	2
86	Any malposition of great vessels, isolated	Major	3
87	Any malposition of great vessels, multiple	Major	26
88	Ductus arteriosus persistens, isolated	Major	29
89	Ductus arteriosus persistens, multiple	Major	16
90	Coarctation of aorta—pre-ductal, isolated	Major	9
91	Coarctation of aorta—pre-ductal, multiple	Major	17
92	Any coarctation of aorta (pre-ductal or post-ductal), isolated	Major	19
93	Any coarctation of aorta (pre-ductal or post-ductal), multiple	Major	17
	Total number of children with cardiovascular malformations		404
	Total number of cardiovascular malformations		567

[1]VSD = Ventricular septal defect; PS = pulmonic stenosis; PPS = peripheral pulmonic stenosis
[2]Anomalous renal artery/vein (1); abnormal origin renal artery (1); vena azygos (1); single pulmonary artery/vein (1); absent pulmonary vein (1); stenosis ductus venosus (1)

449

Malformations of the Musculoskeletal System (MS)

Code			No. of Children
1	Polydactyly	Minor	370
2	Absence of limb or part thereof[1]	Major	32
3	Hypoplasia of limb or part thereof[2]	Major	51
4	Syndactyly	Major	125
5	Arthrogryposis	Major	6
6	Anomalies of vertebrae[3]	Minor	13
7	Hemivertebrae	Major	13
8	Congenital dislocation of hip	Major	92
9	Hemimelia/phocomelia	Major	7
10	Muscle absence/atrophy/hypoplasia	Major	17
11	Absence/atrophy/hypoplasia pectoralis	Major	10
12	Absence/atrophy/hypoplasia rectus abdominis	Major	4
13	Micrognathia/hypoplastic jaw	Major	21
14	Miscellaneous foot abnormalities[4]	Minor	10
15	Anomalies of ribs/sternum[5]	Minor	16
16	Abnormal face/skull[6]	Major	5
17	Abnormal implantation/deformed toes	Minor	12
18	Webbed neck	Minor	10
19	Other musculoskeletal malformations[7]	Major	10
20	Some muscle absence/atrophy/hypoplasia[8]	Major	3
	Total number of children with musculoskeletal malformations		717
	Total number of musculoskeletal malformations		810

Coalition Codes: 10 = 11, 12, 20

[1]Fingers (6); hand (3); left hand (2); finger (2); upper extremity (2); fibula (2); toe (2); phalanx 5th toe (1); right 5th digit (1); metacarpals and phalanges (1); fingers and hand (1); forearm and hand (1); toes (1); innominate bone (1); hand, fingers, toes (1); forearm, hand, fingers (1); ulna, radius (1); foot and toes (1); tibia (1); fingernail (1)

[2]Fingers (12); toes (11); leg (5); forearm (3); femur (3); foot (3); tibia (2); hand (1); humerus and foot (1); left distal phalanx (1); fingers and toes (1); great toes (1); lower extremity (1); radius (1); forearm and fingers (1); humerus (1); femur and fibula (1); humerus and ulna (1); hand and fingers (1)

[3]Fused vertebrae (3); hypoplasia sacrum (1); absence/hypoplasia coccyx (1); ankylosis of spine (1); anomaly of vertebrae, n.o.s. (1); extra vertebrae (1); short thoracic spine (1); absent coccyx (1); absent sacrum (1); absent vertebrae (1); hypoplasia vertebrae (1)

[4]Rocker bottom feet (6); hallux valgus (3); foot deformity (1)

[5]Anomaly of ribs, n.o.s. (5); missing ribs (3); flaring ribs (3); hypoplasia ribs (2); absent ossification of ribs (1); hypoplasia sternum (1); bifid sternum (1)

[6]Hypoplasia skull bones (1); orbital bone defect (1); hypoplasia orbital plate (1); agenesis skull, n.o.s. (1); absent nasal septum (1)

[7]Hypertrophy extremity (2); vertical talus (2); limb/body length disproportion (1); hemihypertrophy (1); coxa valga (1); chondrodysplasia/congenital calcification (1); radial deviation of wrist with dimpling of ulna (1); tail remnant (1)

[8]Absent sternocleidomastoid (1); atrophy muscles upper and lower extremities (1); atrophy caudal muscles (1)

Malformations of the Respiratory Tract (RT)

Code			No. of Children
1	Laryngeal/tracheal malacia	Major	4
2	Malformations of epiglottis/larynx/bronchi	Major	12
3	Malformations of thoracic wall[1]	Major	18
4	Malformations of diaphragm[2]	Major	11
5	Diaphragmatic hernia	Major	13
6	Hypoplasia/agenesis lung	Major	32
7	Bilobed lung	Minor	14
8	Choanal atresia	Major	3
9	Hiatal hernia	Major	8
10	Malformed lung[3]	Minor	26
11	Anomalies of teeth	Minor	19
12	Other respiratory malformations[4]	Major	5
13	Cleft lip only	Major	24
14	Co-existent cleft lip and palate	Major	24
15	Cleft lip with or without cleft palate	Major	48
16	Cleft palate only	Major	31
17	Some epiglottis/bronchi malformations[5]	Major	8
	Total number of children with respiratory malformations		218
	Total number of respiratory malformations		240

Coalition Codes: 2 = 1, 17
                  15 = 13, 14

[1] Pigeon breast (9); shield chest (2); asymmetry of chest (2); displaced mediastinum (1); hypoplasia thorax (1); deformed xiphoid (1); square-shaped thorax (1); deformed thorax (1)
[2] Agenesis diaphragm (7); eventration (2); hypoplasia diaphragm (1); malformation of diaphragm, n.o.s. (1)
[3] Incomplete lobation (10); abnormal lobation (4); incomplete fissure (2); multilobed lung—6 (1); incomplete partition (1); fissure abnormality (1); accessory lobe (1); anomalous lobe (1); fusion of lobes (1); trilobed (1); hypertrophy of lungs (1); anomaly of lobes, n.o.s. (1); abnormal lobes (1)
[4] Macroglossia (4); single nostril (1)
[5] Redundant epiglottis (2); redundant mucosa (1); angulation epiglottis (1); agenesis bronchi (1); absent uvula (1); subglottis stenosis (1); subglottis obstruction (1)

Malformations of the Gastrointestinal Tract (GIT)

Code			No. of Children
1	Omphalocele	Major	22
2	Anal atresia	Major	26
3	Tracheo-esophageal fistula	Major	11
4	Malrotation	Minor	25
5	Hirschsprung's disease	Major	13
6	Duodenal atresia	Major	7
7	Other gastrointestinal malformations[1]	Major	7
8	Other hernias[2]	Minor	5
9	Anomalies of pancreas[3]	Major	6
10	Anomalies of liver[4]	Major	3
11	Anomalies of gallbladder[5]	Major	5
12	Pyloric stenosis	Major	95
13	Meckel's diverticulum	Minor	21
14	Atresia/agenesis colon[6]	Major	3
15	Atresia/hypoplasia small intestine	Major	7
16	Anomalous shaped/lobation of liver[7]	Minor	5
17	Biliary atresia	Major	8
18	Atrophy/hypoplasia intestine	Major	15
19	Accessory spleen	Minor	23
20	Umbilical hernia	Minor	51
21	Asplenia	Major	3
22	Anomalies of pancreas/gallbladder	Major	11
	Total number of children with gastrointestinal malformations		301
	Total number of gastrointestinal malformations		346

Coalition Codes: 18 = 6, 14, 15
22 = 9, 11

[1]Ectopic colon (1); duplication of cecum (1); dextroposition of spleen (1); duodenal diverticulum (1); adhesion bands (1); congenital duodenal bands (1); constricting duodenal bands (1)
[2]Epigastric hernia (3); ventral hernia (1); femoral hernia (1)
[3]Pancreatic rest (2); duplication of pancreas (1); annular pancreas (1); accessory pancreas (1); absent pancreas (1)
[4]Ectopic liver (2); extra-hepatic biliary system (1)
[5]Agenesis gallbladder (2); absent cystic duct (2); hypoplasia gallbladder (1)
[6]Atresia colon (2); agenesis colon (1)
[7]Anomalous lobation (3); anomalous shaped liver (2)

Malformations of the Genitourinary System (GUS)

Code			No. of Children
1	Hypospadias	Minor	188
2	Polycystic kidney	Major	33
3	Single kidney	Major	11
4	Hypoplastic kidney	Major	15
5	Horseshoe kidney	Major	8
6	Other kidney malformations[1]	Major	5
7	Double ureter	Major	9
8	Absent ureter	Major	10
9	Stenotic ureter	Major	26
10	Hypoplasia penis	Major	4
11	Abnormal testes[2]	Major	15
12	Malformed uterus/fallopian tubes	Major	11
13	Abnormal ovary[3]	Major	8
14	Malformations of male genitalia	Coalition	218
15	Rectal fistula	Major	7
16	Malformations of female genitalia	Coalition	35
17	Malposition/ectopic kidney	Major	5
18	Double collecting system	Major	11
19	Mullerian malfusion[4]	Major	4
20	Malformations of bladder/ureter[5]	Major	13
21	Hydronephrosis	Major	23
22	Hydroureter	Major	21
23	Obstructive uropathy	Major	47
24	Ambiguous genitalia[6]	Major	5
25	Hydrocele	Minor	10
26	Malformations of male genitalia—minor[7]	Minor	6
27	Malformations of female genitalia—major[8]	Major	14
28	Malformations of female genitalia—minor[9]	Minor	22
29	Some uterine malformations[10]	Major	7
30	Some double collecting malformations[11]	Major	2
31	Malformations of male genitalia except hypospadias	Coalition	33

Total number of children with genitourinary malformations　　366
Total number of genitourinary malformations　　471

Coalition Codes: 12 = 19, 29
　　　　　　　　14 = 1, 10, 11, 25, 26
　　　　　　　　16 = 27, 28
　　　　　　　　18 = 7, 30
　　　　　　　　23 = 9, 21, 22
　　　　　　　　31 = 10, 11, 25, 26

[1]Absence both kidneys (2); absent glomerulogenesis (1); hypertrophy of kidney (1); double kidney (1)
[2]Undescended testes (12); absent testes (2); aberrant testes (1)
[3]Dysgenesis ovary (4); hypoplasia ovary (1); fibrous dysgenesis (1); agenesis (1); ectopic ovary (1)
[4]Double uterus, separate vagina (1); bicornate uterus (1); bicornate uterus, double cervix, vagina (1); incomplete uterine septum (1)
[5]Hypertrophy of bladder (3); extrophic bladder (2); agenesis bladder (2); dilated bladder (2); hypertrophy (1); ectopic ureter (1); ectopic urethral meatus (1); urachal fistula (1)
[6]Pseudohermaphrodite (2); hypertrophy wolfian ducts—female (1); labia majora and mullerian ducts—male (1); hermaphrodite (1)
[7]Chordee (3); abnormal ventral foreskin (1); absent epididymis (1); hypoplasia prostate (1)
[8]Dysgenesis ovaries (3); imperforate hymen (2); hypoplastic ovaries (1); fibrous dysgenesis (1); dysgenesis ovaries and enlarged clitoris (1); absence vaginal opening (1); agenesis ovaries (1); abnormal vagina (1); ectopic ovaries (1); malformed vulva, absent external genitalia (1); enlarged clitoris (1)
[9]Labial adhesions (10); vaginal tag (7); redundant vaginal mucosa (1); post vaginal web (1); prolapsed vaginal mucosa (1); hypertrophy labia majora (1); vulvar membrane (1)
[10]Malformed uterus, n.o.s. (3); agenesis fallopian tubes (1); absent uterus (1); cloaca, absent vagina (1); uterus attached to bowel, tubes adherent to side of uterus (1)
[11]Double collecting system (1); duplication renal pelvis (1)

Malformations of the Eye and Ear

Code			No. of Children
1	Anophthalmia/microphthalmia	Major	11
2	Coloboma	Minor	13
3	Cataract	Major	44
4	Glaucoma/buphthalmos	Major	10
5	Corneal opacity	Major	8
6	Other eye malformations[1]	Major	4
7	Absent/abnormal external meatus	Major	9
8	Pre-auricular skin tag	Minor	38
	Total number of children with eye/ear malformations		121
	Total number of eye/ear malformations		137

Coalition Codes: None

[1]Eye herniation (1); Koeber Salus Elsching (1); megalocornea (1); aniridia (1)

Syndromes

Code			No. of Children
1	Down	Major	61
2	Situs inversus/dextrocardia	Major	12
3	Hypertrophy/enlarged adrenal	Major	5
4	Hypoplasia/atrophy adrenal	Major	26
5	Anomalies thyroid[1]	Major	7
6	Other adrenal syndromes[2]	Major	16
7	Adrenogenital	Major	4
8	Pierre Robin	Major	3
9	Achondroplasia	Major	4
10	Caffey's	Major	6
11	Albinism	Major	5
12	Inborn errors metabolism[3]	Major	9
13	Other syndromes[4]	Major	15
14	Turner's	Major	3
15	Other trisomies[5]	Major	5
16	Any chromosomal	Major	70
17	Klinefelter's	Major	1
	Total number of children with syndromes		176
	Total number of syndromes		182

Coalition Codes: 16 = 1, 14, 15, 17

[1]Ectopic thyroid (2); hypertrophy of thyroid (1); absent thyroid (1); enlarged thymus (1); anomaly thyroid, n.o.s. (1); enlarged thyroid (1)
[2]Malposition (5); necrosis adrenal cortex (3); horseshoe-shaped adrenal (1); involutionary changes adrenal cortex (1); accessory nodule (1); malposition adrenal cortex (1); abnormal shaped cortex (1); cytomegaly (1); cytomegaly adrenal cortex (1); cystic transformation adrenal cortex (1)
[3]Glucose 6 phosphate dehydrogenase deficiency (4); glycogen storage (2); galactosemia (2); congenital metabolic alkalosis (1)
[4]Klippel Feil (2); osteogenesis imperfecta (2); cleidocranial dysostosis (2); Apert's (1); Nail-Patella syndrome (1); Cornelia de Lange (1); Potter's (1); cranial facial dysostosis (1); Poland's syndactyly (1); Crouzon's (1); Lowe's (1); Eagle's Syndrome (1)
[5]Trisomy 18 (2); Trisomy E Group (2); Trisomy 13 (1)

Tumors

Code			No. of Children
1	Any mixed tumors[1]	Mixed	2
2	Any malignant tumors	Malignant	24
3	Wilms' tumor	Malignant	5
4	Leukemias[2]	Malignant	8
5	CNS tumors[3]	Malignant	8
6	Other malignant tumors[4]	Malignant	3
7	Any benign tumors	Benign	138
8	Papillomas/polyps	Benign	12
9	Dermoid cysts	Benign	11
10	Any cyst (except dermoid)[5]	Benign	42
11	Hemangioma/granuloma	Benign	19
12	Hairy nevus	Benign	22
13	Other benign tumors[6]	Benign	24
14	Lymphangioma	Benign	8
	Total number of children with tumors		164
	Total number of tumors		164

Coalition Codes: 2 = 3, 4, 5, 6
    7 = 8, 9, 10, 11, 12, 13, 14

[1]Eosinophilic granuloma, eyelid (1); Letterer-Siwe (1)
[2]Stem cell (2); lymphocytic (2); stem cell, lymphocytic (1); lymphoblastic (1); myelogenous (1); unclassified (1)
[3]Neuroblastoma, adrenal, bilateral (2); retinoblastoma, bilateral, multiple (1); neuroblastoma, adrenal, unilateral (1); neuroblastoma, mediastinal, posterior (1); astrocytoma, spinal medulla (1); medulloblastoma, brain (1); glioma, brain (1)
[4]Granulosa cell tumor, testes (1); hepatoblastoma (1); nephroblastoma, bilateral (1)
[5]Cystic mass, scalp (4); thyroglossal duct cyst (3); pulmonary cyst (3); periurethral cyst (2); cystic testes (2); vaginal cyst (2); cyst, hand (2); inclusion cyst, vaginal (1); cyst, head (1); cyst, eyebrow (1); cyst, scalp (1); cyst, gum (1); subcutaneous cyst, scalp (1); cyst areola (1); cyst, eyelid (1); cyst, lip (1); cyst, nipple (1); cyst, eye (1); Gartners cyst (1); epidermal cyst, face (1); omphalomesenteric cyst (1); branchial cleft cyst (1); mesenteric cyst (1); congenital pancreatic cyst (1); cystic mass, abdominal (1); cystic mass, palate (1); cyst, face (1); cyst, scalp, n.o.s. (1); choledochal cyst (1); sebaceous cyst, skull (1); dental cyst (1)
[6]Teratoma of sacrum (2); ranula (2); lipoma, sacral (1); ganglion, wrist (1); lipomyxoma, lip (1); subcutaneous nodule, back (1); mass, thigh, n.o.s. (1); tumor, scalp, n.o.s. (1); mass, sacral, n.o.s. (1); tumor, parotid n.o.s. (1); neurofibromatosis (1); lipoma, scalp (1); benign tumor spinal cord (1); cortical adenoma kidney (1); facial nodule (1); lipoma, ear (1); adenoma kidney (1); mass, chest, n.o.s. (1); chalazion, lid (1); calcified mass, abdominal (1); benign tumor cranial vault (1); xanthoma, chest (1)

Malformations with Non-Uniform Hospital Distributions

Code		No. of Children
1	Inguinal hernia	683
2	Clubfoot	192
3	Cleft gum	110
4	Pectus excavatum	92
5	Urethral obstruction	68
6	Abnormal hands/fingers	10
	Total number of children with non-uniform malformations	1,128
	Total number of non-uniform malformations	1,155

Complete Listing of Drugs Used by 50,282 Women

The following is a complete listing, by pharmacological group, of all the drugs analyzed in this book. The grouping is the same as that used in Chapters 20 to 33. For each drug group, subgroup, and individual drug, the number of users and percentage of use in the total cohort are given, both for use during the first four lunar months of pregnancy, and for use anytime during pregnancy.

	Use During LM 1-4		Use Anytime During Pregnancy	
	No.	%	No.	%
Analgesics and antipyretics	15,909	31.64	33,841	67.30
Non-addicting analgesics and antipyretics	15,463	30.75	32,856	65.34
Aspirin	14,864	29.56	32,164	63.97
Phenacetin	5,546	11.03	13,031	25.92
Salicylamide	744	1.48	1,623	3.23
Acetaminophen	266	0.45	781	1.55
Analgesic and cold capsules, n.o.s.	152	0.30	644	1.28
Sodium salicylate	54	0.11	162	0.32
Pyrazolon derivatives	17	0.03	45	0.09
Other non-addicting analgesics and antipyretics	10	0.02	34	0.07
Narcotic analgesics	1,564	3.11	6,754	13.41
Propoxyphene	686	1.36	2,914	5.80
Codeine	563	1.12	2,522	5.02
Meperidine	268	0.53	1,100	2.19
Paregoric	90	0.18	562	1.12
Morphine	70	0.14	448	0.89
Ethoheptazine	60	0.12	300	0.60
Opium	36	0.07	181	0.36
Hydromorphone	12	0.02	61	0.12
Hydrocodone	12	0.02	60	0.12
Diphenoxylate	7	0.01	33	0.07
Alphaprodine	1	0.00	33	0.07
Other opium alkaloids	22	0.04	36	0.07
Other narcotic analgesics	5	0.01	25	0.05
Antimicrobial and antiparasitic agents	8.088	16.09	17,538	34.88
Antibiotics	4,444	8.84	9,560	19.01
Tetracycline	341	0.68	1,336	2.66
Antibiotic, n.o.s.	202	0.40	390	0.78
Streptomycin	135	0.27	355	0.71
Chloramphenicol	98	0.19	348	0.69
Oxytetracycline	119	0.24	328	0.65
Demeclocycline	90	0.18	280	0.56
Nystatin	142	0.28	230	0.46
Erythromycin	79	0.16	230	0.46
Tyrothricin	31	0.06	130	0.26
Neomycin	30	0.06	118	0.23
Gramicidin	61	0.12	96	0.19
Bacitracin	18	0.04	83	0.17
Novobiocin	21	0.04	41	0.08
Dihydrostreptomycin	18	0.04	34	0.07
Chlortetracycline	14	0.03	30	0.06
Polymyxin B	7	0.01	22	0.04
Amphotericin B	9	0.02	21	0.04
Penicillin derivatives	3,546	7.05	7,171	14.26
Other antibiotics	19	0.04	48	0.10
Sulfonamides	1,455	2.89	5,689	11.31
Sulfisoxazole	796	1.58	4,287	8.53
Sulfa, n.o.s.	318	0.63	653	1.30
Sulfamethoxypyridazine	61	0.12	358	0.71

	Use During LM 1-4		Use Anytime During Pregnancy	
	No.	%	No.	%
Sulfadiazine	95	0.19	293	0.58
Sulfamethoxazole	46	0.09	210	0.42
Sulfamerazine	48	0.10	156	0.31
Sulfamethazine	47	0.09	151	0.30
Sulfathiazole	100	0.20	124	0.25
Sulfacetamide	93	0.18	102	0.20
Sulfamethizole	37	0.07	93	0.18
Sulfabenzamide	88	0.18	91	0.18
Sulfanilamide	55	0.11	65	0.13
Sulfadimethoxine	16	0.03	52	0.10
Other sulfonamides	13	0.03	32	0.06
Systemic antimicrobial and antiparasitic agents	981	0.95	3,185	6.33
Phenazopyridine	219	0.44	1,109	2.21
Nitrofurantoin	83	0.17	590	1.17
Antimony potassium tartrate	75	0.15	394	0.78
Methenamine	49	0.10	299	0.59
Mandelic acid	30	0.06	224	0.45
Quinine	104	0.21	221	0.44
Diiodohydroxyquin	169	0.34	172	0.34
Hexylresorcinol	20	0.04	151	0.30
Isoniazid	85	0.17	146	0.29
Furazolidone	132	0.26	137	0.27
Metronidazole	31	0.06	95	0.19
Aminosalicylic acid	43	0.09	59	0.12
Methylene blue	9	0.02	46	0.09
Pyrvinium pamoate	7	0.01	43	0.09
Piperazine	3	0.01	30	0.06
Oxyquinoline	21	0.04	26	0.05
Arsenicals	20	0.04	25	0.05
Other systemic antimicrobials and antiparasitics	20	0.04	35	0.07
Topical antimicrobial agents	2,918	5.80	4,792	9.53
Cetalkonium	775	1.54	2,195	4.37
Benzethonium	1,131	2.25	1,134	2.26
Phenylmercuric acetate	889	1.77	930	1.85
Cetylpyridinium	326	0.65	490	0.97
Boric acid	253	0.50	463	0.92
Nitrofurazone	234	0.47	239	0.48
Thymol	52	0.10	117	0.23
Ricinoleic acid	110	0.22	110	0.22
Benzalkonium	50	0.10	103	0.20
Aminacrine	59	0.12	61	0.12
Thiomersal	56	0.11	60	0.12
Gentian violet	40	0.08	57	0.11
Phenol	23	0.05	42	0.08
Chlorobutanol	11	0.02	34	0.07
Povidone iodine	6	0.01	27	0.05
Chlordantoin	24	0.05	26	0.05
Hydrogen peroxide	2	0.00	19	0.04
Other topical antimicrobial agents	71	0.14	117	0.23
Immunizing agents	9,222	18.34	22,707	45.16
Poliomyelitis vaccine, parenteral	6,774	13.47	18,219	36.23

	Use During LM 1-4		Use Anytime During Pregnancy	
	No.	%	No.	%
Polio virus vaccine, live oral	1,628	3.24	3,059	6.08
Influenza virus vaccine	650	1.29	2,283	4.54
Tetanus toxoid	337	0.67	853	1.70
Smallpox vaccine	172	0.34	281	0.56
Diphtheria toxoid	75	0.15	148	0.29
Polio virus vaccine, n.o.s.	39	0.08	136	0.27
Allergy desensitization vaccine	64	0.13	104	0.21
Typhoid vaccine	44	0.09	94	0.19
Measles virus vaccine, live attenuated	37	0.07	80	0.16
Pertussis vaccine	13	0.03	27	0.05
Measles virus vaccine, inactivated	6	0.01	7	0.01
Other virus vaccines	4	0.01	9	0.02
Specific desensitization vaccine	14	0.03	25	0.05
Other bacterial vaccines	15	0.03	34	0.07
Antinauseants, antihistamines, and phenothiazines	6,194	12.32	14,641	29.12
Antihistamines and antinauseants	5,401	10.74	12,678	25.21
Chlorpheniramine	1,070	2.13	3,931	7.82
Diphenhydramine	595	1.18	2,948	5.86
Pheniramine	831	1.65	2,442	4.86
Doxylamine succinate	1,169	2.32	1,700	3.38
Meclizine	1,014	2.02	1,463	2.91
Antinauseant, n.o.s.	596	1.19	774	1.54
Trimethobenzamide	340	0.68	700	1.39
Methapyrilene	263	0.52	525	1.04
Tripelennamine	100	0.20	490	0.97
Thonzylamine	148	0.29	444	0.88
Brompheniramine	65	0.13	412	0.82
Pyrilamine	121	0.24	392	0.78
Antihistamine, n.o.s.	131	0.26	326	0.65
Phenyltoloxamine	45	0.09	142	0.28
Chlorothen	36	0.07	71	0.14
Bromodiphenhydramine	10	0.02	64	0.13
Triprolidine	16	0.03	62	0.12
Buclizine	44	0.09	62	0.12
Chlorcyclizine	13	0.03	57	0.11
Invert sugar	18	0.04	46	0.09
Thenyldiamine	12	0.02	45	0.09
Pyrrobutamine	15	0.03	42	0.08
Dexbrompheniramine	14	0.03	32	0.06
Cyclizine	15	0.03	28	0.06
Phenindamine	12	0.02	28	0.06
Other antihistamines and antinauseants	8	0.02	38	0.08
Phenothiazines	1,309	2.60	3,675	7.31
Prochlorperazine	877	1.74	2,023	4.02
Promethazine	114	0.23	746	1.48
Promazine	50	0.10	347	0.69
Chlorpromazine	142	0.28	284	0.56
Perphenazine	63	0.13	166	0.33
Trimeprazine	14	0.03	140	0.28
Trifluoperazine	42	0.08	95	0.19
Triflupromazine	36	0.07	93	0.18

	Use During LM 1-4		Use Anytime During Pregnancy	
	No.	%	No.	%
Pipamazine	40	0.08	86	0.17
Thiethylperazine	19	0.04	49	0.10
Thioridazine	13	0.03	34	0.07
Fluphenazine	9	0.02	29	0.06
Propiomazine	0	0.00	22	0.04
Other phenothiazines	18	0.04	40	0.08
Sedatives, tranquilizers, and antidepressants	3,122	6.21	14,278	28.40
Barbiturates	2,413	4.80	12,639	25.14
Phenobarbital	1,415	2.81	8,037	15.98
Secobarbital	378	0.75	4,248	8.45
Pentobarbital	250	0.50	1,523	3.03
Amobarbital	298	0.59	867	1.72
Butalbital	112	0.22	325	0.65
Butabarbital	109	0.22	305	0.61
Thiopental	152	0.30	297	0.59
Methohexital	41	0.08	104	0.21
Thiamylal	21	0.04	79	0.16
Other barbiturates	16	0.03	44	0.09
Tranquilizers and nonbarbiturate sedatives	946	1.88	3,231	6.43
Meprobamate	356	0.71	1,204	2.39
Chlordiazepoxide	257	0.51	740	1.47
Glutethimide	67	0.13	640	1.27
Chloral hydrate	71	0.14	358	0.71
Sedative, tranquilizer, n.o.s.	165	0.33	256	0.51
Hydroxyzine	50	0.10	187	0.37
Ethchlorvynol	12	0.02	124	0.25
Methyprylon	8	0.02	47	0.09
Ethinamate	3	0.01	38	0.08
Chlormezanone	5	0.01	26	0.05
Diazepam	10	0.02	23	0.05
Benactyzine	15	0.03	21	0.04
Other tranquilizers and nonbarbiturate sedatives	18	0.04	64	0.13
Antidepressants	59	0.12	152	0.30
Imipramine	19	0.04	55	0.11
Amitriptyline	21	0.04	43	0.09
Tranylcypromine	13	0.03	24	0.05
Nialamide	1	0.00	20	0.04
Other tricyclic antidepressants	1	0.00	1	0.00
Other monoamine oxidase inhibitors	7	0.01	16	0.03
Drugs affecting the autonomic nervous system	4,657	9.26	12,502	24.86
Sympathomimetic drugs	3,082	6.13	9,719	19.33
Phenylephrine	1,249	2.48	4,194	8.34
Phenylpropanolamine	726	1.44	2,489	4.95
Dextroamphetamine	367	0.73	1,069	2.13
Ephedrine	373	0.74	873	1.74
Isoxsuprine	54	0.11	858	1.71
Amphetamines	215	0.43	509	1.01
Epinephrine	189	0.38	508	1.01

	Use During LM 1-4		Use Anytime During Pregnancy	
	No.	%	No.	%
Methamphetamine	89	0.18	320	0.64
Phenmetrazine	58	0.12	257	0.51
Diethylpropion	40	0.08	225	0.45
Pseudoephedrine	39	0.08	194	0.39
Naphazoline	20	0.04	106	0.21
Isoproterenol	31	0.06	95	0.19
Levonordefrin	26	0.05	93	0.18
Levarterenol	18	0.04	42	0.08
Cyclopentamine	17	0.03	41	0.08
Methylphenidate	11	0.02	32	0.06
Methoxyphenamine	3	0.01	24	0.05
Benzphetamine	6	0.01	22	0.04
Xylometazoline	8	0.02	22	0.04
Other sympathomimetic drugs	33	0.07	120	0.24
Parasympatholytic drugs	2,323	4.62	5,623	11.18
Dicyclomine	1,024	2.04	1,593	3.17
Belladonna	554	1.10	1,355	2.69
Atropine	401	0.80	1,198	2.38
Isopropamide iodide	180	0.36	1,071	2.13
Hyoscyamus	41	0.08	117	0.23
Piperidolate	16	0.03	111	0.22
Propantheline bromide	33	0.07	81	0.16
Homatropine	26	0.05	86	0.17
Scopolamine aminoxide hydrobromide	79	0.16	172	0.34
Scopolamine	309	0.61	881	1.75
Hyoscyamine	322	0.64	1,067	2.12
Other parasympatholytics	44	0.09	97	0.19
Parasympathomimetic drugs	30	0.06	44	0.09
Neostigmine bromide	22	0.04	29	0.06
Other parasympathomimetic drugs	8	0.02	16	0.03
Anesthetics, anticonvulsants, muscle relaxants, and stimulants	2,657	5.28	6,990	13.90
Local anesthetics	2,165	4.31	5,703	11.34
Local anesthetic, n.o.s.	386	0.77	998	1.98
Lidocaine	293	0.58	947	1.88
Benzocaine	47	0.09	238	0.47
Mepivacaine	82	0.16	224	0.45
Propoxycaine	41	0.08	90	0.18
Tetracaine	23	0.05	76	0.15
Dibucaine	9	0.02	76	0.15
Procaine	1,340	2.66	3,395	6.75
Other local anesthetics	21	0.04	49	0.10
General anesthetics and oxygen	218	0.43	492	0.98
Nitrous oxide	76	0.15	187	0.37
General anesthetic, n.o.s.	98	0.19	169	0.34
Oxygen	52	0.10	146	0.29
Halothane	25	0.05	50	0.10
Cyclopropane	17	0.03	50	0.10
Ether	8	0.02	23	0.05
Other general anesthetics	16	0.03	33	0.07

	Use During LM 1-4		Use Anytime During Pregnancy	
	No.	%	No.	%
Nonbarbiturate anticonvulsants	151	0.30	425	0.85
Phenytoin	132	0.26	273	0.54
Magnesium sulfate	6	0.01	141	0.28
Primidone	15	0.03	26	0.05
Other nonbarbiturate anticonvulsants	17	0.03	18	0.04
Central nervous system stimulants	60	0.12	228	0.45
Lobelia	38	0.08	149	0.30
Gelsemium	8	0.02	40	0.08
Ammonia spirit	14	0.03	35	0.07
Other central nervous system stimulants	0	0.00	5	0.01
Muscle relaxants	83	0.17	266	0.53
Methocarbamol	22	0.04	119	0.24
Succinylcholine	26	0.05	49	0.10
Carisoprodol	14	0.03	45	0.09
Other neuromuscular blockers	13	0.03	17	0.03
Other centrally acting muscle relaxants	15	0.03	46	0.09
Smooth muscle stimulants	57	0.11	196	0.39
Sparteine	1	0.00	96	0.19
Ergotamine	25	0.05	37	0.07
Ergonovine	18	0.04	33	0.07
Other ergot derivatives	14	0.03	31	0.06
Caffeine and other xanthine derivatives	5,773	11.48	13,509	26.87
Caffeine	5,378	10.70	12,696	25.25
Theophylline	117	0.23	394	0.78
Aminophylline	76	0.15	259	0.52
Chlorotheophylline (Dimenhydrinate)	319	0.63	697	1.39
Other xanthine derivatives	4	0.01	17	0.03
Diuretics and drugs taken for cardiovascular disorders	392	0.78	15,887	31.60
Diuretics	280	0.56	15,671	31.17
Hydrochlorothiazide	107	0.21	7,575	15.07
Chlorothiazide	63	0.13	5,283	10.51
Chlorthalidone	20	0.04	1,310	2.61
Bendroflumethiazide	13	0.03	1,156	2.30
Acetazolamide	12	0.02	1,024	2.04
Methyclothiazide	3	0.01	942	1.87
Diuretic, n.o.s.	38	0.08	735	1.46
Polythiazide	10	0.02	505	1.00
Trichlormethiazide	2	0.00	405	0.81
Meralluride	5	0.01	390	0.78
Quinethazone	8	0.02	316	0.63
Triamterene	5	0.01	271	0.54
Benzthiazide	5	0.01	142	0.28
Mercaptomerin	7	0.01	121	0.24
Cyclothiazide	1	0.00	108	0.21
Carbonic anhydrase inhibitors	14	0.03	1	0.00
Other mercury diuretics	2	0.00	2	0.00
Other miscellaneous diuretics	0	0.00	7	0.01
Other thiazide diuretics	2	0.00	14	0.03

	Use During LM 1-4		Use Anytime During Pregnancy	
	No.	%	No.	%
Antihypertensive agents	53	0.11	525	1.04
Hydralazine	8	0.02	136	0.27
Reserpine and other rauwolfia alkaloids	48	0.10	475	0.94
Other antihypertensive agents	7	0.01	40	0.08
Vasodilators	39	0.08	129	0.26
Ethyl nitrite	24	0.05	98	0.19
Other vasodilators	15	0.03	32	0.06
Digitalis glycosides	52	0.10	129	0.26
Cough medicines	948	1.89	7,941	15.79
Expectorants	864	1.72	6,277	12.48
Ammonium chloride	365	0.73	3,401	6.76
Chloroform, p.o.	421	0.84	2,181	4.34
Elixir terpin hydrate	146	0.29	1,762	3.50
Glyceryl guaiacolate	197	0.39	1,336	2.66
Ipecac	68	0.14	379	0.75
Potassium iodide	56	0.11	221	0.44
Pine tar	14	0.03	93	0.18
Scilla	7	0.01	68	0.14
Desmethylemetine	7	0.01	68	0.14
Cocillana	2	0.00	38	0.08
Euphorbia pilulifera	6	0.01	22	0.04
Other expectorants	1	0.00	8	0.02
Antitussives	344	0.68	867	1.72
Dextromethorphan hydrobromide	300	0.60	580	1.15
Caramiphen	38	0.08	236	0.47
Levopropoxyphene	2	0.00	31	0.06
Other antitussives	6	0.01	32	0.06
Unspecified cough medicines	55	0.11	1,789	3.56
Drugs taken for gastrointestinal disorders	440	0.88	1,500	2.98
Phenolphthalein	236	0.47	806	1.60
Cascara	53	0.11	188	0.37
Bismuth subgallate	13	0.03	144	0.29
Dioctyl sodium sulfosuccinate	30	0.06	116	0.23
Casanthranol	21	0.04	109	0.22
Black draught	39	0.08	100	0.20
Taka-Diastase	33	0.07	97	0.19
Podophyllin	14	0.03	29	0.06
Papain	14	0.03	27	0.05
Bile salts	11	0.02	25	0.05
Dehydrocholic acid	6	0.01	20	0.04
Other peroral enzymes	7	0.01	26	0.05
Miscellaneous gastrointestinal drugs	8	0.02	15	0.03
Hormones, hormone antagonists, and contraceptives	2,327	4.63	3,506	6.97
Progestational agents	866	1.72	1,399	2.78
Progesterone	253	0.50	527	1.05
Hydroxyprogesterone	162	0.32	495	0.98

	Use During LM 1-4		Use Anytime During Pregnancy	
	No.	**%**	**No.**	**%**
Medroxyprogesterone	130	0.26	217	0.43
Norethynodrel	154	0.31	180	0.36
Norethindrone	132	0.26	148	0.29
Progestational agent, n.o.s.	96	0.19	99	0.20
Ethisterone	29	0.06	38	0.08
Other progestational agents	10	0.02	11	0.02
Estrogenic agents	614	1.22	761	1.51
Diethylstilbestrol	164	0.33	233	0.46
Mestranol	179	0.36	206	0.41
Estrogen, n.o.s.	110	0.22	118	0.23
Estradiol	48	0.10	98	0.19
Ethinyl estradiol	89	0.18	98	0.19
Dienestrol	36	0.07	39	0.08
Estrogens, conjugated	11	0.02	24	0.05
Other estrogenic agents	3	0.01	8	0.02
Thyroid hormones	560	1.11	825	1.64
Thyroxin and thyroid	537	1.07	780	1.55
Liothyronine	34	0.07	76	0.15
Corticosteroids and corticotropins	145	0.29	275	0.55
Prednisone	43	0.09	75	0.15
Hydrocortisone	21	0.04	74	0.15
Cortisone	34	0.07	56	0.11
Methylprednisolone	16	0.03	26	0.05
Dexamethasone	8	0.02	23	0.05
Prednisolone	15	0.03	21	0.04
Other corticosteroids and corticotropins	21	0.04	40	0.08
Antidiabetic drugs	139	0.28	234	0.47
Insulin	121	0.24	198	0.39
Tolbutamide	13	0.03	42	0.08
Oral hypoglycemic agents	8	0.02	16	0.03
Miscellaneous hormones	131	0.26	433	0.86
Oxytocin	6	0.01	255	0.51
Hormone, n.o.s.	105	0.21	119	0.24
Lututrin	5	0.01	26	0.05
Infrequently used hormones	15	0.03	37	0.07
Thyroid suppressants	25	0.05	38	0.08
Propylthiouracil	16	0.03	26	0.05
Other thyroid suppressants	10	0.02	14	0.03
Oral contraceptives	278	0.55	309	0.61
Mestranol and norethynodrel	154	0.31	180	0.36
Oral contraceptives, n.o.s.	96	0.19	99	0.20
Mestranol and norethindrone	25	0.05	26	0.05
Other oral contraceptives	5	0.01	7	0.01
Local contraceptives	462	0.92	466	0.93
Nonoxynol 9	342	0.68	346	0.69
P-diisobutylphenoxy-polyethoxy E	84	0.17	84	0.17
Local contraceptive, n.o.s.	37	0.07	37	0.07

	Use During LM 1-4		Use Anytime During Pregnancy	
	No.	%	No.	%
Inorganic compounds and certain vitamins	2,542	5.06	10,116	20.12
Bromides, fluorides, and iodides	1,526	3.03	5,312	10.56
Fluorides	122	0.24	1,422	2.83
Iodides	489	0.97	1,635	3.25
Bromides	986	1.96	2,610	5.19
Calcium, parenteral iron, and vitamins	1,091	2.17	5,598	11.13
Iron, i.m.	66	0.13	1,864	3.71
Vitamins B_{12} and K	28	0.06	219	0.44
Calcium compounds	1,007	2.00	3,739	7.44
Diagnostic aids	108	0.21	313	0.62
Radiopaque media	69	0.14	150	0.30
Intravenous dilution test agent	22	0.04	127	0.25
Radioactive material	21	0.04	50	0.10
Technical aids	431	0.86	1,736	3.45
Local irritants and keratolytics	386	0.77	1,661	3.30
Sodium tetradecyl sulfate	95	0.19	606	1.21
Resorcinol	8	0.02	118	0.23
Methyl salicylate	19	0.04	85	0.17
Allantoin	51	0.10	53	0.11
Pulsatilla nigra	38	0.08	41	0.08
Camphor	168	0.33	763	1.52
Other local irritants and keratolytics	9	0.02	26	0.05
Enzymes	19	0.04	51	0.10
Agents for wound protection (aluminum powder)	27	0.05	31	0.06
Rare drugs	300	0.60	777	1.55
Miscellaneous infrequently used drugs	50	0.10	148	0.29
Hallucinogenic drugs	2	0.00	2	0.00
Antineoplastic agents	2	0.00	3	0.01
Uricosuric agents	4	0.01	7	0.01
Narcotic antagonists	4	0.01	9	0.02
Chelating agents	8	0.02	9	0.02
Intravenous nutrients	3	0.01	17	0.03
Infrequently used IV drugs	7	0.01	17	0.03
Antiarrythmic drugs	7	0.01	22	0.04
Asthma medication, n.o.s.	7	0.01	26	0.05
Anticoagulants	10	0.02	39	0.08
Drugs with unknown ingredients	250	0.50	632	1.26

Drug Exposure During the First Four Lunar Months of Pregnancy in Relation to Specific Malformation Entities

This appendix is designed to display relationships between individual drugs taken during the first four lunar months of pregnancy and individual malformations. The measure of association given in each instance is the relative risk estimate standardized for hospital variability by the Mantel-Haenszel method. With simple arithmetic, the crude relative risk can also be estimated. For example, the first row of the appendix shows that there were 14,864 mother-child pairs exposed to aspirin; 10 exposed children had anencephaly (0.67 per 1,000). By subtraction, there were 35,418 non-exposed pairs, among which there were 16 children with anencephaly (0.45 per 1,000). The unadjusted relative risk is 1.5 (0.67/ 0.45). The adjusted relative risk after standardization for hospital variability is 1.6.

The individual drugs are arranged in the same sequence as they have been presented elsewhere in this book; the malformations are also arranged in sequence.

For present purposes, the malformations listed in Appendix 2 have been slightly modified in the following ways:

Central Nervous Malformations In addition to individual deformities, craniospinal fusion defects with and without anencephaly are also evaluated as outcomes; any cranial nerve malformation, any brain malformation, and any spinal malformation are not evaluated as outcomes because they are too non-specific.

Cardiovascular Malformations In all instances in which a malformation has been classified as "isolated," "multiple," or "any," the outcome "any" (e.g., any ventricular septal defect) is evaluated. In addition to individual deformities, conus arteriosus syndrome, endocardial cushion defect, hypoplastic left heart syndrome, and Tetralogy of Fallot are each evaluated as outcomes.

Musculoskeletal Malformations In addition to individual deformities, muscle absence and/or atrophy and/or hypoplasia is evaluated as an outcome.

Respiratory Malformations In addition to individual deformities, cleft lip with or without cleft palate is evaluated as an outcome; any malformation of the thoracic wall or cavity is not evaluated as an outcome because it is too non-specific.

Gastrointestinal Malformations In addition to individual malformations, atrophy or hypoplasia of the intestine and anomalies affecting the pancreas or gall bladder are evaluated as outcomes.

Genitourinary Malformations In addition to individual deformities, malformed uterus, malformations of the female genitalia, double collecting system, obstructive uropathy, and malformations of the male genitalia (other than hypospadias) are evaluated as outcomes.

Malformations of the Eye and Ear All malformations are evaluated.

Syndromes Klinefelter's syndrome (one affected child) is ignored.

Tumors In addition to individual lesions, any malignant tumors and any benign tumors are evaluated as outcomes.

In this study, the relationship of every recorded drug exposure to every recorded malformation has been determined. It is impractical to present the data on all the relationships. To reduce the number to a practical size, certain arbitrary rules have been adopted:

First, data are not presented when there were fewer than three exposed children with any given malformation, since we judged that any positive association, regardless of its magnitude, would not be informative with such sparse data.

Second, when there were three or more exposed and malformed children, data are only presented if the criteria given below are met.

No. of Exposed Children With the Malformation	Hospital-Standardized Relative Risk
3–4	≥ 5.0 or < 0.5
5	≥ 2.0 or < 0.7
6–9	≥ 1.5 or < 0.8
≥ 10	all estimates

The appendix has been deliberately designed to show that in the context of multiple comparisons there will inevitably be a range of positive and negative associations occurring by chance. The positive associations, even when striking, are uninterpretable without independent confirmatory evidence. Also, estimates of "statistical significance" are improper, and none are presented.

Even with the above-mentioned rules, the appendix still tends to give more emphasis to positive associations than to absence of association or to negative associations: apart from instances in which there were exposed and malformed children, but the relative risks did not meet the criteria for inclusion, there were also many thousands of instances in which none of the children with a given deformity were exposed to particular drugs. It is impractical to list all of these instances. This is, perhaps, not of major importance since the assumption has been made

467

throughout this study that there are no drugs that prevent malformations. Readers wishing to gain insight into anomalies that gave no evidence of positive association with exposure to any particular drug should consult this appendix and Appendix 2 at the same time. Malformations listed in Appendix 2 which do not appear here obviously did not meet the criteria for inclusion cited above.

If any individual drug does not appear in this appendix, it was not associated with any individual malformation in terms of the criteria given here.

Finally, it must be re-emphasized that the data presented in this appendix cannot be used to infer that a particular drug causes a particular malformation, or group of malformations, without independent confirmation.

Analgesics and antipyretics

Non-addicting analgesics and antipyretics

No. of Mother-Child Pairs Exposed	Malformation Class*		Total No. of Malformed Children	No. of Exposed Children with Malformations	Hospital Standardized Relative Risk
14,864	Aspirin				
	CNS	Anencephaly	26	10	1.6
		Meningomylocele	36	14	1.4
		Hydrocephaly	75	20	0.8
		Microcephaly	77	16	0.6
		Hypoplasia/atrophy brain	10	5	2.3
		Craniosynostosis	26	9	1.5
		Rachischisis/cranioschisis	8	5	5.5
		Craniospinal fusion defects	53	18	1.1
		Union anencephaly, craniospinal fusion defects	69	22	1.1
	CVS	Any ventricular septal defect (open or closing)	171	54	1.0
		Transposition of great arteries	17	7	1.5
		Ductus arteriosus persistens	45	13	1.0
		Any coarctation of aorta (pre or post)	36	17	2.1
		Coarctation of aorta—preductal	26	12	1.9
		Coarctation of aorta—postductal	10	5	2.8
		Tetralogy of Fallot	15	8	3.0
		Atrial septal defect—secundum	38	13	1.2
		Aortic stenosis	16	8	2.4
		Conus arteriosus syndrome	44	17	1.5
		Endocardial cushion defect	34	10	1.0
		Pulmonic valvular or unspecified stenosis	56	16	1.0
	MS	Polydactyly	370	116	1.0
		Absence of limb or part thereof	32	11	1.5
		Hypoplasia of limb or part thereof	51	9	0.5
		Syndactyly	125	37	0.9
		Congenital dislocation of hip	92	32	1.1
		Miscellaneous foot abnormalities	10	7	6.2

*CNS = Central Nervous System; CVS = Cardiovascular System; MS = Musculoskeletal System; RT = Respiratory Tract; GIT = Gastrointestinal Tract; GUS = Genitourinary System; E/E = Eye/Ear; SYN = Syndromes; TUM = Tumors; NU = Non-Uniform

469

No. of Mother-Child Pairs Exposed	Malformation Class*		Total No. of Malformed Children	No. of Exposed Children with Malformations	Hospital Standardized Relative Risk
	RT	Malformations of epiglottis/larynx/bronchi	12	6	2.4
		Hypoplasia/agenesis lung	32	10	1.2
		Malformed lung	26	11	1.5
		Cleft lip with or without cleft palate	48	12	0.8
		Cleft palate only	31	4	0.4
	GIT	Omphalocele	22	10	2.1
		Anal atresia	26	13	2.4
		Malrotation	25	10	1.4
		Pyloric stenosis	95	31	1.2
		Meckel's diverticulum	21	3	0.5
		Umbilical hernia	51	17	1.2
	GUS	Hypospadias	188	59	1.1
		Polycystic kidney	33	11	1.2
		Malformations of female genitalia	36	12	1.3
		Obstructive uropathy	47	16	1.2
	E/E	Anophthalmia/microphthalmia	11	5	2.0
		Cataract	44	17	1.9
		Pre-auricular skin tag	38	7	0.6
	SYN	Down syndrome	61	15	0.8
		Situs inversus/dextrocardia	12	7	3.1
		Hypoplasia/atrophy adrenal	26	12	2.4
		Other adrenal syndromes	16	11	6.3
	TUM	Any malignant tumors	24	9	1.6
		Any benign tumors	138	41	1.0
		Any cyst (except dermoid)	42	16	1.4
	NU	Clubfoot	192	67	1.2
		Abnormal hands/fingers	10	7	4.3
		Pectus excavatum	92	33	0.9
		Cleft gum only	110	30	0.9
		Inguinal hernia	683	227	1.2
		Urethral obstruction	68	25	1.1

Drug	Total	System	Defect	N	n	%
Phenacetin	5,546	CNS	Microcephaly	77	5	0.5
			Craniosynostosis	26	6	3.1
		CVS	Any ventricular septal defect (open or closing)	171	17	0.8
		MS	Polydactyly	370	48	1.0
			Syndactyly	125	18	1.4
			Congenital dislocation of hip	92	12	1.1
		GIT	Anal atresia	26	7	2.8
			Pyloric stenosis	95	13	1.4
			Accessory spleen	23	5	2.1
		GUS	Hypospadias	188	19	0.9
		SYN	Other adrenal	16	5	3.6
		TUM	Any benign tumors	138	11	0.7
		NU	Clubfoot	192	26	1.2
			Pectus excavatum	92	14	1.1
			Cleft gum only	110	14	1.1
			Inguinal hernia	683	72	0.9
Salicylamide	744	RT	Malformed lung	26	3	7.1
		NU	Inguinal hernia	683	7	0.7
Acetaminophen	226	MS	Congenital dislocation of hip	92	3	5.6
Narcotic analgesics						
Propoxyphene	686	NU	Clubfoot	192	6	2.2
			Inguinal hernia	683	7	0.7
Codeine	563	GIT	Umbilical hernia	51	3	5.9
		NU	Inguinal hernia	683	12	1.5
Meperidine	268	NU	Inguinal hernia	683	6	1.6

*CNS = Central Nervous System; CVS = Cardiovascular System; MS = Musculoskeletal System; RT = Respiratory Tract; GIT = Gastrointestinal Tract; GUS = Genitourinary System; E/E = Eye/Ear; SYN = Syndromes; TUM = Tumors; NU = Non-Uniform

No. of Mother-Child Pairs Exposed	Malformation Class*		Total No. of Malformed Children	No. of Exposed Children with Malformations	Hospital Standardized Relative Risk
Antimicrobial and antiparasitic agents					
Antibiotics					
Tetracycline 341	GUS	Hypospadias	188	5	3.9
	NU	Inguinal hernia	683	9	1.9
Oxytetracycline 119	NU	Inguinal hernia	683	7	4.3
Demeclocycline 90	NU	Clubfoot	192	3	7.4
Penicillin derivative 3,546	CVS	Any ventricular septal defect (open or closing)	171	13	1.1
		Tricuspid valve malformation	10	4	9.4
	MS	Polydactyly	370	27	0.9
		Syndactyly	125	10	1.2
	GUS	Hypospadias	188	15	1.1
	E/E	Pre-auricular skin tag	38	5	2.0
	TUM	Any benign tumors	138	11	1.2
		Any cyst (except dermoid)	42	6	2.4
	NU	Clubfoot	192	16	1.2
		Pectus excavatum	92	11	2.0
		Cleft gum only	110	11	1.3
		Inguinal hernia	683	55	1.1
Sulfonamides					
Sulfisoxazole 796	CVS	Any coarctation of aorta (pre or post)	36	3	5.3
		Coarctation of aorta—preductal	26	3	7.5
	NU	Inguinal hernia	683	16	1.5

Drug group / agent	N	System	Malformation	n	Obs	Rate
Miscellaneous anti-microbial-antiparasitic agents						
Phenazopyridine	219	NU	Inguinal hernia	683	6	2.0
Diiodohydroxyquin	169	MS	Congenital dislocation of hip	92	3	6.6
Antimicrobial agents for topical use						
Benzethonium	1,131	CVS	Atrial septal defect—secundum	38	4	5.4
		MS	Polydactyly	370	11	0.8
		NU	Inguinal hernia	683	16	1.1
Phenylmercuric acetate	889	MS	Polydactyly	370	5	0.4
		NU	Inguinal hernia	683	13	1.2
Cetalkonium	775	E/E	Pre-auricular skin tag	38	3	6.5
		NU	Clubfoot	192	9	3.3
			Inguinal hernia	683	15	1.4
Cetylpyridinium	326	GIT	Pyloric stenosis	95	3	7.0
Boric acid	253	E/E	Cataract	44	3	13.6
Immunizing agents						
Poliomyelitis vaccine	6,774	CNS	Hydrocephaly	75	5	0.6
			Microcephaly	77	7	0.6
			Craniosynostosis	26	6	2.1
			Craniospinal fusion defects	53	5	0.7
			Union anencephaly, craniospinal fusion defects	69	8	0.7
		CVS	Any ventricular septal defect (open or closing)	171	24	1.0
			Atrial septal defect—primum	15	6	4.0
			Conus arteriosus syndrome	44	5	0.6
			Pulmonic valvular or unspecified stenosis	56	5	0.5

*CNS = Central Nervous System; CVS = Cardiovascular System; MS = Musculoskeletal System; RT = Respiratory Tract; GIT = Gastrointestinal Tract; GUS = Genitourinary System; E/E = Eye/Ear; SYN = Syndromes; TUM = Tumors; NU = Non-Uniform

473

No. of Mother-Child Pairs Exposed	Malformation Class*		Total No. of Malformed Children	No. of Exposed Children with Malformations	Hospital Standardized Relative Risk
	MS	Polydactyly	370	31	1.2
		Absence of limb or part thereof	32	3	0.5
		Syndactyly	125	29	1.3
		Congenital dislocation of hip	92	22	1.3
	RT	Hypoplasia/agenesis lung	32	5	0.6
		Cleft lip with or without cleft palate	48	9	1.6
	GIT	Omphalocele	22	5	2.4
		Pyloric stenosis	95	16	0.8
	GUS	Hypospadias	188	20	0.6
	TUM	Any malignant tumors	24	7	3.3
		Any benign tumors	138	21	1.0
	NU	Clubfoot	192	27	1.1
		Pectus excavatum	92	25	1.3
		Cleft gum only	110	11	1.1
		Inguinal hernia	683	86	0.9
Polio virus vaccine, live oral	1,628				
	MS	Polydactyly	370	20	1.4
	GIT	Omphalocele	22	3	5.4
		Malrotation	25	5	7.9
	TUM	Any benign tumors	138	7	1.8
	NU	Inguinal hernia	683	27	1.3
Influenza virus vaccine	650				
	RT	Cleft palate only	31	3	7.1
Tetanus toxoid	337				
	MS	Polydactyly	370	7	3.2
Antinauseants, antihistamines, and phenothiazines					
Antihistamines and antinauseants					
Doxylamine succinate	1,169				
	CNS	Macrocephaly	18	3	8.2

Drug	N	System	Malformation	N	Obs	Rate
		RT	Diaphragmatic hernia	13	3	11.0
		NU	Clubfoot	192	9	2.0
			Inguinal hernia	683	12	0.7
Chlorpheniramine	1,070	MS	Polydactyly	370	8	1.7
		GIT	Anal atresia	26	3	6.0
		NU	Inguinal hernia	683	22	1.5
Meclizine	1,014	CVS	Hypoplasia cordis	19	3	8.2
			Hypoplastic left heart syndrome	24	3	7.8
		NU	Inguinal hernia	683	18	1.2
Pheniramine	831	E/E	Pre-auricular skin tag	38	3	6.3
		NU	Clubfoot	192	10	3.3
			Inguinal hernia	683	15	1.3
Diphenhydramine	595	CVS	Any ventricular septal defect (open or closing)	171	5	2.2
		RT	Malformations of diaphragm	11	3	29.6
		NU	Clubfoot	192	5	2.1
			Inguinal hernia	683	13	1.7
Thonzylamine	148	MS	Syndactyly	125	3	7.0
Antihistamine, n.o.s.	131	NU	Inguinal hernia	683	7	4.1
Brompheniramine	65	MS	Syndactyly	125	3	12.4
Phenothiazines						
Prochlorperazine	877	CVS	Any ventricular septal defect (open or closing)	171	8	2.4
		RT	Malformations of diaphragm	11	3	21.0
		NU	Inguinal hernia	683	16	1.3
Sedatives, tranquilizers, and antidepressants						
Barbiturates						
Phenobarbital	1,415	CNS	Microcephaly	77	5	2.2

*CNS = Central Nervous System; CVS = Cardiovascular System; MS = Musculoskeletal System; RT = Respiratory Tract; GIT = Gastrointestinal Tract; GUS = Genitourinary System; E/E = Eye/Ear; SYN = Syndromes; TUM = Tumors; NU = Non-Uniform

	No. of Mother-Child Pairs Exposed	Malformation Class*		Total No. of Malformed Children	No. of Exposed Children with Malformations	Hospital Standardized Relative Risk
		CVS	Any ventricular septal defect (open or closing)	171	9	1.9
			Coarctation of aorta—preductal	26	4	5.6
		MS	Polydactyly	370	13	1.2
		NU	Inguinal hernia	683	22	1.2
Secobarbital	378	CNS	Microcephaly	77	3	5.9
		CVS	Any coarctation of aorta (pre or post)	36	3	11.7
			Coarctation of aorta—preductal	26	3	15.6
		NU	Inguinal hernia	683	8	1.5
Amobarbital	298	NU	Inguinal hernia	683	9	2.1
Pentobarbital	250	NU	Inguinal hernia	683	6	1.7
Tranquilizers, nonbarbiturate sedatives						
Meprobamate	356	GUS	Hypospadias	188	5	3.8
		NU	Inguinal hernia	683	8	1.6
Glutethimide	67	NU	Inguinal hernia	683	5	5.4
Drugs affecting the autonomic nervous system						
Sympathomimetic drugs						
Phenylephrine	1,249	MS	Polydactyly	370	12	1.4
			Syndactyly	125	6	1.7
		E/E	Pre-auricular skin tag	38	4	5.7
		NU	Clubfoot	192	14	3.0
			Inguinal hernia	683	22	1.3

Phenylpropanolamine	726	MS	Polydactyly	370	6	1.7
		E/E	Cataract	44	3	6.9
		NU	Pectus excavatum	92	7	2.2
			Inguinal hernia	683	15	1.4
Epinephrine	189	NU	Inguinal hernia	683	6	2.3
Parasympatholytic drugs						
Dicyclomine	1,024	CNS	Macrocephaly	18	3	8.8
		MS	Polydactyly	370	7	1.5
		RT	Diaphragmatic hernia	13	3	12.0
		NU	Clubfoot	192	7	1.8
			Inguinal hernia	683	9	0.6
Belladonna	554	NU	Inguinal hernia	683	10	1.3
Atropine	401	CVS	Any coarctation of aorta (pre or post)	36	3	9.9
			Coarctation of aorta—preductal	26	3	13.6
Anesthetics, anticonvulsants, muscle relaxants, and stimulants						
Local anesthetics						
Local anesthetic, n.o.s.	386	NU	Urethral obstruction	68	4	5.7
Lidocaine	293	NU	Inguinal hernia	683	8	2.0
Procaine	1,340	NU	Inguinal hernia	683	23	1.3
Caffeine and other xanthine derivatives						
Caffeine	5,378	CNS	Microcephaly	77	5	0.5
			Craniosynostosis	26	6	3.2
		CVS	Any ventricular septal defect (open or closing)	171	16	0.8
		MS	Polydactyly	370	46	1.0
			Hypoplasia of limb or part thereof	51	3	0.5
			Syndactyly	125	18	1.4

*CNS = Central Nervous System; CVS = Cardiovascular System; MS = Musculoskeletal System; RT = Respiratory Tract; GIT = Gastrointestinal Tract; GUS = Genitourinary System; E/E = Eye/Ear; SYN = Syndromes; TUM = Tumors; NU = Non-Uniform

No. of Mother-Child Pairs Exposed	Malformation Class*		Total No. of Malformed Children	No. of Exposed Children with Malformations	Hospital Standardized Relative Risk
	GIT	Anal atresia	26	7	2.9
		Pyloric stenosis	95	12	1.3
		Accessory spleen	23	5	2.2
	GUS	Hypospadias	188	20	1.0
		Horsehoe kidney	8	3	5.2
	SYN	Other adrenal	16	5	3.8
	TUM	Any benign tumors	138	11	0.7
	NU	Clubfoot	192	26	1.3
		Pectus excavatum	92	14	1.2
		Cleft gum only	110	14	1.2
		Inguinal hernia	683	68	0.9
Aminophylline	76	MS	Polydactyly	370	3	5.1
Chlorotheophylline (dimenhydrinate)	319	NU	Inguinal hernia	683	8	1.9
Cough medicines					
Expectorants					
Chloroform, p.o.	421	NU	Inguinal hernia	683	14	2.5
Ammonium chloride	365	NU	Inguinal hernia	683	11	2.2
Glyceryl guaiacolate	197	NU	Inguinal hernia	683	7	2.6
Hormones, hormone antagonists and contraceptives					
Progestational agents					
Progesterone	253	NU	Inguinal hernia	683	8	2.2
Medroxyprogesterone	130	NU	Inguinal hernia	683	7	3.8

Thyroid hormones						
Thyroxin and thyroid	537	CVS	Any ventricular septal defect (open or closing)	171	5	2.5
		NU	Inguinal hernia	683	10	1.3
Antidiabetic drugs						
Insulin	121	NU	Inguinal hernia	683	5	3.2
Local contraceptives						
Nonoxynol 9	342	MS	Polydactyly	370	7	2.1
Inorganic compounds and some vitamins						
Bromides, fluorides, and iodides						
Iodides	489	CNS	Hydrocephaly	75	3	5.0
		E/E	Cataract	44	4	11.1
Bromides	986	MS	Polydactyly	370	11	1.5
		NU	Clubfoot	192	7	1.8
			Inguinal hernia	683	16	1.1
Calcium, parenteral iron, and vitamins						
Calcium compounds	1,007	MS	Polydactyly	370	13	1.3
		NU	Inguinal hernia	683	19	1.3

*CNS = Central Nervous System; CVS = Cardiovascular System; MS = Musculoskeletal System; RT = Respiratory Tract; GIT = Gastrointestinal Tract; GUS = Genitourinary System; E/E = Eye/Ear; SYN = Syndromes; TUM = Tumors; NU = Non-Uniform

Drug Exposure Anytime During Pregnancy in Relation to Specific Malformation Entities

This appendix is designed to display relationships between individual drugs taken anytime during pregnancy and each of the malformation entities listed in Appendix 1 (Table 1). The measure of association given in each instance is the relative risk estimate standardized for hospital variability by the Mantel-Haenszel method. With simple arithmetic, the crude relative risk can also be estimated. For example, the first row of the appendix shows that there were 32,164 mother-child pairs exposed to aspirin; 40 exposed children had hydrocephaly (1.2 per 1,000). By subtraction, there were 18,118 non-exposed pairs, among which there were 35 children with hydrocephaly (1.9 per 1,000). The unadjusted relative risk is 0.6 (1.2/1.9). In this instance, the adjusted relative risk after standardization for hospital variability is unchanged and is also 0.6.

The individual drugs are arranged in the same sequence as they have been presented elsewhere in this book; the malformations are also arranged in sequence.

480

In this study, the relationship of every recorded drug exposure at anytime in pregnancy to every recorded "anytime" malformation has been determined. It is impractical to present the data on all the relationships. To reduce the number to a practical size, certain arbitrary rules have been adopted:

First, data are not presented when there were fewer than three exposed children with any given malformation, since we judged that any positive association, regardless of its magnitude, would not be informative with such sparse data.

Second, when there were three or more exposed and malformed children, data are only presented if the criteria given below are met.

No. of Exposed Children With the Malformation	Hospital-Standardized Relative Risk
3–4	≥5.0 or <0.5
5	≥2.0 or <0.7
6–9	≥1.5 or <0.8
≥10	all estimates

The appendix has been deliberately designed to show that in the context of multiple comparisons there will inevitably be a range of positive and negative associations occurring by chance. The positive associations, even when striking, are uninterpretable without independent confirmatory evidence. Also, estimates of "statistical significance" are improper, and none are presented.

Even with the above-mentioned rules, the appendix still tends to give more emphasis to positive associations than to absence of association or to negative associations: apart from instances in which there were exposed and malformed children, but the relative risks did not meet the criteria for inclusion, there were also many thousands of instances in which none of the children with a given deformity were exposed to particular drugs. It is impractical to list all of these instances. This is, perhaps, not of major importance since the assumption has been made throughout this study that there are no drugs that prevent malformations. Readers wishing to gain insight into anomalies that gave no evidence of positive association with exposure to any particular drug should consult this appendix and Appendix 1 at the same time. Malformations listed in Appendix 1 which do not appear here obviously did not meet the criteria for inclusion cited above.

If any individual drug does not appear in this appendix, it was not associated with any individual malformation in terms of the criteria given here.

Finally, two points must be re-emphasized: first, the data presented in this appendix cannot be used to infer that a particular drug causes a particular malformation, or group of malformations, without independent confirmation. Second, the idea that there may be drugs that can cause malformations arising after the first trimester of pregnancy is relatively unexplored. This consideration requires that even greater caution should be used in interpreting the data presented here.

No. of Mother-Child Pairs Exposed	Malformation Class*		Total No. of Malformed Children	No. of Exposed Children with Malformations	Hospital Standardized Relative Risk
Analgesics and antipyretics					
Non-addicting analgesics and antipyretics					
Aspirin 32,164	CNS	Hydrocephaly	75	40	0.6
		Microcephaly	77	42	0.6
		Hypoplasia/atrophy of brain	10	9	4.4
		Macrocephaly	18	13	1.4
		Anomalous pituitary	7	6	3.4
	CVS	Ductus arteriosus persistens	45	27	0.8
	MS	Hypoplasia of limb or part thereof	51	30	0.8
		Congenital dislocation of hip	92	66	1.3
		Miscellaneous foot abnormality	10	9	4.9
	RT	Malformations of thoracic wall	18	9	0.4
		Hiatal hernia	8	6	1.7
		Anomalies of teeth	19	12	1.0
	GIT	Hirschsprung's disease	13	8	0.8
		Pyloric stenosis	95	55	0.8
		Umbilical hernia	51	34	1.1
	GUS	Stenotic ureter	26	15	0.7
		Abnormal ovary	8	3	0.4
		Hydronephrosis	23	17	1.5
		Hydroureter	21	13	0.9
		Malformations of the female genitalia	36	23	1.1
	E/E	Coloboma	13	4	0.2
		Cataract	44	25	0.8
		Corneal opacity	8	5	0.6

	SYN	Hypoplasia/atrophy of adrenals	26	21	2.8
		Other adrenal anomalies	16	13	2.3
		Adrenogenital syndrome	4	4	—
	TUM	Any malignant tumors	24	14	0.8
		Any benign tumors	138	90	1.0
		Any cyst (except dermoid)	42	29	1.2
		Hemangioma/granuloma	19	16	2.5
		Hairy nevus	22	13	0.9
		Other benign	24	12	0.6
	NU	Clubfoot	192	125	0.9
		Pectus excavatum	92	60	0.8
		Inguinal hernia	683	448	1.0
		Urethral obstruction	68	46	1.0
Phenacetin 13,031	CNS	Hydrocephaly	75	20	1.0
		Microcephaly	77	15	0.6
	CVS	Ductus arteriosus persistens	45	14	1.2
	MS	Hypoplasia of limb or part thereof	51	6	0.4
		Congenital dislocation of hip	92	28	1.2
		Other musculoskeletal	10	6	4.7
	RT	Anomalies of teeth	19	3	0.5
	GIT	Pyloric stenosis	95	23	1.0
		Umbilical hernia	51	11	0.8
	GUS	Stenotic ureter	26	5	0.6
		Hydronephrosis	23	8	1.6
		Malformations of the female genitalia	36	6	0.6
	SYN	Other adrenal anomalies	16	8	2.7
	TUM	Any benign tumors	138	38	1.1
		Any cyst (except dermoid)	42	12	1.1
		Hemangioma/granuloma	19	8	1.8
	NU	Clubfoot	192	52	1.0
		Pectus excavatum	92	28	1.1
		Inguinal hernia	683	180	1.0
		Urethral obstruction	68	20	1.0

*CNS = Central Nervous System; CVS = Cardiovascular System; MS = Musculoskeletal System; RT = Respiratory Tract; GIT = Gastrointestinal Tract; GUS = Genitourinary System; E/E = Eye/Ear; SYN = Syndromes; TUM = Tumors; NU = Non-Uniform

483

	No. of Mother-Child Pairs Exposed	Malformation Class*		Total No. of Malformed Children	No. of Exposed Children with Malformations	Hospital Standardized Relative Risk
Salicylamide	1,623	CNS	Hydrocephaly	75	5	2.2
			Macrocephaly	18	3	6.0
		NU	Inguinal hernia	683	17	0.7
Acetaminophen	781	MS	Congenital dislocation of hip	92	8	5.8
		NU	Clubfoot	192	6	1.7
			Inguinal hernia	683	8	0.7
Analgesic and cold capsules, n.o.s.	644	NU	Inguinal hernia	683	6	0.6
Narcotic analgesics						
Propoxyphene	2,914	CNS	Microcephaly	77	6	1.5
		CVS	Ductus arteriosus persistens	45	5	2.2
		E/E	Cataract	44	5	2.5
		TUM	Any benign tumors	138	12	1.5
		NU	Clubfoot	192	18	1.6
			Inguinal hernia	683	51	1.3
Codeine	2,522	CNS	Hydrocephaly	75	7	2.1
		GIT	Pyloric stenosis	95	8	1.5
			Umbilical hernia	51	7	3.3
		TUM	Any benign tumors	138	10	1.3
		NU	Clubfoot	192	15	1.4
			Inguinal hernia	683	51	1.5
Meperidine	1,100	NU	Inguinal hernia	683	19	1.3
Morphine	448	NU	Inguinal hernia	683	10	1.7

Drug	Total	System	Malformation	N	Cases	Rate
Ethoheptazine	300	MS	Congenital dislocation of hip	92	3	5.0
		GIT	Umbilical hernia	51	3	13.4
		NU	Inguinal hernia	683	8	1.9
Opium	181	NU	Inguinal hernia	683	7	2.9
Antimicrobial and antiparasitic agents						
Antibiotics						
Tetracycline	1,336	MS	Hypoplasia of limb or part thereof	51	6	5.1
		NU	Inguinal hernia	683	25	1.4
Oxytetracycline	328	NU	Inguinal hernia	683	7	1.6
Demeclocycline	280	NU	Inguinal hernia	683	8	2.0
Penicillin derivative	7,171	MS	Congenital dislocation of hip	92	11	0.9
		GIT	Pyloric stenosis	95	18	1.5
			Umbilical hernia	51	5	0.6
		E/E	Cataract	44	3	0.4
		TUM	Any benign tumors	138	19	1.0
		NU	Clubfoot	192	31	1.1
			Pectus excavatum	92	18	1.6
			Inguinal hernia	683	104	1.1
			Urethral obstruction	68	9	0.8
Sulfonamides						
Sulfisoxazole	4,287	CVS	Ductus arteriosus persistens	45	8	2.2
		MS	Hypoplasia of limb or part thereof	51	7	1.8
			Miscellaneous foot abnormalities	10	4	11.4
		E/E	Coloboma	13	4	5.5
		SYN	Hypoplasia/atropy of adrenals	26	6	3.9
		TUM	Any benign tumors	138	12	1.2

*CNS = Central Nervous System; CVS = Cardiovascular System; MS = Musculoskeletal System; RT = Respiratory Tract; GIT = Gastrointestinal Tract; GUS = Genitourinary System; E/E = Eye/Ear; SYN = Syndromes; TUM = Tumors; NU = Non-Uniform

485

	No. of Mother-Child Pairs Exposed	Malformation Class*		Total No. of Malformed Children	No. of Exposed Children with Malformations	Hospital Standardized Relative Risk
		NU	Clubfoot	192	19	1.2
			Inguinal hernia	683	51	0.9
			Urethral obstruction	68	13	2.4
Sulfa, n.o.s.	653	NU	Inguinal hernia	683	12	1.4
Miscellaneous antimicrobial-antiparasitic agents						
Phenazopyridine	1,109	NU	Inguinal hernia	683	20	1.4
Nitrofurantoin	590	CVS	Ductus arteriosus persistens	45	3	5.2
Diiodohydroxyquin	172	MS	Congenital dislocation of hip	92	3	6.5
Antimicrobial agents for topical use						
Cetalkonium	2,195	MS	Congenital dislocation of hip	92	10	2.4
		NU	Clubfoot	192	11	1.3
			Inguinal hernia	683	34	1.1
Benzethonium	1,134	NU	Inguinal hernia	683	16	1.1
Phenylmercuric acetate	930	NU	Inguinal hernia	683	14	1.2
Boric acid	463	E/E	Cataract	44	3	7.9
Immunizing agents						
Poliomyelitis vaccine	18,219	CNS	Hydrocephaly	75	16	0.5
			Microcephaly	77	22	0.6
			Macrocephaly	18	8	0.5
		CVS	Ductus arteriosus persistens	45	15	1.1

Code	Condition			
MS	Hypoplasia of limb or part thereof	51	24	1.6
	Congenital dislocation of hip	92	44	1.2
	Miscellaneous foot abnormality	10	3	0.2
RT	Malformations of thoracic wall	18	9	2.4
	Anomalies of teeth	19	8	2.0
GIT	Hirschsprung's disease	13	3	0.4
	Pyloric stenosis	95	45	0.9
	Umbilical hernia	51	19	1.1
GUS	Stenotic ureter	26	8	0.5
	Abnormal ovary	8	3	0.4
	Hydronephrosis	23	5	0.4
	Hydroureter	21	6	0.6
	Malformations of the female genitalia	36	17	0.8
E/E	Coloboma	13	7	1.6
	Cataract	44	22	1.2
	Corneal opacity	8	5	3.5
SYN	Hypoplasia/atrophy of adrenals	26	10	0.8
	Other adrenal anomalies	16	8	0.7
TUM	Any malignant tumors	24	14	4.1
	CNS tumors	8	7	17.9
	Any benign tumors	138	53	0.9
	Papillomas/polyps	12	5	0.7
	Any cyst (except dermoid)	42	19	1.1
	Hairy nevus	22	5	0.5
NU	Clubfoot	192	67	0.9
	Pectus excavatum	92	47	1.2
	Inguinal hernia	683	222	0.8
	Urethral obstruction	68	20	0.9
Polio virus vaccine, live oral		3,059		
GIT	Hirschsprung's disease	13	4	8.8
TUM	Any benign tumors	138	12	1.7
NU	Clubfoot	192	10	0.9
	Pectus excavatum	92	8	2.0
	Inguinal hernia	683	47	1.2

*CNS = Central Nervous System; CVS = Cardiovascular System; MS = Musculoskeletal System; RT = Respiratory Tract; GIT = Gastrointestinal Tract; GUS = Genitourinary System; E/E = Eye/Ear; SYN = Syndromes; TUM = Tumors; NU = Non-Uniform

No. of Mother-Child Pairs Exposed	Malformation Class*		Total No. of Malformed Children	No. of Exposed Children with Malformations	Hospital Standardized Relative Risk
Influenza virus vaccine 2,283	CNS	Microcephaly	77	5	2.6
	GIT	Pyloric stenosis	95	12	2.0
	NU	Clubfoot	192	7	0.7
		Inguinal hernia	683	34	1.1
Tetanus toxoid 853	NU	Inguinal hernia	683	13	1.1
Antinauseants, antihistamines, and phenothiazines					
Antihistamines and antinauseants					
Chlorpheniramine 3,931	CNS	Hydrocephaly	75	8	1.6
	MS	Congenital dislocation of hip	92	16	1.5
	GIT	Pyloric stenosis	95	8	0.8
	GUS	Malformations of the female genitalia	36	6	2.0
	TUM	Any benign tumors	138	11	0.8
	NU	Clubfoot	192	10	0.6
		Pectus excavatum	92	11	0.7
		Inguinal hernia	683	65	1.2
Diphenhydramine 2,948	TUM	Any benign tumors	138	5	0.6
	NU	Pectus excavatum	92	10	1.4
		Inguinal hernia	683	38	1.0
Pheniramine 2,442	MS	Congenital dislocation of hip	92	10	2.0
	GIT	Umbilical hernia	51	5	2.3
	NU	Clubfoot	192	12	1.3
		Inguinal hernia	683	35	1.0

Drug	N	System	Condition	n	Value
Doxylamine succinate	1,700	CNS	Macrocephaly	18	5.8
		GIT	Pyloric stenosis	95	1.9
		NU	Clubfoot	192	1.6
			Inguinal hernia	683	0.9
Meclizine	1,463	NU	Inguinal hernia	683	1.1
Antinauseant, n.o.s.	774	NU	Inguinal hernia	683	1.0
Trimethobenzamide	700	NU	Inguinal hernia	683	0.6
Methapyrilene	525	NU	Clubfoot	192	2.5
			Inguinal hernia	683	1.5
Pyrilamine	392	TUM	Any benign tumors	138	5.3
Antihistamine, n.o.s.	326	NU	Inguinal hernia	683	1.8
Phenothiazines					
Prochlorperazine	2,023	NU	Clubfoot	192	1.3
			Inguinal hernia	683	1.3
			Urethral obstruction	68	2.3
Promethazine	746	NU	Inguinal hernia	683	1.1
Promazine	347	NU	Inguinal hernia	683	1.9
Sedatives, tranquilizers, and antidepressants					
Barbiturates					
Phenobarbital	8,037	CNS	Hydrocephaly	75	0.8
			Microcephaly	77	1.7
		CVS	Ductus arteriosus persistens	45	1.8
		MS	Hypoplasia of limb or part thereof	51	1.7
			Congenital dislocation of hip	92	0.8
		GIT	Pyloric stenosis	95	0.5
			Umbilical hernia	51	1.4

*CNS = Central Nervous System; CVS = Cardiovascular System; MS = Musculoskeletal System; RT = Respiratory Tract; GIT = Gastrointestinal Tract; GUS = Genitourinary System; E/E = Eye/Ear; SYN = Syndromes; TUM = Tumors; NU = Non-Uniform

No. of Mother-Child Pairs Exposed	Malformation Class*		Total No. of Malformed Children	No. of Exposed Children with Malformations	Hospital Standardized Relative Risk
	GUS	Stenotic ureter	26	7	1.8
		Hydronephrosis	23	10	4.3
		Hydroureter	21	9	4.6
	E/E	Coloboma	13	5	2.9
	SYN	Hypoplasia/atrophy of adrenals	26	8	2.4
	TUM	Any malignant tumors	24	6	1.7
		Any benign tumors	138	20	0.8
	NU	Clubfoot	192	29	1.0
		Pectus excavatum	92	8	0.6
		Inguinal hernia	683	108	1.0
		Urethral obstruction	68	5	0.6
Secobarbital 4,248	CNS	Microcephaly	77	13	2.1
	MS	Hypoplasia of limb or part thereof	51	6	1.6
		Congenital dislocation of hip	92	7	0.7
	GIT	Pyloric stenosis	95	7	0.7
	GUS	Stenotic ureter	26	5	2.8
	E/E	Coloboma	13	5	5.8
		Corneal opacity	8	5	22.1
	TUM	Any benign tumors	138	8	0.6
	NU	Clubfoot	192	18	1.0
		Pectus excavatum	92	12	1.5
		Inguinal hernia	683	77	1.4
		Urethral obstruction	68	8	1.8
Pentobarbital 1,523	CNS	Microcephaly	77	6	3.2
	MS	Hypoplasia of limb or part thereof	51	5	2.9
	GU	Stenotic ureter	26	3	5.4

Drug	Total	System	Defect			
		NU	Clubfoot	192	10	1.7
			Inguinal hernia	683	23	1.1
Amobarbital	867	NU	Inguinal hernia	683	23	1.9
Tranquilizers and nonbarbiturate sedatives						
Meprobamate	1,204	NU	Inguinal hernia	683	19	1.1
Chlordiazepoxide	740	NU	Clubfoot	192	6	2.1
			Pectus excavatum	92	7	2.7
			Inguinal hernia	683	16	1.6
Glutethimide	640	NU	Pectus excavatum	92	6	1.9
			Inguinal hernia	683	11	1.2
Drugs affecting the autonomic nervous system						
Sympathomimetic drugs						
Phenylephrine	4,194	MS	Congenital dislocation of hip	92	15	1.8
			Other musculoskeletal	10	4	7.8
		GIT	Umbilical hernia	51	6	1.5
		TUM	Any benign tumors	138	12	1.0
		NU	Clubfoot	192	20	1.2
			Inguinal hernia	683	56	1.0
Phenylpropanolamine	2,489	MS	Congenital dislocation of hip	92	12	1.8
		NU	Clubfoot	192	10	0.9
			Pectus excavatum	92	10	1.0
			Inguinal hernia	683	37	1.1
Dextroamphetamine	1,069	GIT	Pyloric stenosis	95	6	2.1
		NU	Inguinal hernia	683	21	1.4
Ephedrine	873	NU	Inguinal hernia	683	14	1.2

*CNS = Central Nervous System; CVS = Cardiovascular System; MS = Musculoskeletal System; RT = Respiratory Tract; GIT = Gastrointestinal Tract; GUS = Genitourinary System; E/E = Eye/Ear; SYN = Syndromes; TUM = Tumors; NU = Non-Uniform

491

	No. of Mother-Child Pairs Exposed	Malformation Class*		Total No. of Malformed Children	No. of Exposed Children with Malformations	Hospital Standardized Relative Risk
Isoxsuprine	858	NU	Inguinal hernia	683	14	1.0
Epinephrine	508	NU	Inguinal hernia	683	11	1.6
Pseudoephedrine	194	NU	Inguinal hernia	683	8	3.3
Naphazoline	106	NU	Clubfoot	192	3	6.7
Parasympatholytic drugs						
Dicyclomine	1,593	CNS	Macrocephaly	18	3	6.2
		NU	Pectus excavatum	92	9	1.8
			Inguinal hernia	683	18	0.8
Belladonna	1,355	MS	Congenital dislocation of hip	92	6	1.8
		NU	Inguinal hernia	683	20	1.1
Atropine	1,198	NU	Clubfoot	192	8	1.8
			Inguinal hernia	683	20	1.2
Isopropamide iodide	1,071	NU	Inguinal hernia	683	15	1.0
Scopolamine	881	NU	Clubfoot	192	6	1.8
			Inguinal hernia	683	13	1.1
Homatropine	1,067	NU	Inguinal hernia	683	19	1.4
Anesthetics, anticonvulsants, muscle relaxants, and stimulants						
Local anesthetics						
Local anesthetic, n.o.s.	998	GUS	Malformations of the female genitalia	36	3	6.5
		NU	Inguinal hernia	683	14	1.0
			Urethral obstruction	68	5	3.1

492

Drug	Total	System	Condition			
Lidocaine	947	NU	Clubfoot	192	6	1.5
			Inguinal hernia	683	18	1.4
Procaine	3,395	CNS	Hydrocephaly	75	7	1.6
		E/E	Cataract	44	6	1.8
		SYN	Hypoplasia/atrophy of adrenals	26	5	2.6
		TUM	Any malignant tumors	24	5	2.9
			CNS tumors	8	4	8.8
		NU	Clubfoot	192	15	1.3
			Pectus excavatum	92	13	1.6
			Inguinal hernia	683	46	1.0
Muscle relaxants						
Methocarbamol	119	NU	Inguinal hernia	683	6	4.0
Smooth muscle stimulants						
Other ergot derivatives	31	NU	Inguinal hernia	683	3	7.6
Caffeine and other xanthine derivatives						
Caffeine	12,696	CNS	Hydrocephaly	75	19	1.0
			Microcephaly	77	15	0.6
		CVS	Ductus arteriosus persistens	45	14	1.3
		MS	Hypoplasia of limb or part thereof	51	5	0.3
			Congenital dislocation of hip	92	28	1.3
			Other musculoskeletal	10	6	4.9
		RT	Anomalies of the teeth	19	3	0.5
		GIT	Pyloric stenosis	95	23	1.0
			Umbilical hernia	51	12	0.9
		GUS	Stenotic ureter	26	5	0.7
			Hydronephrosis	23	9	2.0
			Hydroureter	21	7	1.5
			Malformations of the female genitalia	36	6	0.6

*CNS = Central Nervous System; CVS = Cardiovascular System; MS = Musculoskeletal System; RT = Respiratory Tract; GIT = Gastrointestinal Tract; GUS = Genitourinary System; E/E = Eye/Ear; SYN = Syndromes; TUM = Tumors; NU = Non-Uniform

No. of Mother-Child Pairs Exposed	Malformation Class*		Total No. of Malformed Children	No. of Exposed Children with Malformations	Hospital Standardized Relative Risk
	E/E	Cataract	44	8	0.8
	SYN	Other adrenal anomaly	16	8	2.8
	TUM	Any benign tumors	138	38	1.1
		Any cyst (except dermoid)	42	11	1.0
		Hemangioma/granuloma	19	9	2.3
		Hairy nevus	22	7	1.5
	NU	Clubfoot	192	51	1.0
		Pectus excavatum	92	27	1.0
		Inguinal hernia	683	177	1.0
		Urethral obstruction	68	20	1.1
Chlorotheophylline (dimenhydrinate) 697	NU	Inguinal hernia	683	10	1.1
Diuretics and drugs taken for cardiovascular disorders					
Diuretics					
Hydrochlorothiazide 7,575	CNS	Hydrocephaly	75	12	0.9
		Microcephaly	77	10	0.9
	CVS	Ductus arteriosus persistens	45	9	1.6
	MS	Congenital dislocation of hip	92	17	1.1
	GIT	Pyloric stenosis	95	20	1.6
		Umbilical hernia	51	6	0.7
	GUS	Malformations of the female genitalia	36	8	1.8
	SYN	Other adrenal anomalies	16	5	3.0
	TUM	Any benign tumors	138	23	1.2
		Hairy nevus	22	9	5.7

Drug	Total	System	Condition	n	Obs	Rate
		NU	Clubfoot	192	27	1.1
			Pectus excavatum	92	18	1.2
			Inguinal hernia	683	90	0.9
			Urethral obstruction	68	3	0.3
Chlorothiazide	5,283	CNS	Hydrocephaly	75	11	1.4
		MS	Congenital dislocation of hip	92	10	1.4
		GIT	Pyloric stenosis	95	10	1.2
		TUM	Any benign tumors	138	12	0.9
		NU	Clubfoot	192	30	1.3
			Pectus excavatum	92	11	1.6
			Inguinal hernia	683	67	0.9
			Urethral obstruction	68	5	0.5
Chlorthalidone	1,310	MS	Congenital dislocation of hip	92	7	1.9
		NU	Inguinal hernia	683	20	1.1
Bendroflumethiazide	1,156	GUS	Hydroureter	21	3	7.8
		TUM	Any benign tumors	138	7	2.6
		NU	Inguinal hernia	683	16	0.9
			Urethral obstruction	68	5	2.0
Acetazolamide	1,024	NU	Inguinal hernia	683	11	0.7
Methyclothiazide	942	CVS	Ductus arteriosus persistens	45	5	6.2
		NU	Inguinal hernia	683	11	0.9
Diuretic, n.o.s.	735	NU	Inguinal hernia	683	10	0.9
Meralluride	390	CNS	Hydrocephaly	75	3	5.9
Antihypertensive agents						
Hydralazine	136	CNS	Microcephaly	77	3	8.4
Reserpine and other rauwolfia alkaloids	475	CNS	Microcephaly	77	7	8.0
		GUS	Hydronephrosis	23	3	18.3
			Hydroureter	21	3	19.4
		NU	Inguinal hernia	683	12	1.9

*CNS = Central Nervous System; CVS = Cardiovascular System; MS = Musculoskeletal System; RT = Respiratory Tract; GIT = Gastrointestinal Tract; GUS = Genitourinary System; E/E = Eye/Ear; SYN = Syndromes; TUM = Tumors; NU = Non-Uniform

495

	No. of Mother-Child Pairs Exposed	Malformation Class*		Total No. of Malformed Children	No. of Exposed Children with Malformations	Hospital Standardized Relative Risk
Digitalis glycosides						
Digitalis glycosides	129	NU	Inguinal hernia	683	6	3.5
Cough medicines						
Expectorants						
Ammonium chloride	3,401	MS	Congenital dislocation of hip	92	5	0.6
		E/E	Cataract	44	6	1.8
		TUM	Any benign tumors	138	17	1.7
		NU	Clubfoot	192	9	0.8
			Pectus excavatum	92	5	0.6
			Inguinal hernia	683	47	1.1
Chloroform, p.o.	2,181	NU	Inguinal hernia	683	36	1.3
Elixir terpin hydrate	1,762	TUM	Any benign tumors	138	9	1.9
		NU	Clubfoot	192	11	1.2
			Inguinal hernia	683	34	1.4
Glyceryl guaiacolate	1,336	NU	Inguinal hernia	683	20	1.1
Potassium iodide	221	NU	Pectus excavatum	92	4	9.1
			Inguinal hernia	683	7	2.4
Antitussives						
Dextromethorphan hydrobromide	580	NU	Inguinal hernia	683	10	1.3
Unspecified cough medicines						
Cough medicine, n.o.s.	1,789	NU	Inguinal hernia	683	29	1.2

Drug						
Drugs taken for gastrointestinal disturbances						
Phenolphthalein	806	NU	Inguinal hernia	683	5	0.4
Cascara	188	TUM	Any benign tumors	138	3	6.5
Bismuth subgallate	144	NU	Inguinal hernia	683	5	2.6
Hormones, hormone antagonists and contraceptives						
Progestational agents						
Progesterone	527	NU	Inguinal hernia	683	18	2.6
Hydroxyprogesterone	495	CNS	Microcephaly	77	4	5.1
		NU	Inguinal hernia	683	15	2.4
Medroxyprogesterone	217	NU	Inguinal hernia	683	8	2.6
Thyroid hormones						
Thyroxin and thyroid	780	NU	Inguinal hernia	683	15	1.4
Antidiabetic drugs						
Insulin	198	NU	Inguinal hernia	683	6	2.3
Miscellaneous hormones						
Oxytocin	255	NU	Inguinal hernia	683	10	2.7
Lututrin	26	NU	Inguinal hernia	683	3	8.2
Inorganic compounds and some vitamins						
Bromides, fluorides and iodides						
Fluorides	1,422	GUS	Hydroureter	21	4	9.3

*CNS = Central Nervous System; CVS = Cardiovascular System; MS = Musculoskeletal System; RT = Respiratory Tract; GIT = Gastrointestinal Tract; GUS = Genitourinary System; E/E = Eye/Ear; SYN = Syndromes; TUM = Tumors; NU = Non-Uniform

No. of Mother-Child Pairs Exposed	Malformation Class*		Total No. of Malformed Children	No. of Exposed Children with Malformations	Hospital Standardized Relative Risk
	TUM	Any benign tumors	138	7	2.0
	NU	Inguinal hernia	683	20	1.0
		Urethral obstruction	68	6	2.2
Iodides 1,635	MS	Congenital dislocation of hip	92	10	2.1
	E/E	Cataract	44	5	4.5
	NU	Pectus excavatum	92	10	1.6
		Inguinal hernia	683	27	1.2
Bromides 2,610	MS	Congenital dislocation of hip	92	9	1.8
	TUM	Any benign tumors	138	10	1.4
	NU	Clubfoot	192	15	1.5
		Inguinal hernia	683	39	1.1
Calcium, parenteral iron and vitamins					
Iron, i.m. 1,864	MS	Hypoplasia of limb or part thereof	51	5	3.5
		Congenital dislocation of hip	92	7	2.7
	NU	Clubfoot	192	10	1.5
		Inguinal hernia	683	23	0.8
Calcium compounds 3,739	CNS	Microcephaly	77	5	0.7
	GIT	Umbilical hernia	51	8	2.3
	E/E	Cataract	44	5	2.2
	NU	Clubfoot	192	18	1.1
		Inguinal hernia	683	54	1.0
		Urethral obstruction	68	3	0.4

498

Technical aids

Local irritants
and keratolytics

Resorcinol	118	NU	Inguinal hernia	683	5	3.2
Camphor	763	NU	Inguinal hernia	683	11	1.1

Rare drugs

Drugs with unknown ingredients	632	NU	Clubfoot	192	5	2.0

*CNS = Central Nervous System; CVS = Cardiovascular System; MS = Musculoskeletal System; RT = Respiratory Tract; GIT = Gastrointestinal Tract; GUS = Genitourinary System; E/E = Eye/Ear; SYN = Syndromes; TUM = Tumors; NU = Non-Uniform

References

Chapter 1

1. Gregg, N.M. Congenital cataract following German measles in the mother. *Trans. Ophthalmol. Soc. Aust.* 3:35, 1941.

2. Wilson, J.G. *Environment and Birth Defects.* New York: Academic Press, 1973.

3. McBride, W.G. Thalidomide and congenital malformations. *Lancet* 2:1358, 1961.

4. Lenz, W. Kindliche Missbildungen nach Medikament während der Draviditat? *Deutsch Med. Wochenschr.* 86:2555, 1961.

5. Leck, I. The etiology of human malformations: insights from epidemiology. *Teratology* 5:303, 1972.

6. Niswander, K.R. and Gordon, M. (eds.). *The Women and Their Pregnancies.* Philadelphia: W.B. Saunders Company, 1972.

7. Warkany, J. *Congenital Malformations: Notes and Comments.* Chicago: Year Book Medical Publishers, Inc., 1971.

8. Murphy, D.P. Outcome of 625 pregnancies in women subjected to pelvic radium or roentgen irradiation. *Am. J. Obstet. Gynecol.* 18:179, 1929.

9. Goldstein, L. and Murphy, D.P. Microcephalic idiocy following radium therapy for uterine cancer during pregnancy. *Am. J. Obstet. Gynecol.* 18:189, 1929.

10. Wood, J.W., Johnson, K.G., and Omori, Y. *In utero* exposure to the Hiroshima atomic bomb. An evaluation of head size and mental retardation twenty years later. *Pediatrics* 39:385, 1967.

11. Satow, W.U., and West, E. Studies on Nagasaki (Japan) children exposed *in utero* to atomic bomb: Roentgenographic survey of skeletal system. *Am. J. Roentgenol.* 74:493, 1955.

12. Stewart, A. and Barber, R. Epidemiological importance of childhood cancers. *Br. Med. Bull.* 27:64, 1971.

13. Harada, Y. Congenital Minamata disease. *Minamata Disease.* Kumanoto University Study Group of Minamata Disease, 1968.

14. Tuchmann-Duplessis, H. *Drug Effects on the Fetus.* Sydney: Adis Press. Acton, Mass.: Publishing Sciences Group, Inc., 1975.

15. Herbst, A.L., Ulfelder, H., and Poskanzer, D.C. Adenocarcinoma of the vagina. *N. Engl. J. Med.* 284:878, 1971.

16. Greenwald, P., Barlow, J.J., Masca, C., and Burnett, W.S. Vaginal cancer after maternal treatment with synthetic estrogens. *N. Engl. J. Med.* 285:390, 1971.

17. Milunsky, A., Graef, J.W., and Gaynor, M.F. Methotrexate-induced congenital malformations, with a review of the literature. *J. Pediatr.* 72:790, 1968.

18. Baden, E. Environmental pathology of the teeth. (Goslin, R.J. and Goldman, H.M., eds.) *Thomas' Oral Pathology.* St. Louis: C.V. Mosby Co., 1970.

19. Shepard, T.H. *Catalog of Teratogenic Agents.* Baltimore: Johns Hopkins University Press, 1973.

Chapter 2

1. Niswander, K.R., and Gordon, M. (eds.) *The Women and Their Pregnancies.* Philadelphia: W.B. Saunders Co., 1972.

2. Broman, S.H., Nichols, P.L., and Kennedy, W.A. *Preschool I.Q., Prenatal and Early Developmental Correlates.* New York: John Wiley & Sons, 1975.

3. *The United States Pharmacopeia,* 18th Revision. Bethesda, Md.: United States Pharmacopeial Convention, Inc., 1970.

4. *U.S.A.N. 10, 1961–1971 Cumulative List,* and *1974 Supplement.* Rockville, Md.: United States Pharmacopeial Convention, Inc., 1972, 1974.

5. *The National Formulary,* 13th Edition. Washington, D.C.: American Pharmaceutical Association, 1970.

6. *Specifications for the Quality Control of Pharmaceutical Preparations,* 2nd Edition of the International Pharmacopeia, and *Supplement,* World Health Organization, Geneva, 1967, 1971.

7. *International Nonproprietary Names for Pharmaceutical Substances, Cumulative List No. 3.* World Health Organization, Geneva, 1971, and *Lists No. 26–34,* published as supplements to WHO Chronicle, 1971–1975.

8. Wilson, C.O. and Jones, T.E. *American Drug Index.* Philadelphia: J.B. Lippincott Co., 1975.

9. *The Merck Index,* 8th Edition. Rahway, N.J.: Merck & Co., Inc., 1968.

10. Heinonen, O.P. Risk factors for congenital heart disease: A prospective study. *Birth Defects: Risks and Consequences.* (Kelly, S., Hook, E.B., Janerich, D.T., and Porter, I.H., eds.). New York: Academic Press, 1976.

Chapter 3

1. Slone, D., Heinonen, O.P., Monson, R.R., Shapiro, S., Hartz, S.C., and Rosenberg, L. Maternal drug exposure and fetal abnormalities. *Clin. Pharmacol. Ther.* 14:648, 1973.

2. Monson, R.R., Rosenberg, L., Hartz, S.C., Shapiro, S., Heinonen, O.P., and Slone, D. Diphenylhydantoin and selected congenital malformations. *N. Engl. J. Med.* 289: 1049, 1973.

3. Shapiro, S., Slone, D., Hartz, S.C., Rosenberg, L., Siskind, V., Monson, R.R., Mitchell, A.A., Heinonen, O.P., Idänpään-Heikilä, J., Härö, S., and Saxén, L. Anticonvulsants and parental epilepsy in the development of birth defects. *Lancet* 1:272, 1976.

4. Fisher, L., and Patil, K. Matching and unrelatedness. *Am. J. Epidemiol.* 100: 347, 1974.

5. Miettinen, O.S. Confounding and effect-modification. *Am. J. Epidemiol.* 100: 350, 1974.

6. Cox, D.R. *Analysis of Binary Data.* London: Methuen, 1970.

7. Armitage, P. *Statistical Methods in Medical Research.* New York: Wiley, 1971.

8. Fleiss, J.L. *Statistical Methods for Rates and Proportions.* New York: Wiley, 1973.

9. Cornfield, J., Gordon, T., and Smith, W.W. Quantal response curves for experimentally controlled variables. *Bull. Int. Statist. Inst.* 38 III: 97, 1961.

10. Hartz, S.C., Rosenberg, L., Heinonen, O.P., Slone, D., and Shapiro, S. Epidemiological screening of multiple risk factors in relation to multiple congenital malformations. *Teratology* 10: 311, 1974.

11. Armitage, P. and Gehan, E.A. Statistical methods for the identification and use of prognostic factors. *Int. J. Cancer* 13: 16, 1974.

12. Walker, S.H., and Duncan, D.B. Estimation of the probability of an event as a function of several independent variables. *Biometrika* 54: 167, 1967.

13. Heinonen, O.P. Risk factors for congenital heart disease. A prospective study. *Birth Defects: Risks and Consequences.* (Kelly, S., Hook, E.B., Janerich, D.T., and Porter, I.H., eds.), New York: Academic Press, 1976.

14. Pearson, H.O. and Hartley, H.O. *Biometrika Tables for Statisticians, Vol. I.* London: Cambridge University Press, 1958.

15. Truett, J., Cornfield, J. and Kamel, W. A multivariate analysis of the risk of coronary heart disease in Framingham. *J. Chron. Dis.* 20: 511, 1967.

16. Brunk, H.D., Thomas, D.R., Elashoff, R.M., and Zippin, C. Computer-aided prognosis. Oregon State University Technical Report No. 40, 1973.

17. Kendall, M.G. and Stuart, A. *The Advanced Theory of Statistics.* Vol. I. London: Griffin, 1963, p. 232.

18. Meyer, M.B. and Comstock, G.W. Maternal cigarette smoking and perinatal mortality. *Am. J. Epidemiol.* 96: 1, 1972.

19. Susser, M. *Causal Thinking in the Health Sciences.* New York: Oxford University Press, 1973.

20. Campbell, G.A. Probability curves showing Poisson's exponential summation. *Bell System Tech. J.* 2: 95, 1923.

Chapter 4

1. United States Bureau of the Census. *Methodology and Scores of Socioeconomic Index.* (Working Paper No. 15) Washington, D.C., 1963.

2. Myrianthopoulos, N.C. and French, K.S. An application of the U.S. Bureau of the Census Socioeconomic Index to a large, diversified patient population. *Social Science and Medicine* 2:283, 1968.

3. Warkany, J. *Congenital Malformations: Notes and Comments.* Chicago: Year Book Medical Publishers, Inc., 1971.

Chapter 5

1. Myrianthopoulos, N.C., and French, K.S. An application of the U.S. Bureau of the Census Socioeconomic Index to a large, diversified patient population. *Social Science and Medicine* 2: 283, 1968.

2. Eastman, N.J. and Hellman, L.M. (eds.). *William's Obstetrics.* 13th Ed. New York: Appleton-Century-Crofts, 1966.

3. Davies, A.M. Geographical epidemiology of the toxemias of pregnancy. *Is. J. Med. Sci.* 7: 751, 1971.

Chapter 9

1. Heinonen, O.P. Risk factors for congenital heart disease. A prospective study. *Birth Defects: Risks and Consequences.* (Kelly, S., Hook, E.B., Janerich,

D.T., and Porter, I.H., eds.) New York: Academic Press, 1976.

Chapter 19

1. McCall, J.D., Globus, M., and Robinson, J. Drug induced skeletal malformations in the rat. *Experientia* 19:183, 1963.

2. Tuchmann-Duplessis, H. and Mercier-Parot, L. Repercussion d'un somnifere, le glutethemide, sur la gestation et le developpement foetal du rat, de la souris et du lapin. *C.R. Acad. Sci.* (Paris) 256:1841, 1963.

3. Wilson, J.G. *Environment and Birth Defects.* New York: Academic Press, 1973.

4. Tuchmann-Duplessis, H. *Drug Effects on the Fetus.* Sydney: Adis Press, Acton, Mass.: Publishing Sciences Group, Inc., 1975.

Chapter 20

1. Richards, I.D.G. Congenital malformations and environmental influences in pregnancy. *Br. J. Prev. Soc. Med.* 23:218, 1969.

2. Nelson, M.M. and Forfar, J.O. Associations between drugs administered during pregnancy and congenital abnormalities of the fetus. *Br. Med. J.* 1:523, 1971.

3. Wilson, J.G. *Environment and Birth Defects.* New York: Academic Press, 1973.

Chapter 21

1. Baden, E. Environmental pathology of the teeth. (Gorlin, R.J. and Goldman, H.M., eds.) *Thomas' Oral Pathology.* St. Louis: C.V. Mosby Co., 1970.

Chapter 22

1. Heinonen, O.P., Shapiro, S., Monson, R., Hartz, S.C., Rosenberg, L., and Slone, D. Immunization during pregnancy against poliomyelitis and in-

fluenza in relation to childhood malignancy. *Int. J. Epidemiol.* 2:229, 1973.

2. Kirschstein, R.L. and Gerber, P. Ependymomas produced after intercerebral innoculation of SV 40 into newborn hamsters. *Nature* (London) 195:299, 1962.

Chapter 23

1. Tuchmann-Duplessis, H. *Drug Effects on the Fetus.* Sydney: Adis Press, Acton, Mass.: Publishing Sciences Group, Inc., 1975.

2. Lenz, W. Malformations caused by drugs in pregnancy. *Am. J. Dis. Childhood* 112:99, 1966.

3. Yerushalmy, J. and Milkovich, L. Evaluation of teratogenic effect of meclizine in man. *Am. J. Obstet. Gynecol.* 93:553, 1965.

4. McBride, W.G. An aetiological study of drug ingestion by women who gave birth to babies with cleft palate. *Australian and New Zealand J. Obstet. Gynecol.* 9:103, 1969.

5. Milkovich, L. and van den Berg, B.J. An evaluation of the teratogenicity of certain antinauseant drugs. *Am. J. Obstet. Gynecol.* 125: 244, 1976.

Chapter 24

1. Hartz, S.C., Heinonen, O.P., Shapiro, S., Siskind, V., and Slone, D. Antenatal exposure to meprobamate and chlordiazepoxide in relation to malformations, mental development and childhood mortality. *N. Engl. J. Med.* 292:726, 1975.

2. Milkovich, L. and van den Berg, B.J. Effects of prenatal meprobamate and chlordiazepoxide hydrochloride on human embryonic and fetal development. *N. Engl. J. Med.* 291:1268, 1974.

3. McCall, J.D., Globus, M., and Robinson, S. Drug-induced skeletal malformations in the rat. *Experientia* 19:183, 1963.

4. Tuchmann-Duplessis, H. and

Mercier-Parot, L. Repercussion d'un somnifere, le glutethimide, sur la gestation et le developpement foetal du rat, de la souris et du lapin. *C.R. Acad. Sci.* (Paris), 256:1841, 1963.

5. Tuchmann-Duplessis, H. *Drug Effects on the Fetus.* Sydney: Adis Press. Acton, Mass.: Publishing Sciences Group, Inc., 1975.

Chapter 25

1. Shepard, T.H. *Catalog of Teratogenic Agents.* Baltimore: Johns Hopkins University Press, 1973.

Chapter 26

1. Shapiro, S., Slone, D., Hartz, S.C., Rosenberg, L., Siskind, V., Monson, R.R., Mitchell, A.A., Heinonen, O.P., Idänpäan-Heikilä, J., Härö, S., and Saxén, L. Anticonvulsants and parental epilepsy in the development of birth defects. *Lancet* 1:272, 1976.

2. Tuchmann-Duplessis, H. *Drug Effects on the Fetus.* Sydney: Adis Press. Acton, Mass.: Publishing Sciences Group, Inc., 1975.

3. Shepard, T.H. *Catalog of Teratogenic Agents.* Baltimore: Johns Hopkins University Press, 1973.

4. Monson, R., Rosenberg, L., Hartz, S.C., Shapiro, S., Heinonen, O.P., and Slone, D. Diphenylhydantoin and selected congenital malformations. *N. Engl. J. Med.* 289:1049, 1973.

Chapter 28

1. Goldman, A.S. and Yakorae, W.C. Teratogenic action in rats of reserpine alone and in combination with salicylate and immobilization. *Proc. Soc. Exp. Biol. Med.* 118:857, 1965.

2. Kalter, H. *Teratology of the Central Nervous System.* Chicago: University of Chicago Press, 1968.

Chapter 31

1. Heinonen, O.P., Slone, D., Monson, R., Hook, E.B., and Shapiro, S. Cardiovascular birth defects and antenatal exposure to female sex hormones. Submitted for publication.

2. Synthetic sex hormones and infants. Editorial. *Br. Med. J.* 2:485, 1974.

3. Are sex hormones teratogenic? Editorial. *Lancet* 2:1489, 1974.

4. Nora, J.J., and Nora, A.H. Can the pill cause birth defects? *N. Engl. J. Med.* 291:731, 1974.

5. Harlap, S., Prywes, R., and Davies, A.M. Birth defects and oestrogens and progesterones in pregnancy. *Lancet* 1:682, 1975.

6. Janerich, D.T., Piper, J.M., and Alexatis, D.M. Oral contraceptives and congenital limb reduction defects. *N. Engl. J. Med.* 291:697, 1974.

7. Tuchmann-Duplessis, H. *Drug Effects on the Fetus.* Sydney: Adis Press. Acton, Mass.: Publishing Sciences Group, Inc., 1975.

8. Landauer, W. Is insulin a teratogen? *Teratology* 5:129, 1972.

9. Milham, S. and Elledge, W. Maternal methimazole and congenital defects in children. *Teratology* 5:125, 1972.

Chapter 33

1. Shirkey, H.C. Human experiences related to adverse drug reactions to the fetus or neonate from some maternally administered drugs. *Drugs and Fetal Development.* (Klingberg, M.A., Abramovici, A., and Clarke, J., eds.) New York: Plenum Press, 1972.

Chapter 35

1. Herbst, A.L., Ulfelder, H., and Poskanzer, D.C. Adenocarcinoma of the vagina: Association of maternal stilbestrol therapy with tumor appearance in young women. *N. Engl. J. Med.* 284:878, 1971.

2. Greenwald, P., Barlow, J.J., Masca, C., and Burnett, W.S. Vaginal cancer after maternal treatment with synthetic estrogens. *N. Engl. J. Med.* 285:390, 1971.

Appendix 1

1. Heinonen, O.P., Shapiro, S., Monson, R., Hartz, S.C., Rosenberg, L., and Slone, D. Immunization during pregnancy against poliomyelitis and influenza in relation to childhood malignancy. *Int. J. Epidemiol.* 2:229, 1973.

2. Eddy, E.B., Borman, G.S., Berkeley, W.H., and Young, R.D. Tumours induced in hamsters by injection of rhesus monkey kidney cell extracts. *Proc. Soc. Exp. Biol. Med.* 107:191, 1961.

3. Fraumeni, Jr., J.F., Stark, C.R., Gold, E., and Lepow, M.L. Simian virus 40 in polio vaccine follow-up of newborn recipients. *Science* 167:59, 1970.

4. Goldman, A.S. and Yakovac, W.C. Teratogenic action in rats of reserpine alone and in combination with salicylate and immobilization. *Proc. Soc. Exp. Biol. Med.* 118:857, 1965.

5. Kalter, H. *Teratology of the Central Nervous System.* Chicago: University of Chicago Press, 1968.

Index of Drug Names

Page references which appear in bold type refer to the "Comments" sections which summarize the findings with respect to drugs of each of Chapters 20–33 and of Appendix 1. It should also be noted that a list of the drugs analyzed in this study appears in Appendix 3 (page 456).

Analgesic and cold capsules, 287, 288, **356,** 434, 484
Analgesic drugs, 286–295, 434, 469, 482
Anesthetics, 357–365, 436, 440, 477, 492
Anileridine, 287
Anisotropine methylbromide, 346
Antacids, 263
Antiarrythmic drugs, 410
Antibiotics, 297–299, 301, 303, 305, **312,** 434, 445, 472, 485
Anticoagulants, 410
Anticonvulsants, 17, 18, 357–365, 436, 440, 477, 492
Antidepressants, 335–344, 436, 438, 475, 489
Antidiabetic drugs, 388–391, 393, 397, **398,** 443, 479, 497
Antihistamines, 11, 322–334, **344,** 436, 437, **445,** 474, 488
Antihypertensive agents, 17, 371–375, 436, 441, **445,** 495
Antimicrobial agents, 296–313, 434, 435, 472, 485
Antimony potassium tartrate, 299, 302, 435
Antinauseants, 322–334, 436, 437, 474, 488
Antineoplastic agents, 3, 410
Antiparasitic agents, 296–313, 434, 435, 472, 485
Antipyretic drugs, 286–295, 434, 469, 482
Antipyrine, 287
Antitussives, 378–381, **383,** 438, 442, 496
Apomorphine, 378
Arsenicals, 298, 299, 302
Aspirin, 11, 276, 279, 287–289, 291, **294, 295,** 370, 434, 466, 469, 480, 482
Asthma medications, 410

Atropine, 346, 347, 350, 354, 439, 477, 492
Acetamidoeugenol, 359
Acetaminophen, 287, 288, 434, 471, 484
Acetanilide, 287
Acetarsone, 299
Acetazolamide, 372, 441, 495
Acetohexamide, 390
Adiphenine, 346
Albumin, iodinated I 131 serum, 410, **415**
Aldosterone, 390
Allantoin, 410, 411
Allergy desensitization vaccine, 315
Alphaprodine, 287
Aluminum powder, 410, 411
Ambenonium, 346
Ambuphylline, 367
Ambutonium bromide, 346
Aminacrine, 300, 302
Aminophylline, 367, **370,** 440, 478
Aminopterin, 281
Aminopyrine, 287
Aminosalicylic acid, 298, 299, 302, **313**
Amitriptyline, 336, 337
Ammonia spirit, 359
Ammonium chloride, 378–381, 442, 478, 496
Amobarbital, 336–338, 340, 341, **344,** 438, 476, 491
Amphetamines, 346, 347, 439
Amphotericin B, 297

Bacitracin, 297
Bacterial protein, I.V., 315
Bacterial vaccine, 315
Barbital, 336
Barbiturates, 11, 335–340, 344, 436, 438, 475, 489
Benactyzine, 336
Bendroflumethiazide, 372, 441, 495
Belladonna, 346, 347, 350, 353, 439, 477, 492
Betamethasone, 390
Bethanechol, 346
Benzalkonium, 300, 302
Benzethonium, 300, 302, 309, 435, 473, 486
Benzocaine, 357–360, 440
Benzonatate, 378
Benzphetamine, 346
Benzthiazide, 372
Benztropine mesylate, 346
Bile salts, 385
Bismuth subcarbonate, 385
Bismuth subgallate, 385, 497
Black draught, 385
Boric acid, 300, 302, 309, 311, 435, 473, 486
Bromelain, 385
Bromides, 402–406, **408,** 444, 479, 498
Bromodiphenhydramine, 323
Brompheniramine, 322–325, 437, 475
Buclizine, 323, 324, 436, 437
Bunamiodyl, 410
Butabarbital, 335–337, 438

Butalbital, 336, 337
Butethamine, 359

Caffeine, 11, 366–370, 436, 440, 477, 493
Calcium, 402, 404, 407, **408,** 444, 479, 498
Camphor, 410, 411, 444, 499
Camphor, monobromated, 410
Caprylate sodium, 299
Capsicum, 410
Caramiphen, 377–379, 438, 442
Carbazochrome salicylate, 287
Carbinoxamine, 323
Carbonic anhydrase inhibitors, 372, 373
Carbromal, 336
Carisoprodol, 359
Carphenazine, 323
Casanthranol, 384, 385, 442
Cascara, 385, 438, 442, 497
Central nervous system stimulants, 357–360, **365,** 436, 440
Cephalothin, 297
Cetalkonium, 300, 302, 309, 310, 312, 435, 473, 486
Cetylpyridinium, 300, 302, 309, 311, 434, 435, 473
Chelating agents, 410
Chlophedianol, 378
Chloral betaine, 336
Chloral hydrate, 335–337, 438
Chloramphenicol, 297, 301, 435
Chlorcyclizine, 323
Chlordantoin, 300, 302
Chlordiazepoxide, 336, 337, 341, 343, **344,** 438, 491
Chlorhexidine, 300
Chlorindanol, 390
Chlormezanone, 336, 436, 438
Chlorobutanol, 300
Chloroform, 359
Chloroform, p.o., 378–380, 442, 478, 496
Chloroquine, 299
Chlorothen, 323, 324
Chlorotheophylline, 367–370, 440, 478, 494
Chlorothiazide, 372, 373, 441, 495
Chlorpheniramine, 323, 324, 326, 328, 332, 437, 475, 488
Chlorpromazine, 323, 324, 437
Chlorpropamide, 390
Chlorprothixene, 323
Chlortetracycline, 297
Chlorthalidone, 371–373, 436, 441, 495
Chlorzoxazone, 359
Cholera vaccine, 315
Clidinium bromide, 346
Clomiphene, 390
Cocaine, 359
Cocillana, 378
Codeine, 287, 288, 292, 293, **294,** 434, 471
"Cold tablets," **350, 383**
Contraceptives, 388–400, 438, 443, 478, 497

507

Methsuximide, 359
Methyclothiazide, 372, 495
Methyl salicylate, 410
Methylatropine, 346
Methyldopa, 372
Methylene blue, 299, 434, 435
Methylergonovine maleate, 359
Methylphenidate, 346
Methylprednisolone, 390
Methyltestosterone, 390
Methylthiouracil, 390
Methyprylon, 336
Methysergide, 359
Metronidazole, 298, 299, 302
Milk of bismuth, 385
Monoamine oxidase inhibitors, 335–337
Morphine, 287, 288, 434, 484
Muscle relaxants, 357–365, 436, 440, 477, 492, 493

Nalidixic acid, 299
Naphazoline, 346, 347
Narcotic analgesics, 287, 288, 289, 292, **445,** 471, 484
Narcotic antagonists, 410
Neomycin, 297, 301
Neostigmine bromide, 346, 347
Nialamide, 336
Nicotinyl alcohol, 372
Nitrofurantoin, 299, 302, 435, 486
Nitrofurazone, 300, 302, 309, 311
Nitroglycerin and amyl nitrite, 372
Nitrous oxide, 358, 360
Non-addicting analgesics, 286–288, 290, 469, 482
Non-barbiturate anticonvulsants, 357–361, **364,** 436, 440
Non-barbiturate sedatives, 335–337, 341, 436, 438, **445,** 476, 491
Nonoxynol 9, 390, 392, 393, 443, 479
Norethindrone, 389–391, 438, 443
Norethynodrel, 389, 391, 443
Nortriptylene, 336
Novobiocin, 297, 301
Nutrients, intravenous, 410
Nystatin, 297, 301, 305, **313,** 435

Oleandomycin, 297
Opium, 287, 288, 434, 485
Opium alkaloids, 287, 288
Orphenadrine, 359
Oxazepam, 336
Oxethazine, 359
Oxycodone, 287
Oxygen, 358, 361, 364, 440
Oxymetazoline, 346
Oxyphencyclimine, 346
Oxyquinoline, 299, 302
Oxytetracycline, 297, 298, 301, **313,** 435, 472, 485

Oxytocin, 390, 497

Pancreatin, 385
Pantopon, 287
Papain, 385
Papaverine, 372
Paraformaldehyde, 300
Paraldehyde, 336
Paramethasone, 390
Parasympatholytic drugs, 345, 347, **356,** 439, 477, 492
Parasympathomimetic drugs, 346–348, **356**
Paratyphoid vaccine, 315
Paregoric, 40, 287, 288, 434
P-Diisobutylphenoxy-Polyethoxy E, 390, 392
Penicillin derivatives, 276, 297, 299, 301, 304, **312, 313,** 435, 472, 485
Pentaerythritol tetranitrate, 372
Pentobarbital, 336, 337, 341, 438, 476, 490
Perphenazine, 323, 324, 437
Pertussis vaccine, 315
Phenacemide, 359
Phenacetin, 11, 287, 289, 291, **294, 295,** 370, 434, 471, 483
Phenaglycodol, 336
Phenazopyridine, 299, 302, 305, 308, 435, 473, 486
Phendimetrazine, 346
Phenelzine, 336
Phenformin, 390
Phenindamine, 323
Pheniramine, 323, 324, 326, 329, **332,** 437, 475, 488
Phenmetrazine, 346, 347, 439
Phenobarbital, 336–339, **344,** 438, 475, 489
Phenocoll-p-pheneditine, 287
Phenol, 298, 300, 302
Phenolphthalein, 384–387, 442, 497
Phenosulfonphthalein, 410
Phenothiazines, 322–334, **344,** 436, 437, 474, 488
Phentolamine, 372
Phenylbutazone, 287
Phenylephrine, 345–347, 349, 350, 439, 476, 491
Phenylmercuric acetate, 300, 302, 309, 310, 435
Phenylpropanolamine, 346, 347, 349, 351, 439, 477, 491
Phenyltoloxamine, 323–325, 436, 437
Phenytoin, 276, 277, 357, 358, 360, **364,** 440
Phthalysulfathiazole, 298
Phytonadione, 402
Pine tar, 378
Pipamazine, 323, 324
Pipazethate, 378
Piperazine, 299
Piperidolate, 346
Piperocaine, 359
Pipradol, 346
Podophyllum, 385

General Index

It should be noted that a complete listing, by anatomic class, of the malformations analyzed in this study appears in Appendix 2 (page 446).